CURRENT
CARDIOVASCULAR
DRUGS

Fourth Edition

CURRENT CARDIOVASCULAR DRUGS

Fourth Edition

Edited by

William H. Frishman
Rosenthal Professor and Chairman of Medicine
Professor of Pharmacology
New York Medical College
Director of Medicine
Westchester Medical Center
Valhalla, New York

Angela Cheng-Lai
Clinical Pharmacy Manager/Cardiology
Montefiore Medical Center
Assistant Professor of Medicine
Albert Einstein College of Medicine
Bronx, New York

James Nawarskas
Associate Professor of Pharmacy
University of New Mexico College of Pharmacy
Albuquerque, New Mexico

Developed by Current Medicine LLC, Philadelphia

Current Medicine LLC
400 Market Street, Suite 700
Philadelphia, PA 19106

CURRENT MEDICINE LLC

400 Market Street, Suite 700 • Philadelphia, PA 19106

Director of Editorial, Design, Production ....Wendy Vetter
Senior Developmental Editor...Elizabeth Rexon
Commissioning Supervisor Books..Annmarie D'Ortona
Cover Design ....Christine Keller-Quirk
Design and Layout...Christine Keller-Quirk
Illustrator ....Wieslawa Langenfeld and Maureen Looney
Production Manager ....Lori Holland
Assistant Production Manager ....Margaret La Mare
Indexer ....Holly Lukens

Library of Congress Cataloging-in-Publication Data

ISBN 1-57340-221-4

Although every effort has been made to ensure that drug doses and other information are presented accurately in this publication, the ultimate responsibility rests with the prescribing physician. Neither the publishers nor the author can be held responsible for errors or for any consequences arising from the use of the information contained therein. Any product mentioned in this publication should be used in accordance with the prescribing information prepared by the manufacturers. No claims or endorsements are made for any drug or compound at present under clinical investigation.

Printed in the US by Edwards Brothers, Inc.

10 9 8 7 6 5 4 3 2 1

For more information please call 1 (800) 427-1796 or (215) 574-2266.

www.current-science-group.com

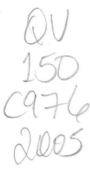

PREFACE

Advances in the areas of cardiovascular physiology, molecular biology, diagnostics, and therapeutics have been occurring at a rapid rate over the past 35 years. This incredible growth in knowledge has made it difficult, if not impossible, for health care providers to integrate all this new information into their clinical practices. Of immediate relevance has been the introduction of a large number of drugs and drug combinations for use in the prevention and treatment of ischemic vascular disease, systemic hypertension, myocardial failure, and arrhythmias. For each new drug entity that becomes available, clinicians must become familiar with its pharmacokinetic and pharmacodynamic profiles, especially when prescribing for patients having various medical conditions. The prescriber must also be aware of potential drug-drug interactions that may cause a loss of treatment efficacy and/or toxicity.

This fourth edition of Current Cardiovascular Drugs is designed to provide an updated practical compendium of current knowledge regarding cardiovascular drug therapy in a concise, easily readable format. The book is organized into chapters by drug class, and details the pharmacologic characteristics of specific treatment entities. The clinical efficacy and limitations of the various drug therapies are discussed using supportive reference material from the most authoritative sources and published clinical trials.

Current Cardiovascular Drugs is not designed to replace traditional textbooks of cardiovascular medicine, or to resolve ongoing controversies in patient management. Rather, its purpose is to provide a user-friendly source to aid in clinical treatment. Only those drugs and drug combinations that are available in the United States are discussed. Appendices are also included that summarize recommendations for cardiovascular drug use in special clinical situations (*eg*, pregnancy, renal disease, hepatic disease), and in specific patient populations (*eg*, the elderly). This book will continue to be updated in future editions on a frequent basis to provide the most current information to practicing physicians, physicians-in-training, pharmacists, nurses, physician assistants, and medical students.

The authors wish to acknowledge the editorial contributions of Joanne Pryor to both this and all the previous editions of the book, and the efforts of Elizabeth Rexon of Current Medicine for her editorial guidance. Finally, the authors wish to thank our colleagues and students for the inspiration to prepare this book, and our respective families whose love, support, and encouragement have provided the impetus to complete this work.

William H. Frishman, MD
Angela Cheng-Lai, PharmD
James Nawarskas, PharmD

DEDICATION

To our clinical colleagues and
their ongoing health care missions

CONTRIBUTORS

Judy W.M. Cheng, PharmD, BCPS

Associate Professor of Pharmacy Practice and Health Sciences
Long Island University
Brooklyn, New York
Clinical Pharmacy Specialist in Cardiology
Mt. Sinai Medical Center
New York, New York

Angela Cheng-Lai, PharmD

Clinical Pharmacy Manager/Cardiology
Montefiore Medical Center
Assistant Professor of Medicine
Albert Einstein College of Medicine
Bronx, New York

William H. Frishman, MD, MACP

Rosenthal Professor and Chairman of Medicine
Professor of Pharmacology
New York Medical College
Director of Medicine
Westchester Medical Center
Valhalla, New York

James Nawarskas, PharmD

Associate Professor of Pharmacy
University of New Mexico College of Pharmacy
Albuquerque, New Mexico

Cynthia A. Sanoski, BS, PharmD

Associate Professor of Clinical Pharmacy
Philadelphia College of Pharmacy
University of the Sciences in Philadelphia
Clinical Pharmacy Specialist in Cardiology
Presbyterian Medical Center
Philadelphia, Pennsylvania

CONTENTS

Current Cardiovascular Drugs is a quick and easy reference for the prescriber. The information in it is drawn from a number of sources, chiefly the manufacturers' data sheets and the international published literature. The recommendations also reflect current prescribing practice among physicians.

The information has been rigorously checked by the authors, the publishers, and qualified pharmacists. However, the book is intended as a memory aid rather than a substi-

tute for the data sheets. **The information in this book must always be used in conjunction with the manufacturers' prescribing information.**

Each chapter is devoted to a different drug class. The first pages of the chapter, the introductory pages, briefly describe the development of drugs in that class, report the results of recent major clinical trials, and provide tabular summaries of the current use and actions of the drugs.

INTRODUCTORY PAGES

The tables on the introductory pages bring together the information given on the individual drug pages in that chapter and give additional guidelines: the reasons for contraindications and warnings, the nature of drug interactions, and the action to be taken in the event of adverse reactions.

INDIVIDUAL DRUG PAGES

Note: There are apparent differences in the incidence of adverse reactions and interactions between drugs of the same class. These differences are due to factors such as variations in the level of reporting by different manufacturers. Many effects are not well validated and a causal connection between drug use and effect has not always been proved.

Doses reflect the manufacturers' data sheets and the authors' recommendations, based on current clinical practice. Dosage requirements for special patient groups may be listed separately.

Guidelines for treating overdosage are given but the prescriber should always consult the manufacturer's data sheet.

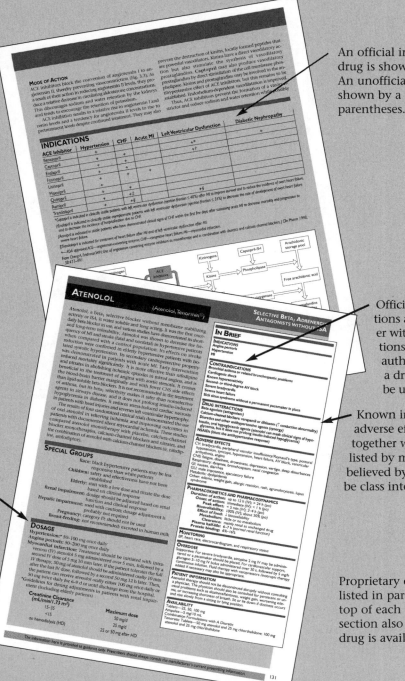

An official indication for a drug is shown by a plus sign. An unofficial indication is shown by a plus sign in parentheses.

Official contraindications are given together with other situations in which the authors believe that a drug should not be used.

Known interactions and adverse effects are listed together with others not listed by manufacturers but believed by the authors to be class interactions.

Proprietary drug names are listed in parentheses at the top of each drug page. This section also indicates if the drug is available generically.

ALPHA-ADRENERGIC BLOCKERS (PERIPHERALLY ACTING ANTIHYPERTENSIVE AGENTS)

The alpha-receptor blockers were the first adrenergic receptor antagonists to be developed for cardiovascular therapy. This occurred shortly after Alquist suggested the alpha/beta classification scheme to explain differences between the pharmacologic actions of adrenergic agonists. The alpha-receptor blockers, **phenoxybenzamine** and **phentolamine** (now recognized as antagonists for both alpha$_1$- and alpha$_2$-receptors), have been in use since the 1960s, primarily for the management of massive catecholamine excess in pheochromocytoma. Subsequently, the quinazoline derivatives (**doxazosin**, **prazosin**, and **terazosin**) were found to have antagonism for a set of alpha receptors primarily found on postsynaptic sites, thus characterized as alpha$_1$. With regard to the cardiovascular system, alpha$_1$-receptors are found in vascular smooth muscle. These receptors mediate the action of norepinephrine released from presynaptic adrenergic nerve terminals, thus causing vasoconstriction, as shown in Figure 1.1. Two subtypes of alpha$_1$-receptors have been identified—alpha$_{1a}$ and alpha$_{1b}$. The former regulates transmembrane calcium entry channels, whereas the latter, through its intracellular action on phospholipase-C and the phosphoinositol system, controls intracellular sequestration of free calcium.

Alpha$_2$-receptors are located within the regulatory centers of the central nervous system (CNS) that control the outflow of the autonomic nervous system. These receptors are also found on presynaptic autonomic nerve terminals (Figure 1.1) where, when activated by a released neurotransmitter, they inhibit neurosecretion. Other locations for alpha$_2$-receptors include platelets, pancreatic islet cells, and nonsynaptic locations of vascular smooth muscle. In vascular tissue, alpha$_2$-receptors mediate the effect of circulating catecholamines. The major actions and characteristics of the alpha-receptors are shown in Table 1.1.

The alpha-receptor antagonists may be divided into two categories—those that block both alpha$_1$- and alpha$_2$-receptors (phenoxybenzamine and phentolamine), and those that selectively block the alpha$_1$-receptor (doxazosin, prazosin, and terazosin). Most adrenergic receptor blocking drugs are competitive antagonists that bind reversibly to their specific receptors and can be displaced by high concentrations of competing agonists. Phenoxybenzamine is the exception, as it bonds irreversibly to alpha-receptors as an alkylating agent. Both phenoxybenzamine and phentolamine reduce

FIGURE 1.1 Site of action of alpha-blockers.

TABLE 1.1 COMPARISON OF THE ALPHA RECEPTORS		
	Alpha$_1$ receptors	**Alpha$_2$ receptors**
Prototype agonist	Norepinephrine	Clonidine
Prototype antagonist	Prazosin	Yohimbine
Presynaptic location	No	Yes
Postsynaptic location	Yes	No
Nonsynaptic location	?	Yes
In the CNS cardiovascular centers	?	Yes
Vascular smooth muscle location	Yes	Yes
Pancreatic islet cells	No	Yes
Platelets	?	Yes
Intracellular signaling system	Alpha$_{1a}$-calcium entry via channels; alpha$_{1b}$-phospholipase-C system- intracellular calcium	Inhibition of adenylcyclase

CNS—central nervous system.

vasoconstriction and decrease blood pressure. However, these drugs cause tachycardia. This is probably because of their antagonism of inhibitory presynaptic alpha$_2$-receptors, which leads to increased release of norepinephrine to postsynaptic cardiac beta-receptors, increasing the heart rate. The effectiveness of these two drugs in pheochromocytoma may be a result of their ability to antagonize both postsynaptic alpha$_1$- and nonsynaptic alpha$_2$-receptors on vascular tissue. **Phentolamine** is available for intravenous bolus injection or infusion to be used in controlling the hypertensive crises of pheochromocytoma. The major use of **phenoxybenzamine** is as an oral agent for the treatment of hypertension in pheochromocytoma.

EFFICACY OF ALPHA$_1$-ANTAGONISTS

The quinazoline alpha$_1$-antagonists—**prazosin**, **terazosin**, and **doxazosin**—are effective antihypertensive agents. They reduce systemic vascular resistance with little change in heart rate, fluid retention, or activation of the renin-angiotensin system. The differences among these drugs are primarily related to their pharmacokinetic profiles and dosing schedule, as shown in Table 1.2. **Prazosin** has the shortest half-life and must be given two to three times daily for effective blood pressure reduction. **Terazosin** and **doxazosin** have longer half-lives; **terazosin** may be given once or twice daily, and **doxazosin** is given once daily. The alpha$_1$-antagonists are metabolized almost entirely by hepatic routes and, as such, do not require dosage adjustment with renal insufficiency.

The alpha$_1$-antagonists are no longer recommended as initial antihypertensive therapy because of the findings of the Antihypertensive and Lipid-Lowering Treatment to Prevent Heart Attack Trial (ALLHAT). The results of this study demonstrated **doxazosin** to be 1) less effective than **chlorthalidone** in reducing blood pressure and 2) associated with a higher incidence of cardiovascular morbidity (eg, stroke, heart failure) compared with **chlorthalidone**. The current role of these drugs for the treatment of hypertension has been relegated primarily to treating high blood pressure in men with benign prostatic hyperplasia (BPH),

although even in this situation these drugs are not the preferred first-line agents. The alpha$_1$-blockers may also be useful as add-on therapy for treating hypertension in patients with high blood pressure refractory to a variety of other antihypertensive drugs.

OTHER EFFECTS

All three quinazoline alpha$_1$-blockers have similar and favorable effects on serum lipid fractions, tending to modestly reduce total and low-density-lipoprotein cholesterol, and slightly increase high-density-lipoprotein cholesterol (Table 1.3). **Prazosin** and **doxazosin** have been shown to reduce blood glucose and serum insulin concentrations. This effect has potential, but unproven, benefit for noninsulin-dependent diabetic hypertensive patients or those with insulin-resistance syndrome.

Perhaps the most significant advantage of the alpha$_1$-antagonists compared with other antihypertensive agents is their ability to antagonize alpha$_1$-receptors in the ureters, prostate, and urinary bladder trigone and sphincters, thereby decreasing resistance to urinary outflow. This has been the basis for their successful use (**terazosin**, in particular) in treating the symptoms of BPH. **Tamsulosin** (Flomax [Boehringer Ingelheim]), an alpha$_1$-receptor antagonist with selectivity for the alpha$_{1A}$-receptors in prostatic tissue, is indicated only for alleviating symptoms associated with BPH. **Tamsulosin** is not recommended for use as an antihypertensive drug because of its specificity for prostatic tissue and limited systemic effect. However, orthostatic hypotension remains a problem with **tamsulosin** therapy, especially when higher doses are administered.

The vasodilating effect of the alpha$_1$-receptor antagonists reduces afterload, which is of theoretic benefit in patients with reduced left ventricular systolic function. On that basis, **prazosin** was studied in a randomized clinical trial (VHeFT) for possible efficacy in congestive heart failure (CHF). However, when compared with placebo, **prazosin** had no effect, whereas a combination of **hydralazine** and **isosorbide** was beneficial in decreasing cumulative mortality. At

TABLE 1.2 PHARMACOKINETICS AND USUAL DOSE RANGE FOR THE ALPHA$_1$-RECEPTOR ANTAGONISTS		
Drug	**Approximate half-life**	**Usual initial dose and dose range**
Prazosin	2–4 h	1 mg 2–3 times daily; 2–20 mg/d in 2–3 divided doses
Terazosin	10–12 h	1 mg at bedtime; 1–20 mg/d in 1–2 divided doses
Doxazosin	20–22 h	1 mg once daily; 1–16 mg once daily

TABLE 1.3 EFFECTS OF ALPHA-BLOCKERS ON PLASMA LIPID PROFILE	
	Effect
Total cholesterol	↓2%–5%
High-density lipoprotein cholesterol	↑2%–4%
Low-density lipoprotein cholesterol	↓4%–10%
Triglycerides	↓3%–10%
Lipoprotein lipase activity	Increased

↑—increased; ↓—decreased.

It has been suggested that the effects of alpha-blockers may be attributable to their stimulation of lipoprotein lipase activity.

present, CHF is not considered an indication for use of the alpha$_1$-receptor antagonists.

ADVERSE EFFECTS

All three alpha$_1$-antagonists share the same adverse effect profile. Most problematic is first-dose orthostatic hypotension, defined as dizziness or syncope caused by a sudden reduction in blood pressure when upright, ocurring shortly after either the initial dose or the first dose of a dosage increase. It is suggested, but not thoroughly evaluated, that this effect is less likely with those drugs having a slower onset and longer half-life (**terazosin** and **doxazosin**). First-dose hypotension should be anticipated when any alpha$_1$-antagonist is given to older patients or to those already taking other antihypertensive agents, especially diuretics and angiotensin-converting enzyme (ACE) inhibitors. Postural hypotension and dizziness are thought to be a consequence of reduced activation of normal alpha$_1$-adrenergic receptor function. Patients receiving alpha$_1$-antagonists (particularly the elderly) should be routinely monitored for postural changes in blood pressure. Other adverse effects of alpha$_1$-antagonists, such as fatigue, nausea, edema, dyspnea, and asthenia, are nonspecific and difficult to relate to specific drug action. Nasal congestion is probably a specific adverse effect of alpha-receptor blockade. Other reported adverse effects are listed with each agent.

COMBINATION THERAPY WITH OTHER ANTIHYPERTENSIVE AGENTS

As mentioned earlier, the alpha$_1$-blockers are no longer considered first-line antihypertensive drugs but may be useful in certain situations as add-on therapy for patients with resistant hypertension. Caution is urged when alpha$_1$-antagonists are prescribed with other antihypertensive agents, because of an increased likelihood of first-dose or postural hypotension. Diuretics (especially high dose), centrally acting agents, or sympatholytics are to be used with caution. With careful monitoring, alpha$_1$-receptor antagonists may be effective when used in combination with beta-receptor antagonists. For example, **doxazosin** and **atenolol** may be effective as a once-daily alpha-/beta-receptor blocker combination in selected patients. **Labetalol**, a nonselective beta-blocker with alpha$_1$-receptor antagonism, is effective as both an oral and an intravenous agent for the treatment of chronic and acute hypertension, respectively. Combinations of ACE inhibitors and alpha$_1$-receptor antagonists may be useful in the absence of reduced blood volume or impaired cardiovascular reflexes. Theoretically, alpha$_1$-blockers may add to the antihypertensive action of calcium channel antagonists because of the effect of alpha$_1$-receptors on transmembrane calcium entry channels.

INDICATIONS

	Doxazosin	Prazosin	Terazosin
Benign prostatic hyperplasia	+	–	+
Hypertension	+	+	+

+—FDA approved; – —not FDA approved.

DOXAZOSIN (Doxazosin, Cardura®)

Doxazosin is structurally related to prazosin. Its long half-life, however, enables it to be used once daily. It is highly selective for alpha$_1$-adrenoceptors, with a ratio of affinities for alpha$_1$/alpha$_2$ of just less than 600. As mentioned earlier in this chapter, it also has beneficial effects on plasma lipids (Table 1.3). In the ALLHAT study, chlorthalidone reduced systolic blood pressure by 3 mm Hg more than doxazosin and was associated with fewer cardiovascular complications (especially stroke and heart failure) compared with doxazosin. As a result of this study, alpha$_1$-receptor antagonists are no longer considered first-line antihypertensive therapy.

By blocking the alpha$_1$-receptors in the urinary bladder neck and prostatic urethra, doxazosin is effective in increasing urinary flow rates and alleviating outflow obstruction and irritation symptoms associated with BPH in both hypertensive and normotensive men. It is important to remember that doxazosin does not reverse the underlying pathophysiology of the disease. Also, prior to initiating doxazosin therapy for BPH, the patient should be examined to rule out the presence of prostatic malignancy.

SPECIAL GROUPS

Race: no differences in response
Children: safety and effectiveness have not been established in children under 18 years of age
Elderly: more sensitive to hypotensive effect; begin with lower dosages and titrate based on clinical response
Renal impairment: no dosage adjustment necessary
Hepatic impairment: use with caution because the drug is hepatically metabolized; begin with lower dosages and titrate based on clinical response
Pregnancy: category C; use only if potential benefit justifies the potential risk to the fetus
Breast-feeding: not recommended; not known if the drug is excreted in human milk

DOSAGE

Benign prostatic hyperplasia: 1–8 mg once daily
Hypertension: 1–16 mg once daily
Doxazosin should be initiated at 1 mg once daily (0.5 mg once daily for the elderly). The dosage may be increased every 1–2 wk based on response. Careful BP monitoring for hypotension and orthostasis is recommended, especially for the elderly. The maintenance dosage may be divided and administered twice daily to minimize an excessive hypotensive response. If therapy is discontinued for several days, it should be reinstituted with a low dosage and slowly increased based on the clinical response.

IN BRIEF

INDICATIONS
Benign prostatic hyperplasia (BPH)
Hypertension

CONTRAINDICATIONS
Known hypersensitivity to quinazolines, such as prazosin and terazosin
Use with tadalafil or vardenafil

DRUG INTERACTIONS
Alcohol[1]
Antihypertensive agents[1,2]
Cimetidine[1,4]
Clonidine[3]
Sildenafil[1]
Tadalafil[1,5]
Vardenafil[1,5]

1 Effect/toxicity of doxazosin may increase.
2 Doxazosin may increase the effect/toxicity of this drug.
3 Doxazosin may decrease the effect of this drug.
4 The clinical significance of this interaction is unclear.
5 Concurrent treatment with doxazosin is contraindicated.

ADVERSE EFFECTS
CV: orthostatic or postural hypotension, syncope, palpitations, chest pain, edema, dyspnea
CNS: dizziness, drowsiness, fatigue, headache, vertigo, somnolence
GU: impotence, priapism, urinary frequency
Skin: rash, pruritus, facial edema
Other: leukopenia/neutropenia, flulike syndrome, rhinitis, hypersensitivity reaction

PHARMACOKINETICS AND PHARMACODYNAMICS
Duration of action: 24 h
Onset of action: 1–2 h
Peak effect: 2–6 h
Bioavailability: 65%
Effect of food: decrease peak concentration by 18% and the extent of absorption by 12%
Protein binding: 98%–99%
Volume of distribution: 1.5 L/kg
Metabolism: metabolized by the liver extensively; several active metabolites
Elimination: 9% in the urine and 63% in the feces; mainly as metabolites (4.8% unchanged)
Elimination half-life: 19–22 h

MONITORING
Supine and sitting/standing BP, complete blood count (CBC) with differential, urinary flow and dysuria (for BPH).

OVERDOSE
Supportive—consider fluid therapy, with vasopressor added if necessary for profound hypotension.

PATIENT INFORMATION
Doxazosin may cause syncope, orthostatic problems, and drowsiness; avoid driving or performing hazardous tasks, especially within 24 h after the first dose or a dosage increment. Sit or lie down if dizziness occurs, and rise slowly from a sitting or lying position. Alcohol may exacerbate these side effects.

AVAILABILITY
Tablets—1, 2, 4, 8 mg

PRAZOSIN (Prazosin, Minipress®)

Prazosin is a selective alpha$_1$-adrenoceptor blocker. Because its bioavailability is unpredicatable and its half-life is relatively short, twice- to thrice-daily dosing is required. It is an effective antihypertensive agent, but its propensity to cause first-dose syncope and postural hypotension, its frequent dosing schedule, and the results of the ALLHAT study (see Doxazosin) have severely limited its clinical usage.

The failure of the VHeFT study to demonstrate a beneficial effect of prazosin on mortality when compared with placebo in the treatment of CHF argues against using prazosin for the treatment of heart failure. It is suspected that prazosin may induce tachyphylaxis in patients with CHF, even after short periods of treatment.

Prazosin has been used to successfully treat symptoms (*eg*, urinary frequency, nocturia) in men with BPH, although it is not FDA approved for this indication.

SPECIAL GROUPS

Race: no differences in response
Children: safety and effectiveness have not been established
Elderly: more sensitive to hypotensive effect; begin with lower dosages and titrate based on clinical response
Renal impairment: begin treatment with 1 mg twice daily, and titrate dosage based on clinical response
Hepatic impairment: use with caution because the drug is hepatically metabolized; begin with lower dosages and titrate based on clinical response
Pregnancy: category C; use only if potential benefit justifies the potential risk to the fetus
Breast-feeding: use with caution; excreted in human milk in small amounts

DOSAGE

Prazosin should be initiated at 1 mg two to three times daily and slowly increased to the usual maintenance dose of 6–15 mg daily in 2–3 divided doses. Most patients can be maintained on twice-daily dosing after initial titration.

Maximum daily dose—40 mg; limited gain in efficacy for dosages above 20 mg/d.

When adding a new antihypertensive agent or a diuretic, the dose of prazosin should be reduced to 1–2 mg 3 times daily and slowly increased based on blood pressure response.

If therapy is discontinued for several days, it should be reinstituted with a low dosage and slowly increased based on the clinical response.

IN BRIEF

INDICATIONS
Hypertension

CONTRAINDICATIONS
Known hypersensitivity to quinazolines, such as doxazosin and terazosin
Use with tadalafil or vardenafil

DRUG INTERACTIONS
Alcohol[1]
Antihypertensive agents[1,3]
Beta-blockers[1]
Clonidine[4]
NSAIDs[2]
Verapamil[1]
Sildenafil[1]
Tadalafil[1,5]
Vardenafil[1,5]

1 Effect/toxicity of prazosin may increase.
2 Effect of prazosin may decrease.
3 Prazosin may increase the effect/toxicity of this drug.
4 Prazosin may decrease the effect of this drug.
5 Concurrent treatment with prazosin is contraindicated.

ADVERSE EFFECTS
CV: orthostatic or postural hypotension, syncope, palpitations, chest pain, edema, dyspnea
CNS: dizziness, drowsiness, fatigue, headache, vertigo, depression
GI: nausea, vomiting, diarrhea
GU: impotence, priapism, urinary frequency
Skin: rash, pruritus
Other: fever, positive antinuclear antibody (ANA) titer, nasal congestion, hypersensitivity reaction

PHARMACOKINETICS AND PHARMACODYNAMICS
Duration of action: 6–12 h
Onset of action: 1–2 h
Peak plasma concentrations: 3 h
Bioavailability: 43%–82% (mean 60%)
Effect of food: delayed absorption but no effect on the extent of absorption
Protein binding: 97%
Volume of distribution: 0.63 (young)–0.89 (elderly) L/kg
Metabolism: metabolized by the liver extensively, several modestly active metabolites
Elimination: mainly via bile and feces as metabolites
Elimination half-life: 2–3 h

MONITORING
Supine and sitting/standing BP.

OVERDOSE
Supportive—consider fluid therapy, with vasopressor added if necessary for profound hypotension.

PATIENT INFORMATION
Prazosin may cause syncope, orthostatic problems, and drowsiness; avoid driving or performing hazardous tasks, especially within 24 h after the first dose or a dosage increment. Sit or lie down if dizziness occurs, and rise slowly from a sitting or lying position. Alcohol may exacerbate these side effects.

AVAILABILITY
Capsules—1, 2, 5 mg
Combination with polythiazide (Minizide): 1, 2, 5 mg capsules each with 0.5 mg polythiazide

TERAZOSIN (Terazosin, Hytrin®)

Terazosin is a selective alpha$_1$-adrenoceptor blocker with an alpha$_1$/alpha$_2$ affinity ratio of 200. Compared with prazosin, terazosin is approximately 25 times more water soluble and has 25 times less affinity for alpha$_1$-receptors. Compared with doxazosin, terazosin has four times the alpha$_1$-receptor selectivity in human prostate tissue. Similar to other alpha$_1$-blockers, terazosin reduces both vascular resistance and capacitance, which results in concurrent afterload and preload reduction. When administered once or twice daily, it is an effective antihypertensive agent with a beneficial effect on the plasma lipid profile. In clinical practice, terazosin is often preferred to prazosin because of its more gradual onset of action and potential for once-daily dosing, although orthostatic hypotension remains a problem. Terazosin is also effective in the management of symptomatic BPH. As with the other alpha$_1$-receptor antagonists, however, it is not a first-line antihypertensive because of its ability to cause orthostatic hypotension and because of the results of the ALLHAT trial (see Doxazosin).

SPECIAL GROUPS

Race: no differences in response

Children: safety and effectiveness have not been established

Elderly: more sensitive to the hypotensive effect; begin with lower dosages and titrate based on clinical response

Renal impairment: no dosage adjustment is necessary

Hepatic impairment: use with caution because the drug is hepatically metabolized; begin with lower dosages and titrate based on clinical response

Pregnancy: category C; use only if potential benefit justifies the potential risk to the fetus

Breast-feeding: not recommended; not known if the drug is excreted in human milk

DOSAGE

BPH: Usual dosage range—up to 10 mg once daily, administered at bedtime. Starting with 1 mg at bedtime, slowly increase the dose to achieve desired response; dosages of 10 mg daily should be continued for a minimum of 4–6 wk to assess/determine the response. Rarely, 20 mg/d may be needed.

Hypertension: Usual dose range—1–5 mg/d at bedtime. Starting with 1 mg at bedtime, slowly increase the dose to achieve desired BP response. Maximum daily dosage is 40 mg; limited gain in efficacy for dosages above 20 mg/d.

If therapy is discontinued for several days, it should be reinstituted with a low dosage (1 mg once daily) and slowly increased based on the clinical response. The maintenance dosage may be divided and administered twice daily to minimize an excessive hypotensive response.

IN BRIEF

INDICATIONS
BPH

Hypertension

CONTRAINDICATIONS
Known hypersensitivity to quinazolines, such as doxazosin and prazosin

Use with tadalafil or vardenafil

DRUG INTERACTIONS
Alcohol[1]

Antihypertensive agents[1,2]

Clonidine[3]

Verapamil[1]

Sildenafil[1]

Tadalafil[1,4]

Vardenafil[1,4]

1 Effect/toxicity of terazosin may increase.

2 Terazosin may increase the effect/toxicity of this drug.

3 Terazosin may decrease the effect of this drug.

4 Concurrent treatment with terazosin is contraindicated.

ADVERSE EFFECTS
CV: orthostatic or postural hypotension, syncope, palpitations, tachycardia, chest pain, edema

CNS: dizziness, headache, drowsiness, fatigue, vertigo, paresthesia, depression

GI: nausea

GU: impotence, priapism, urinary frequency

Other: weight gain, fever, nasal congestion/rhinitis, flulike syndrome, hypersensitivity reaction

PHARMACOKINETICS AND PHARMACODYNAMICS
Duration of action: >24 h

Onset of action: 15 min

Peak effect: 2–3 h

Bioavailability: about 100%

Effect of food: delayed absorption, but no effect on the extent of absorption

Protein binding: 90%–94%

Volume of distribution: 0.8 L/kg

Metabolism: mainly metabolized in the liver

Elimination: urine—40% (10% as unchanged drug); feces—60% (20% as unchanged drug)

Elimination half-life: 12 h

MONITORING
Supine and sitting/standing BP, urinary flow or dysuria (for BPH).

OVERDOSE
Supportive—consider fluid therapy, with vasopressor added if necessary for profound hypotension.

PATIENT INFORMATION
Terazosin may cause syncope and orthostatic problems; avoid driving or performing hazardous tasks, especially within 12–24 h after the first dose or a dosage increment. Sit or lie down if dizziness occurs, and rise slowly from a sitting or lying position. Alcohol may exacerbate these side effects.

AVAILABILITY
Capsules—1, 2, 5, 10 mg

The information here is provided as guidance only. Prescribers should always consult the manufacturer's current prescribing information.

7

PHENOXYBENZAMINE
(Phenoxybenzamine, Dibenzyline®)

Phenoxybenzamine is a long-acting alpha-adrenergic blocker that can produce a "chemical sympathectomy" with oral use. It blocks alpha-adrenergic responses to epinephrine and norepinephrine, resulting in vasodilation and a reflex tachycardia. Unlike phentolamine, it has a relatively slow onset of action, has a long duration of effect (days), and lacks any appreciable direct effect on beta-adrenergic receptors. It is used in patients with pheochromocytoma to control episodes of hypertension and sweating. It is also used in the preoperative management of patients with pheochromocytoma who are being prepared for surgery and in the chronic management of patients with malignant pheochromocytoma. The drug may induce a tachycardia, which may require the concomitant use of a beta-blocker. The possibility of a tachycardia prohibits the routine use of phenoxybenzamine for systemic hypertension. Phenoxybenzamine has also been used to treat dysuria associated with neurogenic bladder, functional outlet obstruction, BPH, and postoperative urinary retention associated with the use of epidural morphine.

SPECIAL GROUPS

Race: no differences in response

Children: safety and effectiveness have not been established

Elderly: use with caution; dosage is adjusted based on clinical response

Renal impairment: use with caution; dosage is adjusted based on clinical response

Hepatic impairment: use with caution, dosage is adjusted based on clinical response

Pregnancy: category C; use only if potential benefit justifies the potential risk to the fetus

Breast-feeding: not recommended; not known if the drug is excreted in human milk

DOSAGE

Initial dose is 10 mg twice daily. Dose should be increased every other day by 10 mg until the desired response is achieved without significant side effects. Usual dose range is 20–40 mg 2–3 times daily.

Note: May be used concurrently with a beta-blocker if troublesome tachycardia coexists.

IN BRIEF

INDICATIONS
Pheochromocytoma, to control hypertensive episodes and excessive sweating

CONTRAINDICATIONS
Hypersensitivity
Any condition in which a decrease in BP is undesirable
Use with tadalafil or vardenafil

DRUG INTERACTIONS
Any agents that may affect BP or heart rate, such as sympathomimetic agents, may cause excessive hypotension or tachycardia.
Phenoxybenzamine blocks the hyperthermia produced by levarterenol and blocks the hypothermia induced by reserpine.
Sildenafil[1]
Tadalafil[1,2]
Vardenafil[1,2]

[1] Effect/toxicity of phenoxybenzamine may increase.
[2] Concurrent treatment with phenoxybenzamine is contraindicated.

ADVERSE EFFECTS
CV: hypotension, tachycardia, arrhythmias, orthostatic hypotension
CNS: drowsiness, fatigue
GI: irritation, dyspepsia
GU: inhibition of ejaculation
Other: nasal congestion, miosis

PHARMACOKINETICS AND PHARMACODYNAMICS
Duration of action: 3–4 d (single dose)
Onset of action: few hours
Peak effect: 7 d after repeated dosing
Bioavailability: 20%–30%
Effect of food: not known
Protein binding: not known
Volume of distribution: not known; highly lipid soluble
Metabolism: mainly in the liver
Elimination: urine and bile
Elimination half-life: 24 h

MONITORING
BP, pulse rate, sweat reduction.

OVERDOSE
Supportive—fluid therapy or norepinephrine may be used in severe hypotension. Other vasopressors are not effective, and epinephrine is contraindicated.

PATIENT INFORMATION
Phenoxybenzamine may cause a significant lowering of BP. Sit or lie down if dizziness occurs, and rise slowly from a sitting or lying position.

AVAILABILITY
Capsules—10 mg

PHENTOLAMINE
(Phentolamine, Regitine®)

Phentolamine is a short-acting, nonselective alpha-adrenergic blocking agent. Its effect is derived by antagonizing the effects of circulating epinephrine or norepinephrine. Phentolamine causes peripheral vasodilation and a reduction in peripheral vascular resistance. It also exhibits some beta-adrenergic activity that contributes to its positive inotropic and chronotropic effect. Phentolamine is not useful for treating chronic hypertension because of the development of tolerance to the antihypertensive effects of the drug and also because of the high incidence of gastrointestinal side effects. Rather, it is used mainly in the management of pheochromocytoma to control or prevent paroxysmal hypertension prior to and during pheochromocytomectomy. It is also used to prevent or treat extravasation associated with intravenous norepinephrine. In addition, phentolamine may be used to treat hypertensive crises caused by sympathomimetic amines or catecholamine excess associated with monoamine oxidase inhibitors. A mixture of phentolamine and papaverine injected into the corpus cavernosum of the penis has been effective in patients with erectile dysfunction.

SPECIAL GROUPS

Race: no differences in response
Children: may be used safely in children with pheochromocytoma (reduce dosage)
Elderly: no dosage adjustment is required
Renal impairment: dosage adjustment is not required
Hepatic impairment: dosage adjustment is not required
Pregnancy: category C; use only if potential benefit justifies the potential risk to the fetus
Breast-feeding: not recommended; not known if the drug is excreted in human milk

DOSAGE

Prevention/control of hypertensive episodes associated with pheochromocytoma:

Management of hypertensive crises associated with pheochromocytoma—5–15 mg intravenously (IV)

Preoperative (pheochromocytomectomy)—5 mg administered IV or intramuscularly (IM) 1–2 h before surgery and repeated if indicated.

Intraoperative—5 mg IV and repeat as indicated to prevent or control hypertension, tachycardia, respiratory depression, convulsions, or other effects related to epinephrine intoxication.

Prevention/treatment of dermal necrosis and sloughing associated with IV norepinephrine:

Prevention—10 mg of phentolamine is added to each liter of norepinephrine solution.

Treatment—initiate within 12 h (as soon as possible) of extravasation; 5–10 mg of phentolamine in 10–15 mL of saline is infiltrated into the area using a small-needle syringe.

Diagnosis of pheochromocytoma (not the first test of choice; all nonessential medications should be withheld for at least 24 h prior to the test): 5 mg IV (preferred) or IM is administered; after the IV dose, BP should be monitored immediately, every 30 s for the first 3 min, and every minute for the next 7 min; after IM dose, BP should be monitored every 5 min for 30–45 min. A BP decrease of at least 35 mm Hg systolic and 25 mm Hg diastolic within 2 min after IV or 20 min after IM administration of phentolamine is considered a positive test for pheochromocytoma.

IN BRIEF

INDICATIONS
Pheochromocytoma—prevention or control of hypertensive episodes; diagnostic test
Prevention or treatment of dermal necrosis and sloughing associated with intravenous administration or extravasation of norepinephrine

CONTRAINDICATIONS
Coronary artery disease
Hypersensitivity
Myocardial infarction
Use with tadalafil or vardenafil

DRUG INTERACTIONS
Epinephrine[1]
Ephedrine[1]
Norepinephrine[1]
Sildenafil[2]
Tadalafil[2,3]
Vardenafil[2,3]

1 Phentolamine may decrease the effect of this drug.
2 Effect/toxicity of phentolamine may increase.
3 Concurrent treatment with phentolamine is contraindicated.

ADVERSE EFFECTS
CV: hypotension, tachycardia, arrhythmias, orthostatic hypotension
CNS: weakness, dizziness
GI: nausea, vomiting, diarrhea, abdominal pain, peptic ulcer exacerbation
Other: nasal congestion, flushing

PHARMACOKINETICS AND PHARMACODYNAMICS
Duration of action: 15–30 min (IV); 30–45 min (IM)
Onset of action: immediate
Peak effect: <2 min (IV); 20 min (IM)
Bioavailability: 100%
Effect of food: not applicable
Protein binding: not known
Volume of distribution: not known
Metabolism: hepatic
Elimination: metabolized in liver; 13% is excreted in urine unchanged
Elimination half-life: 19 min (IV)

MONITORING
BP, pulse rate, and specific clinical response as per indication.

OVERDOSE
Supportive—phentolamine has a short duration of action. Fluid therapy or norepinephrine may be used in severe hypotension. Other vasopressors are not effective, and epinephrine is contraindicated because it may cause a paradoxic reduction in blood pressure.

PATIENT INFORMATION
Phentolamine may cause a significant lowering of BP. Sit or lie down if dizziness occurs, and rise slowly from a sitting or lying position.

AVAILABILITY
Vials—5 mg

The information here is provided as guidance only. Prescribers should always consult the manufacturer's current prescribing information.

9

SELECTED BIBLIOGRAPHY

ALLHAT Officers and Coordinators for the ALLHAT Collaborative Research Group: Major cardiovascular events in hypertensive patients randomized to doxazosin vs chlorthalidone. The Antihypertensive and Lipid-Lowering Treatment to Prevent Heart Attack Trial (ALLHAT). *JAMA* 2000, 283:1967–1975.

Axelrod FB, Krey L, Glickstein JS, *et al.*: Preliminary observations on the use of midodrine in treating orthostatic hypotension in familial dysautonomia. *J Auton Nerv Syst* 1995, 55:29–35.

Baba T, Tomiyama T, Takebe K: Enhancement by an ACE inhibitor of first-dose hypotension caused by an alpha-1 blocker. *N Engl J Med* 1990, 322:1237.

Chobanian AV, Bakris GL, Black HR, for the National High Blood Pressure Education Program Coordinating Committee. The seventh report of the Joint National Committee on Prevention, Detection, Evaluation, and Treatment of High Blood Pressure. The JNC 7 Report. *JAMA* 2003, 289:2560–2572.

Cohn JN, Archibald DG, Ziesche S, *et al.*: Effect of vasodilator therapy on mortality in chronic congestive heart failure: results of a Veterans Administration Cooperative Study. *N Engl J Med* 1986, 314:1547–1552.

Fouad-Tarazi FM, Okabe M, Goren J: Alpha sympathomimetic treatment of autonomic insufficiency with orthostatic hypotension. *Am J Med* 1995, 90:604–610.

Frishman WH: Alpha- and beta-adrenergic blocking drugs. In *Cardiovascular Pharmacotherapeutics Manual.* Edited by Frishman WH, Sonnenblick EH, Sica DA. New York: McGraw Hill; 2004:19–57.

Frishman WH: Alpha- and beta-adrenergic blocking drugs. In *Cardiovascular Pharmacotherapeutics*, edn 2. Edited by Frishman WH, Sonnenblick EH, Sica DA. New York: McGraw Hill; 2003:67–97.

Frishman WH, Azer V, Sica D: Drug treatment of orthostatic hypotension and vasovagal syncope. *Heart Dis* 2003; 5:49–64.

Frishman WH, Kotob F: α-Adrenergic blocking drugs in clinical medicine. *J Clin Pharmacol* 1999, 39:7–16.

Hoffman BB: Catecholamines, sympathomimetic drugs, and adrenergic receptor antagonists. In *Goodman and Gilman's The Pharmacologic Basis of Therapeutics*, edn 10. Edited by Hardman JG, Limbird LE. New York: McGraw Hill; 2001:215–268.

Kaplan NM: Treatment of hypertension: drug therapy. In *Kaplan's Clinical Hypertension*, edn 8. Philadelphia: Lippincott Williams & Wilkins; 2002:237–338.

Lepor H, Meretyk S, Knapp-Maloney G: The safety, efficacy and compliance of terazosin therapy for benign prostatic hypertrophy. *J Urol* 1992, 147:1554–1557.

Minneman KP: Alpha 1-adrenergic receptor subtypes, inositol phosphates and sources of cell Ca2+. *Pharm Rev* 1988, 40:87–119.

Mobley DF, Dias N, Levenstein M: Effects of doxazosin in patients with mild, intermediate and severe benign prostatic hyperplasia. *Clin Ther* 1998, 20:101–109.

Mobley DF, Kaplain SA, Ice K, *et al.*: Effect of doxazosin on the symptoms of benign prostatic hyperplasia: results from three double-blind placebo-controlling studies. *Int J Clin Pract* 1997, 51:282–288.

Neaton JD, Grimm RH Jr, Prineas RJ, *et al.*: Treatment of mild hypertension study: final results. *JAMA* 1993, 207:713–724.

Pollare T, Lithell H, Selinus I, Berne C: Application of prazosin is associated with an increase of insulin sensitivity in obese patients with hypertension. *Diabetologia* 1988, 31:415–420.

Pool JL: α-Adrenergic antagonists. In *Hypertension Primer*, edn 3. Edited by Izzo JR Jr, Black HR. Dallas: American Heart Association; 2003:421–423.

Pool JL: α-Adrenoceptor blockers. In *Hypertension: A Companion to Brenner & Rector's The Kidney*. Edited by Oparil S, Weber MA. Philadelphia: WB Saunders Co.; 2003:495–499.

Shieh S-M, Sheu WH-H, Shen DD-C, *et al.*: Glucose, insulin and lipid metabolism in doxazosin-treated patients with hypertension. *Am J Hypertens* 1992, 5:827–831.

Terazosin for benign prostatic hyperplasia. *Med Lett Drugs Ther* 1994, 36:15–16.

ALPHA₂-ADRENERGIC AGONISTS (CENTRALLY ACTING ANTIHYPERTENSIVE AGENTS)

Centrally acting inhibitors of the sympathetic nervous system are some of the oldest drugs currently used for the treatment of systemic hypertension. Although effective in reducing blood pressure (BP), the clinical use of these agents is limited because of the central sedative and depressive effects associated with their use. This class of drugs is therefore typically reserved as third- or fourth-line drug therapy for the treatment of hypertension.

EFFICACY AND USE

The centrally acting antihypertensive agents may be highly effective when used alone. They are equally effective in treating hypertension in the young and in the elderly. They are especially effective in treating isolated systolic hypertension, which usually occurs in the elderly. These agents appear to be equally effective in treating hypertension in black and white patients. They appear to have little or no deleterious effect on glucose tolerance, renal function, or plasma lipids, making them attractive options for use in the treatment of hypertensive patients with coexisting diabetes or renal dysfunction. Thus, these drugs may be used in a wide range of hypertensive patients, and contraindications to their use are few.

These drugs work synergistically with diuretics for reducing BP and may also be used with other antihyper-tensive drugs as add-on therapy. These agents may reduce left ventricular hypertrophy and enhance diastolic function to some extent. The main limitation to their use is their central nervous system effects, which may impair quality of life for some patients.

Abrupt drug withdrawal, especially with **clonidine**, may actually exacerbate hypertension because of a rebound increase in BP. If cessation of therapy is desired, the dosage of drug should be tapered down gradually before discontinuation.

MODE OF ACTION

Clonidine, **methyldopa**, **guanabenz**, and **guanfacine** appear to have a common mechanism of action. By various means, they stimulate the alpha₂-adrenoceptors in the vasomotor center of the medulla oblongata, resulting in reduced sympathetic outflow from the brain (Fig. 2.1). In the case of **methyldopa**, this does not occur directly. Instead, **methyldopa** is metabolized to alpha-methylnoradrenaline in the brain. The production of this false neurotransmitter at peripheral sites in the body may be responsible for some of the antihypertensive effects of **methyldopa**. The other centrally acting antihypertensives do not appear to require biotransformation for activity, but rather act as direct central

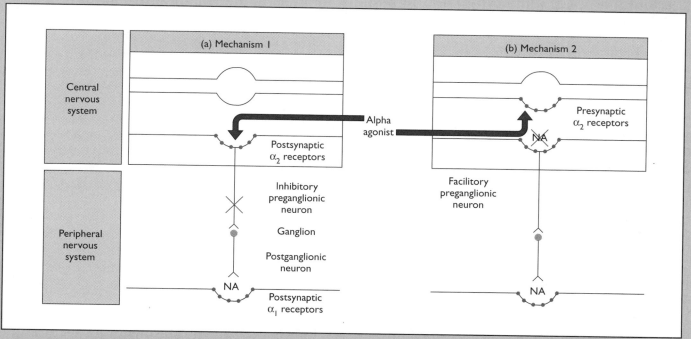

FIGURE 2.1 The interaction of clonidine and related drugs with post- and presynaptic alpha-receptors in the brainstem as a basis for their central hypotensive effect. Two possible mechanisms are shown: (a) Clonidine stimulates postsynaptic alpha₂-receptors; the inhibitory bulbospinal neuron is activated and peripheral sympathetic nervous activity is diminished, which causes a hypotensive effect; and (b) clonidine stimulates presynaptic alpha₂-receptors, diminishing release of central noradrenaline (NA); the facilitatory neuron is activated less and peripheral sympathetic activity is diminished, causing a hypotensive effect. The first mechanism, (a), is most likely correct. (*Adapted from* Van Zwieten PA: The role of adrenoceptors in circulatory and metabolic regulation. *Am Heart J* 1988, 116:1384–1392.)

alpha$_2$-adrenoceptor stimulants. Stimulation of presynaptic alpha$_2$-receptors on peripheral adrenergic neurons may also contribute to the antihypertensive action of these drugs.

These pharmacologic actions ultimately lead to a reduction in peripheral vascular resistance, heart rate, and BP (Table 2.1). After bolus intravenous administration, **clonidine** tends to produce a transient rise in BP. This response is a result of stimulation of peripheral alpha$_2$-receptors on blood vessels. Thereafter, BP falls as central alpha$_2$-receptors are stimulated.

TABLE 2.1 HEMODYNAMIC EFFECTS OF CENTRALLY ACTING AGENTS

Agent	Cardiac output	Plasma volume	Glomerular filtration rate	Orthostasis	Total peripheral vascular resistance	Plasma renin activity
Clonidine	↑	← →	← →	no	↓	↓ or ← →
Guanabenz	↓	← →	← →	mild	↓	↓ or ← →
Guanfacine	↓	← →	← →	mild	↓	↓ or ← →
Methyldopa	—	↑	← →	mild	↓	↓

↑—increase; ↓—decrease; ← →—no change.

INDICATIONS

	Clonidine	Guanabenz	Guanfacine	Methyldopa
Hypertension	+	+	+	+

+—FDA approved.

CLONIDINE
(Clonidine, Catapres®, Duraclon®)

Clonidine stimulates alpha$_2$-adrenergic receptors in the central nervous system (CNS), which results in a decrease in sympathetic outflow from the brain. This, in turn, results in reduced peripheral sympathetic nervous system activity, lowered BP, and bradycardia. The alpha$_2$-agonist activity of clonidine is also responsible for its side effects, such as sedation and dry mouth. Clonidine has been used as an adjunct to alleviate withdrawal symptoms in individuals with opioid or nicotine dependence. By stimulating central presynaptic alpha$_2$-adrenergic receptors, clonidine causes a reduction in adrenergic activity in the CNS, which may be responsible for the withdrawal symptoms. Clonidine is usually administered as oral tablets or as a transdermal system. The latter formulation is applied to the skin once weekly, which may provide more consistent BP control and improve patient compliance. Clonidine is also available as an injectable for the management of severe cancer pain only. For this indication, clonidine is used in combination with an opiate and is administered via an epidural infusion device.

SPECIAL GROUPS

Race: no differences in response
Children: safety and effectiveness have not been established
Elderly: use with caution because these patients may be more sensitive to the hypotensive and sedative effects of the drug; start with a low dosage and titrate based on clinical response. Higher transdermal dosages may be needed because of decreased skin permeability.
Renal impairment: creatinine clearance ≥10 mL/min: no dosage adjustment necessary
creatinine clearance <10 mL/min: reduce dosage by 25%–50%
Hepatic impairment: no dosage adjustment is required
Pregnancy: category C; use only if potential benefit justifies the potential risk to the fetus
Breast-feeding: administration not recommended; drug is excreted in human milk

DOSAGE

Oral: Usual dose range: 0.2–2.4 mg/d in two to three divided doses. Initial dose is 0.05–0.1 mg twice a day; the dose may be increased by 0.1–0.2 mg daily every few days until the desired response is achieved. For rapid BP reduction in patients with severe hypertension, clonidine 0.1–0.2 mg may be given, followed by 0.05–0.2 mg every hour until a total dose of 0.5–0.7 mg or adequate BP control is achieved. Then, a maintenance dose of clonidine is administered and adjusted based on clinical assessment.

IN BRIEF

INDICATIONS
Hypertension (oral and transdermal)

CONTRAINDICATIONS
Known hypersensitivity

DRUG INTERACTIONS
Beta-blockers[1,3]
Calcium channel blockers[3]
CNS depressants, such as alcohol, opiates, barbiturates[3]
Digoxin[3]
Levodopa[4]
Monoamine oxidase (MAO) inhibitors[3]
Other antihypertensive agents[1,3]
Tricyclic antidepressants, such as imipramine, desipramine[2]

[1] Effect/toxicity of clonidine may increase.
[2] Effect of clonidine may decrease.
[3] Clonidine may increase the effect/toxicity of this drug.
[4] Clonidine may decrease the effect of this drug.

ADVERSE EFFECTS
CV: hypotension, tachycardia, bradycardia, Raynaud's symptoms, heart failure, AV block, arrhythmias, orthostatic symptoms, syncope, rebound hypertension
CNS: sedation, dizziness, headache, nervousness, agitation, depression, sleep disturbances, hallucinations, delirium
GI: dry mouth, constipation, nausea, vomiting, anorexia, liver function abnormalities
GU: impotence, ↓libido, urinary frequency
Skin: rash, pruritus, hives, angioedema, contact dermatitis (transdermal system only)
Other: ↑sensitivity to alcohol, dry eyes, blurred vision, dry nasal mucosa, weight gain

PHARMACOKINETICS AND PHARMACODYNAMICS
Duration of action: (po) >8–12 h; (IV) 4 h; (topical) few days
Onset of action: (po/IV) 30–60 min
Peak effect: (po/IV) 2–4 h; (topical) 2–3 d
Bioavailability: (po) 75%–100%
Effect of food: not known
Protein binding: 20%–40%
Volume of distribution: 2.1 L/kg
Metabolism: hepatic
Elimination: renal—65%–72% (40%–60% unchanged); feces—20%
Elimination half-life: 12–16 h (up to 41 h in end-stage renal disease)

MONITORING
BP and medication adherence.

OVERDOSE
Supportive—atropine for bradycardia; fluid therapy and vasopressor therapy, such as dopamine, for profound hypotension; vasodilators, such as phentolamine, as needed for severe hypertension.

PATIENT INFORMATION
Clonidine therapy should not be discontinued abruptly without consulting a physician. Sedation associated with the therapy may impair the ability to perform hazardous activities requiring mental alertness or physical coordination. Concurrent alcohol intake may enhance the sedative effect. Sit or lie down if dizziness occurs, and rise slowly from a sitting or lying position.

CLONIDINE (continued)

DOSAGE (continued)

Transdermal: 0.1–0.6 mg/d, applied weekly to a hairless area of intact skin on the upper outer arm or chest. There is no predictable relationship between the effective oral dose and transdermal dose of clonidine. All patients, including those who have been receiving oral clonidine, should be started with one 0.1 mg/d system applied to a hairless skin area on the upper outer arm or chest every 7 d. If the desired BP control is not achieved, the dose may be increased every 1–2 wk by 0.1 mg/d up to a maximum of 0.6 mg/d (two transdermal 0.3 mg/d systems). Each new transdermal system should be applied to a different site from the previous location.

Note: For patients who are already on oral clonidine, it is recommended that the oral dose be continued for 1–2 d after the first transdermal system is applied.

Intravenous: For hypertensive crisis (not an FDA-approved indication), clonidine 0.15–0.3 mg has been given intravenously over 5 min* with an initial goal of reducing mean arterial BP by ≤25% within the first 2 h, followed by further reduction toward the target BP of 160/100 mm Hg within 2–6 h.

*Slow intravenous administration can minimize the possible hypertension that may precede its hypotensive effect.

AVAILABILITY
Tablets—0.1, 0.2, 0.3 mg
Transdermal system—
  TTS-1: 0.1 mg/24 h (2.5 mg/3.5 cm^2)
  TTS-2: 0.2 mg/24 h (5 mg/7 cm^2)
  TTS-3: 0.3 mg/24 h (7.5 mg/10.5 cm^2)
Parenteral—100 µg/mL and 500 µg/mL (concentrated); both preservative-free
Combination formulations (with a diuretic):
  Combipres Tablets, Clorpres Tablets—
      0.1 mg clonidine and 15 mg chlorthalidone
      0.2 mg clonidine and 15 mg chlorthalidone
      0.3 mg clonidine and 15 mg chlorthalidone

GUANABENZ (Guanabenz, Wytensin®)

Guanabenz is a central alpha$_2$-adrenergic agonist similar to clonidine. Its antihypertensive effect is mediated via stimulation of alpha$_2$-adrenergic receptors in the central nervous system, which results in a decrease in sympathetic outflow. Chronic guanabenz therapy is associated with a decrease in peripheral resistance and heart rate while cardiac output and left ventricular ejection fraction remain unchanged. Similar BP reduction is observed in both supine and standing positions. This may account for fewer orthostatic problems reported with guanabenz therapy. Guanabenz has been used in a limited capacity as an adjunct for the treatment of chronic pain and for the management of opiate withdrawal (not FDA-approved indications).

SPECIAL GROUPS

Race: no differences in response

Children: safety and effectiveness have not been established

Elderly: use with caution because these patients may be more sensitive to the hypotensive and sedative effects of the drug; start with a low dosage and titrate based on clinical response

Renal impairment: use with caution because drug clearance may be reduced; titrate based on clinical response

Hepatic impairment: use with caution because drug metabolism may be reduced; start with low dose and titrate based on clinical response

Pregnancy: category C; use only if potential benefit justifies the potential risk to the fetus

Breast-feeding: not recommended; not known if the drug is excreted in human milk

DOSAGE

Usual dose range: 8–32 mg/d, in two divided doses.

The initial dose is 2–4 mg twice daily. The dosage may be increased in increments of 4–8 mg/d every 1–2 wk (or longer) based on BP response.

IN BRIEF

INDICATIONS
Hypertension

CONTRAINDICATIONS
Known hypersensitivity

DRUG INTERACTIONS
Beta-blockers[3]
Calcium channel blockers[3]
CNS depressants, such as alcohol, opiates, barbiturates[3]
Digoxin[3]
Other antihypertensive agents[1,3]
Tricyclic antidepressants, such as imipramine, desipramine[2]

[1] Effect/toxicity of guanabenz may increase.
[2] Effect of guanabenz may decrease.
[3] Guanabenz may increase the effect/toxicity of this drug.

ADVERSE EFFECTS
CV: hypotension, tachycardia, bradycardia, chest pain, heart failure, edema, AV block, arrhythmias, orthostatic symptoms, rebound hypertension
CNS: sedation, dizziness, weakness, headache, nervousness, agitation, depression, tremor, sleep disturbances, confusion
GI: dry mouth, constipation, nausea, vomiting, anorexia, abnormal liver function tests
GU: urinary frequency, sexual dysfunction
Skin: rash, pruritus
Other: ↑ sensitivity to alcohol, dry eyes, blurred vision, nasal congestion, weight gain

PHARMACOKINETICS AND PHARMACODYNAMICS
Duration of action: 10–12 h or longer
Onset of action: <1 h
Peak effect: 2–7 h
Bioavailability: 70%–80%
Effect of food: not known
Protein binding: 90%
Volume of distribution: large: 93–147 L/kg
Metabolism: unclear, but likely undergoes extensive hepatic metabolism
Elimination: urine—70%–80% (1% unchanged) feces—10%–30%
Elimination half-life: 12–14 h

MONITORING
BP and medication adherence.

OVERDOSE
Supportive—atropine for bradycardia; fluid therapy and vasopressor therapy, such as dopamine, for profound hypotension if necessary.

PATIENT INFORMATION
Guanabenz therapy should not be discontinued abruptly without consulting a physician. Sedation associated with the therapy may impair the ability to perform hazardous activities requiring mental alertness or physical coordination. Concurrent alcohol intake may enhance the sedative effect. Sit or lie down if dizziness occurs, and rise slowly from a sitting or lying position.

AVAILABILITY
Tablets—4, 8 mg

GUANFACINE (Guanfacine, Tenex®)

Guanfacine is a long-acting, central alpha$_2$-adrenergic agonist. Its mechanism of action is similar to that of clonidine and guanabenz. With chronic guanfacine therapy, peripheral vascular resistance is reduced and heart rate is slightly decreased, with minimal effect on cardiac output. Abrupt withdrawal of guanfacine therapy has been associated with less rebound hypertension than clonidine secondary to its long half-life and longer duration of action. The BP usually increases slowly back to pretreatment baseline level over 2–4 d after discontinuation of guanfacine.

SPECIAL GROUPS

Race: no differences in response

Children: safety and effectiveness have not been established

Elderly: use with caution because these patients may be more sensitive to the hypotensive and sedative effects of the drug; start with a low dosage and titrate based on clinical response

Renal impairment: use with caution because drug clearance may be reduced; titrate based on clinical response

Hepatic impairment: use with caution because drug metabolism may be reduced; start with low dose and titrate based on clinical response

Pregnancy: category B; should only be used if clearly indicated

Breast-feeding: not recommended; not known if the drug is excreted in human milk

DOSAGE

Usual dose range: 1–3 mg once daily at bedtime.

The initial dose is 1 mg administered at bedtime to minimize somnolence. The dose may be increased in 1 mg increments every 3–4 wk if adequate BP control is not achieved, up to the maximum of 3 mg/d.

IN BRIEF

INDICATIONS
Hypertension

CONTRAINDICATIONS
Known hypersensitivity

DRUG INTERACTIONS
Beta-blockers[3]
Calcium channel blockers[3]
CNS depressants, such as alcohol, opiates, barbiturates[3]
Digoxin[3]
Other antihypertensive agents[1,3]
Phenobarbital[2]
Phenytoin[2]
Tricyclic antidepressants, such as imipramine, desipramine[2]

1 Effect/toxicity of guanfacine may increase.
2 Effect of guanfacine may decrease.
3 Guanfacine may increase the effect/toxicity of this drug.

ADVERSE EFFECTS
CV: hypotension, tachycardia, bradycardia, chest pain, heart failure, edema, AV block, arrhythmias, orthostatic symptoms, rebound hypertension
CNS: sedation, dizziness, weakness, headache, nervousness, agitation, depression, tremor, sleep disturbances, confusion
GI: dry mouth, constipation, nausea, vomiting, anorexia, abnormal liver function tests, taste alteration
GU: urinary incontinence/frequency, sexual dysfunction
Skin: rash, pruritus, dermatitis, conjunctivitis
Other: ↑ sensitivity to alcohol, dry eyes, blurred vision, weight gain

PHARMACOKINETICS AND PHARMACODYNAMICS
Duration of action: 24 h or longer
Onset of action: 2 h
Peak effect: 6 h
Bioavailability: 80%
Effect of food: not known
Protein binding: 70%
Volume of distribution: 6.3 L/kg
Metabolism: 50% eliminated as conjugation of metabolites
Elimination: urine (40%–75% as unchanged)
Elimination half-life: average 17 h (range 10–30 h)

MONITORING
BP and medication adherence.

OVERDOSE
Supportive—atropine for bradycardia; fluid therapy and vasopressor therapy, such as dopamine, for profound hypotension if necessary.

PATIENT INFORMATION
Guanfacine therapy should not be discontinued abruptly without consulting a physician. Sedation associated with the therapy may impair the ability to perform hazardous activities requiring mental alertness or physical coordination. Concurrent alcohol intake may enhance the sedative effect. Sit or lie down if dizziness occurs, and rise slowly from a sitting or lying position.

AVAILABILITY
Tablets—1, 2 mg

METHYLDOPA, METHYLDOPATE HCL
(Methyldopa, Methyldopate HCl, Aldomet®)

Methyldopa is converted to alpha-methylnorepinephrine, an alpha$_2$-adrenergic agonist, in the CNS. This indirect central alpha$_2$-adrenergic stimulation has been proposed as the major mechanism responsible for the antihypertensive effect of chronic methyldopa therapy. In addition, methyldopa inhibits decarboxylase, which is responsible for the conversion of norepinephrine and serotonin from their precursors in the CNS and peripheral tissues. Plasma methyldopa concentrations do not correlate well with its therapeutic effect. The onset and maximum decrease in BP occur 3–6 h after oral administration. Similar to oral methyldopa, intravenous methyldopate has a relatively slow onset of hypotensive action (3–6 h). Although intravenous methyldopate has been used in hypertensive emergencies, other antihypertensive agents with more rapid onsets of action are preferred when a rapid BP reduction is indicated. Methyldopa is a preferred agent for the management of hypertension during pregnancy because it has minimal adverse effects on the fetus.

SPECIAL GROUPS

Race: no differences in response

Children: safety and effectiveness have not been established

Elderly: use with caution because these patients may be more sensitive to the hypotensive and sedative effects of the drug; start with a low dosage and titrate based on clinical response

Renal impairment: use with caution because drug clearance may be reduced; titrate based on clinical response

Hepatic impairment: contraindicated with active liver disease; use with caution in other forms of hepatic insufficiency; start with low dose, and titrate based on clinical response

Pregnancy: category B (po) and C (IV); although it has been used safely in the third trimester, use only if clearly indicated

Breast-feeding: use with caution; excreted in human milk in negligible amounts

IN BRIEF

INDICATIONS
Hypertension

CONTRAINDICATIONS
Active hepatitis/cirrhosis
Known hypersensitivity to methyldopa or sulfites
Concurrent MAO inhibitor therapy

DRUG INTERACTIONS
Amphetamines[2]
General anesthetics[3]
Iron supplements[2]
Levodopa[1,3]
Lithium carbonate[3]
MAO inhibitors[3]
Norepinephrine[3]
Other antihypertensive agents[1,3]
Phenothiazines[2,3]
Tricyclic antidepressants[2]

[1] Effect/toxicity of methyldopa may increase.
[2] Effect of methyldopa may decrease.
[3] Methyldopa may increase the effect/toxicity of this drug.

ADVERSE EFFECTS
CV: hypotension, orthostatic symptoms, syncope, bradycardia, chest pain, heart failure, edema, rebound hypertension
CNS: sedation, ↓ mental acuity, paresthesia, Parkinsonism, sleep disorders, psychosis, depression, abnormal choreoathetotic movements
GI: dry mouth, nausea, vomiting, diarrhea, constipation, abnormal liver function tests, drug-induced hepatitis, pancreatitis, tongue ulceration
GU: sexual dysfunction
Blood: positive Coombs' test (10%–20% incidence), hemolytic anemia (rare), hemolysis (in glucose-6-phosphate dehydrogenase deficiency)
Skin: rash, urticaria, eczema, ulceration
Other: weight gain, drug-induced fever, flulike syndrome, nasal congestion

PHARMACOKINETICS AND PHARMACODYNAMICS
Duration of action: (po) 24–48 h; (IV) 10–16 h
Onset of action: 3–6 h
Peak effect: 4–6 h
Bioavailability: (po) 25%–50%; (IV) 100%
Effect of food: not known
Protein binding: negligible
Volume of distribution: 0.46 L/kg
Metabolism: extensively metabolized in the liver and GI tract
Elimination: urine—70% as parent drug and metabolites
feces—30%–50%
Elimination half-life: 90–127 min

MONITORING
BP (both supine and sitting/standing);
Lab—direct Coombs' test initially and at 6 and 12 mo of therapy; baseline and periodic CBC and liver function tests.

OVERDOSE
Supportive—fluid therapy and perhaps vasopressor therapy with sympathomimetic drugs if profound hypotension develops; atropine may be used for bradycardia; methyldopa is dialyzable.

PATIENT INFORMATION
Methyldopa therapy should not be discontinued abruptly without consulting a physician. Sedation associated with the therapy may impair the ability to perform hazardous activities requiring mental alertness or physical coordination (especially within the first 2–3 d of therapy or dose increase). Concurrent alcohol intake may enhance the sedative effect. Sit or lie down if dizziness occurs, and rise slowly from a sitting or lying position. Patients should be instructed to report any changes in mood, yellowing of eyes/skin, or unexplained loss of appetite, fever, or joint pains.

METHYLDOPA, METHYLDOPATE HCL (continued)

DOSAGE

Oral (methyldopa): Usual dose range: 500–3000 mg/d in two to four divided doses. The initial dose is 250 mg two to three times daily for 2 d. The dose is then adjusted at intervals of at least 2 d until a desired response is achieved.

Intravenous (methyldopate): Usual dose range: 250–500 mg every 6 h; maximum dosage is 1000 mg every 6 h

AVAILABILITY

Tablets—125, 250, 500 mg
Suspension—250 mg/5 mL, 473 mL
Parenteral—250 mg/5 mL, injectable (methyldopate HCl)
Combination formulations (with a diuretic):
  Aldoclor Tablets—
    250 mg methyldopa
    250 mg chlorothiazide
  Aldoril Tablets—
    250 mg methyldopa
    15 mg hydrochlorothiazide
    250 mg methyldopa
    25 mg hydrochlorothiazide
  Aldoril D Tablets—
    500 mg methyldopa
    30 mg hydrochlorothiazide
    500 mg methyldopa
    50 mg hydrochlorothiazide

SELECTED BIBLIOGRAPHY

Chobanian AV, Bakris GL, Black HR, for the National High Blood Pressure Education Program Coordinating Committee: The seventh report of the Joint National Committee on Prevention, Detection, Evaluation, and Treatment of High Blood Pressure. The JNC 7 Report. *JAMA* 2003, 289:2560–2572.

Cressman MD, Vlasses PH: Recent issues in antihypertensive drug therapy. *Med Clin North Am* 1988, 72:373–398.

Croog SH, Levine S, Testa MA, *et al.*: The effects of antihypertensive therapy on the quality of life. *N Engl J Med* 1986, 314:1657–1664.

Farsang CS: Update on methyldopa. *Ther Hung* 1986, 34:139–149.

Frishman WH, Katz B: Controlled-release drug delivery system in cardiovascular disease treatment. In *Cardiovascular Pharmacotherapeutics*. Edited by Frishman WH, Sonnenblick EH. New York: McGraw-Hill; 1997:1363–1373.

Frishman WH, Schlocker SJ, Awad K, Tejani N: Pathophysiology and medical management of systemic hypertension in pregnancy. *Cardiol in Rev*, in press.

Frohlich ED: Other adrenergic inhibitors and the direct-acting smooth muscle vasodilators. In *Hypertension: A Companion to Brenner and Rector's The Kidney*. Edited by Oparil S, Weber MA. Philadelphia: WB Saunders Co.; 2000:637–643.

Kaplan NM: Treatment of hypertension: drug therapy. In *Kaplan's Clinical Hypertension*. Edited by Kaplan NM. Philadelphia: Lippincott Williams & Wilkins; 2002:237–338.

Krakoff LR: Antiadrenergic drugs with central action, and neuron depletors. In *Cardiovascular Pharmacotherapeutics*, edn 2. Edited by Frishman WH, Sonnenblick EH, Sica DA. New York: McGraw-Hill; 2003:215–219.

Leonetti G: Centrally acting antihypertensive agents. *J Cardiovasc Pharmacol* 1988, 12(Suppl 8):S68–S73.

Lowenthal DT, Matzek KM, MacGregor TR: Clinical pharmacokinetics of clonidine. *Clin Pharmacokinet* 1988, 14:287–310.

Materson BJ: Central and peripheral sympatholytics. In *Hypertension Primer*, edn 3. Edited by Izzo JL Jr, Black HR. Dallas: American Heart Association; 2003:423–425.

Sorkin BM, Heel RC: Guanfacine. *Drugs* 1986, 31:301–306.

Struthers AD, Dollery CT: Central nervous system mechanism in blood pressure control. *Eur J Clin Pharmacol* 1985, 28(Suppl):3–11.

Van Zwieten PA: The role of adrenoceptors in circulatory and metabolic regulation. *Am Heart J* 1988, 116:1384–1392.

Weber MA: Clinical pharmacology of centrally acting antihypertensive agents. *J Clin Pharmacol* 1989, 29:698–602.

Weber MA, Draye JIM: Centrally acting antihypertensive agents: a brief overview. *J Cardiovasc Pharmacol* 1984, 6(Suppl):S803–S807.

Angiotensin-converting enzyme (ACE) inhibitors have been available for more than two decades for clinical use to treat hypertension and congestive heart failure (CHF). An intravenous agent, **enalaprilat**, has been approved by the Food and Drug Administration (FDA) for use in hypertension, and ten oral agents—**benazepril**, **captopril**, **enalapril**, **fosinopril**, **lisinopril**, **moexipril**, **perindopril**, **quinapril**, **ramipril**, and **trandolapril**—are approved and available in the United States.

EFFICACY AND USE

Hypertension

ACE inhibitors offer an important therapeutic option for hypertension: they serve as first-line treatment when thiazide diuretics alone do not provide the desired effect (Table 3.1). According to the seventh report of the Joint National Committee on Prevention, Detection, Evaluation, and Treatment of High Blood Pressure, ACE inhibitors should be considered as initial therapy for hypertension when one or more of the following compelling indications exist: heart failure, post–myocardial infarction (MI), high coronary disease risk, diabetes, chronic kidney disease, and recurrent stroke prevention. Repeated clinical studies have demonstrated the efficacy of ACE inhibitors in lowering blood pressure (BP) and their ability to reduce left ventricular hypertrophy. They are effective and particularly well tolerated in mild to moderate hypertension (both primary and secondary). They do not disturb plasma lipid concentrations and may improve insulin sensitivity and glucose tolerance.

As monotherapy, ACE inhibitors have similar efficacy to beta-blockers and diuretics. Long-acting ACE inhibitors may provide better blood pressure control than short-acting ones. ACE inhibitors are particularly effective when combined with a low dose of a thiazide diuretic, in which case they offset hypokalemia; however, they may increase potassium levels in the presence of potassium-sparing agents. They have additive antihypertensive effects with calcium antagonists and (less so) with beta-blockers.

Heart Failure

ACE inhibitors are also used to treat CHF. By removing renin-angiotensin–mediated vasoconstriction (which frequently underlies the increased afterload on the heart associated with this syndrome), they produce favorable and sustained hemodynamic changes. The CONSENSUS I study demonstrated that the addition of **enalapril** to the treatment of patients with severe heart failure (New York Heart Association class IV) who were already treated with digitalis, diuretics, and (in some cases) other vasodilators produced a significant reduction in mortality compared with addition of placebo (Fig. 3.1). ACE inhibition reduced death caused by progression of heart failure but had no impact on the rate of sudden death.

ACE inhibitors also benefit patients with mild to moderate CHF (class II–III). The treatment arm of the SOLVD study showed that **enalapril** significantly reduced all-cause mortality by 16%, with a 22% reduction in deaths due to progressive heart failure and a significant reduction in hospital admissions (Fig. 3.2). In addition, the SOLVD-Prevention and SAVE studies showed that intervention with **enalapril** and **captopril** reduced the development of severe heart failure and hospital admissions in patients with asymptomatic left ventricular dysfunction. Favorable findings with the use of ACE inhibitors in patients with heart failure were also observed in the V-HeFT II study, where **enalapril** was shown to reduce both total mortality and sudden death over the combination of **hydralazine** and **isosorbide dinitrate**.

Although the benefits associated with ACE inhibition mostly have been illustrated with **captopril** and **enalapril** in patients with CHF, this is probably a class effect. **Ramipril** reduced mortality when therapy was initiated between 3 and 10 days after an acute MI in patients with heart failure in the AIRE study. **Quinapril** and **fosinopril** have been demonstrated to improve exercise tolerance and symptoms in patients with heart failure. At this time, seven of ten ACE inhibitors available in the United States possess FDA-approved labeling for heart failure: **captopril**, **enalapril**, **fosinopril**, **lisinopril**, **quinapril**, **ramipril**, and **trandolapril**. **Captopril**, **enalapril**, **lisinopril**, **ramipril**, and **trandolapril** have been studied for their impact on mortality in patients with heart failure.

TABLE 3.1 COMPLICATED HYPERTENSIVE PATIENTS PARTICULARLY SUITED TO TREATMENT WITH ANGIOTENSIN-CONVERTING ENZYME INHIBITORS	
Concurrent condition	**Reason for use of angiotensin-converting enzyme inhibitor**
Asthma	No effect on airway resistance
Diabetes	No important effect on glycemic control or insulin resistance; reduces signs of progression of diabetic nephropathy
Gout	Reduces uric acid levels
Chronic heart failure	Improves symptoms, hemodynamics, and survival
Post-MI	Reduces morbidity and mortality caused by cardiovascular events
High coronary disease risk	Reduces risk of MI, stroke, and death from cardiovascular causes (as demonstrated by the HOPE study)
Chronic kidney disease	Reduces proteinuria and the rate of GFR decline
Recurrent stroke	Reduces risk of stroke in patients with a history of stroke or TIAs (as demonstrated by PROGRESS when perindopril was used in combination with indapamide)

GFR—glomerular filtration rate; MI—myocardial infarction; TIA—transient ischemic attack.

Unless contraindicated, ACE inhibitor therapy is recommended for all patients with a significantly reduced left ventricular ejection fraction. If possible, the dosage should be titrated to the dosage used in major clinical trials. Once ACE inhibitor therapy is started for the treatment of heart failure, it should be continued for an indefinite period of time unless unbearable side effects occur.

Post–Myocardial Infarction

Immediately following MI, the renin-angiotensin system is activated and progression of ventricular dysfunction (ventricular remodeling) begins to take place. Based on this observation, investigations were initiated to evaluate the possible benefits of ACE inhibitor therapy on mortality and progression to heart failure in patients after MI. Favorable effects from ACE inhibitor therapy were found when **captopril**, **ramipril**, and **trandolapril** were started at least 3 days after MI in the SAVE, AIRE, and TRACE trials, respectively.

The SAVE trial recruited patients with an ejection fraction of 40% or less but without overt heart failure or symptoms of myocardial ischemia after MI. Patients were assigned in randomized fashion to begin treatment with either **captopril** or placebo on days 3 through 16 after MI. Follow-up evaluation for a mean of 3.5 years revealed a reduction in morbidity and mortality caused by major cardiovascular events in the captopril group. The AIRE trial enrolled patients with clinical evidence of heart failure after MI; **ramipril** or placebo was initiated in these patients 3–10 days after MI. Treatment with

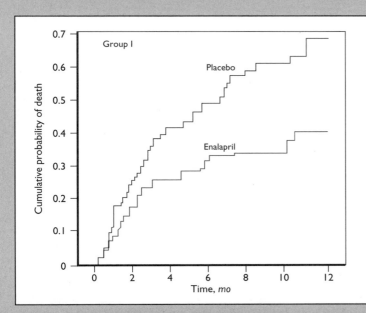

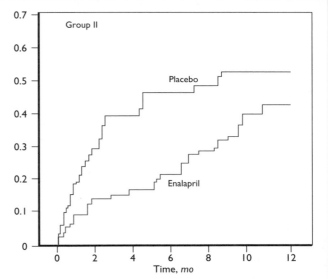

FIGURE 3.1 Cumulative probability of death in CONSENSUS I in patients not taking vasodilators (group I) and those taking vasodilators (group II) at the time of random assignment. (*Adapted from* the CONSENSUS Trial Study Group: Effects of enalapril on mortality in severe congestive heart failure: results of the cooperative North Scandinavian Enalapril Survival Study [CONSENSUS]. *N Engl J Med* 1987, 316:1429–1435.)

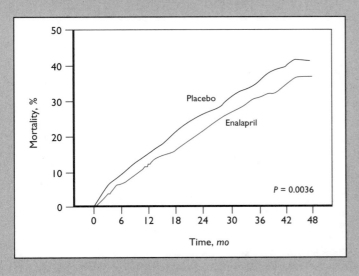

FIGURE 3.2 Cumulative mortality in the SOLVD treatment study. (*Adapted from* the SOLVD Investigators: Effects of enalapril on survival in patients with reduced left ventricular ejection fractions and congestive heart failure. *N Engl J Med* 1991, 325:293–302.)

ramipril was associated with a 27% reduction in all-cause mortality. In the TRACE trial, patients with left ventricular dysfunction on echocardiogram after acute MI were recruited. **Trandolapril** or placebo was randomly assigned to patients 3–7 days after the onset of MI. After a follow-up period of 24–50 months, an 18% reduction in overall mortality was demonstrated in the **trandolapril** group.

Trials of ACE inhibitors as early intervention after MI have shown conflicting results. The CONSENSUS II study involving the use of intravenous **enalaprilat** early postinfarction (within 24 hours) was stopped prematurely, with a 10% excess in deaths in the treatment group. In contrast, ACE inhibitor therapy with **lisinopril** started within 24 hours of acute infarction produced a small but statistically significant reduction in overall mortality in the GISSI-3 study. Similar benefits were observed when **captopril** was initiated within 24 hours of acute MI in the ISIS-4 study.

For many patients who have an acute MI, evidence from clinical trials has confirmed that ACE inhibitors are a valuable addition to standard therapy. Following timely and careful observation of the patient's hemodynamic and clinical status and following administration of routinely recommended treatments (thrombolysis, aspirin, and beta-blockers), ACE inhibitor therapy may be initiated in patients within 24 hours of acute MI. Because simple criteria of efficacy (especially in the early phase) are not available, the starting dose of ACE inhibitors may be individualized on the basis of safety measures, such as hemodynamic response. The target dose should be that used in the clinical trials (Table 3.2).

In patients with left ventricular dysfunction or heart failure after acute MI, therapy should be continued indefinitely. Recently, investigations have been initiated to evaluate the effects of long-term ACE inhibition in survivors of acute MI who have minimal impairment of ventricular function. The HOPE trial showed that **ramipril** significantly reduced the rates of death, MI, and stroke in high-risk patients (including those with a history of MI) who were not known to have a low ejection fraction or heart failure. In addition, the EUROPA investigators found that **perindopril** significantly reduced cardiovascular events in patients with stable coronary heart disease (65% of patients had previous MI) and no apparent heart failure. The HOPE and EUROPA studies have provided strong evidence that regardless of left ventricular function, all patients with coronary artery disease (and without contraindications to ACE inhibitors) should be treated with an ACE inhibitor in addition to aspirin, a beta-blocker, a statin, and aggressive risk-factor modification.

On the basis of the SAVE, AIRE, and TRACE studies, the ACE inhibitors **captopril**, **ramipril**, and **trandolapril** have received FDA approval for the management of patients with left ventricular dysfunction and/or heart failure after sustaining MI. **Lisinopril** is FDA approved for the treatment of hemodynamically stable patients within 24 hours of acute MI to improve survival.

Diabetic Nephropathy

ACE inhibitors have been shown to reduce intraglomerular pressure in diabetic patients, resulting in a reduction in proteinuria and a slight but important reduction in the rate of decline in glomerular filtration rate and prevention of nephropathy. In a randomized placebo-controlled trial of **captopril** (25 mg three times daily) in patients with insulin-dependent diabetes and diabetic nephropathy (proteinuria ≥ 500 mg/d and serum creatinine ≤ 2.5 mg/dL or 221 µmol/L), it was demonstrated that **captopril** could protect against deterioration in renal function and was significantly more effective than in BP control alone. **Captopril** treatment was associated with a 50% reduction in the risk of combined end points of death, need for dialysis, or renal transplantation. Based on this study, **captopril** was approved for use in the treatment of diabetic nephropathy (proteinuria ≥ 500 mg/d) to slow the progression of diabetic kidney disease.

Vascular Disease

The HOPE study evaluated more than 9000 high-risk patients, 55 years of age or older, who had evidence of vascular disease or diabetes plus one other cardiovascular risk factor and who were not known to have a low ejection fraction or heart failure. Patients were randomized to receive **ramipril** 10 mg once daily or matching placebo for a mean of 5 years. Follow-up evaluation showed that a significantly smaller proportion of patients in the **ramipril** group reached a composite end point of MI, stroke, or death from cardiovascular causes compared with the placebo group (14% vs 17.8%). Thus, **ramipril** has gained FDA approval for the reduction in risk of MI, stroke, and death from cardiovascular causes in patients at high risk of developing a major cardiovascular event.

MODE OF ACTION

ACE inhibitors block the conversion of angiotensin I to angiotensin II, thereby preventing vasoconstriction (Fig. 3.3). As a result of their action in reducing angiotensin II levels, they produce a relative decrease in circulating aldosterone concentrations. This discourages sodium and water retention by the kidneys and tends to encourage the retention of potassium.

ACE inhibition results in a relative rise in angiotensin I and renin levels and a tendency for angiotensin II levels to rise to pretreatment levels despite continued treatment. Alternative pathways, including chymase, also result in angiotensin II formation during treatment with ACE inhibitors. They may also prevent the destruction of kinins, locally formed peptides that are powerful vasodilators. Kinins have a direct vasodilatory action but also stimulate the synthesis of vasodilatory prostaglandins. **Captopril** may also produce vasodilatory prostaglandins by direct stimulation of the cell membrane phospholipase. Kinins and prostaglandins may be involved in the antihypertensive effect of ACE inhibitors, but this remains to be established. Endothelium-dependent vasodilatation is improved.

TABLE 3.2 SUMMARY OF RANDOMIZED CLINICAL TRIALS OF ANGIOTENSIN-CONVERTING ENZYME INHIBITORS IN PATIENTS WITH ACUTE MYOCARDIAL INFARCTION

Trial	No. randomized/no. screened, (%)*	Population	Exclusion criteria	Drug initiation from MI	Drug and dose (mg)	Follow-up duration	Overall mortality (control/treated), %	Reduction in mortality, %	p
Trials in High-Risk Acute MI Patients									
SAVE	2231/36,630 (6)	MI, EF ≤40%	ACE inhibitor for CHF or HBP, age >80 yr, SCr >221 μmol/L	3–16 d (mean, 11 d)	Captopril 12.5–50 tid	24–60 mo (mean, 42 mo)	24.6/20.4	19	0.019
AIRE	2006/30,717 (6.5)	MI, clinical HF	NYHA IV, clinical severe RF	3–10 d (mean, 5.4 d)	Ramipril 2.5–5 bid	6–30 mo (mean, 15 mo)	23/17	27	0.002
TRACE	1749/7010 (25)	MI, WMI ≤1.2	0.5 mg trandolapril not tolerated, SCr >200 μmol/L	3–7 d (median, 4 d)	Trandolapril 1–4/d	24–50 mo	42.3/34.7	18	0.001
SMILE	1556/20,261 (8)	Anterior MI, nonthrombolyzed	SBP <100 mm Hg, Killip 4, SCr >221 μmol/L	6–24 h (mean, 15 h)	Zofenopril 7.5–30 bid	12 mo	14.1/10.0	29	0.011
CATS	298	Anterior MI, thrombolyzed	BP <100/55 mm Hg, >200/120 mm Hg, RF	≤6 h	Captopril 6.25–25 tid	3 mo	4.0/6.0	—	—
CONSENSUS-II	6090/10,387 (59)	MI	BP <100/60 mm Hg, <105/65 mm Hg, clinical severe RF	≤1 d	Enalaprilat IV, oral 2.5 bid–20 daily	41–180 d (mean, 6 mo; 2952 patients)	9.4/10.2	—	0.26
Trials in Relatively Unselected Acute MI Patients									
GISSI-3	19,394/43,047 (45)	MI	Severe heart failure, Killip 4, SBP ≤100 mm Hg, SCr >177 μmol/L	≤1 d	Lisinopril 2.5–10 once daily	6 wk	7.1/6.3	11	0.03
ISIS-4	58,050	MI	SBP <90–100 mm Hg, Killip 4	≤1 d	Captopril 6.25–50 bid	5 wk	7.7/7.2	7.0	0.02
CCS-1	13,634	MI	SBP <90 mm Hg, chronic diuretic therapy	≤36 h	Captopril 6.25–12.5 tid	4 wk	9.6/9.1	6.0	0.3

*Figures are not comparable with post-acute MI trials because of different screening procedures.

ACE—angiotensin-converting enzyme; AIRE—Acute Infarction Ramipril Efficacy Study; bid—twice a day; CATS—Captopril and Thrombolysis Study; CCS—Chinese Cardiac Study; CHF—congestive heart failure; CONSENSUS—Cooperative New Scandinavian Enalapril Survival Study; EF—ejection fraction; GISSI-3—Gruppo Italiano per lo Studio della Sopravvivenza nell'Infarto Miocardico-3; HBP—high blood pressure; HF—heart failure; ISIS-4—International Study of Infarct Survival-4; IV—intravenous; MI—myocardial infarction; NYHA—New York Heart Association class; RF—renal failure; SAVE—Survival and Ventricular Enlargement Trial; SBP—systolic blood pressure; SCr—serum creatinine; SMILE—Survival of Myocardial Infarction: Long-term Evaluation; tid—three times a day; TRACE—Trandolapril Cardiac Evaluation Study; WMI—wall motion index.

Adapted from Latini R, Maggioni AP, Flather M, et al. for the meeting participants: ACE inhibitor use in patients with myocardial infarction: summary of evidence from clinical trials. *Circulation* 1995, 92:3132–3137.

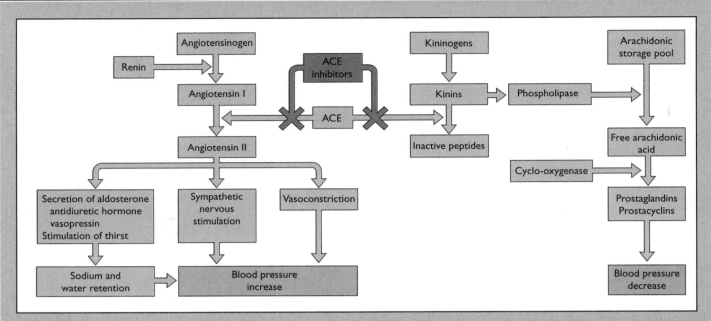

Figure 3.3 Angiotensin-converting enzyme (ACE) inhibitors block the formation of vaso-constrictive sodium-retaining factors, while enhancing accumulation of vasodilatory factors.

Tissue	Effect of angiotensin-converting enzyme inhibitor
TABLE 3.3	**Tissue effects of angiotensin-converting enzyme inhibitors**
Lung	High concentration of ACE. It is possible that ACE inhibitor–induced cough is related to marked ACE inhibition in this tissue.
Central nervous system	Reduced sympathetic outflow with ACE inhibitors could be due to an effect in the CNS.
Arterial wall	Increased arterial compliance and decreased myointimal proliferation, and reduced adverse effects of hypertension on vascular wall structure
Heart	Possible reduction in hypertrophy, partly by direct action on cardiac ACE as well by blood pressure reduction. Possible reduction in cardiac arrhythmias by direct cardiac action.
Kidney	Reduces intraglomerular pressure mainly by dilatation of the efferent arteriole. Reduced albuminuria in patients with nephropathy and also slowing of progressive decline in glomerular filtration rate regardless of cause (although acute renal failure may occur in the presence of low renal perfusion and high plasma renin activity, eg, renal artery stenosis or severe heart failure).

ACE—angiotensin-converting enzyme; CNS—central nervous system; NSAIDs—nonsteroidal anti-inflammatory drugs.

Thus, ACE inhibitors prevent the formation of a vasoconstrictor and reduce sodium and water retention while possibly enhancing the activity of natural vasodilators. A central mechanism has also been postulated because naloxone blunts the antihypertensive effects of ACE inhibitors.

ACE appears to be almost ubiquitous, found in many if not all body tissues. All ACE inhibitors appear capable of inhibiting the enzyme in all tissues, but their effects in different tissues (Table 3.3) may reflect their relative tissue penetration and the relative concentration of ACE in that tissue. ACE inhibition in different tissues may account for some of the effects of these drugs over and above their vasodilatory activity.

Clinical pharmacologic studies suggest that the reason ACE inhibitors do not induce a reflex increase in heart rate may be either a decrease in sympathetic tone or a rise in vagal activity. In uncomplicated hypertension, there appears to be no adverse effects on organ perfusion; indeed, renal blood flow characteristically increases. In heart failure, renal perfusion pressure may decline to critical levels, particularly in patients with severe forms of the syndrome.

INDICATIONS

ACE Inhibitor	HTN	HF	LVD, Post-MI	LVD, Asymptomatic	Improve Survival Post-MI	Reduce Risk of MI, Stroke, and Death From Cardiovascular Causes	Diabetic Nephropathy
Benazepril	+						
Captopril	+	+	+				+
Enalapril	+	+		+			
Enalaprilat	+						
Fosinopril	+	+					
Lisinopril	+	+			+		
Moexipril	+						
Perindopril	+						
Quinapril	+	+					
Ramipril	+	+*				+	
Trandolapril	+	+*	+				

*For treatment of heart failure post-MI.

+—FDA approved; ACE—angiotensin-converting enzyme; HF—heart failure; HTN—hypertension; LVD—left ventricular dysfunction; MI—myocardial infarction.

BENAZEPRIL (Lotensin®)

Benazepril belongs to the largest group of ACE inhibitors, which contains the carboxyl group. It is a prodrug that is metabolized in the liver and other tissues to produce the active metabolite benazeprilat. The effective accumulation half-life of benazeprilat is estimated to be about 10 to 11 h, thus allowing for once-daily dosing. Benazepril is currently indicated for the treatment of hypertension. It can be used alone or in combination with other antihypertensive agents.

SPECIAL GROUPS

Race: whites may respond better than blacks due to lower renin levels usually found in blacks; however, racial differences in BP responses are greatly reduced by the concurrent use of diuretics

Children: safety and effectiveness have not been established

Elderly: no dosage adjustment is required

Hepatic impairment: dosage adjustment is generally not necessary

Renal impairment: reduction of daily dose is required in patients with creatinine clearance (CrCl) < 30 mL/min/1.73m^2

Patients on hemodialysis: anaphylactoid reactions have been reported in patients dialyzed with high-flux membranes and treated concurrently with an ACE inhibitor. A different type of dialysis membrane or a different class of medication should be considered.

Pregnancy: category C (first trimester); category D (second and third trimesters). Use of ACE inhibitors in the second and third trimesters of pregnancy has been associated with fetal skeletal abnormalities, neonatal renal failure, and neonatal death. Benazepril should be discontinued as soon as possible when pregnancy is detected.

Breast-feeding: not recommended; may be excreted in breast milk

IN BRIEF

INDICATIONS
Hypertension. Benazepril can be used alone or in combination with other antihypertensive agents.

CONTRAINDICATIONS/WARNINGS
Hypersensitivity, pregnancy, history of angioedema related to ACE inhibitors, patients dialyzed with high-flux membranes.

DRUG INTERACTIONS
Adrenergic-blocking agents[1,3]
Anesthetics[3]
Antacids[2]
Aspirin[2,5]
Digoxin[3,4]
Diuretics[1,3]
Hypoglycemic agents/insulin[3]
Lithium[3]
NSAIDs (indomethacin)[2]
Potassium supplements[3]
Potassium-sparing diuretics[1,3]

1 Effect/toxicity of benazepril may increase.
2 Effect of benazepril may decrease.
3 Benazepril may increase the effect/toxicity of this drug.
4 Benazepril may decrease the effect of this drug.
5 The clinical significance of this interaction is unclear.

ADVERSE EFFECTS
Cardiovascular: hypotension (<1%), orthostatic hypotension (<1%)
CNS: headache (6%), dizziness (4%), fatigue (2%–3%), somnolence/drowsiness (1%–2%)
GI/GU: abdominal pain (<1%), nausea (1%–2%), pancreatitis (<1%), UTI (<1%)
Respiratory: cough (2%–4%), dyspnea (<1%)
Dermatologic: rash, pruritus, photosensitivity (<1%), flushing (<1%)
Renal: increased BUN and serum creatinine (<1%), increased serum creatinine to >150% of baseline values (2%)
Others: angioedema (0.5%), neutropenia (rare), anemia, syncope (0.1%), asthenia (<1%), impotence (<1%), elevations of liver function tests, hyperkalemia (1%)

PHARMACOKINETICS AND PHARMACODYNAMICS
Duration of action: up to 24 h
Onset of action: 1 h
Peak effect: 2–4 h
Bioavailability: ≈ 37%
Effect of food: none
Protein binding: 96.7% benazepril; 95.3% benazeprilat
Volume of distribution: ≈ 8.7 L
Metabolism: cleavage of the ester group (primarily in the liver) converts benazepril to its active metabolite, benazeprilat
Elimination: renal (benazeprilat), 20%; bile (benazeprilat), 11%–12%
Half-life: 10–11 h (benazeprilat)

MONITORING
BP—Observe carefully for first-dose hypotension, especially in patients with heart failure, patients with renovascular hypertension, and patients who are sodium or volume depleted.
Renal function—Acute renal failure may occur on initiation of ACE inhibitor therapy if the kidneys are dependent on angiotensin II for perfusion. This affects patients with bilateral renal artery stenosis or stenosis of the artery to a solitary kidney, patients with heart failure, or patients who are in hypovolemic states. Rises in serum creatinine or BUN should be an indication to reduce diuretic or benazepril dosage.
Suspect renal artery stenosis if there is a substantial increase in serum creatinine.
Electrolytes, CBC.

DOSAGE

Usual initial dose is 10 mg once daily. Dose can be titrated up to 40 mg/d (in one or two divided doses.) A dose of 80 mg gives an increased response, but experience with this dose is limited. A lower initial dose of 5 mg once daily should be given to patients with renal impairment (CrCl of < 30 mL/min/1.73m^2) or to patients in whom diuretics have not been discontinued.

OVERDOSE

Treatment should be symptomatic and supportive. The patient's BP may be maintained with infusion of normal saline solution. Benazepril is only slightly dialyzable, but dialysis may be considered in overdosed patients with severe renal impairment.

PATIENT INFORMATION

Benazepril may be taken with or without food. Benazepril may cause dizziness, fainting, or lightheadedness, especially during the first few days of therapy; avoid abrupt changes in posture. Use caution when driving or doing other things that require alertness. Consult with physician immediately if pregnancy is detected. Notify physician if persistent side effects occur. Do not discontinue therapy without your physician's advice. Do not use salt substitute unless advised by physician.

AVAILABILITY

Tablets—5 mg, 10 mg, 20 mg, 40 mg
Combination formulations:
Lotensin HCT—benazepril hydrochloride/hydrochlorothiazide combination tablets
  5 mg/6.25 mg
  10 mg/12.5 mg
  20 mg/12.5 mg
  20 mg/25 mg
Lotrel—amlodipine/benazepril hydrochloride combination capsules
  2.5 mg/10 mg
  5 mg/10 mg
  5 mg/20 mg
  10 mg/20 mg

The information here is provided as guidance only. Prescribers should always consult the manufacturer's current prescribing information.

27

CAPTOPRIL (Captopril, Capoten®)

Captopril was the first clinically useful ACE inhibitor. Early severe reactions were related to the very high doses used in high-risk patients. It is directly active and rapidly absorbed. It is about as effective as beta-blockers and diuretics and combines well with diuretics and calcium antagonists (and to a lesser extent, with beta-blockers) to lower BP. Quality of life was reported to be good with captopril. Captopril seems to be as effective as digoxin in controlling heart failure in patients without atrial fibrillation. It modifies postinfarction heart enlargement (remodeling). In the SAVE study, intervention with captopril started on days 3 through 16 after MI demonstrated a reduction in all-cause mortality of 19%. Recurrent MI, development of severe heart failure, and CHF requiring hospitalization were also reduced significantly. Similarly, early intervention with captopril in the ISIS-4 study showed a slight but significant reduction in postinfarction mortality. Captopril also benefits patients with diabetic nephropathy. It is associated with a 51% reduction in the risk of end-stage renal disease or death compared with placebo.

SPECIAL GROUPS

Race: whites may respond better than blacks due to lower renin levels usually found in blacks; however, racial differences in BP responses are greatly reduced by the concurrent use of diuretics

Children: there is limited experience reported in the literature with the use of captopril in the pediatric population. Captopril should be used in children only if other measures for controlling BP have not been effective.

Elderly: usually respond well. Dose should allow for age-related reduction in renal function.

Hepatic impairment: dosage adjustment is generally not necessary

Renal impairment: reduce initial dosage and use smaller or less frequent doses

Patients on hemodialysis: anaphylactoid reactions have been reported in patients dialyzed with high-flux membranes and treated concurrently with an ACE inhibitor. A different type of dialysis membrane or a different class of medication should be considered.

Pregnancy: category C (first trimester); category D (second and third trimesters). Use of ACE inhibitors in the second and third trimesters of pregnancy has been associated with fetal skeletal abnormalities, neonatal renal failure, and neonatal death. Captopril should be discontinued as soon as possible when pregnancy is detected.

Breast-feeding: not recommended; captopril has been detected in breast milk

IN BRIEF

INDICATIONS
Hypertension
Heart failure
Left ventricular dysfunction after MI
Diabetic nephropathy

CONTRAINDICATIONS/WARNINGS
Hypersensitivity, pregnancy, history of angioedema related to ACE inhibitors, patients dialyzed with high-flux membranes.

DRUG INTERACTIONS
Adrenergic-blocking agents[1,3]
Allopurinol[6]
Anesthetics[3]
Antacids[2]
Aspirin[2,5]
Digoxin[3,4]
Diuretics[1,3]
Hypoglycemic agents/insulin[3]
Iron salts[2]
Lithium[3]
NSAIDs (indomethacin)[2]
Potassium-sparing diuretics[1,3]
Potassium supplements[3]

1 Effect/toxicity of captopril may increase.
2 Effect of captopril may decrease.
3 Captopril may increase the effect/toxicity of this drug.
4 Captopril may decrease the effect of this drug.
5 The clinical significance of this interaction is unclear.
6 A higher risk of hypersensitivity reaction may occur.

ADVERSE EFFECTS
Cardiovascular: hypotension, orthostatic hypotension, chest pain (1%), tachycardia (1%)
CNS: headache (0.5%–2%), dizziness (0.5%–2%), fatigue (0.5%–2%), somnolence/drowsiness, insomnia (0.5%–2%), paresthesias (0.5%–2%)
GI/GU: abdominal pain (0.5%–2%), nausea (0.5%–2%), diarrhea (0.5%–2%), dysgeusia (2%–4%), dry mouth (0.5%–2%), hepatitis, pancreatitis
Respiratory: cough (0.5%–2%), dyspnea (0.5%–2%)
Dermatologic: rash (4%–7%), pruritus (2%), photosensitivity, flushing
Renal: proteinuria (<1%), nephrotic syndrome (<0.5%), elevations of BUN or serum creatinine
Others: angioedema (0.1%), anemia, eosinophilia, neutropenia (rare), impotence, syncope, elevations of liver function tests, hyperkalemia

PHARMACOKINETICS AND PHARMACODYNAMICS
Duration of action: 6–12 h
Onset of action: 15 min to 1 h
Peak effect: 1–1.5 h
Bioavailability: 70%
Effect of food: the bioavailability of captopril may be reduced as much as 40% when taken with food. It is not known whether the effects of food on the pharmacokinetics of captopril translate into effects on its clinical efficacy.
Protein binding: 25%–30%
Volume of distribution: 0.7 L/kg
Metabolism: mainly uncharacterized; protein-captopril conjugates formed
Elimination: mostly renal (95%); 40%–50% as unchanged drug; remainder as metabolites
Half-life: 2 h

CAPTOPRIL (continued)

DOSAGE

Hypertension: Initiate with 25 mg two or three times daily. Increase dose if necessary to 150 mg/d (given as three divided doses) depending on severity of hypertension and clinical response. In renovascular hypertension, when diuretics have not been discontinued, or in renal impairment, initial dose should be 6.25 mg, titrated cautiously according to response.

Children: Initiate with 0.3 mg/kg of body weight three times daily. Dosage may be increased in increments of 0.3 mg/kg at intervals of 8–24 h until adequate blood pressure control is achieved.

Elderly: Initiate with the lowest dose possible and titrate according to clinical response.

Congestive heart failure: Initially, 6.25–12.5 mg three times daily, increased according to clinical response. The target dose is 150 mg/d given in three divided doses.

Diabetic nephropathy: 25 mg three times daily.

Left ventricular dysfunction after MI: Initially, 6.25 mg, followed by 12.5 mg three times daily. Then increase dose to 25 mg three times daily during the next several days. Target dose of 50 mg three times daily may be achieved over the next several weeks.

MONITORING

BP—Observe carefully for first-dose hypotension, especially in patients with heart failure, patients with renovascular hypertension, and patients who are sodium or volume depleted.

Renal function—Acute renal failure may occur on initiation of ACE inhibitor therapy if the kidneys are dependent on angiotensin II for perfusion. This affects patients with bilateral renal artery stenosis or stenosis of the artery to a solitary kidney, patients with heart failure, or patients who are in hypovolemic states. Rises in serum creatinine or BUN should be an indication to reduce diuretic or captopril dosage.

Suspect renal artery stenosis if there is a substantial increase in serum creatinine.

Electrolytes, CBC.

OVERDOSE

Treatment should be symptomatic and supportive.

The patient's BP may be maintained with infusion of normal saline solution. Although captopril may be removed from the adult circulation by hemodialysis, there is inadequate data concerning the effectiveness of hemodialysis in removing captopril from the circulation of neonates or children.

PATIENT INFORMATION

Take captopril 1 h before meals. Captopril may cause dizziness, fainting, or lightheadedness, especially during the first few days of therapy; avoid abrupt changes in posture. Use caution when driving or doing other things that require alertness. Consult with physician immediately if pregnancy is detected. Notify physician if persistent side effects occur. Do not discontinue therapy without your physician's advice. Do not use salt substitute unless advised by physician.

AVAILABILITY

Tablets—12.5 mg, 25 mg, 50 mg, 100 mg
Combination formulations:
  Capozide—captopril/hydrochlorothiazide combination tablets
    25 mg/15 mg
    25 mg/25 mg
    50 mg/15 mg
    50 mg/25 mg

ENALAPRIL (Enalapril, Vasotec®)

Enalapril was the first nonsulfhydryl prodrug. It is rapidly absorbed and converted relatively slowly to enalaprilat, the active ACE inhibitor. It has a long duration of action and has been demonstrated to reduce left ventricular hypertrophy. Enalapril reduces systolic blood pressure to a slightly greater extent than do beta-blockers. It has an antihypertensive effect similar to that of the calcium antagonists but is generally better tolerated. In mild to moderate heart failure, enalapril significantly reduced mortality by 16% and death from progressive heart failure by 22% (SOLVD). The prevention arm of SOLVD resulted in delay in the onset of overt heart failure and reduced hospital admissions. Early intervention with intravenous enalaprilat post-MI did not benefit patients in the CONSENSUS II study.

The intravenous form (enalaprilat) is the metabolite of the prodrug enalapril. It is approved for the parenteral treatment of hypertension but should be used with caution in patients with renovascular hypertension.

SPECIAL GROUPS

Race: whites may respond better than blacks due to lower renin levels usually found in blacks; however, racial differences in BP responses are greatly reduced by the concurrent use of diuretics

Children: safety and effectiveness have not been established

Elderly: usually respond well. Dose should allow for age-related reduction in renal function.

Hepatic impairment: dosage adjustment is generally not necessary

Renal impairment: dose must be adjusted according to renal function

Patients on hemodialysis: anaphylactoid reactions have been reported in patients dialyzed with high-flux membranes and treated concurrently with an ACE inhibitor. A different type of dialysis membrane or a different class of medication should be considered.

Pregnancy: category C (1st trimester); category D (second and third trimesters). Use of ACE inhibitors in the second and third trimesters of pregnancy has been associated with fetal skeletal abnormalities, neonatal renal failure, and neonatal death. Enalapril should be discontinued as soon as possible when pregnancy is detected.

Breast-feeding: not recommended; enalapril and enalaprilat have been detected in breast milk

IN BRIEF

INDICATIONS
Hypertension
Heart failure
Asymptomatic left ventricular dysfunction

CONTRAINDICATIONS/WARNINGS
Hypersensitivity, pregnancy, history of angioedema related to ACE inhibitors, patients dialyzed with high-flux membranes.

DRUG INTERACTIONS
Adrenergic-blocking agents[1,3]
Anesthetics[3]
Antacids[2]
Aspirin[2,5]
Digoxin[3,4]
Diuretics[1,3]
Hypoglycemic agents/insulin[3]
NSAIDs (indomethacin)[2]
Lithium[3]
Potassium-sparing diuretics[1,3]
Potassium supplements[3]
Rifampin[2]
Tadalafil[1,3] (additive hypotensive effect)

1 Effect/toxicity of enalapril may increase.
2 Effect of enalapril may decrease.
3 Enalapril may increase the effect/toxicity of this drug.
4 Enalapril may decrease the effect of this drug.
5 The clinical significance of this interaction is unclear.

ADVERSE EFFECTS
Cardiovascular: hypotension (1%–7%), orthostatic hypotension (1%–3%), chest pain (2%), angina pectoris (1%–2%)
CNS: headache (2%–5%), dizziness (4%–7%), fatigue (1%–3%), somnolence/drowsiness, insomnia, paresthesias
GI/GU: abdominal pain (1%–2%), nausea (1%–2%), diarrhea (1%–2%), dysgeusia (≤1%), dry mouth, hepatitis, pancreatitis, UTI (1%–2%)
Respiratory: cough (1%–3%), dyspnea (1%–2%), bronchitis (1%–2%)
Dermatologic: rash (1%–2%), pruritus, photosensitivity, flushing
Renal: elevations of BUN or serum creatinine
Others: angioedema (0.2%), syncope (0.5%–2%), impotence, anemia, eosinophilia, neutropenia (rare), thrombocytopenia (rare), elevations of liver function tests, hyperkalemia (1%)

PHARMACOKINETICS AND PHARMACODYNAMICS
Duration of action: PO, up to 24 h; IV, ≈ 6 h
Onset of action: PO, within 1 h; IV, 15 min
Peak effect: PO, 4–6 h; IV, 1–4 h
Bioavailability: 60%
Effect of food: none
Protein binding: 50%–60%, enalaprilat
Volume of distribution: 1.7 ± 0.7 L/kg
Metabolism: converted to enalaprilat in the liver; no further metabolism known
Elimination: enalapril: 60% renal, 33% fecal; enalaprilat: >90% renal (as unchanged drug)
Half-life: 1.3 h, enalapril; 11 h, enalaprilat

MONITORING
BP—Observe carefully for first-dose hypotension, especially in patients with heart failure, patients with renovascular hypertension, and patients who are sodium or volume depleted.
Renal function—Acute renal failure may occur on initiation of ACE inhibitor therapy if the kidneys are dependent on angiotensin II for perfusion. This affects patients with bilateral renal artery stenosis or stenosis of the artery to a solitary kidney, patients with heart failure, or patients who are in hypovolemic states. Rises in serum creatinine or BUN should be an indication to reduce diuretic or enalapril dosage.
Suspect renal artery stenosis if there is a substantial increase in serum creatinine.
Electrolytes, CBC.

ENALAPRIL (continued)

DOSAGE

Hypertension: Adult—Initial oral dose is 2.5 to 5 mg/d. Increased to the usual effective maintenance dose of 10–20 mg/d (maximum, 40 mg/d can be given in two divided doses) as needed and as tolerated. In renovascular hypertension or in patients in whom diuretics have not been discontinued, the starting dose should be 2.5 mg/d. The usual IV dose in hypertension is 1.25 mg every 6 h administered intravenously over a 5-min period. An initial dose of 0.625 mg over 5 min should be used in patients who are sodium and volume depleted or who have renal impairment (CrCl <30 mL/min). Patients should be observed 1 h after dose to watch for hypotension. If response is inadequate after 1 h, the 0.625 mg dose can be repeated and therapy continued at a dose of 1.25 mg every 6 h. For conversion from intravenous to oral therapy, the recommended initial dose of enalapril tablets is 5 mg once daily for patients with CrCl >30 mL/min and 2.5 mg once daily for patients with CrCl ≤30 mL/min. Dosage should then be adjusted according to BP response.

Elderly—Initially 2.5 mg by mouth. Titrated according to clinical response.

Renal impairment—In patients with moderate to severe renal impairment (CrCl <30 mL/min), the starting oral dose should be 2.5 mg daily, adjusted according to response.

Heart failure: Initially, 2.5 mg by mouth once or twice daily. Titrated according to clinical response. The usual maintenance dose is 5–40 mg/d given in two divided doses.

Asymptomatic left ventricular dysfunction: Initially, 2.5 mg by mouth twice daily. Titrated according to clinical response. Targeted daily dose is 20 mg/d given in two divided doses.

OVERDOSE

Treatment should be symptomatic and supportive. The patient's BP may be maintained with infusion of normal saline solution. Enalaprilat may be removed from general circulation by hemodialysis.

PATIENT INFORMATION

Enalapril may be taken with or without food. Enalapril may cause dizziness, fainting, or lightheadedness, especially during the first few days of therapy; avoid abrupt changes in posture. Use caution when driving or doing other things that require alertness. Consult with physician immediately if pregnancy is detected. Notify physician if persistent side effects occur. Do not discontinue therapy without your physician's advice. Do not use salt substitute unless advised by physician.

AVAILABILITY

Tablets—2.5 mg, 5 mg, 10 mg, 20 mg
Injection—1.25 mg enalaprilat/mL, in 1 and 2 mL vials
Combination formulations:
  Vaseretic—enalapril maleate/ hydrochlorothiazide combination tablets
      5 mg/12.5 mg
      10 mg/25 mg
  Teczem—enalapril maleate/diltiazem malate ER (extended-release) combination tablets
      5 mg/180 mg
  Lexxel—enalapril maleate/felodipine ER (extended-release) combination tablets
      5 mg/2.5 mg
      5 mg/5 mg

The information here is provided as guidance only. Prescribers should always consult the manufacturer's current prescribing information.

31

FOSINOPRIL (Fosinopril, Monopril®)

Fosinopril is a nonsulfhydryl prodrug ACE inhibitor, containing a phosphinic acid rather than a carboxylic acid group. Fosinopril is metabolized by the liver and other tissues to produce the active diacid metabolite fosinoprilat. The elimination half-life of fosinoprilat is longer than that of captopril but similar to that of enalaprilat. This allows for once-daily dosing in the management of hypertension. Fosinopril has also been demonstrated to improve exercise tolerance and symptoms in patients with heart failure. Fosinoprilat is excreted to equal degrees by the liver and kidneys. This feature allows compensatory clearance in either hepatic or renal impairment or old age, suggesting that little dosage adjustment is required in the general population.

SPECIAL GROUPS

Race: whites may respond better than blacks due to lower renin levels usually found in blacks; however, racial differences in BP responses are greatly reduced by the concurrent use of diuretics

Children: safety and effectiveness have not been established

Elderly: usually respond well. Dose reduction generally not required

Hepatic impairment: the apparent total body clearance of fosinoprilat in patients with hepatic insufficiency is approximately one half of that in patients with normal hepatic function. Use usual dose with frequent monitoring.

Renal impairment: due to partial compensatory clearance by the liver, dose reduction is not required

Patients on hemodialysis: anaphylactoid reactions have been reported in patients dialyzed with high-flux membranes and treated concurrently with an ACE inhibitor. A different type of dialysis membrane or a different class of medication should be considered.

Pregnancy: category C (first trimester); category D (second and third trimesters). Use of ACE inhibitors in the second and third trimesters of pregnancy has been associated with fetal skeletal abnormalities, neonatal renal failure, and neonatal death. Fosinopril should be discontinued as soon as possible when pregnancy is detected.

Breast-feeding: not recommended; fosinoprilat has been detected in breast milk

IN BRIEF

INDICATIONS
Hypertension
Heart failure

CONTRAINDICATIONS/WARNINGS
Hypersensitivity, pregnancy, history of angioedema related to ACE inhibitors, patients dialyzed with high-flux membranes.

DRUG INTERACTIONS
Adrenergic-blocking agents[1,3]
Anesthetics[3]
Antacids[2]
Aspirin[2,5]
Digoxin[3,4]
Diuretics[1,3]
Hypoglycemic agents/insulin[3]
Lithium[3]
NSAIDs (indomethacin)[2]
Potassium-sparing diuretics[1,3]
Potassium supplements[3]

1 Effect/toxicity of fosinopril may increase.
2 Effect of fosinopril may decrease.
3 Fosinopril may increase the effect/toxicity of this drug.
4 Fosinopril may decrease the effect of this drug.
5 The clinical significance of this interaction is unclear.

ADVERSE EFFECTS
Cardiovascular: hypotension (≤1%–4.4%), orthostatic hypotension (1%–2%), chest pain (1%–2%), rhythm disturbances (≤1%–1.4%)
CNS: headache (≥1%), dizziness (1%–12%), fatigue (≥1%), somnolence/drowsiness (≤1%), insomnia (≤1%), paresthesias (≤1%)
GI/GU: abdominal pain (≤1%), nausea (1%–2%), diarrhea (>1%), hepatitis (≤1%), pancreatitis (≤1%), dry mouth (≤1%)
Respiratory: cough (2%–10%), dyspnea (≥1%), upper respiratory infection (2%)
Dermatologic: rash (≤1%), pruritus (≤1%), photosensitivity (≤1%), flushing (≤1%)
Renal: elevations of BUN or serum creatinine
Others: angioedema (≤1%), syncope (≤1%), neutropenia (rare), elevations of liver function tests, hyperkalemia (2%–3%)

PHARMACOKINETICS AND PHARMACODYNAMICS
Duration of action: 24 h
Onset of action: 1 h
Peak effect: 2–6 h
Bioavailability: 36%
Effect of food: decreased rate of absorption, unknown clinical significance
Protein binding: 97%–98% (fosinoprilat)
Volume of distribution: 10 L
Metabolism: converted to fosinoprilat in the liver; fosinoprilat is also conjugated to the beta-glucuronide.
Elimination: cleared equally by renal and hepatic routes
Half-life: 12 h (fosinoprilat)

MONITORING
BP—Observe carefully for first-dose hypotension, especially in patients with heart failure, patients with renovascular hypertension, and patients who are sodium or volume depleted.
Renal function—Acute renal failure may occur on initiation of ACE inhibitor therapy if the kidneys are dependent on angiotensin II for perfusion. This affects patients with bilateral renal artery stenosis or stenosis of the artery to a solitary kidney, patients with heart failure, or patients who are in hypovolemic states. Rises in serum creatinine or BUN should be an indication to reduce diuretic or fosinopril dosage.
Suspect renal artery stenosis if there is a substantial increase in serum creatinine.
Electrolytes, CBC.

DOSAGE

Hypertension: Initial dose is 10 mg/d, increased to the usual effective dose of 20–40 mg/d. Some patients appear to have a further response to 80 mg. Total daily doses may be divided into two if trough effect is inadequate.

Heart failure: The usual initial dose is 10 mg/d. Following the initial dose of fosinopril, the patient should be observed under medical supervision for at least 2 h for the presence of hypotension or orthostasis and, if present, until BP stabilizes. An initial dose of 5 mg is preferred in patients with moderate to severe renal failure or in those who have been vigorously diuresed. Dosage should be increased, over a period of several weeks, to a dose that is maximal and tolerated but not exceeding 40 mg/d. The usual effective dosage range is 20–40 mg once daily.

OVERDOSE

Treatment should be symptomatic and supportive. The patient's BP may be maintained with infusion of normal saline solution. Fosinoprilat is poorly removed from the body by both hemodialysis and peritoneal dialysis.

PATIENT INFORMATION

Fosinopril may be taken with or without food. Fosinopril may cause dizziness, fainting, or lightheadedness, especially during the first few days of therapy; avoid abrupt changes in posture. Use caution when driving or doing other things that require alertness. Consult with physician immediately if persistent side effects occur. Do not discontinue therapy without your physician's advice. Do not use salt substitute unless advised by physician.

AVAILABILITY

Tablets—10 mg, 20 mg, 40 mg
Combination formulations:
 Monopril HCT—fosinopril/hydrochlorothiazide combination tablets
  10 mg/12.5 mg
  20 mg/12.5 mg

The information here is provided as guidance only. Prescribers should always consult the manufacturer's current prescribing information.

33

LISINOPRIL (Lisinopril, Prinivil®, Zestril®)

Lisinopril is not a prodrug and is a close analogue of enalaprilat, the active metabolite of enalapril. Because lisinopril does not undergo metabolism and is excreted unchanged entirely in the urine, it can be selected for patients with hepatic impairment. Lisinopril has been shown to be effective in both hypertension and CHF when given once daily. It reduces systolic and diastolic pressure more than diuretics and reduces systolic blood pressure more than atenolol or metoprolol. Lisinopril has similar antihypertensive efficacy when compared with nifedipine but is associated with a lower incidence of side effects. It has an additive antihypertensive effect when added to hydrochlorothiazide, nifedipine, or (less so) a beta-blocker.

In a study comparing the use of lisinopril with captopril in 189 patients with class II to IV CHF, lisinopril 5 to 20 mg/d produced significantly greater improvements in left ventricular ejection fraction than captopril 37.5 to 150 mg/d. Furthermore, lisinopril (but not captopril) was shown to improve exercise duration in patients with impaired renal function. In addition to its established efficacy in the treatment of hypertension and heart failure, lisinopril has been demonstrated to reduce mortality and cardiovascular morbidity in patients with MI when given as early treatment.

SPECIAL GROUPS

Race:	whites may respond better than blacks because of lower renin levels usually found in blacks; however, racial differences in BP responses are greatly reduced by the concurrent use of diuretics
Children:	safety and effectiveness have not been established
Elderly:	usually respond well. Dose should allow for age-related reduction in renal function.
Hepatic impairment:	lisinopril is not metabolized; hepatic impairment is unlikely to be of any clinical importance
Renal impairment:	dose must be adjusted according to renal function
Patients on hemodialysis:	anaphylactoid reactions have been reported in patients dialyzed with high-flux membranes and treated concurrently with an ACE inhibitor. A different type of dialysis membrane or a different class of medication should be considered
Pregnancy:	category C (first trimester); category D (second and third trimesters). Use of ACE inhibitors in the second and third trimesters of pregnancy has been associated with fetal skeletal abnormalities, neonatal renal failure, and neonatal death. Lisinopril should be discontinued as soon as possible when pregnancy is detected.
Breast-feeding:	not recommended; lisinopril may be excreted in breast milk

IN BRIEF

INDICATIONS
Hypertension
Heart failure
Improve survival post-MI

CONTRAINDICATIONS/WARNINGS
Hypersensitivity, pregnancy, history of angioedema related to ACE inhibitors, patients dialyzed with high-flux membranes.

DRUG INTERACTIONS
Adrenergic-blocking agents[1,3]
Anesthetics[3]
Antacids[2]
Aspirin[2,5]
Digoxin[3,4]
Diuretics[1,3]
Hypoglycemic agents/insulin[3]
Lithium[3]
NSAIDs (indomethacin)[2]
Potassium-sparing diuretics[1,3]
Potassium supplements[3]

1 Effect/toxicity of lisinopril may increase.
2 Effect of lisinopril may decrease.
3 Lisinopril may increase the effect/toxicity of this drug.
4 Lisinopril may decrease the effect of this drug.
5 The clinical significance of this interaction is unclear.

ADVERSE EFFECTS
Cardiovascular: hypotension (1%–4.4%), orthostatic hypotension (1%–2%), chest pain (3%–4%), angina pectoris (>1%), rhythm disturbances (≤1%)
CNS: headache (4%–5%), dizziness (5%–11%), fatigue (2%–3%), somnolence/drowsiness (≤1%), insomnia (≤1%), paresthesias (≤1%), depression (>1%)
GI/GU: abdominal pain (2%–3%), nausea (1%–2%), diarrhea (2%–4%), hepatitis (≤1%), pancreatitis (≤1%), dry mouth (≤1%), UTI (≤1%)
Respiratory: cough (>1%), dyspnea (>1%), upper respiratory infection (1%–2%)
Dermatologic: rash (1%–2%), pruritus (>1%), photosensitivity (≤1%), flushing (≤1%)
Renal: elevations of BUN or serum creatinine
Others: angioedema (0.1%), neutropenia (rare), syncope, impotence (1%), asthenia (>1%), myalgia (>1%), elevations of liver function tests (rare), hyperkalemia (2%)

PHARMACOKINETICS AND PHARMACODYNAMICS
Duration of action:	24 h
Onset of action:	1 h
Peak effect:	6 h
Bioavailability:	≈ 25%, widely variable between individuals
Effect of food:	no effect
Protein binding:	none
Volume of distribution:	2.4 ± 1.4 L/kg
Metabolism:	no significant metabolism
Elimination:	100% in urine as unchanged drug
Half-life:	12 h

MONITORING
BP—Observe carefully for first-dose hypotension, especially in patients with heart failure, patients with renovascular hypertension, and patients who are sodium or volume depleted.
Renal function—Acute renal failure may occur on initiation of ACE inhibitor therapy if the kidneys are dependent on angiotensin II for perfusion. This affects patients with bilateral renal artery stenosis or stenosis of the artery to a solitary kidney, patients with heart failure, or patients who are in hypovolemic states. Rises in serum creatinine or BUN should be an indication to reduce diuretic or lisinopril dosage.
Suspect renal artery stenosis if there is a substantial increase in serum creatinine.
Electrolytes, CBC.

LISINOPRIL (continued)

DOSAGE

Hypertension: Initial dose is 10 mg/d, adjusted to usual effective dose range of 10–40 mg/d according to response (maximum daily dose is 40 mg). In patients with moderate to severe renal impairment (CrCl of 10–30 mL/min), the starting dose should be 5 mg/d.

Heart failure: The usual initial dose is 5 mg/d, administered under close medical observation, especially in patients with low BP. The usual effective dosage range is 5–20 mg once daily.

Acute MI: In hemodynamically stable patients within 24 h of the onset of acute MI, the first dose of lisinopril is 5 mg, followed by 5 mg after 24 h, 10 mg after 48 h, and then 10 mg once daily. Patients should receive, as appropriate, the standard recommended treatments, such as thrombolytics, aspirin, and beta-blockers. Patients with a low systolic blood pressure ($\leq$120 mm Hg) when treatment is initiated or during the first 3 days after the infarct should be given a lower dose of 2.5 mg. If hypotension occurs (systolic blood pressure $\leq$100 mm Hg), a daily maintenance dose of 5 mg may be given with temporary reductions to 2.5 mg if needed.

OVERDOSE

Treatment should be symptomatic and supportive. The patient's BP may be maintained with infusion of normal saline solution. Lisinopril can be removed by hemodialysis.

PATIENT INFORMATION

Lisinopril may be taken with or without food. Lisinopril may cause dizziness, fainting, or lightheadedness, especially during the first few days of therapy. Avoid abrupt changes in posture. Use caution when driving or doing other things that require alertness. Consult with physician immediately if pregnancy is detected. Notify physician if persistent side effects occur. Do not discontinue therapy without your physician's advice. Do not use salt substitute unless advised by physician.

AVAILABILITY

Tablets—2.5 mg, 5 mg, 10 mg, 20 mg, 30 mg, 40 mg
Combination formulations:
Prinzide—lisinopril/hydrochlorothiazide combination tablets
 10 mg/12.5 mg
 20 mg/12.5 mg
 20 mg/25 mg
Zestoretic—lisinopril/hydrochlorothiazide combination tablets
 10 mg/12.5 mg
 20 mg/12.5 mg
 20 mg/25 mg

MOEXIPRIL (Univasc®)

Moexipril is a nonsulfhydryl prodrug that is hydrolyzed after oral administration to its active metabolite, moexiprilat. Moexipril has an oral bioavailability of about 13%. Food can affect the rate and extent of absorption of moexipril. The peak concentration (C_{max}) and area under the concentration-time curve (AUC) of moexipril are reduced by approximately 70% and 40%, respectively, after a low-fat breakfast. Greater reductions of C_{max} and AUC have been observed after a high-fat meal. Moexiprilat has an elimination half-life of up to 9 hours, allowing for once-daily dosing in the management of hypertension.

Moexipril administered at 7.5–15 mg once daily has demonstrated similar efficacy in BP control to that of atenolol 25–50 mg once daily, metoprolol 100 mg once daily, verapamil sustained-release 180–240 mg once daily, nitrendipine 20 mg once daily, or captopril 25–50 mg twice daily. Further reductions in BP were achieved when moexipril was added to either hydrochlorothiazide or nifedipine in patients who were inadequately controlled with monotherapy.

SPECIAL GROUPS

Race: the antihypertensive effect is considerably smaller in black patients because of lower renin levels usually found in blacks; however, racial differences in BP responses with ACE inhibitors are greatly reduced by the concurrent use of diuretics

Children: safety and effectiveness have not been established

Elderly: usually respond well. Dose should allow for age-related reduction in renal function.

Hepatic impairment: dosage adjustment is generally not necessary. However, a lower initial dose should be considered.

Renal impairment: dose must be adjusted according to renal function

Patients on hemodialysis: anaphylactoid reactions have been reported in patients dialyzed with high-flux membranes and treated concurrently with an ACE inhibitor. A different type of dialysis membrane or a different class of medication should be considered.

Pregnancy: category C (first trimester); category D (second and third trimesters). Use of ACE inhibitors in the second and third trimesters of pregnancy has been associated with fetal skeletal abnormalities, neonatal renal failure, and neonatal death. Moexipril should be discontinued as soon as possible when pregnancy is detected.

Breast-feeding: not recommended; moexipril may be excreted in breast milk

IN BRIEF

INDICATIONS
Hypertension

CONTRAINDICATIONS/WARNINGS
Hypersensitivity, pregnancy, history of angioedema related to ACE inhibitors, patients dialyzed with high-flux membranes.

DRUG INTERACTIONS
Adrenergic-blocking agents[1,3]
Anesthetics[3]
Antacids[2]
Aspirin[2,5]
Digoxin[3,4]
Diuretics[1,3]
Hypoglycemic agents/insulin[3]
Lithium[3]
NSAIDs (indomethacin)[2]
Potassium-sparing diuretics[1,3]
Potassium supplements[3]

1 Effect/toxicity of moexipril may increase.
2 Effect of moexipril may decrease.
3 Moexipril may increase the effect/toxicity of this drug.
4 Moexipril may decrease the effect of this drug.
5 The clinical significance of this interaction is unclear.

ADVERSE EFFECTS
Cardiovascular: hypotension (<1%), orthostatic hypotension (<1%), chest pain (>1%), angina pectoris (<1%), rhythm disturbances (<1%), peripheral edema (>1%)
CNS: headache (>1%), dizziness (4%), fatigue (2%–3%), somnolence/drowsiness (<1%), insomnia (<1%)
GI/GU: abdominal pain (<1%), nausea (>1%), diarrhea (3%), hepatitis (<1%), pancreatitis (<1%), dry mouth (<1%)
Respiratory: cough (6%), dyspnea (<1%), upper respiratory infection (>1%)
Dermatologic: rash (1%–2%), pruritus (<1%), photosensitivity (<1%), flushing (1%–2%)
Renal: elevations of BUN or serum creatinine
Others: angioedema (<1%), anemia (<1%), syncope (<1%), myalgia (1%–2%), elevations of liver function tests, hyperkalemia (1%)

PHARMACOKINETICS AND PHARMACODYNAMICS
Duration of action: up to 24 h
Onset of action: 1 h
Peak effect: 3–6 h
Bioavailability: 13% as moexiprilat
Effect of food: C_{max} and AUC are markedly reduced when moexipril is taken with food. Therefore, this agent should be taken in a fasting state.
Protein binding: 50% (moexiprilat)
Volume of distribution: 2.8 L/kg (moexiprilat)
Metabolism: both moexipril and moexiprilat are converted to diketopiperazine derivatives and unidentified metabolites
Elimination: 13% in urine (7% as moexiprilat, 1% as moexipril, 5% as other metabolites); 53% in feces (52% as moexiprilat, 1% as moexipril)
Half-life: 2–9 h (moexiprilat)

MONITORING
BP—Observe carefully for first-dose hypotension, especially in patients with heart failure, patients with renovascular hypertension, and patients who are sodium or volume depleted.
Renal function—Acute renal failure may occur on initiation of ACE inhibitor therapy if the kidneys are dependent on angiotensin II for perfusion. This affects patients with bilateral renal artery stenosis or stenosis of the artery to a solitary kidney, patients with heart failure, or patients who are in hypovolemic states. Rises in serum creatinine or BUN should be an indication to reduce diuretic or moexipril dosage.
Suspect renal artery stenosis if there is a substantial increase in serum creatinine.
Electrolytes, CBC.

MOEXIPRIL *(continued)*

DOSAGE

Hypertension: Usual initial dose in patients not receiving diuretics is 7.5 mg once daily, increased gradually to a maximum of 30 mg/d according to response, given as a single daily dose or two divided doses. In renovascular hypertension or in patients in whom diuretics have not been discontinued, the starting dose should be 3.75 mg once daily with close medical supervision. For patients with creatinine clearance $\leq$40 mL/min/1.73 m^2, the initial dose should also be 3.75 mg once daily given cautiously.

OVERDOSE

Treatment should be symptomatic and supportive. The patient's BP may be maintained with infusion of normal saline solution. The dialyzability of moexipril is not known.

PATIENT INFORMATION

Moexipril should be taken 1 h before meals. Moexipril may cause dizziness, fainting, or lightheadedness, especially during the first few days of therapy; avoid abrupt changes in posture. Use caution when driving or doing other things that require alertness. Consult with physician immediately if pregnancy is detected. Notify physician if persistent side effects occur. Do not discontinue therapy without your physician's advice. Do not use salt substitute unless advised by physician.

AVAILABILITY

Tablets—7.5 mg, 15 mg
Combination formulations:
Uniretic—moexipril hydrochloride/hydrochlorothiazide
  combination tablets
  7.5 mg/12.5 mg
  15 mg/25 mg

The information here is provided as guidance only. Prescribers should always consult the manufacturer's current prescribing information.

37

PERINDOPRIL (Aceon®)

Perindopril, a carboxyl-containing ACE inhibitor structurally related to enalapril, is the 10th ACE inhibitor to become available for treatment of hypertension in the United States. Perindopril is a prodrug that is hydrolyzed in the liver to its active metabolite, perindoprilat. Unlike enalapril, perindopril's molecular structure includes a lipophilic perhydroindole group, which may contribute to its longer duration of action. Furthermore, perindoprilat has a high affinity for ACE, which appears to contribute to perindopril's longer ACE inhibitory activity compared with enalapril.

Clinical trials have found perindopril to be effective for the treatment of essential hypertension when given once daily. Several clinical trials also demonstrated that perindopril was as effective as captopril, atenolol, and the combination of amiloride and hydrochlorothiazide for the reduction of blood pressure. Perindopril appears to provide other ACE inhibitor–related advantages, such as reduction of left ventricular hypertrophy, reduction of proteinuria in diabetic renal impairment, and improvement of arterial structure and function. According to a study performed by Reid *et al.* in elderly patients with heart failure, the initial doses of both oral enalapril (2.5 mg) and oral captopril (6.25 mg) significantly decreased blood pressure compared with placebo, whereas the initial dose of oral perindopril (2 mg) did not. Thus, the lack of first-dose hypotension may be an advantage that perindopril has over other ACE inhibitors. Treatment with perindopril was shown to improve functional and clinical status in patients with mild, moderate, and severe congestive heart failure in several small and short-term clinical trials. Further studies are required to clarify perindopril's role in the treatment of heart failure.

The PROGRESS study demonstrated that the combination of perindopril and indapamide reduced the risk of stroke by 43% in patients with a history of stroke or transient ischemic attack. Furthermore, reductions in the risk of stroke were similar in hypertensive and nonhypertensive patients. In a more recent study, EUROPA, perindopril significantly reduced a combined frequency of cardiovascular death, MI, or cardiac arrest within 4.2 years by 20% (9.9% in the placebo group vs 8.0% in the perindopril group) in patients with stable coronary heart disease and no apparent heart failure.

IN BRIEF

INDICATIONS
Hypertension

CONTRAINDICATIONS/WARNINGS
Hypersensitivity, pregnancy, history of angioedema related to ACE inhibitors, patients dialyzed with high-flux membranes.

DRUG INTERACTIONS
Adrenergic-blocking agents[1,3]
Anesthetics[3]
Antacids[2]
Aspirin[2,5]
Digoxin[3,4]
Diuretics[1,3]
Hypoglycemic agents/insulin[3]
Potassium-sparing diuretics[1,3]
Potassium supplements[3]
Lithium[3]
NSAIDs (indomethacin)[2]

1 Effect/toxicity of perindopril may increase.
2 Effect of perindopril may decrease.
3 Perindopril may increase the effect/toxicity of this drug.
4 Perindopril may decrease the effect of this drug.
5 The clinical significance of this interaction is unclear.

ADVERSE EFFECTS
Cardiovascular: hypotension, chest pain, abnormal ECG
CNS: headache, dizziness, somnolence, insomnia, paresthesias, depression
GI: dyspepsia, nausea, vomiting, pancreatitis
Respiratory: cough (6%–12%), upper respiratory infection, sinusitis, pneumonitis
Dermatologic: rash
Renal: elevations of BUN or serum creatinine
Others: small decreases in hemoglobin and hematocrit, hyperkalemia (<2%), tinnitus, lower extremity pain, asthenia, impotence (1%), elevation of liver function tests, neutropenia, angioedema (0.1%)

PHARMACOKINETICS AND PHARMACODYNAMICS
Duration of action: ≈ 24 h
Time to peak
plasma concentration: 1 h (perindopril), 3–7 h (perindoprilat)
Peak effect: 6 h
Bioavailability: ≈ 75% (perindopril), 25% (perindoprilat)
Effect of food: food does not affect the rate or extent of absorption of perindopril but decreases bioavailability of perindoprilat by about 35%
Protein binding: 60% (perindopril), 10%–20% (perindoprilat)
Volume of distribution: 0.22 L/kg (perindopril), 0.16 L/kg (perindoprilat)
Metabolism: perindopril is extensively hydrolyzed in the liver to its active metabolite, perindoprilat
Elimination: perindopril and its metabolites are excreted mostly in the urine with approximately 4%–12% excreted as unchanged drug
Half-life: 1.5–2.9 h (perindopril), 3–10 h (apparent plasma half-life of perindoprilat), 30–120 h (terminal elimination half-life of perindoprilat)

PERINDOPRIL (continued)

SPECIAL GROUPS

Race: whites may respond better than blacks because of lower renin levels usually found in blacks; however, racial differences in BP responses are greatly reduced by the concurrent use of diuretics

Children: safety and effectiveness have not been established

Elderly: lower dose is required. Dose should also allow for age-related reduction in renal function.

Hepatic impairment: dose adjustments may not be necessary in patients with compensated hepatic cirrhosis. Further studies are required to evaluate the need for dose reductions in patients with more severe forms of liver disease.

Renal impairment: dose must be adjusted according to renal function

Patients on hemodialysis: anaphylactoid reactions have been reported in patients dialyzed with high-flux membranes and treated concurrently with an ACE inhibitor. A different type of dialysis membrane or a different class of medication should be considered.

Pregnancy: category C (first trimester); category D (second and third trimesters). Use of ACE inhibitors in the second and third trimesters of pregnancy has been associated with fetal skeletal abnormalities, neonatal renal failure, and neonatal death. Perindopril should be discontinued as soon as possible when pregnancy is detected.

Breast-feeding: not recommended. Perindopril may be excreted in breast milk.

DOSAGE

The recommended initial dose as monotherapy for hypertension is 4 mg once daily. This dose can be titrated according to response to a maximum of 16 mg per day. The usual maintenance dose is 4–8 mg once daily. For patients with CrCl of 30–60 mL/min, initiate with 2 mg once daily and titrate according to response to a maximum of 8 mg daily. The safety and efficacy of perindopril have not been established for patients with CrCl <30 mL/min.

MONITORING

BP.
Renal function—Acute renal failure may occur on initiation of ACE inhibitor therapy if the kidneys are dependent on angiotensin II for perfusion. This affects patients with bilateral renal artery stenosis or stenosis of the artery to a solitary kidney, patients with heart failure, or patients who are in hypovolemic states. Rises in serum creatinine or blood urea nitrogen should be an indication to reduce diuretic or perindopril dosage.
Suspect renal artery stenosis if there is a substantial increase in serum creatinine.
Electrolytes, CBC.

OVERDOSE

Treatment should be symptomatic and supportive. BP may be maintained with infusion of normal saline solution. Perindopril can be removed by hemodialysis.

PATIENT INFORMATION

Perindopril may be taken with or without food. Perindopril may cause headache, dizziness, or lightheadedness. Use caution when driving or doing other things that require alertness. Consult with physician immediately if pregnancy is detected. Notify physician if persistent side effects occur. Do not discontinue therapy without your physician's advice. Do not use salt substitute unless advised by physician.

AVAILABILITY

Tablets: 2 mg, 4 mg, 8 mg

QUINAPRIL (Accupril®)

Quinapril is a nonsulfhydryl prodrug ACE inhibitor. Although quinaprilat has a short elimination half-life of 2 h, its ability to bind strongly with tissue ACE enables this agent to give an antihypertensive effect for as long as 24 h. Similar to other ACE inhibitors, quinapril reduces left ventricular hypertrophy. In patients with mild to severe hypertension, quinapril 10 to 40 mg/d given as a single dose or in two divided doses daily appeared to have similar efficacy to enalapril 10 to 40 mg/d. A further increase in antihypertensive effect was observed when quinapril was combined with hydrochlorothiazide. Administration of quinapril 2.5 to 30 mg/d to patients with CHF improved New York Heart Association class, symptoms of heart failure, exercise tolerance, and workload in these patients. Similar to most of the other agents in this class, quinapril is FDA approved for the treatment of hypertension and heart failure.

SPECIAL GROUPS

Race:	whites may respond better than blacks because of lower renin levels usually found in blacks; however, racial differences in BP responses are greatly reduced by the concurrent use of diuretics
Children:	safety and effectiveness have not been established
Elderly:	usually respond well. Dose should allow for age-related reduction in renal function
Hepatic impairment:	conversion of parent drug into active metabolite may be impaired depending on degree of liver impairment. However, dose adjustment may not be needed.
Renal impairment:	dose must be adjusted according to renal function
Patients on hemodialysis:	anaphylactoid reactions have been reported in patients dialyzed with high-flux membranes and treated concurrently with an ACE inhibitor. A different type of dialysis membrane or a different class of medication should be considered.
Pregnancy:	category C (first trimester); category D (second and third trimesters). Use of ACE inhibitors in the second and third trimesters of pregnancy has been associated with fetal skeletal abnormalities, neonatal renal failure, and neonatal death. Quinapril should be discontinued as soon as possible when pregnancy is detected.
Breast-feeding:	not recommended; quinapril is secreted in breast milk

IN BRIEF

INDICATIONS
Hypertension
Heart failure

CONTRAINDICATIONS/WARNINGS
Hypersensitivity, pregnancy, history of angioedema related to ACE inhibitors, patients dialyzed with high-flux membranes.

DRUG INTERACTIONS
Adrenergic-blocking agents[1,3]
Anesthetics[3]
Antacids[2]
Aspirin[2,5]
Digoxin[3,4]
Diuretics[1,3]
Hypoglycemic agents/insulin[3]
Lithium[3]
NSAIDs (indomethacin)[2]
Potassium-sparing diuretics[1,3]
Potassium supplements[3]
Tetracycline[4]

1 Effect/toxicity of quinapril may increase.
2 Effect of quinapril may decrease.
3 Quinapril may increase the effect/toxicity of this drug.
4 Quinapril may decrease the effect of this drug.
5 The clinical significance of this interaction is unclear.

ADVERSE EFFECTS
Cardiovascular: hypotension (3%), orthostatic hypotension (<1%), chest pain (2%–3%), angina pectoris (<1%), rhythm disturbances (<1%)
CNS: headache (1%–6%), dizziness (4%–8%), fatigue (2%–3%), somnolence/drowsiness (≤1%), insomnia (≤1%)
GI/GU: abdominal pain (1%), nausea (1%–3%), diarrhea (1%–2%), hepatitis (<0.5%), pancreatitis (<0.5%), dry mouth (≤1%)
Respiratory: cough (2%–5%), dyspnea (2%)
Dermatologic: rash (1%–2%), pruritus (≤1%), photosensitivity (<0.5%), flushing (≤1%)
Renal: elevations of BUN or serum creatinine
Others: angioedema (0.1%), neutropenia (rare), anemia (<0.5%), syncope (≤1%), impotence (≤1%), myalgia (1%–2%), elevations of liver function tests, hyperkalemia (2%)

PHARMACOKINETICS AND PHARMACODYNAMICS
Duration of action:	up to 24 h
Onset of action:	1 h
Peak effect:	2–4 h
Bioavailability:	60%
Effect of food:	the rate and extent of quinapril absorption are diminished moderately (about 25%–30%) when administered with a high-fat meal
Protein binding:	97%
Volume of distribution:	0.4 L/kg
Metabolism:	converted to quinaprilat and two minor metabolites in the liver
Elimination:	61% renal; 37% fecal
Half-life:	≈ 2 h (quinaprilat)

MONITORING
BP—Observe carefully for first-dose hypotension, especially in patients with heart failure, patients with renovascular hypertension, and patients who are sodium or volume depleted.
Renal function—Acute renal failure may occur on initiation of ACE inhibitor therapy if the kidneys are dependent on angiotensin II for perfusion. This affects patients with bilateral renal artery stenosis or stenosis of the artery to a solitary kidney, patients with heart failure, or patients who are in hypovolemic states. Rises in serum creatinine or BUN should be an indication to reduce diuretic or quinapril dosage.
Suspect renal artery stenosis if there is a substantial increase in serum creatinine.
Electrolytes, CBC.

QUINAPRIL (continued)

DOSAGE

Hypertension: The recommended initial dose in patients not on diuretics is 10 or 20 mg once daily. Dosage adjustments should be made at intervals of at least 2 weeks. Most patients require dosages of 20, 40, or 80 mg/d given as a single dose or in two equally divided doses. In renovascular hypertension, or in patients in whom diuretics have not been discontinued, the starting dose should be 2.5–5 mg/d. For patients with creatinine clearance of 31–60 mL/min, the initial dose should be 5 mg daily. For patients with creatinine clearance of 10–30 mL/min, the initial dose should be 2.5 mg daily.

Heart failure: The usual initial dose is 5 mg twice daily, administered under close medical observation, especially in patients with low BP. If the initial dosage is well-tolerated, patients should then be titrated as tolerated at weekly intervals until an effective dose, usually 20–40 mg daily given in two equally divided doses, is reached. For patients with creatinine clearance of 31–60 mL/min, the initial dose should be 5 mg daily. For patients with creatinine clearance of 10–30 mL/min, the initial dose should be 2.5 mg daily. If the initial dose is well-tolerated, quinapril may be given as a twice-daily regimen on the following day.

OVERDOSE

Treatment should be symptomatic and supportive. The patient's BP may be maintained with infusion of normal saline solution. Hemodialysis has little effect on the elimination of quinapril and quinaprilat.

PATIENT INFORMATION

Quinapril may be taken with or without food. Quinapril may cause dizziness, fainting, or lightheadedness, especially during the first few days of therapy. Avoid abrupt changes in posture. Use caution when driving or doing other things that require alertness. Consult with physician immediately if pregnancy is detected. Notify physician if persistent side effects occur. Do not discontinue therapy without your physician's advice. Do not use salt substitute unless advised by physician.

AVAILABILITY

Tablets—5 mg, 10 mg, 20 mg, 40 mg
Combination formulations:
Accuretic—quinapril/hydrochlorothiazide combination tablets
 10 mg/12.5 mg
 20 mg/12.5 mg
 20 mg/25 mg

RAMIPRIL

(Altace®)

Ramipril is a nonsulfhydryl prodrug that is hydrolyzed after absorption to form the active metabolite ramiprilat. Ramiprilat has a long elimination half-life of 13–17 h, thus permitting once-daily administration. In patients with mild to moderate essential hypertension, ramipril 10 mg administered once daily demonstrated similar antihypertensive efficacy as atenolol 100 mg once daily or captopril 50 mg twice daily. In addition, ramipril 5 to 10 mg given once daily was shown to be comparable to enalapril 10 to 20 mg once daily. The addition of hydrochlorothiazide may yield adequate BP reduction in those patients who did not respond to ramipril alone. Ramipril has also exhibited beneficial effects in patients with moderate to severe CHF. A significant reduction in mortality was observed when ramipril was initiated between 3 and 10 days after an acute MI in patients with heart failure in the AIRE study. Ramipril presents as a useful ACE inhibitor for use in patients with hypertension and CHF.

The HOPE study showed that ramipril significantly reduced the composite outcome of MI, stroke, or death in patients who were at high risk for cardiovascular events but who did not have left ventricular dysfunction or heart failure. In addition, a subanalysis of the HOPE study showed that ramipril significantly reduced the combined end point of MI, stroke, or cardiovascular death as well as overt nephropathy in diabetic patients with high risk for cardiovascular events.

SPECIAL GROUPS

Race:	whites may respond better than blacks because of lower renin levels usually found in blacks; however, racial differences in BP responses are greatly reduced by the concurrent use of diuretics
Children:	safety and effectiveness have not been established
Elderly:	usually respond well. Dose should allow for age-related reduction in renal function.
Hepatic impairment:	conversion of parent drug into active metabolite may be impaired, depending on degree of liver impairment
Renal impairment:	dose must be adjusted according to renal function
Patients on hemodialysis:	anaphylactoid reactions have been reported in patients dialyzed with high-flux membranes and treated concurrently with an ACE inhibitor. A different type of dialysis membrane or a different class of medication should be considered.
Pregnancy:	category C (first trimester); category D (second and third trimesters). Use of ACE inhibitors in the second and third trimesters of pregnancy has been associated with fetal skeletal abnormalities, neonatal renal failure, and neonatal death. Ramipril should be discontinued as soon as possible when pregnancy is detected.
Breast-feeding:	not recommended; ramipril may be excreted in breast milk

IN BRIEF

INDICATIONS
Hypertension
Heart failure post-MI
Reduction in risk of MI, stroke, and death from cardiovascular causes

CONTRAINDICATIONS/WARNINGS
Hypersensitivity, pregnancy, history of angioedema related to ACE inhibitors, patients dialyzed with high-flux membranes.

DRUG INTERACTIONS
Adrenergic-blocking agents[1,3]
Anesthetics[3]
Antacids[2]
Aspirin[2,5]
Digoxin[3,4]
Diuretics[1,3]
Hypoglycemic agents/insulin[3]
Lithium[3]
NSAIDs (indomethacin)[2]
Potassium-sparing diuretics[1,3]
Potassium supplements[3]

1 Effect/toxicity of ramipril may increase.
2 Effect of ramipril may decrease.
3 Ramipril may increase the effect/toxicity of this drug.
4 Ramipril may decrease the effect of this drug.
5 The clinical significance of this interaction is unclear.

ADVERSE EFFECTS
Cardiovascular: hypotension (0.5%–10%), orthostatic hypotension (2%), chest pain (≤1%), angina pectoris (<1%–3%)
CNS: headache (1%–5%), dizziness (2%–4%), fatigue (2%), somnolence/drowsiness (<1%), insomnia (<1%), vertigo (<1%–1.5%)
GI/GU: abdominal pain (<1%), nausea (<1%–2%), diarrhea (≤1%), hepatitis (<1%), pancreatitis (<1%), dry mouth (<1%)
Respiratory: cough (7%–12%), dyspnea (<1%), upper respiratory infection
Dermatologic: rash, pruritus, photosensitivity (<1%)
Renal: elevations of BUN or serum creatinine
Others: angioedema (0.3%), asthenia (<1%–2%), neutropenia (rare), anemia (<1%), syncope (<1%–2%), impotence (<1%), myalgia (<1%), elevations of liver function tests, hyperkalemia (1%)

PHARMACOKINETICS AND PHARMACODYNAMICS
Duration of action:	up to 24 h
Onset of action:	1–2 h
Peak effect:	3–6 h
Bioavailability:	up to 60%
Effect of food:	the rate, but not extent, of absorption is reduced
Protein binding:	73%, ramipril; 56%, ramiprilat
Metabolism:	ramipril is almost completely metabolized to ramiprilat, which has about six times the ACE inhibitory activity of ramipril, and to the diketopiperazine ester, the diketopiperazine acid, and the glucuronides of ramipril and ramiprilat, all of which are inactive
Elimination:	60% renal; 40% fecal
Half-life:	13–17 h (ramiprilat)

MONITORING
BP—Observe carefully for first-dose hypotension, especially in patients with heart failure, patients with renovascular hypertension, and patients who are sodium or volume depleted.
Renal function—Acute renal failure may occur on initiation of ACE inhibitor therapy if the kidneys are dependent on angiotensin II for perfusion. This affects patients with bilateral renal artery stenosis or stenosis of the artery to a solitary kidney, patients with heart failure, or patients who are in hypovolemic states. Rises in serum creatinine or BUN should be an indication to reduce diuretic or ramipril dosage. Suspect renal artery stenosis if there is a substantial increase in serum creatinine.
Electrolytes, CBC.

RAMIPRIL (continued)

DOSAGE

Hypertension: Usual initial dose is 2.5 mg/d, increased gradually to a maximum of 20 mg/d according to response, given in a single dose or two equally divided doses. In renovascular hypertension or in patients in whom diuretics have not been discontinued, the starting dose should be 1.25 mg/d. For patients with creatinine clearance of <40 mL/min/1.73 m^2, the initial dose should be 1.25 mg/d. Dosage may be titrated upward until BP is controlled or to a maximum of 5 mg/d.

Heart failure post-MI: The usual initial dose is 2.5 mg twice daily. Patients who become hypotensive at this dose may be switched to 1.25 mg twice daily, but all patients should then be titrated toward a target dose of 5 mg twice daily if tolerated. For patients with creatinine clearance of <40 mL/min/1.73 m^2, the initial dose should be 1.25 mg daily. Dosage may then be increased to 1.25 mg twice daily up to a maximum dose of 2.5 mg twice daily, depending on clinical response and tolerance.

Reduction in risk of MI, stroke, and death from cardiovascular causes: Initiate at 2.5 mg once daily for 1 wk, increase dose to 5 mg once daily for the next 3 wk, and then increase dose as tolerated to 10 mg once daily (may be given as two divided doses).

OVERDOSE

Treatment should be symptomatic and supportive. The patient's BP may be maintained with infusion of normal saline solution. It is not known if ramipril or ramiprilat can be usefully removed from the body by hemodialysis.

PATIENT INFORMATION

Ramipril may be taken with or without food. Capsule usually is swallowed whole but may be sprinkled on applesauce or mixed in water or apple juice. The mixture should be consumed in its entirety. Ramipril may cause dizziness, fainting, or lightheadedness, especially during the first few days of therapy; avoid abrupt changes in posture. Use caution when driving or doing other things that require alertness. Consult with physician immediately if pregnancy is detected. Notify physician if persistent side effects occur. Do not discontinue therapy without your physician's advice. Do not use salt substitute unless advised by physician.

AVAILABILITY

Capsules—1.25 mg, 2.5 mg, 5 mg, 10 mg

TRANDOLAPRIL (Mavik®)

Trandolapril is a nonsulfhydryl prodrug and is hydrolyzed in the liver to its active metabolite, trandolaprilat, after oral administration. Trandolaprilat has a high affinity for ACE, which results in a slow dissociation and a long biologic half-life. Near total ACE inhibition 24 h after a single dose and significant ACE inhibition 72 h following drug withdrawal after long-term therapy have been observed with trandolapril. The trough:peak ratio with once-daily administration of trandolapril was found to be higher than 50% (50%–100%). In patients with essential hypertension, trandolapril administered once daily can effectively reduce systolic and diastolic BP throughout the 24-h post-dose period.

The antihypertensive efficacy of trandolapril 0.5–4 mg/d has been demonstrated to be comparable to that of enalapril 2.5–20 mg/d or lisinopril 10 mg/d. Concomitant therapy with a thiazide diuretic or calcium antagonist further enhances the antihypertensive efficacy of trandolapril. In addition, trandolapril 2–4 mg/d appeared to be as effective as atenolol 100–200 mg/d, hydrochlorothiazide 25 mg/d, or sustained-release nifedipine 40 mg/d in BP control. Trandolapril has also exhibited beneficial effects in patients with left ventricular dysfunction. A significant decrease in mortality was observed when trandolapril was initiated between 3 and 7 d after an acute MI in patients with left ventricular dysfunction.

Trandolapril is indicated for the treatment of hypertension and for the management of patients with heart failure or left ventricular dysfunction post MI.

SPECIAL GROUPS

Race: whites may respond better than blacks because of lower renin levels usually found in blacks; however, racial differences in BP responses are greatly reduced by the concurrent use of diuretics

Children: safety and effectiveness have not been established

Elderly: usually respond well; dose should allow for age-related reduction in renal function

Hepatic impairment: lower doses should be considered in patients with hepatic insufficiency

Renal impairment: dose must be adjusted according to renal function

Patients on hemodialysis: anaphylactoid reactions have been reported in patients dialyzed with high-flux membranes and treated concurrently with an ACE inhibitor. A different type of dialysis membrane or a different class of medication should be considered.

Pregnancy: category C (first trimester); category D (second and third trimesters). Use of ACE inhibitors in the second and third trimesters of pregnancy has been associated with fetal skeletal abnormalities, neonatal renal failure, and neonatal death. Trandolapril should be discontinued as soon as possible when pregnancy is detected.

Breast-feeding: not recommended. Trandolapril may be excreted in breast milk.

IN BRIEF

INDICATIONS
Hypertension
Heart failure post-MI
Left ventricular dysfunction post-MI

CONTRAINDICATIONS/WARNINGS
Hypersensitivity, pregnancy, history of angioedema related to ACE inhibitors, patients dialyzed with high-flux membranes.

DRUG INTERACTIONS
Adrenergic-blocking agents[1,3]	Hypoglycemic agents/insulin[3]
Anesthetics[3]	Lithium[3]
Antacids[2]	NSAIDs (indomethacin)[2]
Aspirin[2,5]	Potassium-sparing diuretics[1,3]
Digoxin[3,4]	Potassium supplements[3]
Diuretics[1,3]	

1 Effect/toxicity of trandolapril may increase.
2 Effect of trandolapril may decrease.
3 Trandolapril may increase the effect/toxicity of this drug.
4 Trandolapril may decrease the effect of this drug.
5 The clinical significance of this interaction is unclear.

ADVERSE EFFECTS
Cardiovascular: hypotension (0.3%–11%), chest pain (≤1%), palpitations (≤1%)
CNS: headache (>1%), dizziness (1%–23%), fatigue (>1%), somnolence/drowsiness (≤1%), insomnia (≤1%)
GI/GU: abdominal pain (≤1%), vomiting (≤1%), diarrhea (≤1%), dyspepsia (≤5%), pancreatitis (≤1%), UTI (1%)
Respiratory: cough (2%–35%), dyspnea (≤1%), upper respiratory infection (≤1%)
Dermatologic: rash (≤1%), pruritus (≤1%), flushing (≤1%)
Renal: elevations of BUN or serum creatinine
Others: angioedema (0.1%), neutropenia (rare), asthenia (3%–4%), syncope (≤6%), impotence (≤1%), myalgia (4%–5%), elevations of liver function tests, hyperkalemia (0.4%)

PHARMACOKINETICS AND PHARMACODYNAMICS
Duration of action:	≥24 h
Onset of action:	2 h
Peak effect:	4–8 h
Bioavailability:	10% as trandolapril, 70% as trandolaprilat
Effect of food:	food slows absorption of trandolapril but does not affect AUC or C_{max} of trandolaprilat or C_{max} of trandolapril
Protein binding:	80%, trandolapril; 65%–94%, trandolaprilat
Volume of distribution:	18 L
Metabolism:	in addition to trandolaprilat, at least seven other metabolites have been found, principally glucuronides or de-esterification products
Elimination:	33% in urine (mostly as trandolaprilat); 66% in feces
Half-life:	6 h, trandolapril; 10 h, trandolaprilat

MONITORING
BP—Observe carefully for first-dose hypotension, especially in patients with heart failure, patients with renovascular hypertension, and patients who are sodium or volume depleted.
Renal function—Acute renal failure may occur on initiation of ACE inhibitor therapy if the kidneys are dependent on angiotensin II for perfusion. This affects patients with bilateral renal artery stenosis or stenosis of the artery to a solitary kidney, patients with heart failure, or patients who are in hypovolemic states. Rises in serum creatinine or BUN should be an indication to reduce diuretic or trandolapril dosage.
Suspect renal artery stenosis if there is a substantial increase in serum creatinine.
Electrolytes, CBC.

TRANDOLAPRIL (continued)

DOSAGE

Hypertension: Usual initial dose is 1 mg/d in nonblack patients and 2 mg/d in black patients. Increased (at ≥1-wk intervals) to a maximum of 8 mg/d according to response. Most patients have required dosages of 2–4 mg/d. There is little experience with doses more than 8 mg/d. Patients inadequately treated with once-daily dosing at 4 mg may be treated with twice-daily dosing. In renovascular hypertension or in patients in whom diuretics have not been discontinued, the starting dose should be 0.5 mg/d. For patients with a creatinine clearance <30 mL/min or with hepatic cirrhosis, the recommended initial dose is also 0.5 mg/d.

Heart failure or left ventricular dysfunction post-MI: The usual initial dose is 1 mg/d. Following the initial dose, titrate as tolerated toward a target dose of 4 mg/d. If a 4 mg dose is not tolerated, patients can continue therapy with the greatest tolerated dose. For patients with a creatinine clearance <30 mL/min or with hepatic cirrhosis, the recommended initial dose is 0.5 mg/d.

OVERDOSE

Treatment should be symptomatic and supportive. The patient's BP may be maintained with infusion of normal saline solution. Trandolaprilat is removed by hemodialysis.

PATIENT INFORMATION

Trandolapril may be taken with or without food. Trandolapril may cause dizziness, fainting, or lightheadedness, especially during the first few days of therapy; avoid abrupt changes in posture. Use caution when driving or doing other things that require alertness. Consult with physician immediately if pregnancy is detected. Notify physician if persistent side effects occur. Do not discontinue therapy without your physician's advice. Do not use salt substitute unless advised by physician.

AVAILABILITY

Tablets—1 mg, 2 mg, 4 mg
Combination formulations:
 Tarka—trandolapril/verapamil hydrochloride ER tablets—
  2 mg/180 mg
  1 mg/240 mg
  2 mg/240 mg
  4 mg/240 mg

Al-Khatib SM: Angiotensin-converting enzyme inhibitors: a new therapy for atrial fibrillation [editorial]. *Am Heart J* 2004, 147:751–752.

Björck S, Nyberg G, Mulec H, *et al.*: Beneficial effects of angiotensin converting enzyme inhibition on renal function in patients with diabetic nephropathy. *Br Med J* 1986, 293:471–474.

Brogden RN, Wiseman LR: Moexipril: A review of its use in the management of essential hypertension. *Drugs* 1998, 55:845–860.

Burris JF: The expanding role of angiotensin converting enzyme inhibitors in the management of hypertension. *J Clin Pharmacol* 1995, 35:337–342.

Cheng A, Frishman WH: Use of angiotensin-converting enzyme inhibitors as monotherapy and in combination with diuretics and calcium channel blockers. *J Clin Pharmacol* 1998, 38:477–491.

Cohn JN, Johnson G, Ziesche S, *et al.*: A comparison of enalapril with hydralazine-isosorbide dinitrate in the treatment of chronic congestive heart failure. *N Engl J Med* 1991, 325:303–310.

CONSENSUS Trial Study Group: Effects of enalapril on mortality in severe congestive heart failure. Results of the Cooperative North Scandinavian Enalapril Survival Study (CONSENSUS). *N Engl J Med* 1987, 316:1429–1435.

Croog SM, Levine S, Testa MA, *et al.*: The effects of antihypertensive therapy on the quality of life. *N Engl J Med* 1986, 314:1657–1664.

Dunn A, Chow MSS: Focus on perindopril: a long-acting ACE inhibitor for hypertension that improves arterial distensibility and compliance. *Formulary* 1998, 33:33–43.

EURopean trial On reduction of cardiac events with Perindopril in stable coronary Artery disease investigators: Efficacy of perindopril in reduction of cardiovascular events among patients with stable coronary artery disease: randomised, double-blind, placebo-controlled, multicentre trial (the EUROPA study). *Lancet* 2003, 362:782–788.

Frishman WH, Cheng A: Secondary prevention of myocardial infarction: the role of β-adrenergic blockers and angiotensin converting enzyme inhibitors. *Am Heart J* 1999, 137:S25–S34.

Giles TD: Clinical experience with lisinopril in congestive heart failure: focus on the older patient. *Drugs* 1990, 39(suppl 2):17–22.

GISEN Group: Randomised placebo-controlled trial of effect of ramipril on decline in glomerular filtration rate and risk of terminal renal failure in proteinuric, non-diabetic nephropathy. *Lancet* 1997, 349:1857–1863.

Goa KL, Balfour JA, Zuanetti G: Lisinopril: a review of its pharmacology and clinical efficacy in the early management of acute myocardial infarction. *Drugs* 1996, 52:564–588.

Gosse P, Dallocchio M, Gourgon R: ACE inhibitors in mild to moderate hypertension: comparison of lisinopril and captopril administered once daily. *J Human Hypertens* 1989, 3:23–28.

Gruppo Italiano per lo Studio della Sopravvivenza nell' Infarto Miocardico (GISSI): Six-month effects of early treatment with lisinopril and transdermal glyceryl trinitrate singly and together withdrawn six weeks after acute myocardial infarction: the GISSI-3 trial. *J Am Coll Cardiol* 1996, 27:337–344.

Herman AG: Differences in structure of angiotensin-converting enzyme inhibitors might predict differences in action. *Am J Cardiol* 1992, 70:102C–108C.

Heart Outcomes Prevention Evaluation study investigators: Effects of an angiotensin-converting-enzyme inhibitor, ramipril, on cardiovascular events in high-risk patients. *N Engl J Med* 2000, 342:145–153.

Heart Outcomes Prevention Evaluation (HOPE) study investigators: Effects of ramipril on cardiovascular and microvascular outcomes in people with diabetes mellitus: results of the HOPE study and MICRO-HOPE substudy. *Lancet* 2000, 355:253–259.

Hirooka Y, Imaizumi T, Masaki H, *et al.*: Captopril improves impaired endothelium-dependent vasodilation in hypertensive patients. *Hypertension* 1992, 20:175–180.

Howes LG: Critical assessment of ACE inhibitors: part I. *Aust Fam Physician* 1995, 24:425–429.

Jaffe IA: Adverse effects profile of sulphydryl compounds in man. *Am J Med* 1986, 30:471–476.

Johnston CI: Angiotensin converting enzyme inhibitors. In *Handbook of Hypertension, Vol. 5: Clinical Pharmacology of Antihypertensive Drugs*. Edited by Doyle AE. Amsterdam: Elsevier; 1984:272–311.

Joint National Committee on Prevention, Detection, Evaluation, and Treatment of High Blood Pressure: The seventh report of the Joint National Committee on Prevention, Detection, Evaluation, and Treatment of High Blood Pressure. *JAMA* 2003, 289:2560–2572.

Kaplan HR, Taylor DG, Olson SC, Andrews LK: Quinapril: a preclinical review of the pharmacology, pharmacokinetics, and toxicology. *Angiology* 1989, 40:335–350.

Kober L, Torp-Pedersen C, Carlsen JE, *et al.* for the Trandolapril Cardiac Evaluation (TRACE) study group: A clinical trial of the angiotensin-converting enzyme inhibitor trandolapril in patients with left ventricular dysfunction after myocardial infarction. *N Engl J Med* 1995, 333:1670–1676.

Lancaster SG, Todd PA: Lisinopril: a preliminary review of its pharmacodynamic and pharmacokinetic properties and therapeutic use in hypertension and congestive heart failure. *Drugs* 1988, 35:646–669.

Latini R, Maggioni AP, Flather M, et al.: ACE inhibitor use in patients with myocardial infarction: summary of evidence from clinical trials. *Circulation* 1995, 92:3132–3137.

Leonetti G, Cuspidi C: Choosing the right ACE inhibitor: a guide to selection. *Drugs* 1995, 49:516–535.

Lewis EJ, Hunsicker LG, Bain RP, et al.: The effect of angiotensin converting enzyme inhibition on diabetic nephropathy. *N Engl J Med* 1993, 329:1456–1462.

Loeb HS, Johnson G, Herrick A, et al.: Effect of enalapril, hydralazine plus isosorbide dinitrate, and prazosin, on hospitalization in patients with chronic congestive heart failure: the V-HeFT VA Cooperative Study Group. *Circulation* 1993, 87(suppl 6):V178.

Mathiesen ER, Hommel E, Giese J, Parving HH: Efficacy of captopril in postponing nephropathy in normotensive insulin dependent diabetic patients with microalbuminuria. *Br Med J* 1991, 303:81–87.

Nash DT: Comparative properties of angiotensin-converting enzyme inhibitors: relations with inhibition of tissue angiotensin-converting enzyme and potential clinical implications. *Am J Cardiol* 1992, 69:26C–32C.

Nelson KM, Yeager BF: What is the role of angiotensin-converting enzyme inhibitors in congestive heart failure and after myocardial infarction? *Ann Pharmacother* 1996, 30:986–993.

Pellizzer A-M, Krum H: ACE inhibitors in cardiovascular disease: which patient? Which drug? Which dose? *Aust Fam Physician* 1996, 25:1067–1077.

Pfeffer MA, Braunwald E, Moyé LA, et al., on behalf of the SAVE Investigators: Effect of captopril on mortality and morbidity in patients with left ventricular dysfunction after myocardial infarction: results of the Survival and Ventricular Enlargement (SAVE) trial. *N Engl J Med* 1992, 327:669–677.

Pfeffer MA, Lamas GA, Vaughan DE, et al.: Effect of captopril on progressive ventricular dilatation after anterior myocardial infarction. *N Engl J Med* 1988, 319:80–86.

PROGRESS Collaborative Group: Randomised trial of a perindopril-based blood-pressure-lowering regimen among 6105 individuals with previous stroke or transient ischaemic attack. *Lancet* 2001, 358:1033–1041.

Reid JL, MacFadyen RJ, Squire IB, Lees KR: Blood pressure response to the first dose of angiotensin-converting enzyme inhibitors in congestive heart failure. *Am J Cardiol* 1993, 71:57E–60E.

Santoro D, Natali A, Palombo C, et al.: Effects of chronic angiotensin converting enzyme inhibition on glucose tolerance and insulin sensitivity in essential hypertension. *Hypertension* 1992, 20:181–191.

Sica DA, Gehr TWB, Frishman WH: The renin-angiotensin axis: angiotensin-converting enzyme inhibitors and angiotensin-receptor blockers. In *Cardiovascular Pharmacotherapeutics Manual*. Edited by Frishman WH, Sonnenblick EH, Sica DA. New York: McGraw-Hill; 2004:96–130.

Swedberg K, Held P, Kjekshus J, et al., on behalf of the CONSENSUS II Study Group: Effects of the early administration of enalapril on mortality in patients with acute myocardial infarction: results of the Cooperative New Scandinavian Enalapril Survival Study II (CONSENSUS II). *N Engl J Med* 1992, 327:678–684.

The Acute Infarction Ramipril Efficacy (AIRE) Study Investigators: Effects of ramipril on mortality and morbidity of survivors of acute myocardial infarction with clinical evidence of heart failure. *Lancet* 1993, 342:821–828.

The American College of Cardiology/American Heart Association Task Force on Practice Guidelines (Committee on Evaluation and Management of Heart Failure): Guidelines for the evaluation and management of heart failure. *Circulation* 1995, 92:2764–2784.

The Fourth Internal Study of Infarct Survival (ISIS-4) Collaborative Group: A randomised factorial trial assessing early oral captopril, oral mononitrate, and intravenous magnesium sulphate in 58,050 patients with suspected acute myocardial infarction. *Lancet* 1995, 345:669–685.

The SOLVD Investigators: Effects of enalapril on survival in patients with reduced left ventricular ejection fractions and congestive heart failure. *N Engl J Med* 1991, 325:293–302.

The SOLVD Investigators: Effects of enalapril on mortality and the development of heart failure in asymptomatic patients with reduced left ventricular ejection fractions. *N Engl J Med* 1992, 327:685–691.

Todd PA, Benfield P: Ramipril: a review of its pharmacological properties and therapeutic efficacy in cardiovascular disorders. *Drugs* 1990, 39:110–135.

Voors AA, Herre Kingma J, van Gilst WH: Drug differences between ACE inhibitors in experimental settings and clinical practice. *J Cardiovasc Risk* 1995, 2:413–422.

Wadworth AN, Brogden RN: Quinapril: a review of its pharmacological properties, and therapeutic efficacy in cardiovascular disorders. *Drugs* 1991, 41:378–399.

White HD: Should all patients with coronary disease receive angiotensin converting enzyme inhibitors? *Lancet* 2003, 362:755–757.

Wiseman LR, McTavish D: Trandolapril: a review of its pharmacodynamic and pharmacokinetic properties, and therapeutic use in essential hypertension. *Drugs* 1994, 48:71–90.

Zaman AG, Kearney MT, Schecter C, et al.: Angiotensin-converting enzyme inhibitors as adjunctive therapy in patients with persistent atrial fibrillation. *Am Heart J* 2004, 147:823–827.

Zannad F: Trandolapril: How does it differ from other angiotensin converting enzyme inhibitors? *Drugs* 1993, 46(suppl 2):172–182.

The information here is provided as guidance only. Prescribers should always consult the manufacturer's current prescribing information.

47

As described in the previous chapter, the renin-angiotensin system (RAS) plays an important role in the body's regulation of arterial blood pressure. The effector hormone of the RAS is angiotensin II, which maintains the systemic vascular resistance and extracellular fluid volume through its direct and indirect vasoconstrictive and blood volume expansion effects (Fig. 4.1). In particular, angiotensin II constricts vascular smooth muscle and increases central sympathetic outflow. In addition, angiotensin II stimulates the release of norepinephrine and epinephrine from the sympathetic nervous system and the adrenal medulla. It exerts antinatriuretic and antidiuretic effects in the kidneys and promotes the release of vasopressin from the pituitary gland and the release of aldosterone from the adrenal cortex (sona glomerulosa).

In addition to its effects on cardiovascular homeostasis, angiotensin II contributes to the control of cellular growth and differentiation, and causes ventricular hypertrophy. Its effect on growth may be pathogenic in patients with chronic cardiovascular disease associated with hypertension.

Angiotensin II exerts its effects by binding to plasma membrane receptors. Two distinct angiotensin II receptor subtypes have been characterized by radioligand binding studies, AT_1 and AT_2. Furthermore, isoforms of AT_1 have been cloned and sequenced in mice and subsequently named AT_{1A} and AT_{1B}. The AT_1 receptor mediates the majority, if not all, of the biologic effects of angiotensin II. Stimulation of the AT_1 receptor causes the direct and indirect vasoconstrictive and volume-expanding effects of angiotensin II, as well as cell growth and proliferation and angiogenesis (Table 4.1). The AT_1 receptor can be selectively inhibited by a group of drugs, the angiotensin II receptor blockers (ARBs), which include **candesartan**, **eprosartan**, **irbesartan**, **losartan**, **olmesartan**, **telmisartan**, and **valsartan**.

EFFICACY AND USE

All ARBs are approved for clinical use in the treatment of systemic hypertension. Some drugs in the class may be more efficacious than others in the control of blood pressure (BP). In contrast to the angiotensin-converting enzyme (ACE) inhibitors, ARBs are usually not associated with cough as a complication. The ARBs have demonstrated beneficial effects in patients with type 2 diabetes. In patients with diabetic nephropathy with or without hypertension, **losartan** and **irbesartan** significantly slowed the progression of nephropathy. In patients with diabetes and microalbuminuria with or without hypertension, **irbesartan** and **valsartan** reduced the rate of progression to nephropathy and restored significantly more patients to normoalbuminuria than

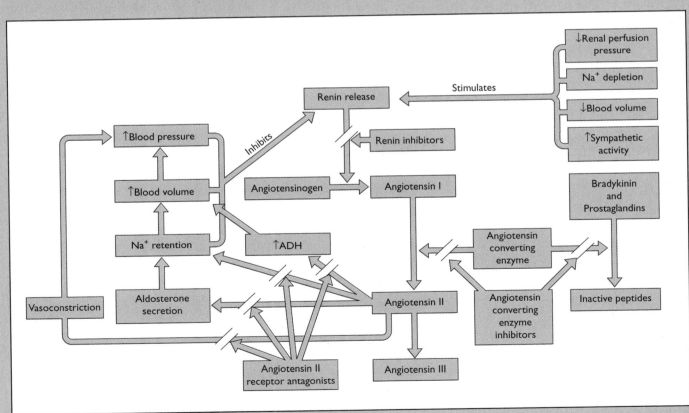

FIGURE 4.1 Schematic representation of renin-angiotensin-aldosterone system. (*Adapted from* Foote EF, Halstenson CE: New therapeutic agents in the management of hypertension: angiotensin-II receptor antagonists and renin inhibitors. *Ann Pharmacother* 1993, 27:1495–1503.)

TABLE 4.1 FUNCTIONS OF AT_1 AND AT_2 RECEPTORS	
Functions of AT_1 receptor	**Functions of AT_2 receptor**
Always expressed	Only expressed during stress or injury
Mediates renal reabsorption of sodium through tubules	Decreases renal reabsorption of sodium
Mediates vasoconstriction	Mediates vasodilatation
Mediates cell growth; inhibits endothelial function, promotes smooth muscle proliferation, stimulates connective tissue deposit in media, facilitates LDL transport to media	Inhibits cell growth (antiproliferation)

AT_1, AT_2—angiotension II subtypes 1 and 2; LDL—low-density lipoprotein.

placebo or **amlodipine**. Results from clinical trials also demonstrate that ARBs, when added to conventional treatment for patients with heart failure, are associated with a reduction in morbidity and mortality as well as an improvement in quality of life. At this time, ARBs are recommended as an alternative for heart failure patients who cannot toler-ate therapy with an ACE inhibitor. The pharmacokinetic and other properties of ARBs are summarized in Table 4.2.

MODE OF ACTION

The ARBs bind selectively to the AT_1 receptor and exert their direct pharmacologic effects on BP by this mechanism. Angiotensin II levels are elevated with ARBs, and the unblocked AT_2 receptor will be stimulated. The AT_2 receptor is expressed at high density during fetal life, and in lesser amounts in the adult heart, adrenal medulla, and brain. These receptors are upregulated during vascular injury and myocardial infarction (MI). The AT_2 receptor mediates an antiproliferative and vasodilator effect of angiotensin II and may potentiate the actions of AT_{1A} blockade, which will have similar effects.

The theoretic benefit of combining ARBs and ACE inhibitors in hypertension and congestive heart failure (CHF) is based on two premises:

1. ACE inhibition does not eliminate angiotensin II production by non-ACE synthetic mechanisms. There may be a gradual loss of pharmacologic action as angiotensin II levels increase.
2. ACE inhibition potentiates the formation of bradykinin, a vasodilator that is not affected by ARBs.

TABLE 4.2 SUMMARY OF ANGIOTENSIN II RECEPTOR ANTAGONISTS AVAILABLE IN THE UNITED STATES

	Losartan potassium	Valsartan	Irbesartan	Candesartan cilexetil	Telmisartan	Eprosartan mesylate	Olmesartan medoxomil
Trade name	Cozaar	Diovan	Avapro	Atacand	Micardis	Teveten	Benicar
Approved indication(s)	HTN HTN with LVH Nephropathy*	HTN Heart failure	HTN Nephropathy*	HTN	HTN	HTN	HTN
Dose							
Initial	25–50 mg/d	80 mg/d	150 mg/d	8–16 mg/d	20–40 mg/d	600 mg/d	20 mg/d
Maintenance	25–100 mg/d†	80–320 mg/d	150–300 mg/d	8–32 mg/d†	20–80 mg/d	400–800 mg/d†	20–40 mg/d
T_{max} (h)	1 (3–4)‡	2–4	1.5–2	3–4	1	1–2	1–2
T:P ratio (%)	58–78	69–76	> 60	80	≥ 97	67	57–70
Dose range (mg)§	50–100	80–160	≥ 150	8–16	20–80	600	5–80
Bioavailability (%)	≈ 33	≈ 25	60–80	≈ 15	42–58	≈ 13	≈ 26
Food effect (AUC/C_{max})¶	↓10%/↓14%	↓40%/↓50%	No effect	No effect	↓6%/↓20% (40 mg AUC/160 mg AUC)	↓15%/↓25%	No effect
Plasma bound (%)	>98 (>99)‡	95	90	>99	>99	≈ 98	99
Volume of distribution (L)	≈ 34 (≈ 12)‡	17**	53–93	0.13 L/kg	500	308	≈ 17
Prodrug	No	No	No	Yes	No	No	Yes
Active metabolite	EXP 3174	—	—	Candesartan	—	—	Olmesartan (RNH-6270)
Metabolism	CYP2C9; CYP3A4	Unknown	CYP2C9	O-deethylation	Conjugation	Glucuronidation	None
Elimination half-life (h)	≈ 2 (6–9)‡	≈ 6**	11–15	≈ 9	≈ 24	5–9	≈ 13
Recovered in the urine (%)	≈ 35	≈ 13	≈ 20	≈ 33	<1%	≈ 7	35–50
Recovered in the feces (%)	≈ 60	≈ 83	≈ 80	≈ 67	>97%	≈ 90	50–65
Initial dosage adjustment							
CrCl <30 mL/min	No	Caution	No	Caution	No	No	No
Hepatic impairment	↓50% dose	Caution	No	No	Caution	No	No
Hemodialyzable	No	No	No	No	No	No	Unknown

*Losartan and irbesartan are indicated for the management of nephropathy in type 2 diabetic patients.

†Total daily dose may be given in two divided doses.

‡Characteristic of active metabolite, EXP 3174.

§This is the dose range that corresponds to the T:P ratio.

¶All agents listed here may be administered with or without food, regardless of food effect.

**Intravenous dosing.

AUC—area under the plasma concentration-time curve; CrCl—creatinine clearance; C_{max}—peak plasma concentration; HTN—hypertension; LVH—left ventricular hypertrophy; T_{max}—time to peak plasma concentration; T:P—trough:peak.

CANDESARTAN CILEXETIL
(Atacand®)

Candesartan binds to angiotensin II subtype 1 (AT_1) receptors selectively and competitively with "insurmountable" binding. Candesartan cilexetil is completely transformed to the active compound candesartan during absorption from the gastrointestinal tract. In contrast to other agents in this class, candesartan has a low bioavailability of about 15%. Candesartan has an elimination half-life of about 9 hours and tight receptor binding, which allows for once-daily dosing.

Ambulatory BP monitoring has shown that the benefits of once-daily candesartan cilexetil persist for 24 h without affecting normal circadian variations. Candesartan cilexetil 8 mg/d was found to be as effective as usual therapeutic dosages of enalapril, losartan potassium, hydrochlorothiazide, or amlodipine in comparative studies. At 16 mg/d, candesartan cilexetil reduced trough diastolic BP significantly more than losartan potassium 50 mg/d in one study, and candesartan cilexetil 16 mg/d titrated as necessary to 32 mg/d more than losartan potassium 50 mg/d titrated as necessary to 100 mg/d in another study. The combination of candesartan cilexetil with either amlodipine or hydrochlorothiazide resulted in further antihypertensive effects.

The CHARM investigators compared candesartan with placebo in three different populations of patients with class II to IV heart failure. The primary outcome of all three trials was the composite of cardiovascular death or hospital admission for CHF. The CHARM-Added study randomized 2548 patients with ejection fractions of 40% or less treated with optimum doses of ACE inhibitors to either candesartan or placebo. At a median follow-up of 41 months, a significantly smaller proportion of patients in the candesartan group compared with the placebo group experienced the primary composite outcome (38% vs 42%). The CHARM-Alternative study randomized 2028 patients with ejection fractions of 40% or less who were intolerant of ACE inhibitors to candesartan or placebo. Similar to results of the CHARM-Added trial, a significantly smaller proportion of patients who received candesartan experienced the primary composite outcome compared with patients who received placebo (33% vs 40%) at a median follow-up of 33.7 months. The CHARM-Preserved study randomized 3023 patients with class II to IV CHF but ejection fractions of more than 40% to additional therapy with candesartan or placebo. At a median follow-up of 36.6 months, the primary outcome was experienced by similar proportions of patients in both groups. However, significantly fewer patients in the candesartan group than in the placebo group (230 vs 279) were admitted to the hospital for CHF once or multiple times. Thus, results from the CHARM studies show that candesartan is beneficial in patients with heart failure as well as in patients with hypertension.

IN BRIEF

INDICATIONS
Treatment of hypertension. Candesartan cilexetil may be used alone or in combination with other antihypertensive agents.

CONTRAINDICATIONS/WARNINGS
Hypersensitivity

Pregnancy

DRUG INTERACTIONS
Because candesartan is not significantly metabolized by the cytochrome P450 system and has no effects on P450 enzymes, interactions with drugs that inhibit or are metabolized by those enzymes would not be anticipated.

Lithium[3]

NSAIDs[2]

Potassium-sparing diuretics[1,3]

Potassium supplements[3]

1 Effect/toxicity of candesartan may increase.

2 Effect of candesartan may decrease.

3 Candesartan may increase the effect/toxicity of this drug.

ADVERSE EFFECTS
CNS: headache (>1%), dizziness (4%), fatigue (>1%)

Respiratory: upper respiratory tract infection (6%), cough (1%–2%, less common than with ACE inhibitors)

GI: diarrhea (>1%), abdominal pain (>1%), nausea/vomiting (>1%)

Hematologic: small decreases in hemoglobin and hematocrit, anemia (rare), leukopenia (rare), thrombocytopenia (rare)

Renal: increased blood urea nitrogen (BUN) or serum creatinine (uncommon)

PHARMACOKINETICS AND PHARMACODYNAMICS
Duration of action: ≥24 h

Time to peak plasma concentration: 3–4 h

Bioavailability: ≈ 15%

Effect of food: no effect

Protein binding: >99%

Volume of distribution: 0.13 L/kg

Metabolism: candesartan undergoes minor hepatic metabolism to form an inactive metabolite

Elimination: ≈ 33% recovered in urine, ≈ 67% recovered in feces

Elimination half-life: ≈ 9 h

MONITORING
BP, electrolytes, serum creatinine, BUN.

OVERDOSE
Treatment should be symptomatic and supportive. Candesartan is not removed by hemodialysis.

The information here is provided as guidance only. Prescribers should always consult the manufacturer's current prescribing information.

51

CANDESARTAN CILEXETIL (continued)

SPECIAL GROUPS

Race: no effect

Children: safety and effectiveness have not been established

Elderly: no initial dosage adjustment is required

Renal impairment: no initial dosage adjustment is required

Hepatic impairment: no initial dosage adjustment is required

Pregnancy: category C (first trimester); category D (second and third trimesters). Candesartan should be discontinued as soon as pregnancy is detected.

Breast-feeding: not recommended; candesartan may be excreted in breast milk

DOSAGE

The usual initial dose is 16 mg once daily when used as monotherapy in patients who are not volume depleted. Candesartan may be administered once or twice daily, with total daily doses ranging from 8 to 32 mg. Hydrochlorothiazide has an additive effect.

PATIENT INFORMATION

Because dizziness may occur in some patients, use caution when driving or doing other things that require alertness. Consult with physician immediately if pregnancy is detected. Notify physician if persistent side effects occur. Do not discontinue therapy without your physician's advice.

AVAILABILITY

Tablets—4 mg, 8 mg, 16 mg, 32 mg
Combination formulation:
Atacand HCT—candesartan cilexetil/hydrochlorothiazide combination tablets
    16 mg/12.5 mg
    32 mg/12.5 mg

EPROSARTAN MESYLATE
(Teveten®)

Eprosartan is a competitive angiotensin II receptor antagonist with a high affinity for the angiotensin II subtype 1 (AT_1) receptor. The antihypertensive efficacy of eprosartan has been examined in a number of placebo-controlled, dose-finding, and comparative trials. Results of these clinical trials have consistently shown statistically significant differences in antihypertensive efficacy favoring eprosartan doses of 400 mg or greater per day over placebo. Eprosartan was also shown to be at least as effective as enalapril at lowering blood pressure in patients with mild to severe hypertension. The frequency of adverse events observed with eprosartan has been similar to that seen with placebo. In addition, there are no clinically significant drug interactions associated with eprosartan. Given the excellent tolerability and drug interaction profiles of eprosartan, the use of this agent may help to improve patient compliance with a drug regimen. Eprosartan may be particularly advantageous when used as a part of combination therapy for the management of hypertension. Further studies are needed to define the effects of eprosartan on other disease states, such as heart failure, myocardial infarction, and cerebral stroke.

SPECIAL GROUPS

Race: no effect
Children: safety and effectiveness have not been established
Elderly: initial dosage adjustment is not required
Renal impairment: initial dosage adjustment is not required; maximum dose should not exceed 600 mg daily
Hepatic impairment: initial dosage adjustment is not required
Pregnancy: category C (first trimester); category D (second and third trimesters). Eprosartan should be discontinued as soon as pregnancy is detected.
Breast-feeding: not recommended; may be excreted in breast milk

DOSAGE

The usual initial dose is 600 mg once daily when used as monotherapy in patients who are not volume depleted. Dosage may be titrated within the range of 400 to 800 mg/d given in one or two divided doses.

IN BRIEF

INDICATIONS
Treatment of hypertension. Eprosartan may be used alone or in combination with other antihypertensives, such as diuretics and calcium channel blockers.

CONTRAINDICATIONS/WARNINGS
Hypersensitivity
Pregnancy

DRUG INTERACTIONS
Because eprosartan is not metabolized by the cytochrome P450 system, inhibitors of CYP450 enzyme would not be expected to affect its metabolism.
NSAIDs[2]
Potassium-sparing diuretics[1,3]
Potassium supplements[3]

1 Effect/toxicity of eprosartan may increase.
2 Effect of eprosartan may decrease.
3 Eprosartan may increase the effect/toxicity of this drug.

ADVERSE EFFECTS
CNS: headache (≥ 1%), dizziness (≥ 1%), fatigue (2%)
GI: abdominal pain (2%), diarrhea (≥ 1%), dyspepsia/heartburn (≥ 1%)
Respiratory: upper respiratory tract infection (8%), cough (4%, not significantly different from placebo), pharyngitis (4%), rhinitis (4%)
Musculoskeletal: arthralgia (2%), myalgia (≥ 1%)
Hematologic: decreased hemoglobin of >20% (0.1%)
Renal: minor elevations in blood urea nitrogen (BUN) and serum creatinine (≈ 1%)
Other: increased potassium level to ≥ 5.6 mmol/L (0.9%)

PHARMACOKINETICS AND PHARMACODYNAMICS
Duration of action: ≈ 24 h
Time to peak plasma concentration: 1–2 h
Bioavailability: ≈ 13%
Effect of food: area under the curve (AUC) decreased by 15%; maximum concentration (C_{max}) decreased by 25%
Protein binding: ≈ 98%
Volume of distribution: 308 L
Metabolism: eprosartan is not metabolized by the cytochrome P450 system
Elimination: eprosartan is eliminated by biliary and renal excretion, primarily as unchanged compound. ≈ 7% recovered in urine, ≈ 90% recovered in feces.
Elimination half-life: 5–9 h

MONITORING
Blood pressure, electrolytes (serum potassium), serum creatinine, BUN, CBC

OVERDOSE
Treatment should be symptomatic and supportive. Eprosartan is not removed by hemodialysis.

PATIENT INFORMATION
Because dizziness may occur in some patients, use caution when driving or doing other things that require alertness. Consult with physician immediately if pregnancy is detected. Notify physician if persistent side effects occur. Do not discontinue therapy without your physician's advice.

AVAILABILITY
Tablets—400 mg, 600 mg
Combination formulation:
Teveten HCT—eprosartan mesylate/hydrochlorothiazide combination tablets
    600 mg/12.5 mg
    600 mg/25 mg

IRBESARTAN (Avapro®)

Irbesartan suppresses the activity of angiotensin II via selective and competitive antagonism of the angiotensin II subtype 1 (AT_1) receptor. Compared with other agents in this class, irbesartan has a high bioavailability of about 60%–80%. Irbesartan has a long elimination half-life of 11–15 h, thus allowing for once-daily dosing.

Irbesartan was demonstrated to reduce BP to an extent comparable to enalapril and atenolol. When compared with losartan 100 mg/d, irbesartan 300 mg/d was found to reduce BP to a greater extent in one study involving patients with mild to moderate hypertension. Similar to losartan and valsartan, the addition of hydrochlorothiazide to irbesartan resulted in additive antihypertensive effects.

The renoprotective effects of irbesartan in hypertensive patients with type 2 diabetes have been demonstrated in large clinical trials. Results from a study conducted by Lewis et al. showed that irbesartan was protective against the individual end point of doubling of serum creatinine. In addition, irbesartan slowed the loss of renal function in patients with overt diabetic nephropathy when compared with non–renin-angiotensin system–blocking antihypertensive medications. In another trial conducted by Parving et al., irbesartan was found to reduce the risk of microalbuminuria progressing to overt diabetic nephropathy in patients with type 2 diabetes. At this time, irbesartan is indicated for the management of nephropathy in type 2 diabetic patients and for the management of hypertension.

SPECIAL GROUPS

Race: the magnitude of BP lowering appeared somewhat less in black patients in some trials

Children: safety and effectiveness have not been established in children less than 6 years of age

Elderly: no dosage adjustment is required

Renal impairment: no dosage adjustment is required

Hepatic impairment: no dosage adjustment is required

Pregnancy: category C (first trimester); category D (second and third trimesters). Irbesartan should be discontinued as soon as pregnancy is detected.

Breast-feeding: not recommended; irbesartan may be excreted in breast milk

DOSAGE

Management of hypertension: In adults and adolescents 13 to 16 years of age, the usual initial dose is 150 mg/d. Dosages may be titrated to 300 mg once daily. Hydrochlorothiazide has an additive effect. Patients not adequately managed by the maximum dose of 300 mg once daily are unlikely to derive additional benefit from a higher dose or twice-daily dosing. For children 6 to 12 years of age, an initial dose of 75 mg once daily is reasonable. For patients requiring further reduction in BP, titrate dosage to 150 mg once daily.

Management of nephropathy in type 2 diabetic adult patients: The recommended target maintenance dose is 300 mg once daily.

IN BRIEF

INDICATIONS
Treatment of hypertension. Irbesartan can be used alone or in combination with other antihypertensive agents.
Management of nephropathy in type 2 diabetic patients

CONTRAINDICATIONS/WARNINGS
Hypersensitivity
Pregnancy

DRUG INTERACTIONS
In vitro studies show appreciable inhibition of the formation of oxidized irbesartan metabolites with the known cytochrome CYP2C9 substrates/inhibitors, tolbutamide, and nifedipine; however, clinical consequences were insignificant.
Potassium-sparing diuretics[1,3]
Potassium supplements[3]
NSAIDs[2]

[1] Effect/toxicity of irbesartan may increase.
[2] Effect of irbesartan may decrease.
[3] Irbesartan may increase the effect/toxicity of this drug.

ADVERSE EFFECTS
CNS: headache ($\geq$1%), dizziness ($\geq$1%), fatigue (4%)
Respiratory: upper respiratory tract infection (9%), cough (3%, less than with ACE inhibitors)
GI: diarrhea (3%), dyspepsia (2%), nausea/vomiting ($\geq$1%)
Hematologic: decreased hemoglobin of 0.2 g/dL (0.2%), neutropenia (0.3%)
Renal: increased BUN or serum creatinine (<1%)

PHARMACOKINETICS AND PHARMACODYNAMICS
Duration of action: 24 h
Time to peak plasma concentration: 1–2 h
Bioavailability: 60%–80%
Effect of food: no effect
Protein binding: 90%
Volume of distribution: 53–93 L
Metabolism: cytochrome P450 2C9 is the primary enzyme involved in the metabolism of irbesartan. No active metabolites have been identified.
Elimination: $\approx$ 20% recovered in urine, $\approx$ 80% recovered in feces
Elimination half-life: 11–15 h

MONITORING
BP, electrolytes, serum creatinine, BUN, CBC.

OVERDOSE
Treatment should be symptomatic and supportive. Irbesartan is not removed by hemodialysis.

PATIENT INFORMATION
Because dizziness may occur in some patients, use caution when driving or doing other things that require alertness. Consult with physician immediately if pregnancy is detected. Notify physician if persistent side effects occur. Do not discontinue therapy without your physician's advice.

AVAILABILITY
Tablets—75 mg, 150 mg, 300 mg
Combination formulation:
Avalide—irbesartan/hydrochlorothiazide combination tablets
150 mg/12.5 mg
300 mg/12.5 mg

LOSARTAN POTASSIUM
(Cozaar®)

Losartan potassium was the first nonpeptide angiotensin II receptor antagonist available for oral treatment of hypertension in the United States. This agent binds competitively and selectively to the angiotensin II subtype 1 (AT_1) receptor, thus blocking the physiologic effects induced by angiotensin II. Losartan undergoes considerable first-pass metabolism with a bioavailability of about 33%. Approximately 14% of an oral dose of losartan is converted to an active carboxylic acid metabolite, EXP 3174. In contrast to losartan potassium, EXP 3174 is a partial "insurmountable" antagonist of the AT_1 receptor. This active metabolite has a terminal half-life of 6–9 h and contributes substantially to losartan's antihypertensive effect.

Losartan decreases BP to a similar extent as enalapril, atenolol, or felodipine extended release when administered as monotherapy (50–100 mg once daily) in patients with mild to moderate hypertension. Further BP reduction was observed when hydrochlorothiazide was combined with losartan. Approximately 30% of patients with severe hypertension have responded to the combination product.

Losartan has also been studied in patients with type 2 diabetes and nephropathy, heart failure, left ventricular hypertrophy, and in high-risk patients after acute myocardial infarction. The RENAAL study showed that losartan significantly reduced the incidence of a doubling of serum creatinine concentration and end-stage renal disease compared with placebo in patients with type 2 diabetes and nephropathy. The ELITE II Losartan Heart Failure Survival Study was initiated to compare the effects of losartan and captopril in improving survival in elderly heart failure patients. Although losartan was not superior to captopril in improving survival, it was significantly better tolerated.

The LIFE study randomized 9193 patients with essential hypertension and left ventricular hypertrophy to once-daily losartan-based or atenolol-based treatment. A majority of patients in both groups also received additional drugs, such as hydrochlorothiazide; 92% of patients in this study were white. The incidence of cardiovascular mortality and myocardial infarction were not statistically different between the two groups. However, the incidence of stroke was significantly lower in the losartan group compared with the atenolol group (5% vs 7%). The OPTIMAAL investigators compared the effects of losartan and captopril in high-risk patients after acute myocardial infarction. Although losartan was significantly better tolerated than captopril, a nonsignificant difference in total mortality in favor of captopril was observed. Based on the results of these studies, losartan is currently approved for the management of hypertension, of hypertensive patients with left ventricular hypertrophy, and of nephropathy in type 2 diabetic patients.

IN BRIEF

INDICATIONS
Treatment of hypertension. Losartan can be used alone or in combination with other antihypertensive agents.
Management of hypertensive patients with left ventricular hypertrophy to reduce the risk of stroke (but there is evidence that this benefit does not apply to black patients).
Management of nephropathy in type 2 diabetic patients.

CONTRAINDICATIONS/WARNINGS
Hypersensitivity
Pregnancy

DRUG INTERACTIONS
Cimetidine[1,4]
Fluconazole[1]
NSAIDs[2]
Potassium-sparing diuretics[1,3]
Potassium supplements[3]
Phenobarbital[2,4]
Rifampin[2]

1 Effect/toxicity of losartan may increase.
2 Effect of losartan may decrease.
3 Losartan may increase the effect/toxicity of this drug.
4 The clinical significance of this interaction is unclear.

ADVERSE EFFECTS
CNS: headache (>1%), dizziness (4%),
Respiratory: upper respiratory tract infection (7%), cough (3%–4%, less than with ACE inhibitors)
GI: diarrhea (2%–3%), dyspepsia (1%–2%)
Hematologic: slight decreases in hemoglobin and hematocrit.
Renal: increased BUN or serum creatinine (<1%)

PHARMACOKINETICS AND PHARMACODYNAMICS
Duration of action:	≈ 24 h
Time to peak plasma concentration:	losartan, 1 h; EXP 3174, 3–4 h
Bioavailability:	≈ 33%
Effect of food:	AUC decreased by 10%; C_{max} decreased by 14%
Protein binding:	losartan, 98.7%; EXP 3174, 99.8%
Volume of distribution:	losartan, ≈ 34 L; EXP 3174, ≈ 12 L
Metabolism:	≈ 14% of losartan is converted to active metabolite EXP 3174
Elimination:	≈ 35% recovered in urine, ≈ 60% recovered in feces
Elimination half-life:	losartan, ≈ 2 h; EXP 3174, ≈ 6–9 h

MONITORING
BP, electrolytes, serum creatinine, BUN, CBC.

OVERDOSE
Treatment should be symptomatic and supportive. Losartan and EXP 3174 are not removed by hemodialysis.

The information here is provided as guidance only. Prescribers should always consult the manufacturer's current prescribing information.

55

LOSARTAN POTASSIUM (continued)

SPECIAL GROUPS

Race: BP response is notably less in black patients when compared with white patients

Children: safety and effectiveness have not been established

Elderly: no dosage adjustment is required

Renal impairment: no dosage adjustment is required

Hepatic impairment: reduction of the initial dose is required

Pregnancy: category C (first trimester); category D (second and third trimesters). Losartan should be discontinued as soon as pregnancy is detected.

Breast-feeding: not recommended; losartan may be excreted in breast milk

DOSAGE

Hypertension: The usual initial dose is 50 mg once daily. Dosage can be titrated up to 100 mg/d (in one or two divided doses). A lower initial dose of 25 mg once daily should be given to patients at high risk for hypotension or volume depletion, and to those with hepatic dysfunction.

Management of nephropathy in type 2 diabetic patients: The usual starting dose is 50 mg once daily. Dose should be increased to 100 mg once daily based on BP response.

Hypertension with left ventricular hypertrophy: The usual initial dose is 50 mg once daily. Hydrochlorothiazide 12.5 mg/d should be added and/or the dose of losartan should be increased to 100 mg once daily, followed by an increase in hydrochlorothiazide to 25 mg once daily based on blood pressure response.

PATIENT INFORMATION

Because dizziness may occur in some patients, use caution when driving or doing other things that require alertness. Consult with physician immediately if pregnancy is detected. Notify physician if persistent side effects occur. Do not discontinue therapy without your physician's advice.

AVAILABILITY

Tablets, film coated—25 mg, 50 mg, 100 mg
Combination formulation:
Hyzaar—losartan potassium/hydrochlorothiazide combination tablets
    50 mg/12.5 mg
    100 mg/25 mg

OLMESARTAN MEDOXOMIL
(Benicar®)

Olmesartan medoxomil is an ARB that exhibits its effect through selective antagonism of the angiotensin II subtype 1 (AT_1) receptor. It is a prodrug that is de-esterified to the active metabolite olmesartan. Monotherapy with olmesartan medoxomil in once-daily doses of 20–40 mg has produced significant reductions in systolic and diastolic blood pressure in hypertensive patients. Similar to other ARBs, olmesartan medoxomil may be taken once daily without regard to meals. Because olmesartan is not metabolized by the cytochrome P450 enzyme system, it has a low potential for metabolic drug interactions. Olmesartan is also well-tolerated and has a favorable safety profile that is comparable to that of placebo. Results from animal studies suggest that olmesartan medoxomil may prove to be a useful treatment for diabetic nephropathy and atherosclerosis. At this time, olmesartan is indicated for the treatment of hypertension.

SPECIAL GROUPS

Race: no information
Children: safety and effectiveness have not been established
Elderly: initial dosage adjustment is not required
Renal impairment: initial dosage adjustment is not required
Hepatic impairment: initial dosage adjustment is not required
Pregnancy: category C (first trimester); category D (second and third trimesters). Olmesartan should be discontinued as soon as pregnancy is detected.
Breast-feeding: not recommended; may be excreted in breast milk

DOSAGE

The usual recommended initial dose is 20 mg once daily when used as monotherapy in patients who are not volume contracted. If further reduction in BP is required after 2 weeks of therapy, the dose may be increased to 40 mg. Doses above 40 mg do not appear to have greater effect. Twice-daily dosing offers no advantage over the same total dose given once daily. For patients with possible depletion of intravascular volume, olmesartan should be initiated under close medical supervision and consideration should be given to use of a lower starting dose.

IN BRIEF

INDICATIONS
Treatment of hypertension. Olmesartan may be used alone or in combination with other antihypertensive agents.

CONTRAINDICATIONS/WARNINGS
Hypersensitivity
Pregnancy

DRUG INTERACTIONS
Because olmesartan medoxomil is not metabolized by the cytochrome P450 system and has no effects on P450 enzymes, interactions with drugs that inhibit, induce, or are metabolized by those enzymes are not expected.
NSAIDs[2]
Potassium-sparing diuretics[1,3]
Potassium supplements[3]

1 Effect/toxicity of olmesartan may increase.
2 Effect of olmesartan may decrease.
3 Olmesartan may increase the effect/toxicity of this drug.

ADVERSE EFFECTS
CNS: headache (>1%), dizziness (3%), fatigue (>0.5%)
GI: abdominal pain (>0.5%), diarrhea (>1%), dyspepsia/heartburn (>0.5%)
Respiratory: upper respiratory tract infection (>1%), cough (0.9%, not significantly different from placebo), pharyngitis (>1%), rhinitis (>1%)
Musculoskeletal: arthralgia (>0.5%), myalgia (>0.5%), pain (>1%)
Hematologic: small decreases in hemoglobin and hematocrit

PHARMACOKINETICS AND PHARMACODYNAMICS
Duration of action: ≈ 24 h
Time to peak plasma concentration: 1–2 h
Bioavailability: ≈ 26%
Effect of food: no effect
Protein binding: 99%
Volume of distribution: ≈ 17 L
Metabolism: following the rapid and complete conversion of olmesartan medoxomil to olmesartan during absorption, there is virtually no further metabolism of olmesartan
Elimination: ≈ 35%–50% recovered in urine, ≈ 50%–65% recovered in feces
Elimination half-life: ≈ 13 h

MONITORING
Blood pressure, electrolytes (serum potassium)

OVERDOSE
The most likely manifestations of overdosage are hypotension and tachycardia; bradycardia could be encountered if parasympathetic (vagal) stimulation occurs. If symptomatic hypotension should occur, supportive treatment should be initiated. The dialyzability of olmesartan is unknown.

PATIENT INFORMATION
Because dizziness may occur in some patients, use caution when driving or doing other things that require alertness. Consult with physician immediately if pregnancy is detected. Notify physician if persistent side effects occur. Do not discontinue therapy without your physician's advice.

AVAILABILITY
Tablets—5 mg, 20 mg, 40 mg
Combination formulation:
Benicar HCT—olmesartan medoxomil/hydrochlorothiazide combination tablets
20 mg/12.5 mg
40 mg/12.5 mg
40 mg/25 mg

The information here is provided as guidance only. Prescribers should always consult the manufacturer's current prescribing information.

57

TELMISARTAN (Micardis®)

Telmisartan is a nonpeptide angiotensin II receptor antagonist that inhibits the angiotensin II subtype 1 (AT_1) receptor selectively and competitively. Telmisartan has an extended elimination half-life of about 24 h. This allows the agent to have a longer lasting antihypertensive effect.

In two studies that used ambulatory BP monitoring, telmisartan given once daily was shown to provide better diastolic BP control for the full dosing interval than losartan potassium 50 mg or amlodipine 5 or 10 mg. In patients with mild to moderate hypertension, telmisartan 40–160 mg once daily was found to be at least as effective as atenolol 50 or 100 mg and lisinopril 10–40 mg. Telmisartan 80 mg/d was demonstrated to be more effective than enalapril 20 mg/d in one study. Similar to the other agents in this class, telmisartan is approved by the Food and Drug Administration (FDA) for the treatment of hypertension.

SPECIAL GROUPS

Race: BP response in black patients (usually in low-renin population) is noticeably less than that in white patients

Children: safety and effectiveness have not been established

Elderly: no initial dosage adjustment is required

Renal impairment: no dosage adjustments are required in patients with mild to moderate renal impairment

Hepatic impairment: use with caution; an alternative treatment can be considered

Pregnancy: category C (first trimester); category D (second and third trimesters). Telmisartan should be discontinued as soon as pregnancy is detected.

Breast-feeding: not recommended; telmisartan may be excreted in breast milk

DOSAGE

The usual initial dose is 40 mg once daily. The dosage may be titrated within the range of 20–80 mg/d according to response. Initiate treatment under close medical supervision for patients with hepatic impairment or biliary obstructive disorders. Correct the condition of patients with depletion of intravascular volume or initiate therapy under close supervision.

IN BRIEF

INDICATIONS
Treatment of hypertension. Telmisartan can be used alone or in combination with other antihypertensive agents.

CONTRAINDICATIONS/WARNINGS
Hypersensitivity
Pregnancy

DRUG INTERACTIONS
Digoxin[3]
NSAIDs[2]
Potassium-sparing diuretics[1,3]
Potassium supplements[3]
Warfarin[4,5]

1 Effect/toxicity of telmisartan may increase.
2 Effect of telmisartan may decrease.
3 Telmisartan may increase the effect/toxicity of this drug.
4 Telmisartan may decrease the effect of this drug.
5 The clinical significance of this interaction is unclear.

ADVERSE EFFECTS
CNS: headache (1%), dizziness (1%), fatigue (1%)
Respiratory: upper respiratory tract infection (7%), cough (less common than with ACE inhibitors)
GI: diarrhea (3%), abdominal pain (1%), nausea/vomiting (1%)
Hematologic: decreased hemoglobin of >2 g/dL (<1%), anemia (rare)
Renal: increased BUN or serum creatinine (<1%)

PHARMACOKINETICS AND PHARMACODYNAMICS
Duration of action: ≥24 h
Time to peak plasma concentration: 1 h
Bioavailability: 42%–58%
Effect of food: AUC decreased by 6%–20%
Protein binding: >99%
Volume of distribution: 500 L
Metabolism: biotransformation is minimal
Elimination: <1% recovered in urine, >97% recovered in feces
Elimination half-life: ≈ 24 h

MONITORING
BP, electrolytes, serum creatinine, BUN, CBC, serum digoxin concentration.
Note—Patients on dialysis may develop orthostatic hypotension; monitor BP closely.

OVERDOSE
Treatment should be symptomatic and supportive. Telmisartan is not removed by hemodialysis.

PATIENT INFORMATION
Because dizziness may occur in some patients, use caution when driving or doing other things that require alertness. Consult with physician immediately if pregnancy is detected. Notify physician if persistent side effects occur. Do not discontinue therapy without your physician's advice.

AVAILABILITY
Tablets—20 mg, 40 mg, 80 mg
Combination formulation:
Micardis HCT—telmisartan/hydrochlorothiazide combination tablets
  40 mg/12.5 mg
  80 mg/12.5 mg

VALSARTAN

(Diovan®)

Valsartan was the next angiotensin II receptor antagonist that became available for the treatment of hypertension after losartan. Similar to losartan, valsartan binds competitively and selectively to the angiotensin II subtype 1 (AT_1) receptor. Valsartan also undergoes extensive first-pass metabolism with a bioavailability of approximately 25%. Valsartan has an elimination half-life of about 6 h, which allows for once-a-day dosing.

The antihypertensive efficacy of valsartan was demonstrated to be similar to that of losartan, lisinopril, enalapril, amlodipine, and hydrochlorothiazide in patients with mild to moderate essential hypertension. Addition of hydrochlorothiazide was shown to provide BP control in patients who responded inadequately to valsartan monotherapy.

Valsartan has also been studied in patients with type 2 diabetes and microalbuminuria, in patients with heart failure, and in high-risk patients after myocardial infarction. The MARVAL study showed that valsartan lowered elevated urine albumin excretion more effectively than amlodipine in patients with type 2 diabetes and microalbuminuria. The Val-HeFT investigators found that the addition of valsartan to standard therapy in patients with heart failure significantly decreased the need for hospitalization due to heart failure (18.2% in the placebo group vs 13.8% in the valsartan group). In addition, treatment with valsartan resulted in significant improvements in New York Heart Association (NYHA) class, ejection fraction, signs and symptoms of heart failure, and quality of life as compared with placebo.

More recently, the VALIANT investigators compared the effects of valsartan, captopril, and the combination of the two drugs in patients with myocardial infarction complicated by left ventricular systolic dysfunction, heart failure, or both. During a median follow-up of 24.7 months, the incidence of overall mortality was similar among the three treatment groups. The VALIANT investigators concluded that valsartan is as effective as captopril in patients who are at high risk for cardiovascular events after myocardial infarction. Combining valsartan with captopril was shown to increase the rate of adverse events without improving survival. At this time, valsartan is approved by the FDA for the treatment of hypertension and heart failure.

IN BRIEF

INDICATIONS
Treatment of hypertension. Valsartan can be used alone or in combination with other antihypertensive agents.
Treatment of heart failure (NYHA class II to IV) in patients who are intolerant of ACE inhibitors.

CONTRAINDICATIONS/WARNINGS
Hypersensitivity
Pregnancy

DRUG INTERACTIONS
The enzyme(s) responsible for valsartan metabolism have not been identified but do not seem to be CYP 450 isozymes. The inhibitory or induction potential of valsartan on CYP 450 is also unknown.
NSAIDs[2]
Potassium-sparing diuretics[1,3]
Potassium supplements[3]

1 Effect/toxicity of valsartan may increase.
2 Effect of valsartan may decrease.
3 Valsartan may increase the effect/toxicity of this drug.

ADVERSE EFFECTS
CNS: headache (>1%), dizziness (>1%), fatigue (2%)
Respiratory: upper respiratory tract infection (>1%), cough (>1%, less than with ACE inhibitors)
GI: diarrhea (>1%), dyspepsia (>0.2%), abdominal pain (2%), nausea/vomiting (>1%)
Hematologic: decreased hemoglobin and hematocrit of >20% (<1%)
Renal: increased BUN or serum creatinine
Other: increased serum potassium of >20% (4%–10%)

PHARMACOKINETICS AND PHARMACODYNAMICS
Duration of action: ≈ 24 h
Time to peak plasma concentration: 2–4 h
Bioavailability: ≈ 25%
Effect of food: AUC decreased by 40%; C_{max} decreased by 50%
Protein binding: 95%
Volume of distribution: 17 L (IV dosing)
Metabolism: the primary metabolite, valeryl 4-hydroxy valsartan, is inactive
Elimination: ≈ 13% recovered in urine, ≈ 83% recovered in feces
Elimination half-life: ≈ 6 h (IV dosing)

MONITORING
BP, electrolytes, serum creatinine, BUN, CBC, liver function tests.

OVERDOSE
Treatment should be symptomatic and supportive. Valsartan is not removed by hemodialysis.

VALSARTAN (continued)

SPECIAL GROUPS

Race: no information

Children: safety and effectiveness have not been established

Elderly: increased AUC and half-life of valsartan have been observed; however, dosage adjustments are not usually required

Renal impairment: caution is advised when valsartan is administered to patients with severe renal impairment

Hepatic impairment: use with caution; initial dosage adjustments are not required in patients with mild to moderate hepatic insufficiency

Pregnancy: category C (first trimester); category D (second and third trimesters). Valsartan should be discontinued as soon as pregnancy is detected.

Breast-feeding: not recommended; valsartan may be excreted in breast milk

DOSAGE

Hypertension: The usual initial dose is 80 or 160 mg once daily when used as monotherapy in patients who are not volume depleted. Dosage may be increased to 320 mg/d gradually if necessary.

Heart failure: The usual initial dose is 40 mg twice daily. Dosage should be titrated to 80 mg twice daily and then to 160 mg twice daily as tolerated. Maximum daily dose administered in clinical trials was 320 mg in divided doses. Reduction of concomitant diuretic dosage should be considered. Concomitant use with an ACE inhibitor and a beta-blocker is not recommended.

PATIENT INFORMATION

Because dizziness may occur in some patients, use caution when driving or doing other things that require alertness. Consult with physician immediately if pregnancy is detected. Notify physician if persistent side effects occur. Do not discontinue therapy without your physician's advice.

AVAILABILITY

Tablets—40 mg, 80 mg, 160 mg, 320 mg
Combination formulations:
Diovan HCT—valsartan/hydrochlorothiazide combination tablets
80 mg/12.5 mg
160 mg/12.5 mg
160 mg/25 mg

SELECTED BIBLIOGRAPHY

Brenner BM, Cooper ME, de Zeeuw D, *et al.* for the RENAAL Study Investigators: Effects of losartan on renal and cardiovascular outcomes in patients with type 2 diabetes and nephropathy. *N Engl J Med* 2001, 345:861–869.

Brunner HR, Laeis P: Clinical efficacy of olmesartan medoxomil. *J Hypertens* 2003, 21(Suppl 2):S43–S46.

Cheng-Lai A: Eprosartan: an angiotensin-II receptor antagonist for the management of hypertension. *Heart Dis* 2002, 4:54–59.

Cohn JN, Tognoni G, for the Valsartan Heart Failure Trial Investigators: A randomized trial of the angiotensin-receptor blocker valsartan in chronic heart failure. *N Engl J Med* 2001, 345:1667–1675.

Dahlöf B, Devereux RB, Kjeldsen SE, *et al.* for the LIFE study group: Cardiovascular morbidity and mortality in the Losartan Intervention For Endpoint reduction in hypertension study (LIFE): a randomised trial against atenolol. *Lancet* 2002, 359:995–1003.

Dickstein K, Kjekshus J, and the OPTIMAAL steering committee, for the OPTIMAAL Study Group: Effects of losartan and captopril on mortality and morbidity in high-risk patients after acute myocardial infarction: the OPTIMAAL randomised trial. *Lancet* 2002, 360:752–760.

Gardner SF, Franks AM: Olmesartan medoxomil: the seventh angiotensin receptor antagonist. *Ann Pharmacother* 2003, 37:99–105.

Gheorghiade M, Cody RJ, Francis GS, *et al.*: Current medical therapy for advanced heart failure. *Am Heart J* 1998, 135:S231–S248.

Gillis JC, Markham A: Irbesartan: a review of its pharmacodynamic and pharmacokinetic properties and therapeutic use in the management of hypertension. *Drugs* 1997, 54:885–902.

Goa KL, Wagstaff AJ: Losartan potassium: a review of its pharmacology, clinical efficacy and tolerability in the management of hypertension. *Drugs* 1996, 51:820–845.

Granger CB, McMurray JJV, Yusuf S, *et al.* for the CHARM investigators and committees: Effects of candesartan in patients with chronic heart failure and reduced left-ventricular systolic function intolerant to angiotensin-converting-enzyme inhibitors: the CHARM-Alternative trial. *Lancet* 2003, 362:772–776.

Hamroff G, Katz SD, Mancini D, *et al.*: Addition of angiotensin II receptors blockade to maximal angiotensin-converting-enzyme inhibition improves exercise capacity in patients with severe congestive heart failure. *Circulation* 1999; 99:990–992.

Julius S, Kjeldsen SE, Weber M, *et al.* for the VALUE trial group: Outcomes in hypertensive patients at high cardiovascular risk treated with regimens based on valsartan or amlodipine: the VALUE randomised trial. *Lancet* 2004, 363:2022–2031.

Kang PM, Landau AJ, Eberhardt RT, *et al.*: Angiotensin II receptor antagonists: a new approach to blockade of the renin-angiotensin system. *Am Heart J* 1994, 127:1388.

Kostis JB, Frishman WH, Gradman AH: The renin angiotensin system, hypertension, and angiotensin receptor blockers (monograph). Philadelphia: Mosby-Wolfe Med Communications; 1999.

Le Jemtel TH, Sonnenblick EH, Frishman WH: Diagnosis and management of heart failure. In Alexander RW, Schlant RC, Fuster V: *Hurst's the Heart* 11th ed. New York: McGraw-Hill; 2004, in press.

Lewis EJ, Hunsicker LG, Clarke WR, *et al.* for the Collaborative Study Group: Renoprotective effect of the angiotensin-receptor antagonist irbesartan in patients with nephropathy due to type 2 diabetes. *N Engl J Med* 2001, 345:851–860.

Lindholm LH: Valsartan treatment of hypertension: does VALUE add value? *Lancet* 2004, 363:2010–2011.

Markham A, Goa KL: Valsartan: a review of its pharmacology and therapeutic use in essential hypertension. *Drugs* 1997, 54:299–311.

McClellan KJ, Goa KL: Candesartan cilexetil: a review of its use in essential hypertension. *Drugs* 1998, 56:847–869.

McClellan KJ, Markham A: Telmisartan. *Drugs* 1998, 56:1039–1044.

McMurray JJ, Östergren J, Swedberg K, *et al.* for the CHARM investigators and committees: Effects of candesartan in patients with chronic heart failure and reduced left-ventricular systolic function taking angiotensin-converting-enzyme inhibitors: the CHARM-Added trial. *Lancet* 2003; 362:767–771.

Parving HH, Lehnert H, Bröchner-Mortensen J, *et al.* for the Irbesartan in Patients with Type 2 Diabetes and Microalbuminuria Study Group: The effect of irbesartan on the development of diabetic nephropathy in patients with type 2 diabetes. *N Engl J Med* 2001, 345:870–878.

Patterson JH: Angiotensin II receptor blockers in heart failure. *Pharmacotherapy* 2003, 23:173–182.

Pfeffer MA, McMurray JJV, Velazquez EJ, *et al.* for the Valsartan in Acute Myocardial Infarction Trial Investigators: Valsartan, captopril, or both in myocardial infarction complicated by heart failure, left ventricular dysfunction, or both. *N Engl J Med* 2003, 349:1893–1906.

Pitt B, Poole-Wilson PA, Segal R, *et al.* on behalf of the ELITE II investigators: Effect of losartan compared with captopril on mortality in patients with symptomatic heart failure: randomized trial—the Losartan Heart Failure Survival Study ELITE II. *Lancet* 2000, 355:1582–1587.

Pitt B, Segal R, Martinez FA, *et al.* on behalf of the ELITE Study Investigators: Randomised trial of losartan versus captopril in patients over 65 with heart failure (Evaluation of Losartan in the Elderly Study: ELITE). *Lancet* 1997, 349:747–752.

Pohl M, Cooper M, Ulrey J, *et al.*: Safety and efficacy of irbesartan in hypertensive patients with type II diabetes and proteinuria [abstract]. *Am J Hypertens* 1997, 10:105A.

Sica DA, Gehr TWB, Frishman WH: The renin-angiotensin axis: Angiotensin-converting enzyme inhibitors and angiotensin-receptor blockers. In *Cardiovascular Pharmacotherapeutics Manual*. Edited by Frishman WH, Sonnenblick EH, Sica DA. New York: McGraw-Hill; 2004:96–130.

Tonkon M, Awan N, Niazi I, *et al.*: Combination of irbesartan with conventional therapy including angiotensin converting enzyme inhibitors [abstract]. *Heart Failure '97*. May 24–27, 1997, Cologne.

Viberti G, Wheeldon NM, for the MicroAlbuminuria Reduction With VALsartan (MARVAL) Study Investigators: Microalbuminuria reduction with valsartan in patients with type 2 diabetes mellitus: a blood pressure-independent effect. *Circulation* 2002, 106:672–678.

Weber MA, Julius S, Kjeldsen SE, *et al.*: Blood pressure dependent and independent effects of antihypertensive treatment on clinical events in the VALUE trial. *Lancet* 2004, 363:2049–2051.

Yusuf S, Pfeffer MA, Swedberg K, *et al.* for the CHARM investigators and committees: Effects of candesartan in patients with chronic heart failure and preserved left-ventricular ejection fraction: the CHARM-Preserved trial. *Lancet* 2003, 362:777–781.

In recent years, there has not been a great influx of new antiarrhythmic agents for clinical use besides the introduction of **dofetilide**, which is primarily used to treat supraventricular tachyarrhythmias. Despite considerable advances in our understanding of basic and clinical arrhythmia mechanisms and the availability of more than a dozen drugs with antiarrhythmic activity, several factors limit the enthusiasm with which these agents are currently being prescribed. These include

1. The cardiac toxicities of antiarrhythmic drugs, particularly their propensity to cause or exacerbate more severe arrhythmias (*ie*, proarrhythmia), to depress electrical function, including sinus node activity and cardiac conduction, and to depress myocardial contractility.
2. The disappointing results of several clinical trials that have demonstrated an unfavorable risk/benefit ratio and even higher mortality in "high-risk" patients with premature ventricular beats treated with various antiarrhythmic drugs.
3. Evidence for the beneficial role of beta-blockers in post–myocardial infarction (MI) patients along with the lack of benefit and increased risk with the use of antiarrhythmics in this setting.
4. The noncardiac toxicities of antiarrhythmic drugs.
5. The advent and evolution of new antiarrhythmic technologies and procedures, including antiarrhythmic devices (*eg*, implantable cardioverter-defibrillators [ICDs]) and ablation procedures. Based on clinical evidence, the ICD has generally become a standard therapy for the chronic management of ventricular arrhythmias. However, antiarrhythmics still play a role as adjunctive therapy in this setting, to minimize the frequency of ICD discharges.

Because of these factors, the indications for utilizing most antiarrhythmic agents are now more restricted, and the Food and Drug Administration (FDA) recommends that many of these agents be started in a hospital setting, particularly for patients with the most severe arrhythmias or underlying cardiac disease. Thus, therapy for each patient should be individualized, risks and benefits evaluated, and specific therapeutic goals established. Efficacy and toxicity of antiar-

rhythmics are determined by clinical outcomes. For certain antiarrhythmics, obtaining plasma concentrations is sometimes helpful, particularly to check for patient compliance, as any amount of a drug may be sufficient to produce toxicity or proarrhythmia. This fact sometimes makes it very difficult to determine whether an arrhythmia is aggravated by an antiarrhythmic or is caused by an underlying condition.

In this chapter, the antiarrhythmic agents are presented according to the traditional Vaughan Williams classification, with which most physicians are familiar (Table 5.1); however, it is important to realize that this classification has several limitations. It separates the antiarrhythmics on the basis of only one dominant mechanism, although many antiarrhythmic agents exert more than one effect. An example of this is amiodarone, which has electrophysiologic properties of all four Vaughan Williams classes. Another limitation is the great variability and individuality among drugs within a class, which prevents secure substitution of one agent for another. In addition, this system is somewhat incomplete because it excludes such drugs as digoxin, adenosine, and atropine. A new classification, the Sicilian Gambit, has been proposed that takes into account the underlying arrhythmia mechanism, which can include an abnormality in impulse formation (*eg*, automaticity, triggered arrhythmias) and/or an abnormality in impulse conduction (*ie*, reentry phenomena). It also classifies antiarrhythmic agents on the basis of their numerous effects on myocardial cell targets that include cell receptors, ion channels, and electrolyte pumps. However, despite this proposal for an alternative method for categorizing antiarrhythmics, the Vaughan Williams classification system continues to be the most frequently used in clinical practice.

GENERAL CONTRAINDICATIONS AND PRECAUTIONS FOR ANTIARRHYTHMIC THERAPY

Considerable caution should be exercised when starting a patient on an antiarrhythmic agent. It is recommended that class I or III antiarrhythmics be started in a hospital setting, particularly for those patients with life-threatening arrhythmias or structural heart disease. The following contraindications

INDICATIONS

	Diso	Flec	Lido	Mexil	Moric	Procain	Propa	Quin	Tocain
Atrial fibrillation	(+)	+	–	–	–	(+)	+	+	–
Atrial flutter	(+)	+	–	–	–	(+)	(+)	+	–
Atrial tachycardia	(+)	–	–	–	–	(+)	–	+	–
Atrial extrasystoles	(+)	–	–	–	–	–	–	+	–
Supraventricular tachycardia	(+)	+	–	–	–	(+)	(+)	+	–
Life-threatening ventricular tachycardia	+	+	+	+	+	+	+	–	+
Ventricular tachycardia	(+)	–	(+)	(+)	(+)	(+)	–	+	(+)
Wolff-Parkinson-White syndrome	–	(+)	–	–	–	(+)	(+)	+	–

+—FDA approved; – – —not FDA approved; (+)—clinical use not FDA approved. Diso—disopyramide; Flec—flecainide; Lido—lidocaine; Mexil—mexiletine; Moric—moricizine; Procain—procainamide; Propa—propafenone; Quin—quinidine; Tocain—tocainide.

generally apply to the majority of the antiarrhythmic drugs:

Hypersensitivity

Sinus node dysfunction (in the absence of a pacemaker)

Long QT interval

Advanced conduction disease (particularly second- or third-degree heart block in the absence of a pacemaker)

Advanced heart failure or markedly depressed cardiac function (with the exception of amiodarone and dofetilide)

It is important to remember that all antiarrhythmics can potentially cause or exacerbate mechanical or electrical dysfunction, including depression of automaticity and conduction, and all have a potential for causing proarrhythmia. Class I antiarrhythmic agents, known as the sodium (Na^+) channel blockers, may be subdivided into classes Ia, Ib, and Ic (Table 5.1). These agents vary in the rate at which they bind and then dissociate from the Na^+ channel receptor. Class Ia drugs (**quinidine, procainamide, disopyramide**) have binding kinetics that are immediate between those of the class Ib and Ic agents. These drugs also prolong the action potential duration. Class Ib antiarrhythmics (**lidocaine, mexiletine, tocainide**) bind to and dissociate from the Na^+ channel receptor quickly ("fast on–off"). These drugs shorten the action potential duration. The class Ic antiarrhythmics (**flecainide, propafenone**) slowly bind to and dissociate from the Na^+ channel receptor ("slow on–off"). These drugs have little effect on the action potential duration. In addition, class I antiarrhythmics possess rate dependence whereby Na^+ channel blockade is greatest at fast heart rates (ie, tachycardia) and least during slower heart rates (ie, bradycardia). There are other important differences among the three subgroups. For example, the QT interval tends to be prolonged by class Ia drugs, whereas the class Ic drugs have the most potent negative inotropic effects.

EFFICACY AND USE

The class Ia drugs have retained a role in the treatment of arrhythmias despite the development of new types of antiarrhythmic drugs. However, the use of these drugs in the treatment of supraventricular and ventricular arrhythmias is limited by their adverse-effect profiles. All three representatives of this class have similar effects on clinical electrophysiologic parameters (Table 5.1). These drugs have a tendency to increase the QT and His-ventricular intervals. For the treat-

TABLE 5.1 CLASSIFICATION OF ANTIARRHYTHMIC AGENTS

Class	Drug	Main electrophysiologic/pharmacologic effect
Ia	Quinidine	Depression of V_{max}; increased AP duration; increased QT interval; widening of the QRS complex. Moderate effects on phase 0 and ERP
	Procainamide	
	Disopyramide	
Ib	Lidocaine	Depression of V_{max}; decreased AP duration; unchanged QT interval or QRS complex. Minimal effects on phase 0 and little effect on ERP
	Mexiletine	
	Tocainide	
Ic	Flecainide	Marked depression of V_{max}; unchanged AP duration; increased QRS complex without primary change in QT interval. Minimal effects on ERP
	Moricizine	
	Propafenone	
II	Sympathetic inhibitors, eg, beta-blockers	Inhibition of sympathetic activity; decreased QTc interval in congenital long QT syndrome
III	Amiodarone	Increased AP duration; increased QT interval
	Bretylium	
	Sotalol (d,l-sotalol)	
	Ibutilide	
	Dofetilide	
IV	Verapamil	Blocking of slow inward calcium current
	Diltiazem	
Miscellaneous	Digitalis	Inhibition of Na^+/K^+ pump; vagal effect
	Atropine	Antivagal effect
	Adenosine	Vagal-like effect

AP—action potential; ERP—effective refractory period; V_{max}—the maximum rate of depolarization of the cell; it equates with the fast inward sodium current.

ment of atrial fibrillation, **quinidine** and **procainamide** can be useful for restoration and maintenance of sinus rhythm. The clinical use of **disopyramide** for this indication tends to be limited because of its potent anticholinergic and negative inotropic effects. This group of drugs may also be useful in the treatment of life-threatening refractory ventricular arrhythmias. Data from one meta-analysis suggests that these agents do not improve prognosis by suppressing asymptomatic postinfarction ventricular ectopy. In addition, in a separate meta-analysis, the use of **quinidine** for maintenance of sinus rhythm in patients with atrial fibrillation has been associated with an increased risk of mortality. The use of class Ia agents to restore and maintain sinus rhythm in patients with atrial fibrillation has significantly declined over the past decade, primarily because of increasing concern about their proarrhythmic effects.

The class Ib agents primarily exert their electrophysiologic effects on ventricular myocardium, because they have little or no effect on atrial tissue. Therefore, these agents are used only for the treatment of ventricular arrhythmias. When compared with the class Ia agents, the class Ib drugs tend to have more tolerable adverse-effect profiles and are less proarrhythmic. **Lidocaine** is still used in various acute settings for the treatment of ventricular arrhythmias because of its intravenous (IV) formulation and relatively rapid onset of action. **Mexiletine** can be combined with a class Ia or III antiarrhythmic for the treatment of refractory ventricular arrhythmias. Although these drugs have been shown to be effective in the treatment of ventricular arrhythmias, they have not been shown to improve survival.

Class Ic agents are generally very potent in slowing conduction of the cardiac impulse. These drugs can be used for the treatment of supraventricular and ventricular arrhythmias. Their noncardiac side effects appear to be relatively minor, but they may be highly proarrhythmic in patients with structural heart disease. The clinical use of these agents has significantly declined over the past decade, which is likely attributed to the negative results of the Cardiac Arrhythmia Suppression Trial (CAST) (Fig. 5.1). This trial was conducted to determine whether the suppression of asymptomatic or minimally symptomatic premature ventricular contractions (PVCs) with the class Ic antiarrhythmics, **encainide**, **flecainide**, or **moricizine**, would reduce the incidence of arrhythmic death in survivors of an MI. **Encainide** and **flecainide** were associated with a significant increase in mortality. Consequently, the results of this trial have significantly limited the use of **flecainide** in partic-

ular, especially in patients with structural heart disease. Although **propafenone** was not evaluated in CAST, there still tends to be an overall negative perception of this drug's safety in patients with structural heart disease, simply because it is in the same class of antiarrhythmics as **flecainide**. The use of these drugs should be avoided in patients with any form of structural heart disease, which includes coronary artery disease, left ventricular dysfunction, valvular heart disease, and left ventricular hypertrophy. For the treatment of atrial fibrillation, these drugs are considered first-line therapy in patients with structurally normal hearts because they have the most optimal long-term safety profiles.

MODE OF ACTION

Depression of automaticity in pacemaker fibers is a property common to all class I antiarrhythmic agents (Table 5.1). It is fortunate that most antiarrhythmic agents depress subsidiary pacemaker cells to a greater degree than those of the sinoatrial (SA) node, although toxic doses of some can suppress all cardiac pacemaker activity and result in arrest of the heartbeat.

Drugs within this group have a local anesthetic effect on nerve and myocardial cell membranes. They inhibit the fast inward Na^+ current and thus slow the maximum rate of depolarization. Their dominant effect is to slow the rate of rise in the action potential (V_{max}). A reduction in V_{max} has been found to be associated with 1) an increase in the threshold of excitability, 2) a depression of the conduction velocity, and 3) a prolongation of the effective refractory period. These actions are also consistently associated with inhibition of spontaneous diastolic depolarization in automatic myocardial cells.

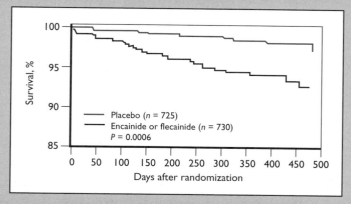

FIGURE 5.1 The effect of flecainide or encainide on survival of patients after myocardial infarction in the CAST study.

DISOPYRAMIDE PHOSPHATE

(Disopyramide phosphate, Disopyramide phosphate extended release, Norpace®, Norpace® CR)

Disopyramide depresses myocardial responsiveness and the electrophysiologic conduction rate. Diastolic depolarization is slowed in tissues with augmented automaticity, and the effective refractory period of the atrium and the ventricles is increased, but conduction in accessory pathways is prolonged. Disopyramide has a direct negative inotropic effect on the myocardium, particularly in patients with abnormal heart function. It also exhibits prominent anticholinergic actions, which is a major factor limiting its usage. Disopyramide is a class Ia antiarrhythmic agent available in conventional and sustained-release formulations.

SPECIAL GROUPS

Race: no differences in response
Children: safety and effectiveness have not been established; some experiences have been published—age specific
Elderly: dosage adjustment is required
Renal impairment: dosage adjustment is required
Hepatic impairment: dosage adjustment is required
Pregnancy: category C; use only if potential benefit justifies the potential risk to the fetus
Breast-feeding: not recommended; drug is excreted in breast milk

DOSAGE

Adults: Loading dose of 300–400 mg po followed by maintenance regimen of 400–800 mg po daily; maximum dose is 1.6 g/d. Daily doses can be given in four divided doses every 6 h with non–sustained-release products, or in two equally divided doses every 12 h with controlled- or extended-release products.

Patients < 50 kg, or with hepatic or renal impairment: Loading dose of 150–200 mg po followed by 400 mg/d in two or four divided doses, depending on the dosage form used.

The controlled- or extended-release formulation of disopyramide should not be used initially if rapid plasma concentrations are desired and is not recommended for patients with severe renal impairment.

Maintenance dose (with non–sustained-release products) in patients with severe renal impairment:

Creatinine Clearance (CrCl), mL/min	Maintenance Dose
30–40	100 mg every 8 h
15–30	100 mg every 12 h
<15	100 mg every 24 h

Children: Use non–sustained-release formulation given in divided doses every 6 h

Age, y	Maintenance Dose, mg/kg/d
<1	10–30
1–4	10–20
4–12	10–15
12–18	6–15

IN BRIEF

INDICATIONS
Life-threatening ventricular arrhythmias
Supraventricular arrhythmias (unlabeled use)

CONTRAINDICATIONS/WARNINGS
Hypersensitivity to disopyramide
Second- or third-degree heart block or sick sinus syndrome in the absence of a pacemaker
Long QT syndrome
Heart failure
Cardiogenic shock
Use with caution in myasthenia gravis, angle-closure glaucoma, renal or hepatic impairment, or urinary retention.

DRUG INTERACTIONS
Warfarin[3]
Beta-blockers[1,3]
Hepatic enzyme inducers (eg, phenytoin, rifampin, phenobarbital)[2]
Anticholinergics[1,3]
Hypoglycemic agents[3]
Class Ia and III antiarrhythmics[1,3]
Alcohol[1]
Macrolides[1]
1 Effect/toxicity of disopyramide may increase.
2 Effect of disopyramide may decrease.
3 Disopyramide may increase the effect/toxicity of this drug.

ADVERSE EFFECTS
Cardiovascular: edema, chest pain, weight gain, syncope, hypotension, heart failure exacerbation, torsades de pointes, QT interval prolongation
CNS: dizziness, headache, fatigue, nervousness
GI: nausea, vomiting, diarrhea, constipation, anorexia, dry mouth, bloating
GU: urinary hesitancy or retention
Ocular: blurred vision

PHARMACOKINETICS AND PHARMACODYNAMICS
Duration of action: 1.5–8.5 h (immediate release)
Onset of action: 30 min–3.5 h
Peak effect: 2–2.5 h
Bioavailability: 60%–80%
Effect of food: not known
Protein binding: approximately 50% (range, 20%–60% depending on serum concentration)
Volume of distribution: 1.4–1.7 L/kg
Metabolism: hepatic; primary metabolite has weak antiarrhythmic and potent anticholinergic actions
Elimination: 80% renal (about 50% unchanged, 30% metabolites); 15% biliary; hemodialyzable
Half-life: 5–7 h (prolonged in renal or hepatic impairment)

MONITORING
ECG, blood pressure (BP), baseline left ventricular function, electrolytes (K^+, Mg++), periodic plasma concentrations (preferably unbound), CNS symptoms, signs and symptoms of heart failure, signs and symptoms of anticholinergic effects on the GI and GU systems.

OVERDOSE
There is no specific antidote; treatment should be supportive and symptomatic. ECG monitoring is essential. A mechanical respirator and endocardial pacer may be helpful. Medications such as digitalis, diuretics, dopamine, isoproterenol, and neostigmine may be used when indicated. Hemodialysis or charcoal hemoperfusion may help.

PATIENT INFORMATION
Report confusion, constipation, blurred vision, syncope, palpitations, urination difficulty, edema, or shortness of breath to your physician. Do not discontinue therapy without your physician's advice.

AVAILABILITY
Capsules (immediate release)—100 mg, 150 mg
Capsules (extended or controlled release)—100 mg, 150 mg

FLECAINIDE ACETATE
(Tambocor®)

Flecainide is a class Ic antiarrhythmic agent. It is a potent blocker of fast Na^+ channels and thereby slows conduction velocity and diminishes automaticity in the atria, ventricles, His-Purkinje system, and atrioventricular (AV) node. Because of the slowed cardiac conduction, increases in the PR interval and QRS duration may be seen. Its relatively selective effects on retrograde pathways of AV nodal and anomalous AV conduction make it effective in terminating paroxysmal reentrant supraventricular tachycardia in most patients.

Flecainide is most commonly used in clinical practice for the treatment of atrial fibrillation/flutter. Although flecainide is approved by the FDA for the treatment of life-threatening ventricular arrhythmias, its utility in this setting has been compromised by the results of the CAST. This trial was conducted to determine if the suppression of asymptomatic or minimally symptomatic PVCs with flecainide, encainide, or moricizine, would decrease the incidence of death from arrhythmia in patients who survived an MI. This trial was terminated prematurely after the discovery that the use of flecainide and encainide was associated with a higher incidence of total mortality and arrhythmic death (Fig. 5.1).

SPECIAL GROUPS

Race: no differences in response
Children: safety and effectiveness have not been established
Elderly: lower doses recommended because of age-related decline in clearance
Renal impairment: dosage adjustment is required
Hepatic impairment: use only if benefit outweighs the risk; then dose to be reduced and serum drug levels recommended
Pregnancy: category C; use only if potential benefit justifies the potential risk to the fetus
Breast-feeding: not recommended; drug is excreted in breast milk

DOSAGE

Sustained ventricular tachycardia: Initiate at 100 mg po every 12 h; increase in increments of 50 mg twice daily every 4 d as needed. Usual maintenance dose is 150 mg po every 12 h. Maximum dose is 400 mg/d.

Paroxysmal supraventricular tachycardia, paroxysmal atrial fibrillation/flutter: For conversion to sinus rhythm, a single oral loading dose of 200–300 mg may be used. For maintenance of sinus rhythm, initiate at 50 mg po every 12 h. Increase in increments of 50 mg twice daily every 4 d as needed. Maximum dose is 300 mg/d.

For patients with severe renal impairment (CrCl <35 mL/min): Decrease initial dose to 50 mg po every 12 h; increase doses at intervals longer than 4 d if needed, and monitor plasma levels closely.

IN BRIEF

INDICATIONS
Life-threatening ventricular arrhythmias
Supraventricular tachyarrhythmias

CONTRAINDICATIONS/WARNINGS
Hypersensitivity to flecainide
Right bundle branch block when associated with a left hemiblock in the absence of a pacemaker
Second- or third-degree heart block in the absence of a pacemaker
Recent MI
Cardiogenic shock
Heart failure
Use with caution in sinus node dysfunction, sick sinus syndrome, severe renal or hepatic impairment, or coronary artery disease.

DRUG INTERACTIONS
Amiodarone[3]
Digoxin[3]
Beta-blockers[3]
Verapamil[3]
Diltiazem[3]
Urinary alkalinizers (eg, high-dose antacids, sodium bicarbonate, carbonic anhydrase inhibitors)[1]
Urinary acidifiers (eg, ammonium chloride)[2]
Cimetidine[1]
Ritonavir[1]

[1] Effect/toxicity of flecainide may increase.
[2] Effect of flecainide may decrease.
[3] Flecainide may increase the effect/toxicity of this drug.

ADVERSE EFFECTS
CV: ventricular tachycardia, cardiac arrest, heart failure exacerbation, sick sinus syndrome, AV block
CNS: somnolence, headache, dizziness, fatigue, tremor, fever
GI: nausea, anorexia, abdominal pain
Ocular: visual disturbances
Respiratory: dyspnea

PHARMACOKINETICS AND PHARMACODYNAMICS
Duration of action: 12–30 h
Onset of action: 1–6 h
Peak effect: 2–3 h
Bioavailability: 85%–90%
Effect of food: no effect
Protein binding: 37%–55%
Volume of distribution: 8–10 L/kg
Metabolism: hepatic; inactive metabolites; metabolized by the CYP2D6 isoenzyme
Elimination: ~ 30% excreted in urine as unchanged drug. Urinary acidification accelerates excretion; alkalinization decreases excretion; poorly dialyzable.
Half-life: 10–20 h (19–39 h in severe renal impairment)

MONITORING
ECG and vital signs daily during initiation period for PR and QRS prolongation and every 3–6 mo on maintenance dose, baseline left ventricular function, electrolytes (K^+, Mg^{++}).

OVERDOSE
Hemodynamic, symptomatic, and supportive care. Vasopressor agents, inotropic agents, and pacing may be useful. Emesis or lavage may be followed by activated charcoal. Sodium bicarbonate may reverse QRS prolongation, bradycardia, and hypotension. Charcoal hemoperfusion may be tried. Hemodialysis may only be effective in patients with renal failure.

PATIENT INFORMATION
Report dizziness, rapid heart rate, shortness of breath, or exercise intolerance to your physician. Do not discontinue therapy without a physician's advice.

AVAILABILITY
Tablets—50, 100, 150 mg

LIDOCAINE HYDROCHLORIDE
(Lidocaine HCl, Xylocaine®)

Lidocaine, a class Ib agent, possesses electrophysiologic effects that differ in healthy and ischemic cardiac tissue. In normal tissues, lidocaine shortens the action potential duration of the His-Purkinje system and ventricular myocardium and has no effect on conduction velocity. However, in ischemic tissue, lidocaine prolongs the action potential duration and decreases conduction velocity. Lidocaine has little effect on the atrial myocardium. Lidocaine also has very little effect on the automaticity of the SA node. However, lidocaine does suppress the automaticity of ectopic ventricular pacemakers and His-Purkinje fibers.

Unlike quinidine and procainamide, lidocaine has little effect on autonomic tone and generally does not significantly reduce BP, myocardial contractility, or cardiac output at the recommended doses; however, it can depress cardiac function when used at higher doses and in patients with baseline cardiac dysfunction. Lidocaine is primarily used for the acute treatment of ventricular arrhythmias, especially those associated with acute MI. However, its use in this setting has not been associated with an improvement in survival. The use of lidocaine as prophylaxis against ventricular tachycardia or ventricular fibrillation in patients with MI is not warranted. Even though prophylactic administration of lidocaine in patients with acute MI has been associated with a reduction in the incidence of ventricular fibrillation, it may be associated with a higher mortality rate. Lidocaine is not effective in the treatment of supraventricular arrhythmias such as atrial fibrillation/flutter. However, lidocaine can be used for the treatment of digitalis-induced atrial and/or ventricular arrhythmias because of its selectivity for depolarized myocardium.

SPECIAL GROUPS
Race: no differences in response
Children: safety and effectiveness have not been established; reduce dosage when used in children
Elderly: dosage adjustment is required because of reduction in patients' capacity to metabolize the drug
Heart failure: dosage adjustment is required
Renal impairment: no dosage adjustment needed
Hepatic impairment: dosage adjustment is required
Pregnancy: category B; should be used only if clearly indicated
Breast-feeding: breast-feed with caution; drug is excreted in breast milk

IN BRIEF

INDICATIONS
IV for life-threatening ventricular arrhythmias

CONTRAINDICATIONS/WARNINGS
Hypersensitivity to any amide-type local anesthetic
Second- or third-degree heart block in the absence of a pacemaker
Severe sinus node dysfunction
Stokes-Adams syndrome
Atrial fibrillation and accessory AV pathway (Wolff-Parkinson-White syndrome)
Use with caution in heart failure, hepatic impairment, sinus bradycardia, and the elderly.

DRUG INTERACTIONS
Amiodarone[1]
Procainamide[1,2]
Succinylcholine[2]
Cimetidine[1]
Beta-blockers[1]

1 Effect/toxicity of lidocaine may increase.
2 Lidocaine may increase the effect/toxicity of this drug.

ADVERSE EFFECTS
CV: hypotension, bradycardia, sinus arrest, AV block
CNS: dizziness, drowsiness, headache, confusion, disorientation, paresthesia, slurred speech, hallucinations, seizures, coma
GI: nausea, vomiting
Musculoskeletal: muscle twitching
Ocular: blurred vision
Respiratory: respiratory depression

PHARMACOKINETICS AND PHARMACODYNAMICS
Duration of action: 10–20 min
Onset of action: immediate
Bioavailability: not applicable
Effect of food: not applicable
Protein binding: 65%–75%
Volume of distribution: 1.3 L/kg (reduced in heart failure and hepatic impairment)
Metabolism: hepatic (90%); the two major metabolites, monoethylglycinexylidide and glycinexylidide, have neurotoxic and antiarrhythmic effects
Elimination: <10% excreted in urine as unchanged drug; poorly dialyzable
Half-life: 2 h; increased with congestive heart failure or liver disease (2–7 h and 6–8h, respectively)

MONITORING
Continuous ECG, vital signs, electrolytes (K^+, Mg^{++}). Serum drug concentrations in patients with heart failure, hepatic impairment, or acute MI (unbound concentration preferred), and in those receiving therapy for >24 h.

LIDOCAINE HYDROCHLORIDE (continued)

DOSAGE

Pulseless ventricular tachycardia/ventricular fibrillation: 1–1.5 mg/kg IV push; may give additional 0.5–0.75 mg/kg IV push in 3–5 min if initial response is inadequate, up to a maximum total dose of 3 mg/kg.

Stable ventricular tachycardia (left ventricular ejection fraction [LVEF] >40%): 1–1.5 mg/kg IV push; may give additional 0.5–0.75 mg/kg IV push in 3–5 min if initial response is inadequate, up to a maximum total dose of 3 mg/kg.

Stable ventricular tachycardia (LVEF ≤40%): 0.5–0.75 mg/kg IV push; may repeat every 5–10 min if initial response is inadequate, up to a maximum total dose of 3 mg/kg.

Maintenance infusion: 1–4 mg/min; a slower infusion rate (1–2 mg/min) should be used for elderly patients, patients <50 kg, or those with heart failure or hepatic impairment.

Lidocaine may also be administered via an endotracheal tube at 2–2.5 times the IV dose.

OVERDOSE

Hemodynamic support; discontinue the drug, especially for CNS toxicity manifestations. Sodium bicarbonate may reverse QRS prolongation, bradycardia, and hypotension. Vasopressor agents may be useful. Benzodiazepines may be used to treat seizures. Hemodialysis is not effective.

AVAILABILITY

For direct IV injection—10, 20 mg/mL
For preparation of IV continuous infusion—40, 100, 200 mg/mL
For IV infusion— 2, 4, 8 mg/mL in 5% dextrose

MEXILETINE HYDROCHLORIDE
(Mexiletine HCl, Mexitil®)

Mexiletine has class Ib antiarrhythmic properties. It is a structurally related oral analogue of lidocaine with similar electrophysiologic effects. By blocking Na^+ channels, mexiletine decreases automaticity and shortens the action potential duration of the His-Purkinje system and ventricular myocardium. As with lidocaine, mexiletine also has very little effect on the atrial myocardium. Mexiletine is effective in the treatment of ventricular arrhythmias; however, its efficacy in this setting is limited when used as a single agent. Combining mexiletine with a second antiarrhythmic agent (class Ia or III) has proven more effective for the treatment of ventricular arrhythmias. Mexiletine does not appear to affect left ventricular function, even in patients with a depressed LVEF.

SPECIAL GROUPS

Race: no differences in response
Children: safety and effectiveness have not been established
Elderly: no dosage adjustment needed
Heart failure: dosage adjustment is required
Renal impairment: no dosage adjustment needed
Hepatic impairment: dosage adjustment is required
Pregnancy: category C; use only if potential benefit justifies the potential risk to the fetus
Breast-feeding: not recommended; drug is excreted in breast milk

DOSAGE

Initiate at 200 mg po every 8 h; increase or decrease in increments of 50–100 mg/dose every 2–3 d as needed. For rapid control of ventricular arrhythmias, a loading dose of 400 mg po may be administered followed by a maintenance dose of 200 mg po every 8 h. Maximum dose is 1200 mg/d. Some patients may tolerate twice-daily dosing.

The maintenance dose should be reduced by 30%–50% in patients with heart failure or hepatic impairment.

IN BRIEF

INDICATIONS
Life-threatening ventricular arrhythmias

CONTRAINDICATIONS/WARNINGS
Second- or third-degree heart block in the absence of a pacemaker
Hypersensitivity to mexiletine
Cardiogenic shock
Use with caution in sinus node dysfunction, heart failure, hepatic impairment, and seizure disorders

DRUG INTERACTIONS
Class I antiarrhythmic agents[1]
Theophylline[3]
Cimetidine[1]
Hepatic enzyme inducers (eg, phenytoin, rifampin, phenobarbital)[2]
Urinary alkalinizers (eg, high-dose antacids, sodium bicarbonate, carbonic anhydrase inhibitors)[1]
Urinary acidifiers (eg, ammonium chloride)[2]
Narcotics[2]
Atropine[2]
Aluminum-magnesium hydroxide[2]
Caffeine[3]
Metoclopramide[1]

1 Effect/toxicity of mexiletine may increase.
2 Effect of mexiletine may decrease.
3 Mexiletine may increase the effect/toxicity of this drug.

ADVERSE EFFECTS
CV: hypotension, bradycardia, palpitations, chest pain, ventricular arrhythmias
CNS: dizziness, lightheadedness, tremor, nervousness, drowsiness, confusion, disorientation, paresthesia, ataxia, seizures
Dermatologic: rash
GI: nausea, vomiting, anorexia, heartburn, constipation, diarrhea
Ocular: blurred vision, nystagmus

PHARMACOKINETICS AND PHARMACODYNAMICS
Duration of action: 8–16 h
Onset of action: 1–4 h (average 2 h)
Peak effect: approximately 2–4 h post administration
Bioavailability: 85%–90%
Effect of food: may delay absorption
Protein binding: 50%–60%
Volume of distribution: 5–7 L/kg
Metabolism: hepatic; mostly inactive metabolites; metabolized by the CYP2D6 isoenzyme
Elimination: 10%–15% excreted in urine as unchanged drug. Urinary acidification accelerates excretion; alkalinization decreases excretion; poorly dialyzable.
Half-life: 10–14 h; increased in patients with heart failure or hepatic impairment

MONITORING
ECG and vital signs daily during initiation period and every 3–6 mo on maintenance dose. Observe for neurologic abnormalities when initiating therapy.

OVERDOSE
Treatment is mainly supportive and symptomatic. Acidification of urine may be performed to accelerate excretion of mexiletine. Atropine may be indicated if hypotension or bradycardia occurs. Hemodialysis is not effective.

PATIENT INFORMATION
Mexiletine may be taken with food to decrease gastrointestinal upset. This medication may cause abdominal pain, nausea, vomiting, dizziness, and tremor. Report side effects to your physician. Do not discontinue therapy without your physician's advice.

AVAILABILITY
Capsules—150, 200, 250 mg

MORICIZINE HYDROCHLORIDE (Ethmozine®)

Moricizine is primarily categorized as a class Ic antiarrhythmic. By blocking the fast inward Na^+ current, moricizine decreases conduction velocity and automaticity. It does not markedly affect the atrial, AV nodal, or ventricular refractory periods and has minimal effect on ventricular repolarization. Moricizine is approved for the treatment of life-threatening ventricular arrhythmias, including sustained ventricular tachycardia. The efficacy of moricizine for the treatment of ventricular arrhythmias was evaluated in the CAST II. This trial enrolled survivors of MI with poor left ventricular function who were asymptomatic or had mildly symptomatic ventricular dysrhythmias. As with CAST I, this study was prematurely terminated because moricizine was found to be ineffective and perhaps even harmful. In the first 2 weeks of the trial, mortality (likely due to proarrhythmia) was significantly higher in the moricizine group compared with the placebo group.

SPECIAL GROUPS

Race: no differences in response
Children: safety and effectiveness have not been established
Elderly: no dosage adjustment needed
Renal impairment: dosage adjustment is required
Hepatic impairment: dosage adjustment is required
Pregnancy: category B; should be used only if clearly indicated
Breast-feeding: not recommended; drug is excreted in breast milk

DOSAGE

Initiate at 200 mg po every 8 h; increase in increments of 150 mg daily every 3 d if necessary. Usual maintenance dose is 200–300 mg every 8 h.
Maintenance dose should not exceed 600 mg/d in patients with renal or hepatic impairment.

IN BRIEF

INDICATIONS
Life-threatening ventricular arrhythmias

CONTRAINDICATIONS/WARNINGS
Hypersensitivity to moricizine
Second- or third-degree heart block in the absence of a pacemaker
Right bundle branch block when associated with left hemiblock in the absence of a pacemaker
Cardiogenic shock
Recent MI
Use with caution in sinus node dysfunction, renal or hepatic impairment, or coronary artery disease.

DRUG INTERACTIONS
Antiarrhythmic agents[1,2]
Theophylline[3]
Cimetidine[1]
Diltiazem[1,3]
Digoxin[1,2]

1 Effect/toxicity of moricizine may increase.
2 Moricizine may increase the effect/toxicity of this drug.
3 Moricizine may decrease the effect of this drug.

ADVERSE EFFECTS
CV: proarrhythmia (eg, ventricular tachycardia), heart failure exacerbation, sick sinus syndrome, AV block
CNS: dizziness (lessened by administering in smaller doses), headache, fatigue, insomnia, fever
GI: nausea, anorexia, abdominal pain, diarrhea
Ocular: blurred vision
Respiratory: dyspnea

PHARMACOKINETICS AND PHARMACODYNAMICS
Duration of action: 10–24 h
Onset of action: 2 h
Peak effect: 0.5–2 h
Bioavailability: well absorbed but limited by high first-pass metabolism (34%–38%)
Effect of food: may delay absorption
Protein binding: 95%
Metabolism: hepatic; extensive with at least 26 metabolites (approximately two are active); appears to induce its own metabolism
Elimination: biliary/fecal, 56%; renal, 39% (<1% of a dose excreted in urine as unchanged drug); poorly dialyzable
Half-life: 3–4 h

MONITORING
ECG daily during initiation period and every 3–6 mo on maintenance dose.

OVERDOSE
Gastric lavage if indicated. Hemodynamic and respiratory support, ventricular pacing, and defibrillation if needed. Sodium bicarbonate may reverse QRS prolongation, bradycardia, and hypotension.

PATIENT INFORMATION
Side effects may include dizziness, palpitations, headache, and nausea. Report side effects to your physician. Do not discontinue therapy without your physician's advice.

AVAILABILITY
Tablets—200 mg, 250 mg, 300 mg

PROCAINAMIDE HYDROCHLORIDE
(Procainamide HCl, Procainamide HCl extended release, Procanbid®, Pronestyl®, Pronestyl-SR®)

Procainamide exhibits the electrophysiologic effects of the class Ia antiarrhythmic drugs. It decreases automaticity, slows conduction velocity, and prolongs refractoriness in the atria, ventricles, and His-Purkinje system. Its weak anticholinergic effects may also increase the conductivity of the AV node. Procainamide may also cause vasodilation, which may lead to hypotension during IV administration. Procainamide widens the QRS complex, lengthens the QT interval, and slightly prolongs the PR interval. N-acetyl-procainamide (NAPA), the major metabolite of procainamide, blocks outward potassium (K^+) currents and thereby has class III electrophysiologic properties. NAPA is responsible for causing prolongation of the QT interval. Procainamide is a broad-spectrum antiarrhythmic drug that may be used to treat supraventricular and ventricular dysrhythmias. Blood cell dyscrasias, including agranulocytosis, occur occasionally with procainamide, and its prolonged use has been associated with lupuslike reactions, a major reason for its decline in use.

SPECIAL GROUPS

Race: no differences in response
Children: safety and effectiveness have not been established
Elderly: dosage adjustment is required for renal impairment
Renal impairment: dosage adjustment is required
Hepatic impairment: dosage adjustment is required
Pregnancy: category C; use only if potential benefit justifies the potential risk to the fetus
Breast-feeding: not recommended; drug is excreted in breast milk

IN BRIEF

INDICATIONS
Ventricular arrhythmias
Supraventricular arrhythmias (unlabeled use)
Atrial fibrillation/atrial flutter (unlabeled use)

CONTRAINDICATIONS/WARNINGS
Systemic lupus erythematosus (SLE)
Second- or third-degree heart block in the absence of a pacemaker
Severe sinus node dysfunction
Long QT syndrome
Torsades de pointes due to other type Ia agents
Hypersensitivity to procaine and related drugs
Use with caution in heart failure, renal or hepatic impairment, or myasthenia gravis

DRUG INTERACTIONS
Class I antiarrhythmics[1,3]
Histamine₂-receptor antagonists (eg, cimetidine, ranitidine)[1]
Neuromuscular blocking agents[3]
Anticholinergic agents (eg, atropine, diphenhydramine, tricyclic antidepressants [TCA])[3]
Cholinergic agents (eg, pyridostigmine)[4]
Amiodarone[1]
Antihypertensive agents[3]
Alcohol[2]
Trimethoprim[1]
Ofloxacin[1]

1 Effect/toxicity of procainamide may increase.
2 Effect of procainamide may decrease.
3 Procainamide may increase the effect/toxicity of this drug.
4 Procainamide may decrease the effect of this drug.

ADVERSE EFFECTS
Blood: agranulocytosis, neutropenia, hemolytic anemia, thrombocytopenia
CNS: dizziness, lightheadedness, confusion, hallucinations
CV: torsades de pointes, hypotension (with IV), tachycardia, QT interval prolongation
GI: anorexia, bitter taste, nausea, vomiting, diarrhea
Skin: pruritus, maculopapular rash
Other: SLE-like syndrome (ie, rash, arthralgias, fever, pericarditis, pleuritis)

PHARMACOKINETICS AND PHARMACODYNAMICS
Duration of action: 3–6 h
Onset of action: 1–2 h (oral); immediate (IV)
Peak effect: 60–90 min (oral), immediate (IV)
Bioavailability: 75%–95% (oral)
Effect of food: not known
Protein binding: 15%–20%
Volume of distribution: 2 L/kg
Metabolism: hepatic, 35% converted to active metabolite NAPA (higher in rapid acetylators)
Elimination: renal, 65% excreted in urine as unchanged drug. NAPA is excreted more slowly in renal impairment; hemodialyzable
Half-life: procainamide—2.5–4.5 h (normal renal function); 5.3–20.7 h (renal impairment); 12.5–14 h (anephric) NAPA—6–8 h (normal renal function), 33–48 h (renal failure)

MONITORING
BP, ECG, plasma concentrations of procainamide and NAPA, signs and symptoms of toxicity, antinuclear antibody (ANA) titers, CBC with differential, electrolytes (K^+, Mg++).

PROCAINAMIDE HYDROCHLORIDE *(continued)*

DOSAGE

Supraventricular arrhythmias:

IV: 15–17 mg/kg over 25–60 min, then continuous infusion of 1–4 mg/min (or can convert to oral therapy after initial loading dose)

Oral: Usual dose is 50 mg/kg/d; for immediate release, give in divided doses every 3–6 h; for extended release (Pronestyl-SR, Procainamide HCl extended release), give in divided doses every 6 h; for extended release (Procanbid), give in divided doses every 12 h

Refractory pulseless ventricular tachycardia/ventricular fibrillation:

IV: 15–17 mg/kg infused at 30 mg/min (maximum total dose is 17 mg/kg); if stable rhythm achieved, can initiate continuous infusion at 1–4 mg/min; convert patient to oral therapy when hemodynamically stable and able to take oral medications

Stable ventricular tachycardia:

IV: 20 mg/min infusion given until arrhythmia suppressed, hypotension occurs, QRS widens by >50%, or total dose of 17 mg/kg is administered; if stable rhythm achieved, can initiate continuous infusion at 1–4 mg/min; convert patient to oral therapy when hemodynamically stable and able to take oral medications

Oral: Usual dose is 50 mg/kg/d; for immediate release, give in divided doses every 3–6 h; for extended release (Pronestyl-SR, Procainamide HCl extended release), give in divided doses every 6 h; for extended release (Procanbid), give in divided doses every 12 h

Maintenance dose should be reduced in patients with renal or hepatic impairment.

OVERDOSE

Treatment is primarily symptomatic and supportive. Gastric lavage, emesis, and activated charcoal may be used if ingestion is recent. Fluid replacement, vasopressors, and mechanical cardiorespiratory support may be indicated. Hemodialysis may also be useful. Peritoneal dialysis is not effective. Sodium bicarbonate may reverse QRS prolongation or hypotension. To manage torsades de pointes, give magnesium sulfate 1–2 g IV push, then a continuous infusion of 8–16 g over 24 h. Direct-current cardioversion should be used if hemodynamically unstable. Replenish K^+ if needed. Overdrive pacing, isoproterenol, phenytoin, and lidocaine may also be used to manage torsades de pointes.

PATIENT INFORMATION

Report symptoms of nausea/vomiting, sore throat, rash, joint pain, or shortness of breath to your physician. Do not chew sustained-release tablets. Some sustained-release tablets contain a wax core that slowly releases the medication; the empty and nonabsorbable wax core is eliminated and may be found in feces. Do not discontinue therapy without your physician's advice.

AVAILABILITY

Capsules or tablets, immediate release (Procainamide, Pronestyl)—250 mg, 375 mg, 500 mg

Tablets, extended release (Procainamide HCl extended release, Pronestyl SR) (dosed every 6 h)—250 mg, 500 mg, 750 mg, 1000 mg

Tablets, extended release (Procanbid) (dosed every 12 h)—500 mg, 1000 mg

Injection—100 mg/mL, 500 mg/mL

The information here is provided as guidance only. Prescribers should always consult the manufacturer's current prescribing information.

73

PROPAFENONE HYDROCHLORIDE
(Propafenone, Rythmol®, Rythmol SR®)

Propafenone has the same ability to block Na⁺ channels, slow conduction velocity, and diminish automaticity in the atria, ventricles, AV node, and His-Purkinje system as flecainide. The drug has little or no effect on the action potential duration. However, propafenone also has a mild, nonselective beta-adrenergic blocking effect. Like flecainide, propafenone causes increases in the PR interval and QRS duration. Propafenone also prolongs the antegrade and retrograde refractory periods and slows conduction in accessory pathways.

SPECIAL GROUPS

Race: no differences in response
Children: safety and effectiveness have not been established
Elderly: no dosage adjustment needed
Renal impairment: no dosage adjustment needed
Hepatic impairment: dosage adjustment is needed
Pregnancy: category C; use only if potential benefit justifies the potential risk to the fetus
Breast-feeding: not recommended; unknown if excreted into breast milk

IN BRIEF

INDICATIONS
Life-threatening ventricular arrhythmias
Maintenance of sinus rhythm in patients with symptomatic atrial fibrillation (Rythmol SR)

CONTRAINDICATIONS/WARNINGS
Second- or third-degree heart block in the absence of a pacemaker
Sinus node dysfunction
Bradycardia
Bronchospastic diseases
Severe hypotension
Cardiogenic shock
Heart failure
Electrolyte imbalance
Hypersensitivity to propafenone
Use with caution in hepatic impairment.

DRUG INTERACTIONS
Quinidine[1]
Anesthetics[3]
Digoxin[3]
Warfarin[3]
Beta-blockers[3]
Cyclosporine[3]
Calcium channel blockers[1]
Rifampin[2]
Cimetidine[1]
Ritonavir[1]
Theophylline[3]

1 Effect/toxicity of propafenone may increase.
2 Effect of propafenone may decrease.
3 Propafenone may increase the effect/toxicity of this drug.

ADVERSE EFFECTS
CNS: dizziness, headache, anxiety, fatigue
CV: ventricular tachycardia, bradycardia, AV block, hypotension, heart failure exacerbation
GI: abnormal taste, nausea, vomiting, constipation
Respiratory: bronchospasm, dyspnea

PHARMACOKINETICS AND PHARMACODYNAMICS
Duration of action: 4–22 h
Onset of action: 2–4 h
Peak effect: 2–6 h
Bioavailability: well absorbed, but limited by its high first-pass metabolism (2%–23%). However, it increases with dose and duration of therapy as hepatic metabolism is saturable.
Effect of food: no effect
Protein binding: 85%–95%
Volume of distribution: 1–6 L/kg
Metabolism: hepatic; undergoes polymorphic metabolism via CYP2D6 isoenzyme that is genetically determined. In ~ 90% of patients (extensive metabolizers), propafenone is extensively metabolized into 5-hydroxypropafenone (active metabolite). The other 10% of patients are poor metabolizers and form little if any 5-hydroxypropafenone. N-depropylpropafenone is another active metabolite of propafenone that is not subject to genetic polymorphism.
Elimination: renal (38% as metabolites, <1% as unchanged drug); fecal (53% as metabolites); poorly dialyzable
Half-life: extensive metabolizer—2–10 h; poor metabolizer—10–32 h

PROPAFENONE HYDROCHLORIDE *(continued)*

DOSAGE

Immediate release (for ventricular and supraventricular arrhythmias): Initiate at 150 mg po every 8 h; increase to 225 mg po every 8 h after 3–4 d if needed. Maximum dose is 300 mg po every 8 h.

For conversion to sinus rhythm in patients with atrial fibrillation/flutter, a single oral loading dose of 450–600 mg may be used.

Sustained release (for maintenance of sinus rhythm in patients with atrial fibrillation): Initiate at 225 mg po every 12 h; increase dose to 325 mg po every 12 h after 5 d if needed. Maximum dose is 425 mg po every 12 h.

MONITORING

ECG and vital signs daily during initiation period and every 3–6 mo on maintenance dose; baseline left ventricular function, electrolytes (K^+, Mg++); CNS symptoms.

OVERDOSE

Hemodynamic, symptomatic, and supportive care. Vasopressor agents, inotropic agents, and pacing may be useful. Sodium bicarbonate may reverse QRS prolongation, bradycardia, and hypotension. Hemodialysis is not effective.

PATIENT INFORMATION

Report dizziness, rapid heart rate, shortness of breath, or exercise intolerance to your physician. Do not discontinue medication without physician's advice.

AVAILABILITY

Tablets, immediate release (propafenone, Rythmol)—150 mg, 225 mg, 300 mg

Capsules, sustained release (Rythmol SR)—225 mg, 325 mg, 425 mg

The information here is provided as guidance only. Prescribers should always consult the manufacturer's current prescribing information.

75

QUINIDINE
(Quinidine gluconate, Quinaglute Dura-Tabs®, Quinidine polygalacturonate, Cardioquin®, Quinidine sulfate, Quinora®, Quinidex Extentabs®)

Quinidine, a class Ia agent, is a broad-spectrum antiarrhythmic that may be used to treat supraventricular and ventricular arrhythmias. Specifically, this drug has been used in the management of atrial flutter or fibrillation, AV nodal reentrant tachycardia, and ventricular tachycardia. This drug decreases automaticity, slows conduction velocity, and prolongs refractoriness. Quinidine widens the QRS complex, prolongs the QT interval, and slightly prolongs the PR interval. Quinidine has potent anticholinergic effects on the SA and AV nodes. Consequently, this antiarrhythmic can increase sinus node discharge and AV nodal conduction, which may lead to an increased ventricular rate in patients with atrial fibrillation or flutter. To minimize the risk of this complication, a beta-blocker, nondihydropyridine calcium channel blocker, or digoxin should be initiated before starting quinidine to adequately block the AV node. When used intravenously, quinidine also blocks alpha$_1$-receptors, which may lead to vasodilation and subsequent dose-related hypotension.

Patients with congenital long QT syndrome or a history of torsades de pointes should not be given quinidine because of the increased risk for arrhythmias. Evidence suggests that although quinidine reduces the recurrence of atrial fibrillation after cardioversion, it may significantly increase the risk of death.

SPECIAL GROUPS

Race: no differences in response

Children: safety and effectiveness have not been established

Elderly: initiate with lowest dose and titrate to response

Renal impairment: dosage adjustment is required in severe renal impairment

Hepatic impairment: dosage adjustment is required

Pregnancy: category C; use only if potential benefit justifies the potential risk to the fetus; quinidine has oxytocic properties; quinine use during pregnancy has caused fetal blindness and congenital deafness

Breast-feeding: not recommended; drug is excreted in breast milk

IN BRIEF

INDICATIONS
Paroxysmal supraventricular tachycardia
Ventricular tachycardia
Atrial fibrillation/flutter
Junctional tachycardia
Premature atrial contractions
Atrial tachycardia

CONTRAINDICATIONS/WARNINGS
Hypersensitivity to quinidine or related cinchona derivatives
Myasthenia gravis
Second- or third-degree heart block in the absence of a pacemaker
Torsades de pointes
Digitalis toxicity with AV conduction disorder
History of thrombocytopenic purpura associated with quinidine
Long QT syndrome
Concurrent use of ritonavir
Intraventricular conduction defects exhibiting marked QRS widening
Use with caution in severe renal impairment or hepatic impairment.

DRUG INTERACTIONS
Hepatic enzyme inducers (eg, phenytoin, rifampin, phenobarbital)[2]
Urinary alkalinizers (eg, high-dose antacids, sodium bicarbonate, carbonic anhydrase inhibitors)[1]
Phenothiazines[1,3]
Anticholinergics[3]
Verapamil[3]
Digoxin[3]
Warfarin[3]
Neuromuscular blocking agents[3]
Amiodarone[1]
Disopyramide[2,3]
Procainamide[3]
Propafenone[3]
Beta-blockers[3]
Cholinergic agents (eg, pyridostigmine, physostigmine)[4]
Cimetidine[1]
Nifedipine[2,3]
TCAs[3]
Ritonavir[1]

[1] Effect/toxicity of quinidine may increase.
[2] Effect of quinidine may decrease.
[3] Quinidine may increase the effect/toxicity of this drug.
[4] Quinidine may decrease the effect of this drug.

ADVERSE EFFECTS
Blood: thrombocytopenia; may cause hemolysis in patients with glucose-6-phosphate dehydrogenase deficiency
CNS: dizziness, vertigo, cinchonism (tinnitus, blurred vision, headache), fever
CV: torsades de pointes, hypotension, widening of QRS complex
GI: diarrhea, bitter taste, anorexia, nausea, vomiting, abdominal pain
Skin: pruritus, urticaria

QUINIDINE (continued)

DOSAGE

The dosage of quinidine is expressed in terms of the salt: 267 mg of quinidine gluconate or 275 mg of quinidine polygalacturonate is equivalent to 200 mg of quinidine sulfate. The following dosages are expressed in terms of the respective salts. Because of the increased risk of adverse effects, loading doses of quinidine are no longer recommended.

Quinidine sulfate:

Maintenance of sinus rhythm in patients with atrial fibrillation or flutter: 200–400 mg po every 6–8 h or 300–600 mg extended-release tablets po every 8–12 h

Suppression of ventricular tachycardia after cardioversion: 200–400 mg po every 6 h or 300–600 mg extended-release tablets po every 8–12 h

Quinidine polygalacturonate: Usual maintenance dose: 275 mg po every 8–12 h

Quinidine gluconate:

Oral: 324–648 mg po every 8–12 h

IV: 5–10 mg/kg at an initial rate up to 0.25 mg/kg/min. There is a high risk for hypotension. Monitor ECG for widening of QRS and prolongation of QT intervals, disappearance of the P wave, symptomatic bradycardia, or tachycardia. Consult quinidine package literature for proper dilution of IV formulation.

In patients with severe renal impairment (CrCl <10 mL/min), 75% of the normal maintenance dose should be administered.

In patients with hepatic impairment, the maintenance dose should be reduced by 50%.

PHARMACOKINETICS AND PHARMACODYNAMICS

Duration of action: 6–8 h (sulfate); 12 h (gluconate)
Onset of action: 1 h (sulfate); 2–4 h (gluconate)
Peak effect: 1–2 h (sulfate); 3–5 h (gluconate)
Bioavailability: 80% (sulfate); 70% (gluconate)
Effect of food: may delay absorption
Protein binding: 80%–90%
Volume of distribution: 2–3.5 L/kg (increased in patients with hepatic impairment)
Metabolism: hepatic; 60%–80% converted to two active metabolites; metabolized via the CYP3A4 isoenzyme
Elimination: 10%–25% excreted in urine as unchanged drug; slightly dialyzable
Half-life: 6–8 h (prolonged in patients with hepatic impairment)

MONITORING

CBC, liver function tests, BP, ECG, electrolytes (K^+, Mg^{++}), and quinidine concentrations with dosage changes and chronic administration.

OVERDOSE

Gastric lavage, emesis, and charcoal administration if recent ingestion. Symptomatic treatment (fluid, norepinephrine), BP and ECG monitoring, and cardiac pacing if necessary. Artificial ventilation if indicated. Hemodialysis or forced diuresis may be effective, but not peritoneal dialysis.

To manage torsades de pointes, give magnesium sulfate 1–2 g IV push, then a continuous infusion of 8–16 g over 24 h. Direct-current cardioversion should be used if hemodynamically unstable. Replenish K^+ if needed. Overdrive pacing, isoproterenol, phenytoin, and lidocaine may also be used to manage torsades de pointes.

PATIENT INFORMATION

Quinidine may be taken with food to reduce gastrointestinal upset. Report any symptoms of blurred vision, dizziness, tinnitus, diarrhea, abnormal bleeding or bruising, rash, or fainting to your physician. Do not crush or chew sustained-release tablets; scored tablets may be cut in half. You may see the core of the tablet in stool. Do not discontinue therapy without your physician's advice.

AVAILABILITY

Tablets (Quinidine sulfate)—200 mg, 300 mg
Tablets, quinidine sulfate sustained release (Quinidex Extentabs)—300 mg
Tablets, quinidine gluconate sustained release (Quinaglute Dura-Tabs)—324 mg
Tablets, quinidine polygalacturonate (Cardioquin)—275 mg
Injection (Quinidine gluconate)—80 mg/mL

The information here is provided as guidance only. Prescribers should always consult the manufacturer's current prescribing information.

77

TOCAINIDE HYDROCHLORIDE (Tonocard®)

Tocainide, like mexiletine, is a class Ib agent. It is an orally active analogue of lidocaine that has only a minimal effect on PR, QRS, and QT intervals. The drug has little impact on atrial rhythm disturbances. It is mainly effective for the treatment of ventricular arrhythmias. However, because of its potential to cause serious pulmonary and hematologic toxicities, the use of tocainide should be limited to the treatment of life-threatening ventricular dysrhythmias that are refractory to other antiarrhythmics.

SPECIAL GROUPS

Race: no differences in response
Children: safety and effectiveness have not been established
Elderly: no dosage adjustment needed
Heart failure: dosage reduction may be required
Renal impairment: dosage adjustment is required
Hepatic impairment: dosage adjustment is required
Pregnancy: category C; use only if potential benefit justifies the potential risk to the fetus
Breast-feeding: not recommended; drug is excreted in breast milk

DOSAGE

Maintenance dose: 400 mg po every 8 h; usual maintenance dose is 1.2–1.8 g daily. Maximum dose is 2.4 g/d in divided doses. Reduce initial maintenance dose by 50% in patients with hepatic impairment. In patients with CrCl 10–30 mL/min, reduce dose by 25%. In patients with CrCl <10 mL/min, reduce dose by 50%.

IN BRIEF

INDICATIONS
Life-threatening ventricular arrhythmias

CONTRAINDICATIONS/WARNINGS
Second- or third-degree heart block in the absence of a pacemaker
Hypersensitivity to lidocaine or other amide-type local anesthetics
Use with caution in heart failure, bone marrow depression, renal or hepatic impairment.

DRUG INTERACTIONS
Class I antiarrhythmic agents[1,3]
Rifampin[2]
Cimetidine[2]
Beta-blockers[3]
Caffeine[3]
Theophylline[3]

1 Effect/toxicity of tocainide may increase.
2 Effect of tocainide may decrease.
3 Tocainide may increase the effect/toxicity of this drug.

ADVERSE EFFECTS
Blood: agranulocytosis, leukopenia, anemia, thrombocytopenia
CNS: vertigo, dizziness, drowsiness, confusion, disorientation, ataxia, paresthesia, tremor
CV: hypotension, bradycardia, ventricular arrhythmias, heart failure exacerbation
GI: nausea, vomiting, diarrhea, anorexia
Lungs: pulmonary fibrosis, interstitial pneumonitis, dyspnea, respiratory arrest
Ocular: blurred vision
Skin: rash

PHARMACOKINETICS AND PHARMACODYNAMICS
Duration of action: 12–24 h
Onset of action: 1–2 h
Peak effect: 0.5–2 h
Bioavailability: well absorbed (90%–95%)
Effect of food: absorption is delayed
Protein binding: 10%–20%
Volume of distribution: 3 L/kg
Metabolism: hepatic (50%–60%); stereo-specific metabolism ((S)-enantiomer eliminated more quickly); inactive metabolites
Elimination: 30%–40% excreted in urine as unchanged drug; moderately dialyzable
Half-life: 11–16 h (normal); 14–19 h in patients with heart failure or ventricular arrhythmias; 20–25 h in patients with severe renal impairment

MONITORING
ECG daily during initiation period and every 3–6 mo on maintenance dose. Observe for neurologic abnormalities when initiating therapy. CBC during the first 3 mo of therapy. Baseline chest radiograph, and follow-up if signs and symptoms of pulmonary fibrosis or interstitial pneumonitis occur.

OVERDOSE
Hemodynamic support. Discontinue the drug, especially for CNS toxicity manifestations. Sodium bicarbonate may reverse bradycardia and hypotension.

PATIENT INFORMATION
Report numbness, drowsiness, dizziness, or tremors of extremities to your physician. Nausea may be common. Side effects may be minimized by taking tocainide with food. Do not discontinue therapy without your physician's advice.

AVAILABILITY
Tablets—400 mg, 600 mg

For many years, it has been known that cardiac arrhythmias could be initiated or worsened by stress or emotion or by the cardiac effects of increased catecholamines. Until the development of the beta-blockers, however, no drugs were capable of controlling tachycardia, which has its origins in increased adrenergic activity. The individual drugs in this category are listed in the chapter on beta-blockers. **Sotalol**, a beta-blocker with additional class III properties, is described in the next section (Antiarrhythmic Agents: Class III).

EFFICACY AND USE

The responsiveness of different arrhythmias to beta-blockade is shown in Table 5.2. In general, beta$_1$-selective and nonselective beta-blockers are equally effective in treating supraventricular and ventricular arrhythmias. Beta$_1$-selective and nonselective drugs appear to be equally effective for ventricular arrhythmias after MI. Beta-blockers have been demonstrated to be effective at reducing sudden death and reinfarction in this setting. The efficacy of beta-blockers in this regard sets them apart from other first-line antiarrhythmic agents.

Beta-blockers may be effective in the treatment of supraventricular tachycardias (Table 5.3). These agents are an effective treatment option for chronic ventricular rate control in patients with atrial fibrillation or flutter (Table 5.3). When compared with digoxin, beta-blockers have the advantage of being able to effectively control heart rate at rest and during exercise or stress. Given their mortality benefits in patients with left ventricular systolic dysfunction, beta-blockers are being increasingly used to control ventricular rate in this particular patient population when atrial fibrillation develops. In patients who require combination therapy in order to achieve an adequately controlled ventricular rate, beta-blockers have been shown to act synergistically with digoxin.

MODE OF ACTION

(For the use of individual beta-blockers in arrhythmias, see individual drug pages).

Increased catecholamines or sympathetic stimulation have insignificant effects on the action potential of ventricular muscle, but their effect on automatic tissue within the heart is different. They increase the diastolic depolarization rate and impulse formation by specialized cardiac fibers that slow pacemaker activity. In the intact heart, sympathetic stimulation leads to increased pacemaker activity, with increased conduction in the AV node but no increase in the Purkinje fibers. This heterogeneous shortening of the refractoriness of the conduction apparatus lowers the threshold for ventricular fibrillation. Beta-blockers can depress the rate of rise of the slow response action potentials, particularly in the presence of high levels of catecholamines and high extra-

TABLE 5.2 EXPECTED RESPONSE OF SUPRAVENTRICULAR AND VENTRICULAR CARDIAC ARRHYTHMIAS TO TREATMENT WITH BETA-BLOCKERS	
Arrhythmia	**Response**
Supraventricular arrhythmia	
Sinus tachycardia	Excellent
Paroxysmal supraventricular tachycardia (including Wolff-Parkinson-White syndrome)	Good
Atrial fibrillation	Ventricular rate reduced; not responsible for restoring sinus rhythm
Atrial flutter	Ventricular rate reduced; not responsible for restoring sinus rhythm
Ventricular arrhythmia	
Ventricular premature beats	Fair to good, but good when it results from digitalis toxicity, exercise or stress, ischemic heart disease, mitral valve prolapse, or long QT syndrome
Ventricular tachycardia (sustained)	Fair to good, but good when it results from digitalis toxicity, exercise or stress, or long QT syndrome, chronic infarction, or acute ischemia
Nonsustained ventricular tachycardia	Fair to good, particularly in cases unresponsive to other antiarrhythmic therapy, depending on mechanism
Ventricular fibrillation refractory to initial defibrillation	Good if 1) it results from digitalis toxicity or sympathomimetic amines, or 2) it is refractory to initial defibrillation

Data from Skluth H, Grauer K, Gums J: Ventricular arrhythmias: an assessment of newer therapeutic agents. *Postgrad Med* 1989, 85:137–153.

The information here is provided as guidance only. Prescribers should always consult the manufacturer's current prescribing information.

79

cellular K^+ concentrations. Beta-blockers also inhibit the enhanced spontaneous diastolic depolarizations induced by catecholamines, and therefore diminish automaticity. AV nodal conduction is generally delayed by beta-blockers, leading to prolongation of the PR interval and the effective refractory period. The refractoriness of both antegrade and retrograde accessory pathways in pre-excitation syndromes (such as Wolff-Parkinson-White syndrome) is generally unaffected by beta-blockers at rest, but beta-blockers can blunt the shortening of refractoriness induced by catecholamines. At rest and during exercise, beta-blockers do not significantly affect conduction and refractoriness of His-Purkinje tissue or normal ventricular muscle, but the QT interval may be slightly shortened, suggesting a slight acceleration of ventricular muscle repolarization. In addition, some of the effects of beta-blockers may be secondary to decreasing myocardial ischemia.

TABLE 5.3 AGENTS FOR CONTROLLING VENTRICULAR RATE IN SUPRAVENTRICULAR TACHYCARDIAS			
Agent	**Loading dose**	**Usual maintenance dose**	**Comments**
Digoxin* (Lanoxin)	10–15 µg/kg ideal body weight, up to 1–1.5 mg IV or PO over 24 h	PO: 0.125–0.5 mg/d	Max response may take several hours and days to achieve steady state; caution in renal dysfunction
Esmolol (Brevibloc)	0.5 mg/kg IV over 1 min	CI: 50–300 µg/kg/min with bolus between increases in dosage	Hypotension; short half-life (8 min); additive effects with Dig, CCB
Propranolol (Inderal)	0.5–1 mg IV over ≤ 1 mg/min, repeat after 2 min if needed (max 0.15 mg/kg)	PO: 10–120 mg TID	Caution with HF and asthma; additive effects with Dig, CCB
Metoprolol (Lopressor)	5 mg IV over 5 min every 5 min × 3 doses	PO: 25–100 mg BID	Caution with HF and asthma; additive effects with Dig, CCB
Verapamil* (Isoptin, Calan)	2.5–5 mg IV over 2 min; can double initial dose (administer over 2 min) 15–30 min after completion of initial dose if needed	CI: 5–10 mg/h; PO: 40–120 mg TID or 120–480 mg ER daily	Hypotension with IV; additive effects with BB, digoxin; may ↑ Dig level
Diltiazem* (Cardizem)	0.25 mg/kg IV over 2 min; may repeat with 0.35 mg/kg IV over 2 min if needed	CI: 5–15 mg/h; PO: 60–90 mg TID or QID or 180–360 mg ER daily	Hypotension with IV; additive effects with Dig, CCB; may ↑ Dig level
Adenosine (Adenocard)	6 mg rapid IV push followed with saline flush; may repeat with 12 mg x 2 at 2 min intervals	Not applicable	Patient may have chest tightness, breathlessness, transient/complete heart block

*Caution not to use calcium channel blockers and digoxin in rapid atrial fibrillation with Wolff-Parkinson-White syndrome.

BB—beta-blockers; BID—twice daily; CCB—calcium channel blockers; CI—continuous infusion; Dig—digoxin; ER—extended release; HF—heart failure; IV—intravenous; Max—maximum; PO—oral; QID—four times daily; TID—thrice daily.

ANTIARRHYTHMIC AGENTS: CLASS III

The class III antiarrhythmic drugs, **amiodarone, bretylium, dofetilide, ibutilide**, and **sotalol**, exert their antiarrhythmic effect by blocking K^+ channels and subsequently prolonging refractoriness in atrial and ventricular tissues.

There are ample data from electrophysiologic studies as well as clinical trials defining the therapeutic efficacy of the class III agents in treating supraventricular and ventricular arrhythmias. In the past decade, there has been a dramatic increase in the use of class III antiarrhythmics, with the use of **amiodarone**, in particular, increasing by 125% between 1995 and 2000. This surge in the use of **amiodarone** can partly be attributed to the trepidation associated with using class Ia and Ic antiarrhythmics, especially in patients with structural heart disease. Because **amiodarone** is one of two antiarrhythmics (**dofetilide** is the other) that has never been shown to increase mortality in patients with structural heart disease, it has clearly become the antiarrhythmic of choice in this particular population, which tends to be the majority of patients who present with cardiac arrhythmias.

EFFICACY AND USE

The major effect of **amiodarone** is to delay repolarization. The primary use of **amiodarone** in clinical practice is in the treatment of atrial fibrillation. Because the proportion of patients with atrial fibrillation who have concomitant structural heart disease appears to be increasing, the use of **amiodarone** for this particular arrhythmia has dramatically increased because of its safety profile in this particular patient population. Oral **amiodarone** may be used to restore and maintain sinus rhythm in patients with atrial fibrillation. It is also being increasingly used intravenously to convert atrial fibrillation to sinus rhythm, especially in postoperative patients. **Amiodarone** also appears to be effective in converting and preventing paroxysmal reentrant supraventricular tachycardias, and may also be used in Wolff-Parkinson-White syndrome. IV **amiodarone** may be used to terminate life-threatening ventricular arrhythmias. Based on the results of the Amiodarone in Out-of-Hospital Resuscitation of Refractory Sustained Ventricular Tachyarrhythmias (ARREST) and Amiodarone Versus Lidocaine in Prehospital Ventricular Fibrillation Evaluation (ALIVE) trials, IV **amiodarone** has replaced **lidocaine** as first-line therapy for the treatment of pulseless ventricular tachycardia/ventricular fibrillation in the most recently published Advanced Cardiac Life Support (ACLS) guidelines. In patients with ventricular arrhythmias, oral **amiodarone** may be used for those who refuse ICD therapy or as adjunctive therapy in patients with an ICD, to minimize the frequency of ICD discharges.

Bretylium has historically been used for the treatment of life-threatening ventricular tachycardia or ventricular fibrillation. Its use in clinical practice has become essentially negligible because it was deleted from the ventricular arrhythmia algorithms in the most recent ACLS guidelines. In addi-

tion to having only marginal efficacy for the treatment of ventricular arrhythmias, **bretylium** is also limited by its adverse-effect profile because it may cause severe hypotension. **Sotalol** has both beta-blocking (class II) and class III actions. Although **sotalol** is essentially devoid of noncardiac toxicities, torsades de pointes is a significant concern with the use of this drug. **Sotalol** is effective for the treatment of supraventricular and ventricular arrhythmias. Although sotalol is not effective for converting atrial fibrillation to sinus rhythm, it does appear to have fairly good efficacy in maintaining sinus rhythm in patients with this arrhythmia. **Sotalol** may also be used as adjunctive therapy in patients who experience frequent ICD discharges. **Dofetilide** is a pure class III oral agent that is approved only for the restoration and maintenance of sinus rhythm in patients with atrial fibrillation or atrial flutter. Because it is only available in IV form, **ibutilide** is approved for the acute termination of atrial fibrillation or atrial flutter.

All class III antiarrhythmic agents have the potential to induce arrhythmias. They can prolong the QT interval, which may predispose to the development of a form of polymorphic ventricular tachycardia known as torsades de pointes. Although **amiodarone** may markedly prolong the QT interval, torsades de pointes is a rare occurrence with this particular drug. Although there are many risk factors for this arrhythmia, electrolyte abnormalities such as hypokalemia, hypomagnesemia, and hypocalcemia, are among the most important. Electrolytes should be routinely monitored in patients on a class III antiarrhythmic (other than **amiodarone**), especially if they are concomitantly receiving diuretics.

CLINICAL SIGNIFICANCE

In clinical trials, **sotalol** has been associated with a 40% to 52% success rate in preventing the recurrence of atrial fibrillation after successful cardioversion. In patients with atrial fibrillation, **amiodarone** is associated with conversion rates ranging from 60% to 89%. **Amiodarone** is also very effective for maintaining these patients in sinus rhythm. Based on clinical trials, 60% to 89% of patients receiving low-dose **amiodarone** (200 mg/d) remained in sinus rhythm at 1 year. Specifically, in the most recent trials for preventing atrial fibrillation in post–coronary artery bypass graft (CABG) patients, IV and orally administered **amiodarone** have demonstrated efficacy while maintaining relatively minimal adverse effect profiles. **Ibutilide** and **dofetilide** also appear to be effective agents for conversion of atrial fibrillation to sinus rhythm. **Dofetilide** is also fairly effective for maintaining these patients in sinus rhythm, with an efficacy rate of approximately 50% being reported at 1 year.

Amiodarone and **sotalol** have been evaluated in numerous clinical trials for the treatment of ventricular arrhythmias. Neither of these drugs is associated with a significant reduction in mortality in this patient population. Given their impressive survival benefits in patients who are at high risk for or have a history of ventricular arrhythmias, ICDs have largely replaced antiarrhythmic agents as prophylactic therapy to prevent sudden cardiac death. However, **sotalol** and **amiodarone** may still have a role in patients with an ICD to prevent frequent discharges, which not only minimizes potential discomfort experienced by the patient but also prolongs the battery life of the device.

MODE OF ACTION

The precise mechanisms underlying the activity of the class III drugs are incompletely understood. Their principal effect on cardiac tissue is to delay repolarization by inhibiting K^+ efflux, which subsequently prolongs the action potential duration and the effective refractory period. **Amiodarone** is a unique member of this group of drugs because it possesses electrophysiologic properties of all four Vaughan Williams classes. Therefore, it also blocks Na^+ channels, beta-receptors (nonselectively), and calcium channels. However, **amiodarone**'s predominant effects are in blocking the rapid and slow components of the delayed rectifier K^+ current. Therefore, its effects on prolonging the action potential and refractory period are believed to be the basis of its activity.

Bretylium acutely produces an initial increase and then a decrease in norepinephrine release from sympathetic nerve endings. Such an indirect beta-blocking effect may contribute to its activity; however, **bretylium**, like **amiodarone**, directly prolongs the action potential duration and refractoriness of cardiac tissue.

In addition to its K^+ channel–blocking properties, **sotalol** also has nonselective beta-blocking effects. Like the other two representatives of this class, it prolongs the action potential duration and refractoriness.

In addition to blocking the rapid component of the delayed rectifier K^+ current, **ibutilide** also increases the slow inward Na^+ current. By these mechanisms, **ibutilide** also prolongs the action potential duration and the refractory period.

Dofetilide is considered to be a pure class III agent in that it only blocks K^+ channels and has no effect on Na^+, calcium, or adrenergic receptors. It specifically blocks the rapid component of the delayed rectifier K^+ current, which results in a prolonged action potential and refractory period.

INDICATIONS

	Amiodarone	Bretylium	Sotalol	Ibutilide	Dofetilide
Life-threatening ventricular arrhythmias	+	+	+	−	−
Ventricular fibrillation	+	+	−	−	−
Refractory ventricular arrhythmias	+	+	+	−	−
Supraventricular arrhythmias	(+)	−	+	+	+

+—FDA approved; −—not FDA approved; (+) clinical uses not FDA approved.

AMIODARONE HYDROCHLORIDE
(Pacerone, Cordarone®)

Amiodarone is a unique drug in that it possesses the electrophysiologic characteristics of all four classes of antiarrhythmic agents. Although amiodarone is primarily a K^+ channel blocker (blocks the rapid and slow component of the delayed rectifier K^+ current), it also blocks Na^+ channels, has nonselective beta-blocking activity, and has weak calcium channel–blocking properties. As a result, amiodarone reduces automaticity and conduction velocity and prolongs refractoriness in all cardiac tissues. When administered intravenously, amiodarone's beta-blocking and calcium channel–blocking activities are more predominant. Amiodarone has minimal to no negative inotropic effects, which makes it one of the few antiarrhythmic drugs that can be safely used in patients with left ventricular dysfunction. It also causes coronary and peripheral vasodilation, and therefore decreases peripheral vascular resistance; however, hypotension usually only occurs with IV administration or with large oral doses. Amiodarone prolongs the PR and QT intervals and widens the QRS complex.

Amiodarone is used to treat both supraventricular and ventricular arrhythmias. Since the proportion of patients with atrial fibrillation who have concomitant structural heart disease appears to be increasing, the use of amiodarone for this particular arrhythmia has significantly increased, because this is one of the few antiarrhythmics that have been proven to be safe in this patient population. Amiodarone is often used intravenously to acutely terminate atrial fibrillation or life-threatening ventricular arrhythmias, such as ventricular tachycardia or ventricular fibrillation. Based on data from the ARREST and ALIVE trials, IV amiodarone has replaced lidocaine as first-line therapy for the treatment of pulseless ventricular tachycardia and ventricular fibrillation. Even though ICDs now play a primary role in the chronic management of ventricular arrhythmias, amiodarone is still used in patients who refuse or are not candidates for these devices and in those who experience frequent ICD discharges.

The general usefulness of amiodarone is limited by its extensive adverse-effect profile. Because of its extremely large volume of distribution and high lipophilicity, amiodarone has the potential to accumulate and cause adverse effects in numerous organs, with the lungs, thyroid, eyes, heart, liver, skin, gastrointestinal tract, and central nervous system being most notably affected. All patients should be routinely monitored for signs and symptoms of pulmonary toxicity and ocular complications as well as for thyroid (amiodarone has a significant iodine moiety) and liver disorders. Patients may also develop photosensitivity and skin discoloration. Because of amiodarone's poor bioavailability, large volume of distribution, and long half-life, its onset of action may not be apparent for several months. Therefore, to achieve efficacy more quickly, loading doses of amiodarone must be initially used to saturate the myocardial stores. Once the patient is appropriately loaded with amiodarone, the dose should be reduced to the recommended maintenance dose to minimize the incidence of adverse events. It is important to realize that amiodarone loading may require several weeks and that its effects persist for weeks and even months after its withdrawal.

IN BRIEF

INDICATIONS
Life-threatening ventricular arrhythmias
Supraventricular arrhythmias (unlabeled use)

CONTRAINDICATIONS
Hypersensitivity to amiodarone
Severe sinus node dysfunction
Second- or third-degree heart block in the absence of a pacemaker
Long QT syndrome

DRUG INTERACTIONS
Anesthetics (inhalation)[3]
Disopyramide[1,3]
Cimetidine[1]
Cyclosporine[3]
Phenytoin[2,3]
Quinidine[3]
Fentanyl[1,3]
Beta-blockers[3]
Lidocaine[3]
Procainamide[3]
Calcium channel blockers (ie, verapamil, diltiazem)[3]
Ritonavir[1]
Theophylline[3]
Flecainide[3]
Cholestyramine[2]
Digoxin[3]
Warfarin[3]
Hydroxymethylglutaryl coenzyme A reductase inhibitors (metabolized by CYP3A4 isoenzyme) (ie, simvastatin, atorvastatin, lovastatin)[3]

1 Effect/toxicity of amiodarone may increase.
2 Effect of amiodarone may decrease.
3 Amiodarone may increase the effect/toxicity of this drug.

ADVERSE EFFECTS
The side-effect profile is quite extensive and involves virtually every organ system. Adverse effects become more prevalent with increasing doses and duration of therapy. With a dosage of 400 mg or more daily, adverse reactions occur in 75% of patients taking amiodarone, and 5%–20% require discontinuation of therapy.
Pulmonary: most severe and potentially fatal adverse reaction associated with amiodarone. The two forms of amiodarone-induced pulmonary toxicity are interstitial pneumonitis (or alveolitis) (more common, later onset, dose dependent) and hypersensitivity pneumonitis (allergic reaction, occurs within first 2 mo of therapy; develops in up to 17% of patients). Fatality has been reported in up to 10% of cases. Worsening of asthma may also occur.
Hepatic: elevation of liver function tests (may occur in up to 25% of patients); clinical hepatitis rarely occurs
CV: hypotension (with IV) (16%), bradycardia (1%–5%), AV block; proarrhythmia is rare (<1%)
CNS: malaise, fatigue, ataxia, tremor, insomnia, headache, peripheral neuropathy
Thyroid: hyperthyroidism (2%), hypothyroidism (2%–4%)
GI: nausea/vomiting (10%–33%, usually occurs during the oral loading phase), anorexia, constipation, abdominal pain
Ocular: asymptomatic corneal microdeposits, optic neuropathy, or optic neuritis
Skin: photosensitivity (10%), blue-gray skin discoloration (2%–5%; associated with long-term therapy), phlebitis (associated with IV use)

AMIODARONE HYDROCHLORIDE (continued)

SPECIAL GROUPS

Race: no differences in response

Children: safety and effectiveness have not been established; limited data suggest that amiodarone may be useful in the management of refractory supraventricular or ventricular arrhythmias in selected cases

Elderly: no dosage adjustment needed

Renal impairment: no dosage adjustment needed

Hepatic impairment: use usual dose with caution; elevation of hepatic enzymes (aspartate aminotransferase, alanine aminotransferase, alkaline phosphatase, bilirubin), as well as cases of hepatic injury (resembling alcoholic hepatitis or cirrhosis), have been reported. Therefore, regular monitoring of liver enzymes is recommended.

Pregnancy: category D; amiodarone has shown embryotoxicity with fetal resorption, and growth retardation. Amiodarone and its metabolite cross the placenta. QT prolongation and transient sinus bradycardia have been reported in neonates in limited cases of pregnant women receiving amiodarone in their second or third trimester of pregnancy.

Breast-feeding: not recommended; amiodarone and its metabolite N-desethylamiodarone are distributed in breast milk in concentrations higher than concurrent maternal plasma level

PHARMACOKINETICS AND PHARMACODYNAMICS

Duration of action: weeks to months
Onset of action: variable (several days to months)
Peak effect: variable, 3–7 h
Bioavailability: 22%–86%
Effect of food: not known
Protein binding: 96%
Volume of distribution: 66 L/kg (range 18–148 L/kg)
Metabolism: extensive hepatic metabolism; at least one active metabolite (N-desethylamiodarone); metabolized via CYP3A4 isoenzyme
Elimination: biliary, may undergo enterohepatic recirculation; no renal excretion occurs; not dialyzable
Half-life: 25–110 d (varies with duration of therapy)

MONITORING

ECG and vital signs daily during initiation period, and then every 3–6 mo while on maintenance dose. Liver and thyroid function tests should be performed every 6 mo. Chest radiograph and ophthalmologic exam should be performed annually. Pulmonary function tests may be performed if patient develops symptoms. All of these tests should also be performed at baseline.

OVERDOSE

For recent ingestion, use emesis or lavage. Administer beta-adrenergic agonists or cardiac pacing for atropine-resistant sinus bradycardia. Positive inotropic agents or vasopressors may be used for hypotension. Hemodialysis is not effective.

PATIENT INFORMATION

Take with food. Patients should be warned about skin discoloration and photosensitivity, and to report any shortness of breath, tiredness, abdominal discomfort, or visual abnormality. Follow up with regular visits to physician's office. Do not discontinue therapy without physician's advice.

AVAILABILITY

Tablets—200 mg
Injection for IV infusion—50 mg/mL

DOSAGE

Atrial fibrillation:

IV: 5–7 mg/kg over 30–60 min, then 1200–1800 mg/d given via continuous infusion; convert to oral therapy when hemodynamically stable and able to take oral medications

Oral: 800–1200 mg/d in 2–3 divided doses for 1 wk until patient receives ~ 10 g total, then 200 mg po daily

Pulseless ventricular tachycardia/ventricular fibrillation:

IV: 300 mg IV push (can be diluted in or followed by 10–20 mL saline); may repeat with 150 mg IV push every 3–5 min if necessary (can be diluted in or followed by 10–20 mL saline); if stable rhythm achieved, can initiate continuous infusion at 1 mg/min for 6 h, then 0.5 mg/min (maximum dose is 2.2 g/24 h); convert to oral therapy when hemodynamically stable and able to take oral medications (see dose under "Stable ventricular tachycardia")

Stable ventricular tachycardia:

IV: 150 mg (diluted in 100 mL of 5% dextrose in water or saline) over 10 min; may repeat dose every 10 min if necessary for breakthrough ventricular tachycardia; if stable rhythm achieved, can initiate continuous infusion at 1 mg/min for 6 h, then 0.5 mg/min (maximum dose is 2.2 g/24 h); convert patient to oral therapy when hemodynamically stable and able to take oral medications

Oral: 800–1600 mg/d in 2–3 divided doses for 1 wk until patient receives ~ 15 g total, then 300–400 mg po daily.

IV amiodarone concentration should not exceed 2 mg/mL unless a central venous catheter is used.

BRETYLIUM TOSYLATE
(Bretylium tosylate, Bretylol®)

NOTE: THIS DRUG HAS BEEN DISCONTINUED BY THE MANUFACTURER AS OF AUGUST 2004. Bretylium has historically been used for the acute treatment of life-threatening ventricular tachyarrhythmias and ventricular fibrillation. However, an overall lack of data to support the efficacy of bretylium in this setting contributed to its deletion from the most recently published ACLS guidelines. Bretylium's electrophysiologic effects are thought to occur at the sympathetic nerve terminals. Bretylium accumulates in the sympathetic ganglionic and postganglionic nerve endings and causes an initial release of norepinephrine. Depletion of norepinephrine stores subsequently occurs, and bretylium blocks further reuptake of catecholamines at these nerve endings. Bretylium causes an initial increase in BP, heart rate, and myocardial contractility, which is likely a result of the initial catecholamine release. However, hypotension, which may be severe, eventually results because of the neuronal blockade (sympatholytic effect).

SPECIAL GROUPS

Race: no differences in response
Children: safety and effectiveness have not been established
Elderly: dosage adjustment may be required based on renal function
Renal impairment: dosage adjustment is required
Hepatic impairment: no dosage adjustment needed
Pregnancy: category C; there is a potential risk for reduced uterine blood flow with fetal hypoxia and bradycardia
Breast-feeding: not recommended; unknown if excreted into breast milk

DOSAGE

Hemodynamically unstable ventricular tachycardia and ventricular fibrillation: 5 mg/kg IV over 1 min; if arrhythmia persists, give 10 mg/kg IV over 1 min and repeat if necessary every 15–30 min. Maximum total dose is 30–35 mg/kg. Once arrhythmia is suppressed, initiate maintenance infusion at 1–2 mg/min.

IN BRIEF

INDICATIONS
Life-threatening ventricular arrhythmias

CONTRAINDICATIONS/WARNINGS
Suspected digitalis-induced ventricular tachycardia (may increase the rate of ventricular tachycardia or induce ventricular fibrillation)
Hypersensitivity to bretylium
Use with caution in aortic stenosis or pulmonary hypertension

DRUG INTERACTIONS
Digitalis[2]
Sympathomimetics (eg, dopamine, epinephrine, norepinephrine)[2]
Other antiarrhythmics, such as procainamide, quinidine, lidocaine[1,2]
1 Effect/toxicity of bretylium may increase.
2 Bretylium may increase the effect/toxicity of this drug.

ADVERSE EFFECTS
CV: hypotension (usually orthostatic and supine; occurs in up to 50% of patients), transient hypertension, ventricular arrhythmias, bradycardia, angina
GI: nausea, vomiting (projectile)

PHARMACOKINETICS AND PHARMACODYNAMICS
Duration of action: 6–24 h
Onset of action: 5–10 min
Peak effect: 6–9 h
Bioavailability: not applicable
Effect of food: not applicable
Protein binding: 1%–6%
Volume of distribution: 6 L/kg
Metabolism: none
Elimination: renal, 77% excreted in the urine as unchanged drug; poorly dialyzable
Half-life: 7–11 h; 16–32 h in patients with renal impairment

MONITORING
Constant ECG monitoring and vital signs.

OVERDOSE
Hypotension usually responds to Trendelenburg positioning and volume expansion with IV fluid or plasma. Dopamine or norepinephrine may also be indicated.

PATIENT INFORMATION
Not applicable.

AVAILABILITY
Injection—50 mg/mL (10 mL, 20 mL)
IV infusion—
 1 mg/mL in 5% dextrose (500 mL)
 2 mg/mL in 5% dextrose (250 mL)
 4 mg/mL in 5% dextrose (250 mL, 500 mL)

DOFETILIDE (Tikosyn®)

Dofetilide is a pure class III agent devoid of properties associated with the class I, II, or IV antiarrhythmics. Dofetilide selectively blocks the rapid component of cardiac delayed rectifier K+ current (IKr) and subsequently prolongs atrial and ventricular refractoriness. However, dofetilide primarily affects the atrial rather than the ventricular tissue. Dofetilide exhibits reverse-use dependence, whereby its action potential–prolonging effects are lessened at higher heart rates and increased at lower heart rates. One of the primary concerns associated with the use of dofetilide is torsades de pointes, which appears to be a dose-dependent effect.

Unlike other antiarrhythmics, dofetilide does not possess negative inotropic properties. Therefore, like amiodarone, dofetilide also appears to be safe to use in patients with atrial fibrillation or flutter and concomitant left ventricular systolic dysfunction.

Dofetilide is approved for the conversion of atrial fibrillation or atrial flutter to sinus rhythm and for the maintenance of sinus rhythm in patients with atrial fibrillation or atrial flutter of greater than 1 week in duration who have been converted to sinus rhythm. In the Symptomatic Atrial Fibrillation Investigative Research on Dofetilide (SAFIRE-D) trial, approximately 50% of the patients receiving dofetilide 500 µg twice daily remained in sinus rhythm.

Unlike other antiarrhythmics, dofetilide has extensive requirements for use that have been specified by the FDA and manufacturer. In order to initiate dofetilide therapy, patients must be hospitalized for a minimum of 3 days in a facility where CrCl can be calculated, heart rhythm can be continuously monitored, and emergency cardiac care can be provided. Dofetilide can only be used by prescribers and institutions that have received the necessary education regarding this antiarrhythmic's dosing, monitoring, and potential drug interactions.

SPECIAL GROUPS

Race: no differences in response
Children: safety and effectiveness have not been established
Elderly: dosage adjustment may be required based on renal function
Renal impairment: dosage adjustment is required
Hepatic impairment: no dosage adjustment needed
Pregnancy: category C; use only if potential benefit justifies the potential risk to the fetus
Breast-feeding: not recommended; unknown if excreted into breast milk

IN BRIEF

INDICATIONS
Restoration and maintenance of sinus rhythm in patients with atrial fibrillation/flutter

CONTRAINDICATIONS
Hypersensitivity to dofetilide
CrCl <20 mL/min
Baseline QTc >440 ms (>500 ms in patients with ventricular conduction abnormalities)
Electrolyte abnormalities (eg, hypokalemia, hypomagnesemia)
Concurrent use of verapamil, ketoconazole, cimetidine, trimethoprim/sulfamethoxazole, prochlorperazine, hydrochlorothiazide/triamterene, or megestrol

DRUG INTERACTIONS
Cimetidine[1]
Ketoconazole[1]
Trimethoprim/sulfamethoxazole[1]
Prochlorperazine[1]
Hydrochlorothiazide/triamterene[1]
Megestrol[1]
Verapamil[1]
Macrolides[1]
Metformin[1]
Fluconazole[1]
Itraconazole[1]
Protease inhibitors[1]
Diltiazem[1]
Nefazodone[1]
Zafirlukast[1]
Phenothiazines[1]
Fluoroquinolones[1]
TCAs[1]
Class Ia and III antiarrhythmics[1]
1 Effect/toxicity of dofetilide may increase.

ADVERSE EFFECTS
CNS: headache, fatigue, dizziness, insomnia
CV: torsades de pointes (4%–8%), chest pain
GI: nausea, diarrhea
Respiratory: dyspnea, respiratory tract infection

PHARMACOKINETICS AND PHARMACODYNAMICS
Duration of action: 4 h
Onset of action: 2 h
Peak concentration: 2.5 h
Bioavailability: 96%
Effect of food: delays absorption
Protein binding: 60%–70%
Volume of distribution: 3 L/kg
Metabolism: hepatic (20%)
Elimination: renal; 80% excreted in urine as unchanged drug
Half-life: 8–10 h; prolonged in patients with renal impairment

MONITORING
ECG after each dose and renal function daily during the initiation period, and then every 3–6 mo while on maintenance dose; electrolytes (K+, Mg++).

OVERDOSE
For recent ingestion, use emesis or lavage.
To manage torsades de pointes, give magnesium sulfate 1–2 g IV push, then a continuous infusion of 8–16 g over 24 h. Direct-current cardioversion should be used if hemodynamically unstable. Replenish potassium if needed. Overdrive pacing, isoproterenol, phenytoin, and lidocaine may also be used to manage torsades de pointes.

DOFETILIDE (continued)

DOSAGE

Initiate at 500 µg po twice daily (if CrCl >60 mL/min)
Dosage adjustment required in patients with renal insufficiency (CrCl ≤60 mL/min):

CrCl, mL/min	Maintenance Dose
40–60	250 µg po twice daily
20–39	125 µg po twice daily
<20	Contraindicated

The QTc interval should be monitored 2–3 h after each dose when initiating dofetilide therapy in the hospital. If the increase in the QTc interval is < 15% of baseline, the current dose may be continued. If the increase in the QTc interval is > 15% of baseline or exceeds 500 ms (550 ms in patients with ventricular conduction abnormalities) after the first dose, the dose should be reduced by 50%. If the QTc interval exceeds 500 ms (550 ms in patients with ventricular conduction abnormalities) at any time after the first dosage adjustment, dofetilide should be discontinued.

PATIENT INFORMATION
Report symptoms of fatigue, headache, and rapid heart rate to your physician.

AVAILABILITY
Capsules—120 µg, 250 µg, 500 µg

IBUTILIDE FUMARATE (Corvert®)

Ibutilide is unique among the class III antiarrhythmics in that it prolongs the action potential by increasing the slow inward Na^+ current and by blocking the rapid component of the delayed rectifier K^+ current. Electrophysiologic studies have demonstrated that ibutilide increases atrial and ventricular effective refractory periods. Ibutilide prolongs the QT interval but has little effect on the PR and QRS intervals. Ibutilide has negligible effects on heart rate, cardiac contractility, and BP.

Ibutilide is an IV drug that is only indicated for the acute termination of atrial fibrillation or atrial flutter. In clinical trials, ibutilide restores sinus rhythm in approximately 50% of patients with these arrhythmias. However, ibutilide is more effective for restoring sinus rhythm in patients with atrial flutter than in those with atrial fibrillation. Ibutilide also appears to be effective for facilitating direct-current cardioversion of atrial fibrillation. The most important adverse effect associated with ibutilide is torsades de pointes, which is more likely to occur in the presence of left ventricular systolic dysfunction or electrolyte abnormalities.

SPECIAL GROUPS

Race: no differences in response
Children: safety and effectiveness have not been established
Elderly: no dosage adjustment needed
Renal impairment: no dosage adjustment needed
Hepatic impairment: no data; dosage adjustment is probably not required
Pregnancy: category C; use only if potential benefit justifies the potential risk to the fetus
Breast-feeding: not recommended; unknown if excreted into breast milk

DOSAGE

≥60 kg: 1 mg IV push over 10 min
<60 kg: 0.01 mg/kg IV push over 10 min
Can give a second dose 10 min after completion of the first infusion if atrial fibrillation or flutter does not terminate.

IN BRIEF

INDICATIONS
Acute termination of recent-onset atrial fibrillation/atrial flutter

CONTRAINDICATIONS
History of polymorphic ventricular tachycardia
Hypersensitivity to ibutilide
Long QT syndrome
Electrolyte abnormalities (eg, hypokalemia, hypomagnesemia)
Concurrent use of other drugs that prolong the QT interval

DRUG INTERACTIONS
Class Ia and III antiarrhythmic agents[1,2]
Phenothiazines[1]
TCAs[1]
Macrolides[1]
Fluoroquinolones[1]

1 Effect/toxicity of ibutilide may increase.
2 Ibutilide may increase the effect/toxicity of this drug.

ADVERSE EFFECTS
CNS: headache
CV: hypotension, torsades de pointes, AV block
GI: nausea

PHARMACOKINETICS AND PHARMACODYNAMICS
Duration of action: Unknown
Onset of action: 20–30 min
Peak effect: ~ 40 min post injection
Bioavailability: not applicable
Effect of food: not applicable
Protein binding: 40%
Volume of distribution: 7–15 L/kg
Metabolism: extensively metabolized in liver
Elimination: renal; both parent drug and metabolites are excreted primarily in the urine; 5%–7% as unchanged drug
Half-life: 6 h (range 2–12 h)

MONITORING
Continuous ECG monitoring up to 4 h after the injection(s) or until the QTc interval has returned to baseline. ECG monitoring for more than 4 h post injection is required in patients with hepatic dysfunction; electrolytes (K^+, Mg^{++}).

OVERDOSE
Treatment is symptomatic and supportive. To manage torsades de pointes, give magnesium sulfate 1–2 g IV push, then a continuous infusion of 8–16 g over 24 h. Direct-current cardioversion should be used if hemodynamically unstable. Replenish potassium if needed. Overdrive pacing, isoproterenol, phenytoin, and lidocaine may also be used to manage torsades de pointes.

PATIENT INFORMATION
Inform about the risks of arrhythmias.

AVAILABILITY
Injection—0.1 mg/mL

SOTALOL HYDROCHLORIDE
(Sotalol, Betapace®, Sorine®, Betapace AF®)

Sotalol is a racemic mixture of two optical isomers, d and l. Both isomers have class III antiarrhythmic effects; however, only the l-isomer has nonselective beta-blocking properties. Sotalol does not have intrinsic sympathomimetic properties. Sotalol selectively inhibits the rapid component of the delayed rectifier K^+ current. Sotalol increases the atrial and ventricular refractory periods and prolongs AV nodal conduction without affecting the atrial, His-Purkinje, or ventricular conduction velocity. Thus, sotalol primarily prolongs the QT interval. One of the primary concerns associated with the use of sotalol is torsades de pointes, which appears to be a dose-dependent effect. Sotalol is effective for the treatment of supraventricular and ventricular arrhythmias. Although sotalol is not effective for conversion of atrial fibrillation, it is an effective agent for maintaining sinus rhythm.

SPECIAL GROUPS

Race: no differences in response
Children: safety and efficacy have not been established in children <18 years of age.
Elderly: dosage adjustment may be required based on renal function
Renal impairment: dosage adjustment is required
Hepatic impairment: no dosage adjustment needed
Pregnancy: category B; crosses placenta; therefore, use of sotalol in pregnant women requires that the benefit clearly outweigh the risk
Breast-feeding: not recommended; excretion in breast milk is 2.5–5.5 times the maternal serum drug concentration

DOSAGE

Atrial fibrillation (Betapace AF):
Initiate at 80 mg po twice daily; increase at 3 d intervals to a maximum dose of 160 mg po twice daily, if necessary
Dosing interval must be adjusted in patients with renal insufficiency:

CrCl, mL/min	Dosing Interval
40–60	Every 24 h
<40	Contraindicated

Life-threatening ventricular arrhythmias (Sotalol, Betapace, Sorine):
Initiate at 80 mg po twice daily; increase at 2–3 d intervals to a maximum dose of 320 mg po twice daily if necessary; higher doses (480–640 mg/d) should be reserved for patients with drug-refractory ventricular arrhythmias
Dosing interval must be adjusted in patients with renal insufficiency:

CrCl, mL/min	Dosing Interval
30–60	Every 24 h
10–29	Every 36–48 h
<10	Individualize dose

IN BRIEF

INDICATIONS
Maintenance of sinus rhythm in patients with atrial fibrillation/flutter (Betapace AF)
Life-threatening ventricular arrhythmias (Sotalol, Betapace, Sorine)

CONTRAINDICATIONS
Hypersensitivity to sotalol
History of polymorphic ventricular tachycardia
Severe sinus node dysfunction
Concurrent use of other drugs that prolong the QT interval
Asthma
Sinus bradycardia
Second- and third-degree heart block in the absence of a pacemaker
Long QT syndrome
Cardiogenic shock
Uncontrolled CHF

DRUG INTERACTIONS
Class Ia and III antiarrhythmic agents[1,2]
Phenothiazines[1]
TCAs[1]
Macrolides[1]
Fluoroquinolones[1]
Beta-blockers[1,2]

1 Effect/toxicity of sotalol may increase.
2 Sotalol may increase the effect/toxicity of this drug.

ADVERSE EFFECTS
CNS: fatigue, dizziness, lightheadedness, weakness
CV: torsades de pointes (1%–4%), heart failure exacerbation, bradycardia, chest pain, palpitations
GI: nausea, vomiting, diarrhea, dyspepsia
Respiratory: dyspnea, bronchospasm

PHARMACOKINETICS AND PHARMACODYNAMICS
Duration of action: 12–18 h
Onset of action: 1–3 h
Peak effect: 2.5–4 h
Bioavailability: 90%–100%
Effect of food: reduces absorption up to 30%
Protein binding: none
Volume of distribution: 1.2–2.4 L/kg
Metabolism: not metabolized
Elimination: renal; 80%–90% excreted in urine as unchanged drug; hemodialyzable
Half-life: 12 h; 18–29 h in moderate renal insufficiency; 37–91 h in severe renal insufficiency

MONITORING
ECG, heart rate, renal function, electrolytes (K^+, Mg^{++}).

OVERDOSE
Gastric lavage if recent ingestion. Supportive therapy. To manage torsades de pointes, give magnesium sulfate 1–2 g IV push, then a continuous infusion of 8–16 g over 24 h. Direct-current cardioversion should be used if hemodynamically unstable. Replenish K^+ if needed. Overdrive pacing, isoproterenol, phenytoin, and lidocaine may also be used to manage torsades de pointes.

PATIENT INFORMATION
To be initiated in the hospital. Side effects may include bradycardia, palpitations, fatigue, dizziness, and shortness of breath. Do not discontinue therapy without your physician's advice.

AVAILABILITY
Tablets (Sotalol, Betapace, Sorine)—80 mg, 120 mg, 160 mg, 240 mg
Tablets (Betapace AF)—80 mg, 120 mg, 160 mg

ANTIARRHYTHMIC AGENTS: CLASS IV

Class IV antiarrhythmic drugs interfere with entry of calcium ions through the slow calcium channel. The nondihydropyridine calcium channel blockers, **verapamil** and **diltiazem**, belong in this class of drugs. The dihydropyridine calcium channel blockers (*eg*, **nifedipine**, **amlodipine**) have no significant antiarrhythmic activity. **Verapamil** and **diltiazem** are profiled in the chapter on calcium antagonists.

EFFICACY AND USE

Calcium antagonists are primarily useful for the treatment of supraventricular arrhythmias (Table 5.3). Because of their effect on conduction through the AV node, they can effectively blunt the ventricular response during atrial fibrillation and are useful in the chronic prevention of paroxysmal supraventricular reentrant tachycardia; however, they are not effective for converting atrial fibrillation to sinus rhythm. In addition, chronic oral use of these agents for the prevention of reentrant supraventricular tachycardias is becoming less prominent as catheter ablative procedures are being performed more frequently.

Digoxin may control the ventricular response to atrial fibrillation at rest, but marked increases in ventricular responsiveness may be seen during exercise, which can limit the exercise capacity of such patients. Exercise-induced tachycardia in patients with atrial fibrillation can be markedly attenuated by the addition of **verapamil** or **diltiazem** in patients receiving **digoxin**.

Paroxysmal supraventricular tachyarrhythmias, which have a reentrant mechanism involving the AV node, can usually be terminated within 1–2 minutes after administration of IV **verapamil** or **diltiazem**. These agents alter the conduction and refractoriness of the AV node and can terminate these reentrant rhythms by interrupting the circuit. The efficacy of **verapamil** and **diltiazem** in this type of arrhythmia is extremely high, with over 80% of such episodes converting to sinus rhythm within minutes. **Verapamil** and **diltiazem** are generally considered second-line alternatives to **adenosine** for the treatment of paroxysmal supraventricular tachyarrhythmias.

Both of these drugs are negative inotropes; however, **verapamil** has more potent negative inotropic effects than **diltiazem**. Nevertheless, use of these agents should be generally avoided in patients with left ventricular systolic dysfunction. Hypotension, bradycardia, and heart block are also important concerns with these agents, and extreme caution should be exercised when attempting to combine them with other negative inotropic and/or chronotropic agents, such as beta-blockers. Constipation is a side effect that limits the use of **verapamil** in some individuals, especially in the elderly population. For information on the use of individual calcium antagonists in the treatment of arrhythmias, see the chapter on calcium antagonists.

In patients with sick sinus syndrome, great caution must be exercised with the use of these agents because of a possibility of prolonged asystole. Nondihydropyridine calcium channel blockers are contraindicated in patients with Wolff-Parkinson-White syndrome because of a potential preferential enhancement of conduction through the bypass tract. Also, these agents are not indicated for the treatment of wide-complex tachycardias unless the clinician is certain that a supraventricular tachycardia without anterograde accessory pathway conduction is present. One exception to this rule is a rare form of ventricular tachycardia that is usually seen in young, healthy individuals and is typically sensitive to **verapamil**.

MODE OF ACTION

Unlike class I antiarrhythmic drugs, whose predominant actions are on the fast Na^+ channel, the calcium antagonists depress SA automaticity and AV nodal depolarization predominantly by their effect on the slow inward calcium current. Blockade of this calcium channel slows the conduction and prolongs the refractoriness within the sinus and AV nodes. These pharmacologic effects result in slowing of the sinus discharge rate, prolongation of the PR interval, and a reduction of ventricular responsiveness to atrial arrhythmias. Calcium antagonists may also terminate arrhythmias that involve the AV node. They have little effect on the His-Purkinje system or the ventricular myocardium.

ANTIARRHYTHMIC AGENTS: OTHER

ADENOSINE

Adenosine is a parenteral agent used for converting paroxysmal supraventricular tachyarrhythmias to sinus rhythm.

ATROPINE

Atropine is used for the parenteral management of symptomatic sinus bradycardia.

CARDIAC GLYCOSIDES (DIGOXIN)

Cardiac glycosides have been in clinical use for more than 200 years. Their value in the management of heart failure has been questioned and reestablished, and they continue to have a role in the treatment of various supraventricular arrhythmias.

Efficacy and Use

Digoxin is commonly used to slow conduction through the AV node, thus slowing the ventricular rate in supraventricular arrhythmias such as atrial fibrillation or atrial flutter (Table 5.3). Digoxin is not effective for converting atrial fibrillation or atrial flutter to sinus rhythm. In patients with left ventricular dysfunction and concomitant atrial fibrillation or atrial flutter, digoxin can provide effective heart rate control without increasing the risk for worsening heart failure symptoms because of its additional positive inotropic effects. The use of digoxin in patients with atrial fibrillation or atrial flutter tends to be limited by its relatively slow onset of action and its inability to control heart rate during exercise and even during normal daily activities. The increased sympathetic tone that is generated during exercise tends to offset the vagal effects of digoxin, which limits its efficacy under these conditions. It is often useful to combine digoxin with a beta-blocker or with a nondihydropyridine calcium channel blocker to provide synergistic control of the ventricular rate. Digoxin may also be used for the treatment and prevention of recurrent episodes of paroxysmal supraventricular tachycardia involving the AV node.

Digoxin should not be used for the treatment of supraventricular tachycardia associated with Wolff-Parkinson-White syndrome because it may enhance the conduction of the accessory pathway and subsequently produce rapid ventricular rates and even ventricular fibrillation.

For information on the use of digitalis preparations in the treatment of arrhythmias, see the chapter on inotropic and vasopressor agents.

Mode of Action

Cardiac glycosides affect the autonomic nervous system by stimulating the parasympathetic division, which increases vagal tone. This vagal effect slows conduction through the AV node and prolongs the AV nodal refractory period. With normal doses, conduction velocity and refractoriness of the His-Purkinje system are not directly affected. Cardiac glycosides shorten the effective refractory period of the atria and decrease conduction velocity by a reflex increase in vagal tone and a direct effect on the atria. With therapeutic doses, prolongation of the PR interval, shortening of the QT interval, and ST segment depression occur.

The therapeutic/toxic window with regard to digoxin's antiarrhythmic actions/electrophysiologic effects is relatively narrow, and digoxin may cause a large variety of atrial, junctional, or ventricular tachyarrhythmias and SA and AV nodal conduction abnormalities, some of which may be life threatening. The tachyarrhythmias are apparently related to a mechanism of so-called triggered arrhythmias caused by after-depolarizations. Arrhythmias are more common in the setting of hypokalemia, hypomagnesemia, or hypercalcemia. Digoxin antibodies may be used to reverse the effects of severe digoxin toxicity.

ADENOSINE (Adenocard®)

Adenosine is an endogenous nucleoside found in all cells of the body. When administered as an IV bolus, it slows conduction through the AV node. Adenosine can interrupt a reentrant pathway involving the AV node and restore sinus rhythm in patients with paroxysmal supraventricular tachycardia, including that associated with the Wolff-Parkinson-White syndrome. A comparative study of patients with narrow-complex tachycardia found that the efficacy of adenosine was 100%, whereas that of verapamil was 73%. Because of its extremely short half-life (<10 sec), it can be given safely to patients with wide-complex tachycardias, poor left ventricular function, or severe hypotension, and those receiving concomitant beta-blockade. It may also be used as an aid in the diagnosis of broad- or narrow-complex supraventricular tachycardias; however, adenosine may cause AV block and is not beneficial in terminating atrial fibrillation/flutter or ventricular arrhythmias. Its short half-life means that most side effects are transient.

SPECIAL GROUPS

Race: no differences in response
Children: safety and effectiveness have not been established; however, studies performed to date have not demonstrated pediatric-specific problems
Elderly: no dosage adjustment needed
Renal impairment: no dosage adjustment needed
Hepatic impairment: no dosage adjustment needed
Pregnancy: category C; use only if potential benefit justifies the potential risk to the fetus
Breast-feeding: drug unlikely to be excreted in breast milk because of its short half-life

DOSAGE

Initiate at 6 mg IV push over 1–2 sec; repeat with 12 mg IV push if sinus rhythm not obtained within 1–2 min after first dose; may repeat 12 mg dose a second time if no response in 1–2 min.
Each dose should be immediately followed by a 10 mL saline flush.
Patients receiving dipyridamole concurrently: 1 mg IV push has been reported as effective.

IN BRIEF

INDICATIONS
Paroxysmal supraventricular tachyarrhythmias, including those associated with Wolff-Parkinson-White syndrome
Aid in diagnosis of wide-complex tachycardia suspected to be of supraventricular origin

CONTRAINDICATIONS/WARNINGS
Second- or third-degree heart block or sick sinus syndrome in the absence of a pacemaker
Hypersensitivity to adenosine
Use with caution in patients with asthma.

DRUG INTERACTIONS
Dipyridamole[1]
Theophylline[2]
Caffeine[2]
Carbamazepine[1]
1 Effect/toxicity of adenosine may increase.
2 Effect of adenosine may decrease.

ADVERSE EFFECTS
CNS: headache, dizziness, apprehension
CV: transient postconversion arrhythmias (AV block, PVCs, sinus bradycardia, atrial fibrillation) or asystole, chest pain, palpitations
GI: nausea
Lungs: dyspnea, bronchospasm with asthmatic patients
Skin: flushing

PHARMACOKINETICS AND PHARMACODYNAMICS
Duration of action: 10–20 sec
Onset of action: approximately 8–10 sec
Bioavailability: not applicable
Effect of food: not applicable
Protein binding: not applicable
Volume of distribution: unknown
Metabolism: blood; rapidly metabolized into two clinically inactive metabolites (inosine and adenosine monophosphate)
Elimination: renally, as inactive metabolites
Half-life: 1–10 sec

MONITORING
ECG and vital signs post administration for signs of AV block, asystole, and bronchospasm.

OVERDOSE
No case report. Not likely to be clinically relevant because of its short half-life.

PATIENT INFORMATION
Not applicable.

AVAILABILITY
Injection—3 mg/mL (2 and 5 mL vials)

ATROPINE SULFATE (Atropine)

Atropine is a parasympatholytic drug that blocks the effects of acetylcholine on the SA and AV nodes. Consequently, through this direct vagolytic action, atropine enhances both SA and AV nodal conduction velocity. It also shortens the effective refractory period of the AV node. This agent is primarily used to increase the heart rate in patients with symptomatic bradyarrhythmias. Atropine has been reported to be harmful in some patients with AV block at the His-Purkinje level (type II AV block and third-degree AV block with a new wide QRS complex). While atropine can still be used in these situations, the patient should be monitored closely for paradoxical slowing of the heart rate.

SPECIAL GROUPS

Race: no differences in response
Children: use with caution, as cases of respiratory distress, seizures, muscular hypotonia, and coma have been reported
Elderly: no dosage adjustment needed
Renal impairment: no dosage adjustment needed
Hepatic impairment: no dosage adjustment needed
Pregnancy: category C; use only if potential benefit justifies the potential risk to the fetus
Breast-feeding: not recommended; drug is excreted in breast milk

DOSAGE

Symptomatic bradycardia: 0.5–1 mg IV push; can repeat every 3–5 min to a maximum total dose of 0.04 mg/kg

Asystole: 1 mg IV push every 3–5 min to a maximum total dose of 0.04 mg/kg

Slow administration and doses < 0.5 mg have been associated with paradoxical bradycardia and should be avoided.

Atropine may also be administered via an endotracheal tube at 2–2.5 times the IV dose (should be diluted in 10 mL saline for adults and in 1–2 mL saline for children).

IN BRIEF

INDICATIONS
Symptomatic sinus bradycardia
Asystole

CONTRAINDICATIONS
Narrow-angle glaucoma
Obstructive disease of GI tract
Intestinal atony or megacolon
Hiatal hernia with reflux esophagitis
Tachycardia
Acute hemorrhage
Myasthenia gravis
Obstructive uropathy
Hypersensitivity to atropine

DRUG INTERACTIONS
Cholinergic agents[2]
Drugs with anticholinergic effects (phenothiazines, amantadine, TCAs, type Ia antiarrhythmics)[1,3]
1 Effect/toxicity of atropine may increase.
2 Effect of atropine may decrease.
3 Atropine may increase the effect/toxicity of this drug.

ADVERSE EFFECTS
CNS: headache, disorientation, delirium, excitement, slurred speech
CV: tachycardia, palpitations, chest pain, MI
GI: dry mouth, impaired GI motility, constipation
Lungs: dyspnea, bronchospasm in asthmatic patients
Ocular: blurred vision, mydriasis

PHARMACOKINETICS AND PHARMACODYNAMICS
Duration of action: 4 h
Onset of action: Immediate
Peak effect: 2–4 min
Bioavailability: well-absorbed from bronchial tree with endotracheal administration
Effect of food: unknown
Protein binding: 18%
Volume of distribution: widely distributed throughout the body
Metabolism: hepatic; metabolized into several metabolites
Elimination: renal; 30%–50% excreted in urine as unchanged drug; poorly dialyzable
Half-life: 12 h

MONITORING
ECG, BP, mental status, and respiratory status.

OVERDOSE
Supportive therapy. Acetylcholinesterase inhibitors, such as physostigmine (1–2 mg subcutaneously or IV), may be used in patients with life-threatening symptoms to reverse atropine's anticholinergic effects.

PATIENT INFORMATION
Report shortness of breath, chest pain, difficulty in urination, flushing, dry skin, nervousness, thirst, and other CNS effects to your physician.

AVAILABILITY
Injection—0.05 mg/mL, 0.1 mg/mL, 0.3 mg/mL, 0.4 mg/mL, 0.5 mg/mL, 0.8 mg/mL, 1 mg/mL

The information here is provided as guidance only. Prescribers should always consult the manufacturer's current prescribing information.

93

Anderson JL, Jolivette DM, Fredell PA: Summary of efficacy and safety of flecainide for supraventricular arrhythmias. *Am J Cardiol* 1988, 62:62D–66D.

Antman EM, Beamer AD, Cantillon C, *et al*.: Long-term oral propafenone therapy for suppression of refractory symptomatic atrial fibrillation and atrial flutter. *J Am Coll Cardiol* 1988,12:1005–1011.

Atrial Fibrillation Follow-Up Investigation of Rhythm Management (AFFIRM) Investigators: A comparison of rate control and rhythm control in patients with atrial fibrillation. *N Engl J Med* 2002, 347:1825–1833.

Benditt DG, Williams JH, Jin J, *et al*.: Maintenance of sinus rhythm with oral d,l-sotalol therapy in patients with symptomatic atrial fibrillation and/or atrial flutter. *Am J Cardiol* 1999, 84:270–277.

Burkart F, Pfisterer M, Kiowski W, *et al*.: Effect of antiarrhythmic therapy on mortality in survivors of myocardial infarction with asymptomatic complex ventricular arrhythmias: Basel Antiarrhythmic Study of Infarct Survival (BASIS). *J Am Coll Cardiol* 1990, 16:1711–1718.

Cairns JA, Connolly SJ, Gent M, Roberts R: Post–myocardial infarction mortality in patients with ventricular premature depolarizations: Canadian Amiodarone Myocardial Infarction Arrhythmia Trial Pilot Study. *Circulation* 1991, 84:550–557.

Cairns JA, Connolly SJ, Roberts R, *et al*., for the Canadian Amiodarone Myocardial Infarction (CAMIAT) Investigators: Randomized trial of outcome after myocardial infarction in patients with frequent or repetitive ventricular premature depolarizations: CAMIAT. *Lancet* 1997, 349:675–682.

Campbell TJ: Clinical use of class Ia antiarrhythmic drugs. In *Handbook of Experimental Pharmacology: Antiarrhythmic Drugs*. Edited by Vaughan Williams EM. Heidelberg: Springer Verlag; 1989:175–200.

Capucci A, Boriani G, Botto GL, *et al*.: Conversion of recent-onset atrial fibrillation by a single oral loading dose of propafenone or flecainide. *Am J Cardiol* 1994, 74:503–505.

Cavusoglu E, Frishman WH: Sotalol: a new β-adrenergic blocker for ventricular arrhythmias. *Prog Cardiovasc Dis* 1995, 37:423–440.

Connolly S, Gent M, Roberts RS, *et al*.: Canadian Implantable Defibrillator Study (CIDS): a randomized trial of the implantable cardioverter defibrillator against amiodarone. *Circulation* 2000, 101:1297–1302.

Coplen SE, Antman EH, Berlin JE, *et al*.: Efficacy and safety of quinidine therapy for maintenance of sinus rhythm after cardioversion: a meta-analysis of randomized control trials. *Circulation* 1990, 82:1106–1116.

Cruickshank JM, Prichard BNC: Arrhythmias. In *Beta Blockers in Clinical Practice*. London: Churchill; 1987:577–636.

Daoud E, Strickberger S, Man K, *et al*.: Preoperative amiodarone as prophylaxis against atrial fibrillation after heart surgery. *N Engl J Med* 1997, 337:1785–1791.

Dolak GL for the CASCADE Investigators: Clinical predictors of implantable cardioverter-defibrillator shocks (results of the CASCADE trial). *Am J Cardiol* 1994, 73:237–241.

Donovan KD, Power BM, Hockings BE, *et al*.: Intravenous flecainide versus amiodarone for recent onset atrial fibrillation. *Am J Cardiol* 1995, 75:693–697.

Dorian P, Cass D, Schwartz B, *et al*.: Amiodarone as compared with lidocaine for shock-resistant ventricular fibrillation. *N Engl J Med* 2002, 346:884–890.

Doval HC, Nul DR, Grancelli HO, *et al*., for Grupo de Estudio de la Sobrevida en la Insuficiencia Cardiaca en Argentina (GESICA): Randomized trial of low-dose amiodarone in severe congestive heart failure. *Lancet* 1994, 344:493–498.

Ellenbogen KA, Stambler BS, Wood MA, *et al*.: Efficacy of intravenous ibutilide for rapid termination of atrial fibrillation and atrial flutter: a dose-response study. *J Am Coll Cardiol* 1996, 28:130–136.

Farshi R, Kistner D, Sarma SM, *et al*.: Ventricular rate control in chronic atrial fibrillation during daily activity and programmed exercise: a crossover open-label study of five drug regimens. *J Am Coll Cardiol* 1999, 33:304–310.

Ferreira E, Sunderji R, Gin K: Is oral sotalol effective in converting atrial fibrillation to sinus rhythm? *Pharmacotherapy* 1997, 17:1233–1237.

Frishman WH, Murthy VS, Strom JA, Hershman DL: Ultrashort-acting beta-adrenoceptor blocking drug: esmolol. In *Cardiovascular Drug Therapy*, edn 2. Edited by Messerli FH. Philadelphia: WB Saunders; 1996:507–516.

Frishman WH, Vahdat S, Bhatta S: Innovative pharmacologic approaches to cardiopulmonary resuscitation. *J Clin Pharmacol* 1998, 38:765–772.

Fuster V, Rydén LE, Asinger RW, *et al*.: ACC/AHA/ESC guidelines for the management of patients with atrial fibrillation: a report of the American College of Cardiology/American Heart Association Task Force on Practice Guidelines and the European Society of Cardiology Committee for Practice Guidelines and Policy Conferences (Committee to Develop Guidelines for the Management of Patients with Atrial Fibrillation). *J Am Coll Cardiol* 2001, 38:1231–1265.

Giri S, White CM, Dunn AB, *et al*.: Oral amiodarone for prevention of atrial fibrillation after open heart surgery, the Atrial Fibrillation Suppression Trial (AFIST): a randomised, placebo controlled trial. *Lancet* 2001, 357:830–836.

Gottlieb CD, Horowitz LN: Potential interactions between antiarrhythmic medication and the automatic implantable cardioverter defibrillator. *Pacing Clin Electrophysiol* 1991, 14:898–904.

Gottlieb SS: The use of antiarrhythmic agents in heart failure: implications of CAST. *Am Heart J* 1989, 118:1074–1077.

Greene HL: The efficacy of amiodarone in the treatment of ventricular tachycardia or ventricular fibrillation. *Prog Cardiovasc Dis* 1989, 31:439–446.

Guarnieri T, Nolan S, Gottlieb SO, *et al*.: Intravenous amiodarone for the prevention of atrial fibrillation after open heart surgery: the Amiodarone Reduction in Coronary Heart (ARCH) Trial. *J Am Coll Cardiol* 1999, 34:343–347.

Hagemeijer F: Verapamil in the management of supraventricular tachyarrhythmias occurring after a recent myocardial infarction. *Circulation* 1978, 57:751–755.

Halinen MO, Huttunen M, Paakkinen S, *et al*.: Comparison of sotalol with digoxin-quinidine for conversion of acute atrial fibrillation to sinus rhythm (the Sotalol-Digoxin-Quinidine Trial). *Am J Cardiol* 1995, 76:495–498.

Harron DWG, Shanks RG: Clinical use of class Ib antiarrhythmic drugs. In *Handbook of Experimental Pharmacology: Antiarrhythmic Drugs*. Edited by Vaughan Williams EM. Heidelberg: Springer Verlag; 1989:201–234.

Hine LK, Laird N, Hewitt P, *et al*.: Meta-analytic evidence against prophylactic use of lidocaine in acute myocardial infarction. *Arch Intern Med* 1989, 149:2694–2698.

Ho RT, Callans DJ: Malignant ventricular arrhythmias. In *Cardiovascular Therapeutics. A Companion to Braunwald's Heart Disease*, edn 2. Edited by Antman EM. Philadelphia: WB Saunders Co.; 2001:477–501.

Hombach V, Braun V, Hopp HW, *et al*.: Electrophysiological effects of cardioselective and non-selective beta-adrenoceptor blockers with and without ISA at rest and during exercise. *Br J Clin Pharmacol* 1982, 13:285S–293S.

Hood MA, Smith WM: Adenosine versus verapamil in the treatment of supraventricular tachycardia: a randomized double-crossover trial. *Am Heart J* 1992, 123:1543–1549.

IMPACT Research Group: International Mexiletine and Placebo Antiarrhythmic Coronary Trial (IMPACT). II: results from 24 hour electrocardiogram. *Eur Heart J* 1986, 7:749–759.

Julian DG, Camm AJ, Frangin G, *et al*., for the European Myocardial Infarct Amiodarone Trial (EMIAT) Investigators: Randomized trial of effect of amiodarone on mortality in patients with left ventricular dysfunction after recent myocardial infarction: EMIAT. *Lancet* 1997, 349:667–674.

Juul-Moller S, Edvardsson N, Rehnqvist-Ahlberg N: Sotalol versus quinidine for the maintenance of sinus rhythm after direct current conversion of atrial fibrillation. *Circulation* 1990, 82:1932–1939.

Kerin NZ, Faitel K, Naini M: The efficacy of intravenous amiodarone for the conversion of chronic atrial fibrillation: amiodarone vs quinidine for conversion of atrial fibrillation. *Arch Intern Med* 1996, 156:49–53.

Køber L, Bloch-Thomsen PE, Møller M, *et al*.: Effect of dofetilide in patients with recent myocardial infarction and left-ventricular dysfunction: a randomised trial. *Lancet* 2000, 356:2052–2058.

Kochiadakis GE, Igoumenidis NE, Marketou ME *et al*.: Low-dose amiodarone versus sotalol for suppression of recurrent symptomatic atrial fibrillation. *Am J Cardiol* 1998, 81:995–998.

Kuck KH, Cappato R, Siebels J, Rüppel R. Randomized comparison of antiarrhythmic drug therapy with implantable defibrillators in patients resuscitated from cardiac arrest: The Cardiac Arrest Study Hamburg (CASH). *Circulation* 2000, 102:748–754.

Kudenchuk PJ, Cobb LA, Copass MK, *et al*.: Amiodarone for resuscitation after out-of-hospital cardiac arrest due to ventricular fibrillation. *N Engl J Med* 1999, 341:871–878.

Kumar A: Intravenous amiodarone for therapy of atrial fibrillation and flutter in critically ill patients with severe depressed left ventricular function. *South Med J* 1996, 89:779–785.

Larbuisson R, Venneman I, Stiels B: The efficacy and safety of intravenous propafenone versus intravenous amiodarone in the conversion of atrial fibrillation or flutter after cardiac surgery. *J Cardiothorac Vasc Anesth* 1996, 10:229–234.

Lee JT, Kroemer HK, Silberstein DJ, *et al*.: The role of genetically determined polymorphic drug metabolism in the beta blockade produced by propafenone. *N Engl J Med* 1990, 322:1764–1768.

Mangrum JM: Acute and chronic pharmacologic management of supraventricular tachyarrhythmias. In *Cardiovascular Therapeutics: A Companion to Braunwald's Heart Disease*, edn 2. Edited by Antman EM. Philadelphia: WB Saunders Co.; 2001:423–444.

Members of the Sicilian Gambit: New approaches to antiarrhythmic therapy. Part I. Emerging therapeutic applications of the cell biology of cardiac arrhythmias. *Circulation* 2001, 104:2865–2873.

Morganroth J, Chen CC, Sturm S, Dreifus LS: Oral verapamil in the treatment of atrial fibrillation/flutter. *Am J Cardiol* 1982, 49:981–985.

Moss AJ, Hall WJ, Cannon DS, *et al*.: Improved survival with an implanted defibrillator in patients with coronary disease at high risk for ventricular arrhythmia: Multicenter Automatic Defibrillator Implantation Trial Investigators. *N Engl J Med* 1996, 335:1933–1940.

Moss AJ, Zareba W, Hall WJ, *et al*.: Prophylactic implantation of a defibrillator in patients with myocardial infarction and reduced ejection fraction. *N Engl J Med* 2002, 346:877–883.

Mounsey JP, DiMarco JP: Dofetilide. *Circulation* 2000, 102:2665–2670.

The information here is provided as guidance only. Prescribers should always consult the manufacturer's current prescribing information.

95

Nicklas JM, McKenna WJ, Stewart RA, *et al.*: Prospective, double-blind, placebo-controlled trial of low-dose amiodarone in patients with severe heart failure and asymptomatic frequent ventricular ectopy. *Am Heart J* 1991, 122:1016–1021.

Parker RB, McCollum PL, Bauman JL: Propafenone: a novel type Ic antiarrhythmic agent. *Drug Intel Clin Pharm* 1989, 23:196–203.

Petersen TR for the Norwegian Multicenter Study Group: Six year follow up of the Norwegian Multicenter Study on timolol after acute myocardial infarction. *N Engl J Med* 1985, 313:1055–1058.

Pfisterer ME, Kiowski W, Brunner H, *et al.*: Long-term benefit of 1 year amiodarone treatment for persistent complex ventricular arrhythmias after myocardial infarction. *Circulation* 1993, 87:309–311.

Roden DM: Antiarrhythmic drugs. In *Goodman & Gilman's The Pharmacological Basis of Therapeutics*, edn 10. Edited by Hardman JG, Limbird LE. New York: McGraw Hill; 2001:933–970.

Roy D, Talajic M, Dorian P, *et al.*: Amiodarone to prevent recurrence of atrial fibrillation. *N Engl J Med* 2000, 342:913–920.

Schofield PM, Reid F, Bennett DH: A comparison of atenolol and sotalol in the treatment of patients with paroxysmal supraventricular tachycardia. *Br Heart J* 1987, 57:105–106.

Siebel J, Cappato R, Rüppel R, *et al.* and the CASH Investigators: ICD versus drugs in cardiac arrest survivors: preliminary results of the Cardiac Arrest Study, Hamburg. *PACE* 1993, 16:552–558.

Singh BN, Ellrodt G, Peters T: Verapamil: a review of its pharmacological properties and therapeutic use. *Drugs* 1978, 15:169–197.

Singh SN, Fletcher RD, Fisher SG, *et al.* for the Survival Trial of Antiarrhythmic Therapy in Congestive Heart Failure: Amiodarone in patients with congestive heart failure and asymptomatic ventricular arrhythmias. *N Engl J Med* 1995, 333:77–82.

Singh S, Zoble RG, Yellen, L, *et al.*: Efficacy and safety of oral dofetilide in converting to and maintaining sinus rhythm in patients with chronic atrial fibrillation or atrial flutter: The Symptomatic Atrial Fibrillation Investigative Research on Dofetilide (SAFIRE-D) Study. *Circulation* 2000, 102:2385–2390.

Skluth H, Grauer K, Gums J: Ventricular arrhythmias: an assessment of newer therapeutic agents. *Postgrad Med* 1989, 85:137–153.

Slavik RS, Tisdale JE, Borzak S. Pharmacologic conversion of atrial fibrillation: a systematic review of available evidence. *Prog Cardiovasc Dis* 2001, 44:121–152.

Sljapic TN, Kowey PR, Michelson EL: Antiarrhythmic drugs. In *Cardiovascular Pharmacotherapeutics*, edn 2. Edited by Frishman WH, Sonnenblick EH, Sica DA. New York: McGraw Hill; 2003:225–257.

Stambler BS, Wood MA, Ellenbogen KA: Comparative efficacy of intravenous ibutilide versus procainamide for enhancing termination of atrial flutter by atrial overdrive pacing. *Am J Cardiol* 1996, 77:960–966.

Stanton MS: Antiarrhythmic drugs: quinidine, procainamide, disopyramide, lidocaine, mexiletine, tocainide, phenytoin, moricizine, flecainide, propafenone. In *Cardiac Electrophysiology: From Cell to Bedside*. Edited by Zipes DP, Jalife J. Philadelphia: WB Saunders Co.; 2000:890.

Steinbeck G, Andersen D, Bach P, *et al.*: A comparison of electrophysiologically and guided antiarrhythmic drug therapy with beta blocker therapy in patients with symptomatic sustained ventricular tachyarrhythmias. *N Engl J Med* 1992, 327:987–992.

Steinberg JS, Sadaniantz A, Kron J, *et al.* for the AFFIRM Investigators: Analysis of cause-specific mortality in the Atrial Fibrillation Follow-Up Investigation of Rhythm Management (AFFIRM) study. *Circulation* 2004, 109:1973–1980.

Strasberg B, Arditti A, Sclarovsky S, *et al.*: Efficacy of intravenous amiodarone in the management of paroxysmal or new atrial fibrillation with fast ventricular response. *Int J Cardiol* 1985, 7:47–58.

Task Force of the Working Group on Arrhythmias of the European Society of Cardiology: The Sicilian Gambit: a new approach to the classification of antiarrhythmic drugs and their actions on arrhythmogenic mechanisms. *Circulation* 1991, 84:1831–1851.

Teo KT, Yusuf S, Furberg CD: Effects of prophylactic antiarrhythmic drug therapy in acute myocardial infarction: an overview of results from randomized controlled trials. *JAMA* 1993, 270:1589–1595.

The American Heart Association in Collaboration with the International Liaison Committee on Resuscitation (ILCOR). Guidelines 2000 for cardiopulmonary resuscitation and emergency cardiovascular care: an international consensus on science. *Circulation* 2000, 102(Suppl I):I-142–I-165.

The AVID Investigators: A comparison of antiarrhythmic drug therapy with implantable defibrillators in patients resuscitated from near fatal ventricular arrhythmias. *N Engl J Med* 1997, 337:1576–1583.

The Canadian Trial of Atrial Fibrillation Investigators: Amiodarone to prevent recurrence of atrial fibrillation. *N Engl J Med* 2000, 342:913–920.

The Cardiac Arrhythmia Suppression Trial (CAST) Investigators: Preliminary report: effect of encainide and flecainide on mortality in a randomized trial of arrhythmia suppression after myocardial infarction. *N Engl J Med* 1989, 321:406–412.

The Cardiac Arrhythmia Suppression Trial II Investigators: Effect of the antiarrhythmic agent moricizine on survival after myocardial infarction. *N Engl J Med* 1992, 327:227–233.

The ESVEM Investigators: Determinants of predicted efficacy of antiarrhythmic drugs in the Electrophysiologic Study Versus Electrocardiographic Monitoring trial. *Circulation* 1993, 87:323–329.

Torp-Pedersen C, Møller M, Bloch-Thomsen PE, *et al.* for the Danish Investigations on Arrhythmia and Mortality on Dofetilide (DIAMOND) Study Group: Dofetilide in patients with congestive heart failure and left ventricular dysfunction. *N Engl J Med* 1999, 341:857–865.

Vaughan Williams EM: Classification of antiarrhythmic action. In *Handbook of Experimental Pharmacology: Antiarrhythmic Drugs*. Edited by Vaughan Williams EM. Heidelberg: Springer Verlag; 1989:45–67.

Waldo AL, Camm AJ, De Ruyter H, *et al.*: Effects of d-sotalol on mortality in patients with left ventricular dysfunction after recent and remote myocardial infarction. *Lancet* 1996, 348:7–12.

Wit AL, Hoffman BF, Rosen MR: Electrophysiology and pharmacology of cardiac arrhythmias. IX: cardiac electrophysiological effects of beta-adrenergic receptor stimulation and blockade. *Am Heart J* 1975, 90:795–803.

Woosley RL: Clinical pharmacology of antiarrhythmic drugs. In *Cardiovascular Therapeutics. A Companion to Braunwald's Heart Disease,* edn 2. Edited by Antman EM. Philadelphia: WB Saunders Co.; 2001:407-421.

Woosley RL, Indik JH: Antiarrhythmic drugs. In *Hurst's The Heart*, edn 11. Edited by Fuster V, Alexander RW, O'Rourke RA. New York: McGraw Hill; 2004:949–973.

Wyse DG, Morganroth J, Leidengham R, *et al.*: New insights into the definition and meaning of proarrhythmia during initiation of antiarrhythmic drug therapy from the Cardiac Arrhythmia Suppression Trial and its pilot study. *J Am Coll Cardiol* 1994, 23:1130–1140.

Zarembski DG, Nolan PE Jr, Slack MK, *et al.*: Treatment of resistant atrial fibrillation: a meta-analysis comparing amiodarone and flecainide. *Arch Intern Med* 1995, 155:1885–1891.

Zehender M, Hohnloser S, Mueller B, *et al.*: Effects of amiodarone versus quinidine and verapamil in patients with chronic atrial fibrillation: results of a comparative study and a 2-year follow-up. *J Am Coll Cardiol* 1992, 19:1054–1059.

Antithrombotic drugs are those that either interfere with the development of a thrombus (antiplatelet and anticoagulant drugs) or act to dissolve an existing thrombus (fibrinolytics). Antiplatelet agents prevent platelets from adhering to damaged vessel walls and to one another, a vital step in the initiation of clot formation, particularly in arteries. Anticoagulant therapy is used to prevent clots from forming or progressing by inhibiting the formation of the fibrin framework of the blood clot. Fibrinolytic therapy activates the enzyme pathways that lyse the fibrin meshwork of the blood clot to restore blood flow after a clot has blocked a vessel. Figure 6.1 illustrates the process of clot formation.

The clinical benefits of antithrombotic drugs, when used appropriately, are substantial. These drugs have been repeatedly shown to reduce morbidity and mortality in a variety of diseases caused by thromboses (*eg*, acute myocardial infarction [MI], unstable angina, deep vein thrombosis [DVT], etc). Antithrombotic therapy may involve more than one type of drug in sequence (*eg*, a fibrinolytic agent to dissolve a clot and an antiplatelet agent with or without an anticoagulant drug to prevent the clot from reforming on the injured artery wall). All antithrombotic drugs increase the risk of bleeding. Combinations of these drugs, particularly fibrinolytics and anticoagulants, may increase this risk. These risks must be balanced against the desired therapeutic goals.

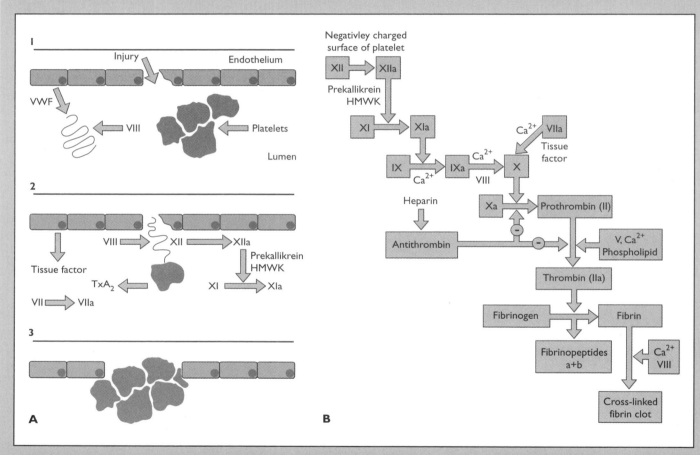

FIGURE 6.1 Stages of hemostasis. **A**, 1) Injury of vascular endothelium; von Willebrand factor (VWF) facilitates the adherence of platelets to the damaged subendothelium. 2) Adherence of platelets and initiation of extrinsic and intrinsic coagulation pathways. The extrinsic pathway is triggered by the release of tissue factor by the damaged subendothelium, which then complexes with activated factor VII, subsequently activating factor X. The activation of factor XII initiates the intrinsic pathway. Thromboxane A_2 (TxA_2) released by platelets pro-

motes platelet aggregation. 3) Aggregated platelets provide a negatively charged surface on which the clotting cascade produces thrombin IIa.

B, The coagulation cascade. Antithrombin interferes with the activation of factors X and II (thrombin). Heparin potentiates the effect of antithrombin. The other anticoagulants work in a similar way by inhibiting the formation of active factors II, VII, IX, and/or X. a—activated clotting factors; HMWK—high molecular weight kininogen.

Anticoagulants are available as rapid-acting parenteral agents (such as **heparin**, low molecular weight **heparins** [LMWHs], **lepirudin**, **desirudin**, **argatroban**, **bivalirudin**, and **fondaparinux**) and oral agents (such as **warfarin**). Anticoagulant therapy is usually initiated with a parenteral agent, followed by long-term oral **warfarin** therapy. **Ximelagatran** (Exanta; AstraZeneca Pharmaceuticals LP, Waltham, MA) is an investigational oral anticoagulant that acts by directly binding to thrombin and inhibiting its action. If approved by the Food and Drug Administration (FDA), it will likely be used in place of **warfarin** in certain situations.

EFFICACY AND USE

In patients with recently diagnosed DVT or thrombophlebitis, anticoagulant therapy can prevent extension and embolization of the thrombus and reduce the risk of pulmonary embolism (PE) or recurrent thromboembolic events. In patients with acute PE, anticoagulation reduces the risk of extension of the thrombus, recurrence, and death.

Anticoagulant therapy is also useful in DVT and PE prophylaxis after major abdominal, gynecologic, orthopedic, or thoracic surgery, especially in high-risk patients. In patients with acute MI, anticoagulant therapy can reduce the risk of systemic thromboembolic complications. **Heparin** and LMWHs are used as adjunct therapy with certain fibrinolytics and antiplatelet drugs in patients with acute MI and as combination therapy with antiplatelet agents in treating unstable angina to help prevent clot progression, prevent reocclusion of the artery, and reduce ischemic events in association with these conditions.

Heparin is used during heart surgery with cardiopulmonary bypass and during coronary angioplasty with and without stent placement. **Bivalirudin** is used during percutaneous coronary intervention (PCI) to reduce the risk of ischemic complications.

In patients with recent cerebral embolism, especially if the heart is the suspected origin of the thrombus, anticoagulation may reduce the risk of recurrence. Cerebral hemorrhage should be ruled out, and the risk of cerebral hemorrhage should be weighed against the risk of recurrent embolic events in a patient before initiating anticoagulant therapy. The treatment is of less value in patients with transient ischemic attacks (TIAs).

LMWHs are sometimes used as "bridge" therapy in patients who have just begun (or re-started) treatment with **warfarin** and are not yet at a therapeutic International Normalized Ratio (INR). In these instances, the LMWH is often given on an outpatient basis for several days until the INR is in the desired range.

Fondaparinux is used primarily to reduce thromboembolic complications following orthopedic surgery. **Argatroban** and **lepirudin** are alternative anticoagulants useful in patients with known or suspected heparin-induced thrombocytopenia (HIT) or a history of HIT. **Desirudin** is indicated for DVT prophylaxis following hip replacement surgery, but may also be used in patients with HIT, although this is an unlabeled indication.

Warfarin may cross the placenta and should therefore be avoided, if possible, during pregnancy. **Heparin** and LMWHs are the anticoagulants of choice during pregnancy.

Some other common indications for anticoagulation include patients with shock, congestive heart failure (CHF), chronic atrial fibrillation or flutter, previous MI, and history of thromboembolism.

MODE OF ACTION

Heparin potentiates the inhibition of antithrombin on activated clotting factors, including IIa (thrombin), IXa, Xa, XIa, and XIIa. Of these, factors IIa and Xa are most responsive to **heparin** inhibition, with thrombin being about 10-fold more sensitive to **heparin** inhibition than factor Xa (Figure 6.1). **Heparin** is not absorbed through the gastrointestinal (GI) tract and should be given either intravenously (IV) or subcutaneously (SC). **Heparin** has a rapid

TABLE 6.1 LOW MOLECULAR WEIGHT HEPARINS APPROVED BY THE U.S. FOOD AND DRUG ADMINISTRATION

Generic (brand) name	Mean molecular weight (D)	Bioavailability (%)	Anti-Xa:Anti IIa	Half-life (h)	Approved dosing for DVT prophylaxis
Dalteparin (Fragmin)	5000	87	2.2–2.8:1	3–5	2500 or 5000 IU once daily*
Enoxaparin (Lovenox)	4500	92	2.7–3.9:1	4.5	30 mg twice daily or 40 mg once daily
Tinzaparin (Innohep)	5500–7500	87	1.5–2.0:1	3–4	Approved only for DVT treatment: 175 IU/kg once daily

*High dose is recommended for high-risk patients.

DVT—deep vein thrombosis.

onset of action and a short duration of action, necessitating administration by either continuous IV infusion or multiple daily SC doses.

LMWHs act primarily through inhibition of factor Xa (Table 6.1). Compared with unfractionated **heparin** (UFH), these agents provide a more predictable dose response with less interpatient variability, making routine monitoring for anticoagulant effect unnecessary. LMWHs have longer half-lives and less of a propensity to cause thrombocytopenia than UFH, with a comparable bleeding risk.

Lepirudin and **desirudin** are direct thrombin inhibitors that are both derived from hirudin, a 65-amino acid peptide found in leech saliva, with all three compounds sharing very similar chemical structures. Unlike **heparin**, which requires antithrombin to elicit its anticoagulant effect and inhibits only free-circulating thrombin, **lepirudin** and **desirudin** act independently of a cofactor and bind to both free and clot-bound thrombin. This may have the advantage

of preventing growth of a clot due to localized fibrin deposition. **Lepirudin** and **desirudin** are structurally very similar. **Lepirudin** is approved only for use in patients with HIT, whereas **desirudin** is indicated only for DVT prophylaxis following hip replacement surgery, although both are probably also effective in the management of other acute thromboembolic problems. **Lepirudin** is administered by continuous IV infusion, whereas **desirudin** is given by SC injection twice daily.

Bivalirudin is a 20–amino acid peptide derivative of hirudin, with a shorter half-life than **desirudin** and **lepirudin**, which is advantageous in reducing bleeding risk.

Warfarin inhibits the synthesis of clotting factors II, VII, IX, and X by competitively inhibiting vitamin K–dependent gamma-carboxylation of the precursor proteins. Following the initiation of **warfarin** therapy, factor VII (plasma half-life of 4–6 h) is depleted first, followed by factors IX, X, and II (plasma half-lives of 20–24 h, 48–72 h,

TABLE 6.2 CHARACTERISTICS OF VARIOUS ANTICOAGULANTS

	Mechanism of action	Main routes of administration	Antidote	Laboratory monitoring
Heparin	Binds to antithrombin and inhibits the actions of coagulation factors II, X, and, to a lesser extent, IX, XI, and XII	IV or SC	Protamine sulfate	aPTT or ACT, platelet count
Low molecular weight heparin	Same as heparin with a predominant effect on inhibition of factor X	SC	Protamine sulfate	Platelet count. Anti-factor Xa concentrations are not necessary but may help guide therapy in certain patients (eg, those with obesity, kidney disease)
Warfarin	Interferes with the production of vitamin K–dependent coagulation factors II, VII, IX, and X	PO	Vitamin K	PT, INR
Lepirudin (Refludan®)	Direct thrombin (factor IIa) inhibitor (rDNA)	IV	None	aPTT
Desirudin (Iprivask®)	Direct thrombin (factor IIa) inhibitor (rDNA)	SC	None	aPTT, especially in patients with renal insufficiency
Bivalirudin (Angiomax®)	Direct thrombin (factor IIa) inhibitor (semisynthetic)	IV	None	ACT or aPTT
Argatroban	Direct thrombin (factor IIa) inhibitor (synthetic)	IV	None	aPTT or ACT
Fondaparinux (Arixtra®)	Direct factor Xa inhibitor (synthetic)	SC	None	Periodic CBC, including platelet count, serum creatinine. Anti–factor Xa concentrations are not necessary but may be obtained if desired

ACT—activated clotting time; aPTT—activated partial thromboplastin time; CBC—complete blood count; INR—International Normalized Ratio; IV—intravenous; PO—oral; PT—prothrombin time; SC—subcutaneous.

and ≥ 60 h, respectively). Although prothrombin time (PT) and INR are prolonged after factor VII depletion, peak antithrombotic effect is not achieved until all four factors are depleted from the circulation, which usually takes several days. Therefore, for more rapid anticoagulation in acute thromboembolic events, therapy with a quicker-acting agent, such as **heparin** or an LMWH, is used. Oral **warfarin** therapy is usually initiated for long-term maintenance with concurrent **heparin** or LMWH (bridge) therapy for the first 5 to 10 days.

Table 6.2 summarizes the characteristics of the currently available anticoagulants.

INDICATIONS

	Heparin	Dalteparin	Enoxaparin	Tinzaparin	Bivalirudin	Desirudin	Lepirudin	Argatroban	Fondaparinux	Warfarin
Venous thrombosis (T/P)	+ (T/P)	(+)(T)+ (P)*	+ (T/P)*	+ (T)	–	+ (P)	–	–	+ (T/P)*	+
Pulmonary embolism (T/P)	+ (T/P)	+ (P)*	+ (T/P)*	+ (T)	–	–	–	–	+ (T/P)*	+
Peripheral arterial embolism (T/P)	+ (T/P)	–	–	–	–	–	–	–	–	–
Atrial fibrillation	+	–	–	–	–	–	–	–	–	+
Disseminated intravascular coagulation	+	–	–	–	–	–	–	–	–	–
Extracorporeal circulation	+	–	–	–	–	–	–	–	–	–
Acute coronary syndrome	(+)	+*	+*	–	–	–	–	–	–	–
Percutaneous coronary angioplasty	(+)	–	–	–	+	–	–	+*	–	–
Heparin-induced thrombocytopenia	–	–	–	–	–	–	+	+	–	–

*Limited indications only (see discussions of each drug).

+—FDA approved; — —not FDA approved; (+)—not FDA approved but commonly used; P—prophylaxis; T—treatment.

HEPARIN SODIUM OR CALCIUM
(Heparin Sodium, Calciparine®)

Heparin acts indirectly at multiple sites in the intrinsic and extrinsic clotting systems by potentiating the inhibitory action of antithrombin on various coagulation factors. Factors IIa and Xa are most responsive to heparin inhibition, with thrombin being about 10-fold more sensitive to heparin inhibition than factor Xa. Heparin also prevents formation of a fibrin clot by inhibiting the thrombin-activated formation of fibrin-stabilized factor. Because heparin does not cross the placenta, it does not affect blood clotting in the fetus. Heparin is therefore the anticoagulant of choice during pregnancy. Although complications in pregnancy have been reported, the incidence seems to be somewhat lower than with coumarin-related oral anticoagulants.

Heparin is used when rapid anticoagulation is desired. It is recommended for use in all patients with acute MI or unstable angina. It is effective in reducing MI and recurrent refractory angina pectoris in patients with unstable angina, although its effect on mortality has not been determined in this population. It can reduce mortality and reinfarction in patients with acute MI (when used alone or as an adjunct to fibrinolytic therapy). Heparin is recommended to be administered in conjunction with alteplase, reteplase, and tenecteplase. Heparin should not be administered for 6 hours after administration of streptokinase, urokinase, or anistreplase (in order to minimize bleeding risk) except in patients at high risk for systemic emboli. It is also useful in the treatment and prevention of venous thrombosis and pulmonary thromboembolism, for reducing clotting during extracorporeal circulation, and after vascular surgery grafts. Low-dose heparin, often given SC, is widely used for patients at high risk of venous thrombosis, such as bedridden patients with severe heart failure, and before surgical arthroplasty of the hip joint.

SPECIAL GROUPS
Race: no differences in response
Children: adjust dosage based on weight, age, and coagulation test results
Elderly: no specific dosage adjustment is required; adjust dosage based on weight and coagulation test results
Renal impairment: no specific dosage adjustment required; adjust dosage based on weight and coagulation test results
Hepatic impairment: no specific dosage adjustment required; adjust dosage based on weight and coagulation test results
Pregnancy: category C; the preferred anticoagulant during pregnancy, but should only be used if clearly indicated
Breast-feeding: not excreted in human milk

IN BRIEF

INDICATIONS
Prophylaxis and treatment:
  Venous thrombosis
  Pulmonary embolism
  Atrial fibrillation with thromboembolism
  Peripheral arterial embolism
  Unstable angina*
  Evolving stroke*
  Acute MI*
Prevention of clotting in:
  Cardiac/ arterial surgery
  Blood transfusion
  Dialysis and other extracorporeal interventions
  Disseminated intravascular coagulation (DIC)
* Not approved by the FDA

CONTRAINDICATIONS
Known hypersensitivity
Active major bleeding
Thrombocytopenia or other blood dyscrasias

DRUG INTERACTIONS
Antibiotics (penicillins and cephalosporins)[1,4]
Anticoagulants[1,3]
Antihistamines[2,4]
Antiplatelet drugs[1,2]
Digoxin[2,4]
Dihydroergotamine mesylate[1]
Fibrinolytics[1,3]
NSAIDs[1]
Tetracycline[2,4]
1 Effect/toxicity of heparin may increase.
2 Effect of heparin may decrease.
3 Heparin may increase the effect/toxicity of this drug.
4 The clinical significance of this interaction is unclear.

ADVERSE EFFECTS
Blood: bleeding/clotting problems, thrombocytopenia
GI: liver function abnormalities
Endocrine: hypoaldosteronism, hyperkalemia, rebound hyperlipidemia (after discontinuation)
Skin: local skin reactions, hematoma, cutaneous necrosis, alopecia
Other: allergic vasospastic reaction, fever, chills, urticaria, anaphylactoid reaction, osteoporosis

PHARMACOKINETICS AND PHARMACODYNAMICS
Duration of action: 1.5 h (IV); >12 h (SC)
Onset of action: immediate (IV); 20–60 min (SC)
Peak effect: 2 min (IV); 2–4 h (SC)
Bioavailability: 100% (IV); variable (SC)
Effect of food: not applicable
Protein binding: extensively bound to plasma proteins
Volume of distribution: approximates blood volume; approximately 60 mL/kg
Metabolism: internalized, desulfated, and depolymerized by macrophages and endothelial cells; partially metabolized by liver heparinase
Elimination: occurs through saturable metabolism (above) and nonsaturable renal clearance, accounting for the dose-dependent half-life
Elimination half-life: increases with increasing dose; average 90 min, range 30–180 min

HEPARIN SODIUM OR CALCIUM (continued)

DOSAGE

Desired activated partial thromboplastin time (aPTT) is usually 1.5–2.5 times control.

Prophylaxis for DVT: SC 5000 U every 8–12 h until the patient is fully ambulatory

Treatment guidelines for thromboembolic events: IV 60–100 U/kg bolus, followed by 12–20 U/kg/h and adjusted based on coagulation test results

SC 10,000–20,000 U loading dose, followed by 8000–10,000 U every 8 h or 15,000–20,000 U every 12 h; dose should be adjusted based on coagulation test results

Open heart and vascular surgery: minimum initial dose is 150 U/kg; usually for procedures <60 min, 300 U/kg is used, and for procedures >60 min, 400 U/kg is used

Heparin lock to maintain IV patency: 10–100 U in the hub and replace after each use

MONITORING

Lab: CBC with platelet count, liver function, serum potassium, and aPTT (1.5–2.5 times control; not required for low-dose heparin). Clinical evidence of active or occult bleeding. Activated clotting time (ACT) should be used with high heparin dosages.

OVERDOSE

Supportive; blood transfusion is indicated for acute, significant blood loss and protamine may be used to neutralize heparin (1 mg protamine/100 U heparin).

PATIENT INFORMATION

Consult physician in the event of bleeding or bruising; hair loss; change in condition of skin; coldness, pain, or color changes in the legs; tingling or sensation loss; or local reactions at the injection site. Elderly patients are at greater risk for hemorrhage. Do not take other drugs without consulting your physician. Aspirin, ibuprofen, or other platelet-active medications should not be taken while on heparin unless prescribed by your physician. Inform all physicians and dentists that heparin is being used. Carry identification stating heparin is being used.

AVAILABILITY (EITHER BOVINE OR PORCINE ORIGIN)

Heparin sodium: syringes, vials, and ampules—2, 10, 40, 50, 100, 1000, 2000, 2500, 5000, 7500, 10000, 20000, 40000 U/mL in various volumes as single-use or multiple-dose packages
Heparin calcium: Syringes—5000 U/0.2 mL

ARGATROBAN

Argatroban is a synthetic direct thrombin inhibitor that selectively and reversibly binds both free and clot-bound thrombin. It is a derivative of L-arginine that does not require a cofactor (eg, antithrombin) for pharmacologic effect. It has a dose-dependent anticoagulant effect, which is monitored using either the aPTT or ACT. It is administered by IV infusion because of its short half-life (39–51 min) and is indicated and primarily used for anticoagulation in patients with HIT. Argatroban has a mechanism of action very similar to that of melagatran, the active metabolite of ximelagatran, an investigational oral direct thrombin inhibitor.

SPECIAL GROUPS

Race: no data
Children: safety and effectiveness have not been established
Elderly: dosage adjustment not required unless liver function is compromised
Renal impairment: dosage adjustment not required because the drug is metabolized and excreted by the liver
Hepatic impairment: use cautiously because of reduced drug clearance; initial dosage should be reduced and titrated based on response
Pregnancy: category B; should only be used if clearly indicated
Breast-feeding: not recommended; unknown if the drug is excreted in human milk

DOSAGE

Prophylaxis or treatment of thrombosis in patients with HIT: 2 µg/kg/min (0.5 µg/kg/min with moderate hepatic impairment) by continuous IV infusion. Check the aPTT 2 h after initiation of therapy and titrate dosage (max. 10 µg/kg/min) to an aPTT of 1.5–3 times control (max. 100 sec)

Patients with or at risk for HIT undergoing PCI: Give a 350 µg/kg IV bolus (over 3–5 min) with a 25 µg/kg/min IV infusion. Check ACT 5–10 min after bolus dose and begin procedure if ACT >300 sec. If ACT <300 sec, administer an additional 150 µg/kg IV bolus and increase infusion to 30 µg/kg/min. The bolus dose may be repeated if ACT remains <300 sec, with the infusion rate increased to 40 µg/kg/min. Recheck aPTT in 5–10 min. If ACT >450 sec, decrease infusion rate to 15 µg/kg/min and check the ACT 5–10 min later. If desired, the argatroban infusion may be continued following the procedure at a lower infusion rate (eg, 2 µg/kg/min with normal liver function).

Conversion to warfarin: Combination therapy results in higher INR values than warfarin alone. Begin warfarin at the expected daily dose (do not use a loading dose) and, if the dosage of argatroban is >2 µg/kg/min, temporarily reduce the dosage to 2 µg/kg/min. Measure the INR daily. Discontinue argatroban once the INR is above 4. Measure the INR 4–6 h after argatroban is discontinued. If INR is subtherapeutic, restart argatroban and repeat this procedure daily until INR is in the desired range.

IN BRIEF

INDICATIONS
Prophylaxis or treatment of thrombosis in patients with HIT
Anticoagulation in patients with or at risk for HIT undergoing PCI

CONTRAINDICATIONS
Known hypersensitivity to argatroban or any of the components in the product
Overt major bleeding

DRUG INTERACTIONS
Anticoagulants[1,2]
Antiplatelet drugs[1,2]
Fibrinolytics[1,2]
1 Effect/toxicity of argatroban may increase.
2 Argatroban may increase the effect/toxicity of this drug.

ADVERSE EFFECTS
Blood: bleeding
GI: nausea, vomiting, abdominal pain, diarrhea
Cardiac: hypotension, bradycardia, dysrhythmias, chest pain
Pulmonary: dyspnea, pneumonia, coughing
Other: hypersensitivity reaction, pain (generalized)

PHARMACOKINETICS AND PHARMACODYNAMICS
Duration of action: 2–4 h
Onset of action: <10 min with bolus administration
Peak plasma concentrations: 1–3 h
Bioavailability: 100%
Protein binding: 54% (20% albumin, 34% alpha$_1$-acid glycoprotein
Volume of distribution: 174 mL/kg
Metabolism: Hepatic, via hydroxylation and aromatization. The primary metabolite (M1) has three- to fivefold less anticoagulant potency than argatroban.
Elimination: primarily in the feces; 16% excreted unchanged in the urine and at least 14% excreted unchanged in the feces
Elimination half-life: 39–51 h

MONITORING
Lab: aPTT (monitored 2 h after initiation or dosage increase, then daily once stable). Monitor ACT for PCI. Monitor for clinical evidence of active or occult bleeding.

OVERDOSE
Supportive; no known antidote.

PATIENT INFORMATION
Argatroban may cause excessive bleeding; report any abnormal bleeding or bruising to your health care provider.

AVAILABILITY
Single-use vials: 250 mg/2.5 mL

BIVALIRUDIN (Angiomax®)

Bivalirudin is a derivative of hirudin, a 65–amino acid thrombin inhibitor produced by the medicinal leech *Hirudo medicinalis*. Bivalirudin is a semisynthetic 20–amino acid derivative of hirudin formed from residues 53 to 64 of the hirudin molecule. Bivalirudin is a direct thrombin inhibitor, which has a lower affinity for thrombin (*ie*, it is a reversible inhibitor) than hirudin, which irreversibly binds this enzyme. The result is a lower bleeding risk with bivalirudin compared with hirudin. Like hirudin, bivalirudin inhibits both free and clot-bound thrombin without reliance on cofactors such as antithrombin. Bivalirudin is indicated only for patients with unstable angina who are undergoing percutaneous transluminal coronary angioplasty, although it has shown efficacy in other settings. The REPLACE-2 (Randomized Evaluation in PCI Linking Angiomax to Reduced Clinical Events) trial demonstrated bivalirudin to be at least as good as combination therapy with heparin and a glycoprotein (GP) IIb/IIIa receptor antagonist in reducing major adverse cardiovascular events in patients undergoing PCI (mostly coronary stent placement). In addition, the risk of major bleeding was lower with bivalirudin in this study.

SPECIAL GROUPS

Race: no data
Children: safety and effectiveness have not been established
Elderly: more sensitive to bleeding; dose should be adjusted based on creatinine clearance
Renal impairment: reduce dosage with creatinine clearance <60 mL/min
Hepatic impairment: no specific dosage adjustments are required, although liver disease may potentiate anticoagulant effects because of impaired production of clotting factors
Pregnancy: category B; should only be used if clearly indicated
Breast-feeding: not recommended; not known if the drug is excreted in human milk

DOSAGE

Use with aspirin and initiate treatment just prior to PCI
Bolus dose: 1.0 mg/kg IV; no adjustment needed for renal insufficiency
Maintenance: 2.5 mg/kg/h IV infusion for 4 h, then 0.2 mg/kg/h for up to 20 h if needed.
The maintenance dose should be reduced in patients with renal insufficiency and the ACT monitored.
REPLACE-2 dosing (clinically used but not FDA approved): 0.75 mg/kg IV bolus immediately before PCI, followed by 1.75 mg/kg/h IV infusion for the duration of the procedure.

IN BRIEF

INDICATIONS
Anticoagulation in conjunction with aspirin in patients with unstable angina undergoing percutaneous transluminal coronary angioplasty.
Anticoagulation in conjunction with aspirin in patients undergoing PCI (eg, coronary stent placement); not an FDA-approved indication

CONTRAINDICATIONS
Known hypersensitivity to bivalirudin or its components
Active major bleeding

DRUG INTERACTIONS
Anticoagulants[1,2]
Antiplatelet drugs[1,2]
NSAIDs[1]
Fibrinolytics[1,2]
1 Effect/toxicity of bivalirudin may increase.
2 Bivalirudin may increase the effect/toxicity of this drug.

ADVERSE EFFECTS
Blood: bleeding
Cardiovascular: hypotension
GI: nausea, abdominal pain
Other: back pain, headache, pain (general), injection site pain

PHARMACOKINETICS AND PHARMACODYNAMICS
Duration of action: 1–2 h
Onset of action: immediate
Peak plasma concentrations: 15–19 min
Protein binding: not significant
Volume of distribution: not clearly defined
Metabolism: proteolytic cleavage of the drug molecule
Elimination: renal
Elimination half-life: about 30 min (1–3.5 h with severe renal insufficiency)

MONITORING
Lab: bivalirudin prolongs coagulation time; ACT is most commonly measured during coronary intervention. ACT monitoring is recommended in all patients with renal insufficiency. Monitor for clinical evidence of active or occult bleeding.

OVERDOSE
Supportive—no specific antidote is available.

PATIENT INFORMATION
Bivalirudin may cause excessive bleeding; report any unexplained bruising or bleeding to your health care provider.

AVAILABILITY
Vials (single use)—250 mg

DALTEPARIN SODIUM (Fragmin®)

Dalteparin, an LMWH, is derived through nitrous acid depolymerization of porcine source heparin. It has an average molecular weight of 5000 D. Similar to other LMWHs, the antithrombotic effect of dalteparin results primarily from its anti–factor Xa activity (anti-Xa/IIa ratio = 2.2–2.8:1). Dalteparin, administered once daily SC starting prior to hip replacement or abdominal surgery and continuing for 5 to 10 days after surgery, is effective in preventing thromboembolic complications in high-risk patients. Although 5000 IU dalteparin is more effective than the 2500 IU dose in patients undergoing abdominal surgery, a higher dose may increase the risk of bleeding. Thus, the higher dose should be used only in patients with a high risk of thromboembolic complications, such as those with underlying malignancy. Dalteparin 2500 IU once daily is at least as effective as heparin 5000 IU given twice daily SC in patients undergoing abdominal surgery. However, it is not clear if dalteparin therapy is more efficacious than heparin 5000 IU every 8 hours or adjusted-dose heparin.

In two large clinical studies, dalteparin 120 IU/kg every 12 hours administered SC with concurrent oral aspirin was effective in reducing death, MI, or recurrent angina in patients with a recent onset of unstable angina or non–Q-wave MI, with comparable efficacy and safety as UFH.

Because of the potential for cross-reactivity (>90%), dalteparin should be avoided, or at most, used only with extreme caution in patients with a history of HIT.

Rare cases of epidural, spinal, and neuraxial hematomas have been reported with the concurrent use of LMWHs and spinal/epidural anesthesia or spinal puncture, which in some cases has resulted in long-term or permanent paralysis. For this reason, these patients should be frequently monitored for signs and symptoms of neurologic impairment; if present, urgent intervention is necessary.

SPECIAL GROUPS

Race: no data
Children: safety and effectiveness have not been established
Elderly: no data, dosage adjustment is probably not required unless renal insufficiency is present
Renal impairment: reduced clearance, use with caution
Hepatic impairment: no data, dosage adjustment not necessary, but use with caution
Pregnancy: category B; should only be used if clearly indicated
Breast-feeding: not recommended; unknown if the drug is excreted in human milk

IN BRIEF

INDICATIONS
Prophylaxis against DVT that may lead to PE in high-risk patients undergoing hip replacement surgery, and also in patients undergoing abdominal surgery who are at risk for thromboembolic complications. Patients at risk include those who are >40 y of age, obese, undergoing surgery under general anesthesia lasting longer than 30 min, or who have additional risk factors, such as malignancy or a history of DVT or PE.
Prevention of ischemic complications in patients with unstable angina or non–Q-wave MI (use with concurrent aspirin)

CONTRAINDICATIONS
Known hypersensitivity to dalteparin, heparin, or pork
Known HIT
Active major bleeding
Patients undergoing regional anesthesia should not receive dalteparin for unstable angina or non–Q-wave MI

DRUG INTERACTIONS
Anticoagulants[1,2]
Antiplatelet drugs[1,2]
NSAIDs[1]
Fibrinolytics[1,2]
1 Effect/toxicity of dalteparin may increase.
2 Dalteparin may increase the effect/toxicity of this drug.

ADVERSE EFFECTS
Blood: hemorrhage, thrombocytopenia
GI: liver function abnormalities
CNS: epidural or spinal hematoma (especially with spinal/epidural anesthesia or spinal puncture)
Skin: local irritation, pruritus, rash, pain, bullous eruption, necrosis
Rare: hypersensitivity reaction, fever, anaphylactoid reaction

PHARMACOKINETICS AND PHARMACODYNAMICS
(based on plasma anti–factor Xa activity)
Duration of action: 10–24 h
Onset of action: <2 h
Peak effect: 2–4 h
Bioavailability: 87%
Protein binding: no specific data; less protein binding than UFH
Volume of distribution: 40–60 mL/kg
Elimination: mainly via kidney as unchanged drug
Elimination half-life: 3–5 h

MONITORING
Lab: CBC with platelet count, anti–factor Xa concentrations if desired (eg, obesity, renal insufficiency), liver transaminases. Monitor for clinical evidence of active or occult bleeding.

OVERDOSE
Supportive; the antithrombotic effect may be partially neutralized with protamine.

PATIENT INFORMATION
Dalteparin may cause excessive bleeding; report any abnormal bleeding or bruising to your health care provider. Rotate injection sites daily to minimize pain and bruising.

DALTEPARIN SODIUM (continued)

DOSAGE

1) **Abdominal surgery (DVT prophylaxis):** Patients with low to moderate risk of thromboembolic complications: 2500 IU SC once daily for 5–10 d starting 1–2 h prior to surgery

   Patients with high risk of thromboembolic complications: 5000 IU SC once daily for 5–10 d starting the evening before surgery; or 2500 IU SC starting 1–2 h prior to surgery with a second 2500 IU dose given 12 h later and followed by 5000 IU SC once daily for 5–10 d

2) **Hip replacement surgery (DVT prophylaxis):** Administer first dose, 2500 IU, SC within 2 h before surgery and second dose of 2500 IU 4–8 h after the surgery (allow at least 6 h between this dose and the first dose on postoperative day 1); dalteparin 5000 IU is then administered SC once daily from first postoperative day and continued for 5–10 d.

   Alternatively, dalteparin 5000 IU may be administered the evening before the surgery, followed by 5000 IU 4–8 h after the surgery (allow about 24 h between doses) and then 5000 IU SC once daily for 5–10 d.

3) **Unstable angina/non–Q-wave MI:** 120 IU/kg (max. 10,000 IU) SC every 12 h with concurrent aspirin therapy for 5–8 d or until the patient is clinically stable.

AVAILABILITY

Syringes:
  2500 anti–factor Xa IU/0.2 mL
  5000 anti–factor Xa IU/0.2 mL
  7500 anti–factor Xa IU/0.3 mL
  10,000 anti–factor Xa IU/1.0 mL
Multiple-dose vials:
  10,000 anti–factor Xa IU/mL, 9.5 mL
  25,000 anti–factor Xa IU/mL, 3.8 mL

DESIRUDIN (Iprivask®)

Desirudin is the most recently approved anticoagulant in the United States (approved April 2003). It is a recombinant hirudin derived from yeast cells. Hirudin is a 65–amino acid thrombin inhibitor produced by the medicinal leech *Hirudo medicinalis*. Desirudin is identical in structure to naturally occurring hirudin except for the absence of a sulfate group on the tyrosine at position 63 of the molecule. Desirudin is an irreversible direct thrombin inhibitor, inhibiting both free and clot-bound thrombin, which leads to a dose-dependent elevation of aPTT. Its antithrombotic effect is not dependent on cofactors such as antithrombin. Desirudin differs from lepirudin and bivalirudin in that it is administered SC. As with other hirudin derivatives, bleeding is the most common adverse effect, with incidence similar to that of enoxaparin. Desirudin is indicated for DVT prophylaxis in patients undergoing hip replacement surgery. In clinical studies, patients undergoing hip replacement surgery had fewer thrombotic events with desirudin compared with either heparin 5000 U SC three times daily or enoxaparin 40 mg SC once daily.

There is a risk of epidural, spinal, and neuraxial hematoma formation with desirudin when spinal/epidural anesthesia or spinal puncture is performed, which can result in long-term or permanent paralysis. For this reason, these patients should be frequently monitored for signs and symptoms of neurologic impairment; if present, urgent intervention is necessary.

SPECIAL GROUPS
Race: no data
Children: safety and effectiveness have not been established
Elderly: no specific dosage adjustment needed unless renal function is compromised
Renal impairment: reduce dosage with creatinine clearance ≤60 mL/min
Hepatic impairment: use with caution; no specific dosage adjustments are required, although liver disease may potentiate anticoagulant effects because of impaired production of clotting factors
Pregnancy: category C; use only if potential benefit justifies the potential risk to the fetus
Breast-feeding: not recommended; not known if the drug is excreted in human milk

DOSAGE
15 mg SC every 12 h given for 9–12 d, with the initial dose given up to 5–15 min before surgery but after induction of regional block anesthesia, if used. Use 5 mg SC every 12 h with creatinine clearance 31–60 mL/min, and use 1.7 mg SC every 12 h with creatinine clearance <31 mL/min.

IN BRIEF

INDICATIONS
DVT prophylaxis in patients undergoing elective hip replacement surgery

CONTRAINDICATIONS
Known hypersensitivity to hirudins
Active major bleeding
Irreversible coagulation disorders

DRUG INTERACTIONS
Anticoagulants[1,2]
Antiplatelet drugs[1,2]
NSAIDs[1]
Fibrinolytics[1,2]
1 Effect/toxicity of desirudin may increase.
2 Desirudin may increase the effect/toxicity of this drug.

ADVERSE EFFECTS
Blood: bleeding and clotting disorders
GI: nausea
Skin: hypersensitivity reactions, wound secretion, injection site mass
Severe/rare: anaphylaxis, anaphylactoid reaction

PHARMACOKINETICS AND PHARMACODYNAMICS
Duration of action: 6–12 h
Onset of action: <1 h
Peak plasma concentrations: 1–3 h
Bioavailability: about 100%
Protein binding: not fully defined
Volume of distribution: 0.25 L/kg
Metabolism: metabolized by the kidney by stepwise degradation
Elimination: renal, with 40%–50% excreted in the urine as unchanged drug
Elimination half-life: about 2 h

MONITORING
Lab: monitor aPTT (peak should not exceed 2 times control) daily in patients at increased risk of bleeding and/or in those with renal impairment. Serum creatinine should be monitored daily in patients with renal impairment. Also monitor for clinical evidence of active or occult bleeding.

OVERDOSE
Supportive; no specific antidote is available. Partial reversal of the anticoagulant effect may be achieved with thrombin-rich plasma concentrates and/or desmopressin.

PATIENT INFORMATION
Desirudin may cause excessive bleeding; report any abnormal bleeding to your health care provider.

AVAILABILITY
Vials (single use)—15 mg

ENOXAPARIN SODIUM
(Lovenox®)

Enoxaparin was the first LMWH available in the United States (FDA approved in 1993). Enoxaparin is produced by alkaline degradation of heparin benzyl ester derived from porcine intestinal mucosa. The average molecular weight is about 4500 D. The antithrombotic effect of enoxaparin is primarily the result of its anti–factor Xa activity (anti-Xa/IIa ratio = 2.7–3.9:1). The approximate anti–factor Xa activity is 1000 IU per 10 mg of enoxaparin.

Enoxaparin therapy, 30 mg twice daily or 40 mg once daily given SC, is effective in reducing the risk for DVT and PE in high-risk surgical patients. It is at least as effective and may be more effective than the conventional heparin therapy, 5000 U SC every 8 hours. Clinical data also indicate that enoxaparin administered 1 mg/kg SC every 12 hours or 1.5 mg/kg SC once daily is as effective as heparin for the treatment of patients with DVT or PE. In addition, clinical data demonstrate that in combination with aspirin, enoxaparin administered 1 mg/kg SC every 12 hours is at least as effective and may be more effective than IV heparin therapy in the reduction of ischemic complications, such as death, MI, or recurrent angina in patients with unstable angina or non–Q-wave MI.

Subcutaneous enoxaparin produces a more rapid and predictable antithrombotic effect with fewer monitoring requirements, and is also more convenient than IV heparin therapy. With these advantages and a convenient route of administration, selected patients with uncomplicated DVT may be discharged early and managed at home. It is important to remember that, similar to heparin, bleeding and thrombocytopenia are problems that may be seen with enoxaparin therapy. Enoxaparin should not be administered to patients with a history of HIT (extensive cross-reactivity).

Rare cases of epidural, spinal, and neuraxial hematomas have been reported with the concurrent use of LMWHs and spinal/epidural anesthesia or spinal puncture, which in some cases have resulted in long-term or permanent paralysis. For this reason, these patients should be frequently monitored for signs and symptoms of neurologic impairment; if present, urgent intervention is necessary.

SPECIAL GROUPS

Race: no data
Children: safety and effectiveness have not been established
Elderly: no dosage adjustment is required
Renal impairment: dosage adjustment is recommended in patients with a creatinine clearance <30 mL/min
Hepatic impairment: no dosage adjustment is necessary
Pregnancy: category B; should be used only if clearly indicated
Breast-feeding: not recommended; unknown if the drug is excreted in human milk

IN BRIEF

INDICATIONS
Prophylaxis against DVT that may lead to PE in patients undergoing hip or knee replacement surgery, in high-risk patients undergoing abdominal surgery, and in patients who are at risk for thrombo-embolic complications due to severely restricted mobility during acute illness

Inpatient treatment of DVT with or without PE when used in conjunction with warfarin

Outpatient treatment of DVT without PE when used in conjunction with warfarin

Prevention of ischemic complications in patients with unstable angina or non–Q-wave MI with concurrent aspirin

CONTRAINDICATIONS
Known hypersensitivity to enoxaparin, heparin, or pork
Known (or history of) HIT
Active major bleeding

DRUG INTERACTIONS
Anticoagulants[1,2]
Antiplatelet drugs[1,2]
NSAIDs[1]
Fibrinolytics[1,2]

1 Effect/toxicity of enoxaparin may increase.
2 Enoxaparin may increase the effect/toxicity of this drug.

ADVERSE EFFECTS
Blood: hemorrhage, thrombocytopenia
GI: liver function abnormalities
CNS: epidural or spinal hematoma (with spinal/epidural anesthesia or spinal puncture)
Skin: local irritation, pain, pruritus, urticaria, hematoma, ecchymosis
Rare: anaphylactoid reaction

PHARMACOKINETICS AND PHARMACODYNAMICS
(based on plasma anti–factor Xa activity)
Duration of action: ≥12 h
Onset of action: <30 min
Peak effect: 3–5 h
Bioavailability: 92%
Protein binding: no specific data; less protein binding than UFH
Volume of distribution: 6 L
Elimination: mainly via kidney
Elimination half-life: 4.5 h (range: 3–6 h)

MONITORING
Lab: CBC with platelet count, liver transaminases, anti–factor Xa concentrations if desired (eg, obesity, renal insufficiency). Monitor for clinical evidence of active or occult bleeding.

OVERDOSE
Supportive; the antithrombotic effect may be partially neutralized with protamine.

ENOXAPARIN SODIUM (continued)

DOSAGE

Knee replacement surgery (DVT prophylaxis): 30 mg every 12 h SC for 7–10 d; start 12–24 h after the surgery

Hip replacement surgery (DVT prophylaxis): 30 mg every 12 h started 12–24 h after surgery and continued for 7–10 d or 40 mg once daily SC started 12 h prior to the surgery and continued for 21 d.

Abdominal surgery (DVT prophylaxis): 40 mg once daily SC for 7–10 d; start 2 h prior to surgery

DVT/PE treatment: 1 mg/kg every 12 h (outpatient or inpatient) or 1.5 mg/kg daily (inpatient only) SC; warfarin therapy should be initiated when appropriate, and enoxaparin should be continued for at least 5 d and until the INR is therapeutic for 2 consecutive days

Unstable angina/non–Q-wave MI: 1 mg/kg every 12 h SC for ≥2 d until the patient is clinically stable (with aspirin)

PATIENT INFORMATION

Enoxaparin may cause excessive bleeding and low platelet problems. Report any abnormal bleeding or bruising to your health care provider. Rotate injection sites daily to minimize pain and bruising.

AVAILABILITY

Ampules—30 mg/0.3 mL
Syringes—30 mg/0.3 mL, 40 mg/0.4 mL, 60 mg/0.6 mL, 80 mg/0.8 mL, 100 mg/1 mL, 120 mg/0.8 mL, 150 mg/1 mL
Multiple-dose vials—300 mg/3 mL

FONDAPARINUX SODIUM
(Arixtra®)

Fondaparinux is a synthetic, specific inhibitor of factor Xa. Much like heparin, fondaparinux requires binding of antithrombin for effect, and is therefore an indirect inhibitor of factor Xa. Fondaparinux potentiates the inhibitory effect of antithrombin on factor Xa by about 300 times. Unlike heparin, fondaparinux binds selectively to antithrombin and not to other plasma proteins or to thrombin itself. Fondaparinux also has no effect on platelet function or aPTT and has greater bioavailability and a longer half-life than heparin after SC administration. Its long half-life (17–21 hours) allows for once-daily SC administration. Fondaparinux is indicated for prevention of venous thrombosis and PE following orthopedic surgery and has recently been approved for the treatment of acute DVT and acute PE when used in conjunction with warfarin.

Fondaparinux therapy (2.5 mg SC once daily) has been shown to result in less venous thromboembolism than enoxaparin therapy (30 mg SC twice daily) in patients undergoing elective major knee surgery, although there was more major bleeding with fondaparinux. Another study demonstrated fondaparinux (2.5 mg SC once daily) treatment to result in fewer thromboembolic events compared with enoxaparin (40 mg SC once daily), but with no increased bleeding risk in patients undergoing surgery for femur fracture. Fondaparinux (5–10 mg SC once daily based on weight) has also been shown to be as effective as UFH (continuous IV infusion; aPTT 1.5–2.5 times control) in preventing symptomatic recurrent venous thromboembolism in patients with acute symptomatic PE. Major bleeding was similar between treatments in this study.

There is a risk of epidural, spinal, and neuraxial hematomas when fondaparinux is administered to a patient undergoing epidural/spinal anesthesia or spinal puncture, which can result in long-term or permanent paralysis. For this reason, these patients should be frequently monitored for signs and symptoms of neurologic impairment; if present, urgent intervention is necessary.

SPECIAL GROUPS

Race: no differences in pharmacokinetics between Asians and whites; no differences in clearance observed between blacks and whites
Children: safety and effectiveness have not been established
Elderly: use with caution; bleeding risk is higher in elderly patients
Renal impairment: clearance is reduced, and bleeding risk increases with a decrease in renal function; fondaparinux is contraindicated with creatinine clearance <30 mL/min; use with caution with creatinine clearance 30–50 mL/min
Hepatic impairment: no data
Pregnancy: category B; should only be used if clearly indicated
Breast-feeding: not recommended; unknown if the drug is excreted in human milk

DOSAGE
2.5 mg SC once daily. The initial dose should be given 6–8 h after surgery and continued for 5–9 d (32 d for hip fracture surgery).

IN BRIEF

INDICATIONS
Prophylaxis of DVT, which may lead to PE in patients undergoing:
Hip fracture surgery
Hip replacement surgery
Knee replacement surgery
Treatment of acute DVT when administered in conjunction with warfarin sodium
Treatment of acute PE when administered in conjunction with warfarin sodium when initial therapy is administered in the hospital

CONTRAINDICATIONS
Severe renal impairment (creatinine clearance <30 mL/min)
Total body weight <50 kg (increased bleeding risk)
Active major bleeding
Bacterial endocarditis
Thrombocytopenia associated with a positive in vitro test for antiplatelet antibody in the presence of fondaparinux
Known hypersensitivity to fondaparinux

DRUG INTERACTIONS
Anticoagulants[1,2]
Antiplatelet drugs[1,2]
Fibrinolytics[1,2]

1 Effect/toxicity of fondaparinux may increase.
2 Fondaparinux may increase the effect/toxicity of this drug.

ADVERSE EFFECTS
Blood: bleeding, thrombocytopenia, anemia
GI: nausea, vomiting, diarrhea, dyspepsia, constipation, elevated serum transaminases
Cardiac: hypotension
CNS: dizziness, confusion, headache, pain
Skin: rash, purpura, bullous eruption, hematoma, surgical site reaction, injection site pain/irritation
Other: hypersensitivity reaction, pain (generalized)

PHARMACOKINETICS AND PHARMACODYNAMICS
(based on plasma anti–factor Xa activity)
Duration of action: 2–4 d
Onset of action: not fully defined; absorption is rapid following SC administration
Peak effect: 3 h
Bioavailability: 100%
Protein binding: minimal
Volume of distribution: 7–11 L
Metabolism: not investigated; excreted unchanged in urine
Elimination: primarily in the urine as unchanged drug (77% of a dose)
Elimination half-life: 17–21 h

MONITORING
Lab: CBC with platelet count, serum creatinine. Anti–factor Xa concentrations may be performed if desired. Monitor for clinical evidence of active or occult bleeding.

OVERDOSE
Supportive; no known antidote.

PATIENT INFORMATION
Fondaparinux may cause excessive bleeding; report any abnormal bleeding or bruising to your health care provider. Inject into fatty tissue and rotate injection sites to minimize bruising and discomfort.

AVAILABILITY
Single-dose prefilled syringe—2.5 mg/0.5 mL

LEPIRUDIN (Refludan®)

Lepirudin is a recombinant hirudin derived from yeast cells. Hirudin is a 65–amino acid thrombin inhibitor produced by the medicinal leech *Hirudo medicinalis*. Lepirudin is identical in structure to naturally occurring hirudin except for the substitution of leucine for isoleucine at the N-terminal end and the absence of a sulfate group on the tyrosine at position 63 of the molecule. Lepirudin is a direct thrombin inhibitor, irreversibly binding and inhibiting both free and clot-bound thrombin. This leads to a dose-dependent elevation of the aPTT. Its antithrombotic effect is not dependent on cofactors such as antithrombin. Lepirudin is not inhibited by activated platelets or other proteins known to neutralize heparin in vivo. As a result, lepirudin provides a more stable and predictable level of anticoagulation than does heparin. However, the irreversible binding of lepirudin to thrombin may increase bleeding risk, thereby limiting the more widespread use of this agent. The OASIS-2 trial demonstrated fewer short-term cardiovascular morbidities in patients with non–ST-segment elevation acute coronary syndromes receiving lepirudin versus heparin, albeit at the cost of more bleeding episodes. Lepirudin is indicated and primarily used for the management of patients with documented type II HIT.

SPECIAL GROUPS

Race: no data
Children: safety and effectiveness have not been established, although it has been safely used in two cases
Elderly: dose should be adjusted based on creatinine clearance
Renal impairment: dose reduction with more frequent monitoring if creatinine clearance is ≤60 mL/min or serum creatinine is >1.5 mg/dL
Hepatic impairment: no specific dosage adjustments are required, although more frequent aPTT monitoring is recommended with serious liver injury
Pregnancy: category B; should only be used if clearly indicated
Breast-feeding: not recommended; not known if the drug is excreted in human milk

DOSAGE

Bolus dose: 0.4 mg/kg (up to 44 mg) over 15–20 sec IV; 0.2 mg/kg with renal insufficiency or with concomitant fibrinolytic therapy.
Maintenance: 0.15 mg/kg/h (up to 16.5 mg/h) IV; adjusted based on aPTT (measured 4 h after bolus and at least once daily). The target aPTT is 1.5–2.5 times control. Treatment should be continued for 2–10 d or longer if indicated. Maintenance dosage should be reduced in patients with concurrent fibrinolytic therapy or renal insufficiency.
Concurrent warfarin therapy: Reduce lepirudin dose to reach an aPTT ratio just above 1.5 before first dose of warfarin. After 4–5 d and once an INR of 2 is achieved, lepirudin therapy should be discontinued.

IN BRIEF

INDICATIONS
Prevention of further thromboembolic complications in patients with HIT and associated thromboembolic disease

CONTRAINDICATIONS
Known hypersensitivity to hirudins
End-stage renal disease
Active major bleeding
Baseline aPTT ratio ≥2.5

DRUG INTERACTIONS
Anticoagulants[1,2]
Antiplatelet drugs[1,2]
NSAIDs[1]
Fibrinolytics[1,2]
1 Effect/toxicity of lepirudin may increase.
2 Lepirudin may increase the effect/toxicity of this drug.

ADVERSE EFFECTS
Blood: bleeding and clotting disorders
GI: liver function abnormalities
Skin: rash, pruritus, urticaria, flushes, chills
Severe/rare: anaphylaxis, anaphylactoid reaction, multiorgan failure

PHARMACOKINETICS AND PHARMACODYNAMICS
Duration of action: no data
Onset of action: rapid
Peak effect: 4 h
Protein binding: no data
Volume of distribution: 12.2–32.1 L
Metabolism: metabolized by release of amino acids via catabolic hydrolysis of the parent drug
Elimination: renal, with 35% excreted in the urine as unchanged drug
Elimination half-life: 1.3 h

MONITORING
Lab: aPTT ratio (1.5–2.5). Clinical evidence of active or occult bleeding.

OVERDOSE
Supportive; no specific antidote is available.

PATIENT INFORMATION
Lepirudin may cause excessive bleeding; blood tests will be monitored frequently to minimize this risk.

AVAILABILITY
Vials—50 mg

TINZAPARIN SODIUM (Innohep®)

Tinzaparin is the most recently approved LMWH in the United States (approved in 2000). It is derived through bacterial enzymatic degradation of UFH of porcine origin. It has an average molecular weight of 5500 to 7500 D and an anti–factor Xa/IIa ratio of 1.5–2.0:1. Tinzaparin is indicated only for the treatment of DVT with or without PE, and is at least as effective, and perhaps more effective, than IV heparin in this regard. Tinzaparin has been studied primarily for inpatient use. Tinzaparin has also been used for DVT prevention, with efficacy comparable to both enoxaparin and heparin, although the risk of bleeding may be higher with tinzaparin. The utility of tinzaparin for the treatment of acute coronary syndromes is unknown. Because of the potential for cross-reactivity, tinzaparin should be avoided in patients with a history of HIT.

Rare cases of epidural, spinal, and neuraxial hematomas have been reported with the concurrent use of LMWHs and spinal/epidural anesthesia or spinal puncture, which in some cases has resulted in long-term or permanent paralysis. For this reason, these patients should be frequently monitored for signs and symptoms of neurologic impairment; if present, urgent intervention is necessary.

SPECIAL GROUPS

Race: no data
Children: safety and effectiveness have not been established
Elderly: no data, dosage adjustment not required unless renal function is compromised
Renal impairment: reduced drug clearance, use with caution
Hepatic impairment: no data, dosage adjustment not necessary, but use with caution
Pregnancy: category B; should be used only if clearly indicated
Breast-feeding: not recommended; unknown if the drug is excreted in human milk

DOSAGE

1) **DVT treatment (inpatient):** 175 IU/kg SC once daily for at least 6 days. Warfarin should be started when appropriate and tinzaparin discontinued when an INR of at least 2.0 has been achieved for 2 consecutive days.
2) **DVT prophylaxis (not FDA approved):** 3500 IU (moderate risk) or 50 IU/kg (high risk) SC once daily for 5–10 d starting 1–2 h prior to surgery.
Alternative regimen for patients undergoing orthopedic surgery (hip or knee replacement): 75 IU/kg SC once daily begun 12–24 h postoperatively or 4500 IU SC given 12 h prior to surgery followed by 4500 IU SC once daily thereafter for 5–10 days.

IN BRIEF

INDICATIONS
Treatment of acute symptomatic DVT with or without PE when administered in conjunction with warfarin. Tinzaparin has primarily been studied in hospitalized patients.

CONTRAINDICATIONS
Known hypersensitivity to tinzaparin, heparin, sulfites, benzyl alcohol, or pork
Known (or history of) HIT
Active major bleeding

DRUG INTERACTIONS
Anticoagulants[1,2]
Antiplatelet drugs[1,2]
NSAIDs[1]
Fibrinolytics[1,2]

1 Effect/toxicity of tinzaparin may increase.
2 Tinzaparin may increase the effect/toxicity of this drug.

ADVERSE EFFECTS
Blood: hemorrhage, thrombocytopenia
GI: liver function abnormalities
CNS: epidural or spinal hematoma (especially with spinal/epidural anesthesia or spinal puncture)
Skin: local irritation, pruritus, rash, pain, bullous eruption, necrosis
Other: hypersensitivity reaction, fever, anaphylactoid reaction, chest pain

PHARMACOKINETICS AND PHARMACODYNAMICS
(based on plasma anti–factor Xa activity)
Duration of action: 12–24 h
Onset of action: 2–3 h
Peak effect: 4–5 h
Bioavailability: 87%
Protein binding: no specific data; less protein binding than UFH
Volume of distribution: 3.1–5.0 L
Elimination: mainly renal
Elimination half-life: 3–4 h

MONITORING
Lab: CBC with platelet count, anti–factor Xa concentrations if desired (eg, obesity, renal insufficiency), liver transaminases. Monitor for clinical evidence of active or occult bleeding.

OVERDOSE
Supportive; the antithrombotic effect may be partially neutralized with protamine.

PATIENT INFORMATION
Tinzaparin may cause excessive bleeding; report any abnormal bleeding or bruising to your health care provider. Rotate injection sites daily to minimize pain and bruising.

AVAILABILITY
Multiple-dose vials: 20,000 anti–factor Xa IU/mL, 2 mL

WARFARIN SODIUM
(Warfarin, Coumadin®)

In the United States, warfarin is used almost exclusively when oral anticoagulation is required. It has a relatively narrow therapeutic index, requiring frequent monitoring for efficacy and safety (bleeding). Because warfarin is almost entirely metabolized in the liver, impaired hepatic function may increase sensitivity to the drug. Hepatic impairment also reduces the synthesis of endogenous clotting factors, further enhancing the therapeutic response to warfarin.

Warfarin is used in a wide variety of clinical situations for preventing complications of thromboembolism, and is a first-line agent in most cases (Table 6.3). Ximelagatran is an investigational oral thrombin inhibitor nearing the end of clinical trials. If approved for use, over time it will compete with warfarin for many of these indications.

Warfarin is available in generic formulations, and close INR monitoring is required when switching a patient from one brand of warfarin to another. Drug interactions with warfarin are plentiful and may be attributed to several mechanisms, such as a reduction in warfarin metabolism or clearance (increases warfarin effect), displacement of warfarin from plasma protein binding sites (increases warfarin effect), or an increase in warfarin metabolism (decreases warfarin effect). Patients on warfarin should be educated on the importance of consulting with a health care provider every time a new medication (even nonprescription) is begun.

The importance of genetics on warfarin metabolism has recently been, and is continuing to be, discovered. Warfarin is metabolized by several cytochrome P-450 (CYP) isoenzymes, and there is great interindividual variability in warfarin metabolism. Genetic variations of the CYP2C9 isoenzyme have recently been implicated in explaining, at least in part, some of the variability in individual responses to this drug.

The most serious risks associated with warfarin are hemorrhage in any tissue or organ and, less frequently, necrosis or gangrene of the skin and other tissues. The risk of hemorrhage is related to the intensity and the duration of anticoagulation. The effect of warfarin may be successfully reversed using exogenous vitamin K. Hemorrhage and tissue necrosis have, in some cases, been reported to result in death or permanent disability. Skin necrosis appears to be associated with local thrombosis and usually appears within a few days of the start of anticoagulant therapy. Anticoagulant therapy with warfarin may also enhance the release of atheromatous plaque emboli. This may increase the risk of systemic cholesterol microembolization, including purple toe syndrome. Some cases have progressed to extensive tissue necrosis or death.

IN BRIEF

INDICATIONS
Prophylaxis and treatment:
  Venous thrombosis
  PE
Prevention of thromboembolic complications:
  Atrial fibrillation
  Cardiac valve replacement
  MI

CONTRAINDICATIONS
Known hypersensitivity
Pregnancy
Recent surgery or trauma involving brain, eye, or spinal cord
Active major bleeding
Blood dyscrasias/hemorrhagic tendencies
Arterial aneurysm
Severe hypertension
Endocarditis, pericarditis, or pericardial effusions
Threatened abortion, eclampsia, and preeclampsia
Inadequate laboratory facilities
Unsupervised patients who cannot take care of themselves, or other lack of patient cooperation
Spinal puncture and other procedures with potential for uncontrollable bleeding
Major regional, lumbar block anesthesia

DRUG INTERACTIONS
Many drugs may affect the response to warfarin. It is important to monitor the patient closely when any alterations in a patient medication profile occur. All patients on warfarin should be educated as to the importance of informing their health care providers when new medications (even nonprescription and herbal products) are being started.
Agents that may increase warfarin's effect:

Acetaminophen	Methylphenidate
Alcohol (acute)	Metronidazole
Allopurinol	Miconazole
Amiodarone	Nalidixic acid
Aminoglycosides	Neomycin, oral
Anabolic steroids	NSAIDs
Antiplatelet drugs	Omeprazole
Cimetidine	Paroxetine
Clarithromycin	Pentoxifylline
Clofibrate	Propafenone
COX-2 inhibitors	Propoxyphene
Disulfiram	Propranolol
Erythromycin	Propylthiouracil
Ethacrynic acid	Quinidine
Fibrinolytics	Quinine
Fluoroquinolones	Sertraline
Fluoxetine	Sulfamethoxazole-trimethoprim
Fluvoxamine	Sulfonamides
Furosemide	Tamoxifen
Gemfibrozil	Tetracycline
Glucagon	Thiazides
Heparin	Thyroid drugs
Hydroxy-methylglutaryl coenzyme A (HMG-CoA) reductase inhibitors	Tricyclic antidepressants Valproate Vitamin E
Influenza virus vaccine	Zafirlukast
Isoniazid	Zileuton
Methyldopa	

WARFARIN SODIUM (continued)

Special Note: The Sixth American College of Chest Physicians (ACCP) Consensus Conference on Antithrombotic Therapy (2001) provides recommendations for therapeutic ranges for oral anticoagulant therapy. An INR of 2.5 is recommended for all indications, with the exception of mechanical prosthetic heart valves and recurrent MI, for which an INR of 3.0 is recommended (Table 6.3). The recommendations for therapeutic ranges are provided as INR values instead of prothrombin time (PT) ratios because the variations in responsiveness of commercial thromboplastins are so wide that the term *typical North American thromboplastin* is no longer valid. The INR is calculated as the (observed patient PT/normal PT) ^{ISI}, where ISI is the International Sensitivity Index for the relevant thromboplastin used in the test. All laboratories today should report the INR value of each measured PT.

SPECIAL GROUPS

Race: Asians appear to be more sensitive than whites to the effect of warfarin

Children: safety and effectiveness have not been established, although warfarin has been successfully given to children. In these cases, more frequent INR determinations are recommended.

Elderly: tend to be more sensitive to warfarin effect; dose based on INR results; may require smaller initial doses

Renal impairment: renal function does not significantly affect warfarin clearance; nonetheless, use with caution and dose based on INR results

Hepatic impairment: liver dysfunction may intensify the effects of warfarin through inhibition of metabolism and reduced production of clotting factors; therefore, use with caution and dose based on INR results

Pregnancy: category X; should not be used

Breast-feeding: excreted in human milk as inactive metabolites; infants nursed by warfarin-treated mothers have slight elevations in PT/INR, although this is of unknown consequence; use warfarin cautiously in this situation, with more frequent INR monitoring to help ensure that recommended INRs are not exceeded.

DRUG INTERACTIONS (CONTINUED)

Agents that may decrease warfarin's effect:

Alcohol (chronic use)	Glutethimide
Aminoglutethimide	Haloperidol
Barbiturates	Mercaptopurine
Carbamazepine	Nafcillin
Chlordiazepoxide	Rifampin
Cholestyramine	Spironolactone
Clozapine	Sucralfate
Corticotropin	Thiazide diuretics
Cyclosporine	Trazodone
Estrogen-containing products	Vitamin K

Agents that may either increase or decrease warfarin's effect:

Corticosteroids	Phenytoin
Cyclophosphamide	Propylthiouracil
Methimazole	Ranitidine

ADVERSE EFFECTS

Blood: bleeding, leukopenia, agranulocytosis, cholesterol microembolization, purple toe syndrome

GI: nausea, vomiting, anorexia, diarrhea, abdominal pain, elevated liver function tests

Skin: dermatitis, urticaria, alopecia, skin necrosis or gangrene, subcutaneous infarction, vasculitis, and local thrombosis

Other: fever, hypersensitivity

PHARMACOKINETICS AND PHARMACODYNAMICS

Duration of action: 4–5 d
Onset of action: 1–3 d
Peak effect: 3–6 d
Bioavailability: 78%–100%
Effect of food: food may decrease the rate but not the extent of absorption; foods rich in vitamin K may interfere with the effect of warfarin
Protein binding: 97%–99%
Volume of distribution: small; about 0.14 L/kg
Metabolism: metabolized by hepatic microsomal enzymes to metabolites with little or no anticoagulant effect
Elimination: excreted in the urine mainly as inactive metabolites
Elimination half-life: 20–60 h

MONITORING

Lab: CBC, liver function, PT, and INR. Monitor for clinical evidence of active or occult bleeding.

OVERDOSE

Supportive; for major bleeding, vitamin K may be used to reverse the effect of warfarin (Table 6.4). For significant blood loss, whole blood transfusion, fresh frozen plasma, or clotting factor concentrates may be administered.

WARFARIN SODIUM *(continued)*

DOSAGE

Adults: Dosage is highly individualized; initiate with 2–5 mg/d for 2–4 d; adjust dose to maintain desired therapeutic INRs per recommendation by the ACCP (Tables 6.3 and 6.4).

The dose of warfarin injection is the same as the oral dose and should only be administered IV. The dose should be given as a slow bolus over 1–2 min.

TABLE 6.3 RECOMMENDED INTERNATIONAL NORMALIZED RATIO (INR) RANGES FOR PATIENTS RECEIVING WARFARIN

Indication	INR range
Prophylaxis of venous thrombosis (high-risk surgery)	2.0–3.0
Treatment of venous thrombosis	
Treatment of PE	
Prevention of systemic embolism	
Tissue heart valves	
Acute MI	
Valvular heart disease	
Atrial fibrillation	
Mechanical prosthetic valves (high risk)	2.5–3.5
Bileaflet mechanical valve in the aortic position	2.0–3.0
Certain patients with thrombosis and the antiphospholipid syndrome	>2.0–3.0
Recurrent MI	2.5–3.5

MI—myocardial infarction; PE—pulmonary embolism.

From The Sixth ACCP Consensus Conference on Antithrombotic Therapy: *Quick Reference Guide for Clinicians.* Northbrook, IL: American College of Chest Physicians; 2001.

TABLE 6.4 MANAGEMENT OF PATIENTS WITH HIGH INTERNATIONAL NORMALIZED RATIO (INR) VALUES

Situation	Recommendation
INR >therapeutic range but <5.0; no significant bleeding	Lower the dose or omit the next dose, and resume therapy at a lower dose when the INR is within therapeutic range; if the INR is only slightly above therapeutic range, dose reduction may not be necessary.
INR >5.0 but <9.0; no significant bleeding	Omit the next dose or two, monitor INR more frequently, and resume therapy at a lower dose when the INR is within therapeutic range.
	Alternatively, omit a dose and give vitamin K (1–2.5 mg PO), especially if the patient is at increased risk for bleeding.
	Patients requiring more rapid reversal before urgent surgery: vitamin K (2–4 mg PO); if INR remains high after 24 h, give an additional dose of vitamin K (1–2 mg PO).
INR >9.0; no significant bleeding	Omit warfarin; give vitamin K (3–5 mg PO); closely monitor INR; if the INR is not substantially reduced in 24–48 h, monitor the INR more often, giving additional vitamin K if necessary.
	Resume therapy at a lower dose when the INR is within therapeutic range.
INR >20; serious bleeding	Omit warfarin; give vitamin K (10 mg by slow IV infusion) supplemented with fresh plasma or prothrombin complex concentrate, depending on urgency; repeat vitamin K if necessary, depending on the INR.
Life-threatening bleeding	Omit warfarin; give prothrombin complex concentrate with vitamin K (10 mg by slow IV infusion); repeat if necessary, depending on the INR.

IV—intravenous; PO—by mouth.

From The Sixth ACCP Consensus Conference on Antithrombotic Therapy: *Quick Reference Guide for Clinicians.* Northbrook, IL: American College of Chest Physicians; 2001.

The information here is provided as guidance only. Prescribers should always consult the manufacturer's current prescribing information.

With the increased awareness that blood platelets play an important role in the pathogenesis of arterial vaso-occlusive conditions (Figure 6.1), interest in antiplatelet therapy has increased markedly. The chief function of platelets is to interact with vascular endothelium and soluble plasma factors in the hemostatic process. Under normal physiologic conditions, platelets are mostly inert. Their adhesion to the subendothelial matrix is prevented by an intact vascular wall. In response to vessel trauma, platelets adhere to newly exposed adhesive proteins, forming a protective monolayer of cells. Within seconds, these platelets are activated by agonists such as thrombin, collagen, and adenosine diphosphate (ADP), causing them to change shape and release stored vesicles. The constituents of the vesicles are mostly involved in the further activation of platelets and the propagation of the hemostatic process. Ultimately these activated platelets aggregate to form a hemostatic plug—closing the lesion in the endothelium and preventing further loss of blood from the site. Under certain pathologic conditions (*ie*, rupture of an atherosclerotic plaque), these platelet aggregates can form thrombi leading to cardiovascular ischemic events, including unstable angina and MI.

Aspirin, the ADP receptor blockers (**ticlopidine, clopidogrel**), and the GP IIb/IIIa integrin receptor antagonists (**abciximab, eptifibatide, tirofiban**), are the major antiplatelet agents used clinically. **Dipyridamole** and **cilostazol** have limited indications and are used less frequently.

EFFICACY AND USE

The value of antiplatelet therapy on cardiovascular morbidity and mortality has been established largely through the clinical use of **aspirin**. The long-acting antiplatelet effect of **aspirin** can be achieved with low doses that avoid many of the side effects associated with its use in inflammatory disorders. **Aspirin** is recommended as prophylaxis against thrombotic events in patients with TIA, ischemic stroke, coronary artery disease (CAD), atrial fibrillation, prosthetic heart valves, and/or hip fracture surgery, as well as in patients undergoing revascularization procedures.

The antithrombotic activity of **dipyridamole** is more evident when artificial surfaces (prosthetic heart valves, grafts, cannulae) are involved. **Dipyridamole**'s effects are more obvious on synthetic surfaces than on biologic ones, and so, despite a beneficial trend in decreasing vascular events after MI and in reducing occlusion rates in coronary artery grafts, it has no proven benefit in CAD or stroke. **Dipyridamole** may work synergistically with **warfarin** or **aspirin**. There is little role for **dipyridamole** in cardiovascular medicine, with the major use of this drug being in combination with **aspirin** for secondary stroke prevention.

Cilostazol has been studied primarily in patients with intermittent claudication, and is only approved for alleviating symptoms in patients with this condition. **Ticlopidine** and **clopidogrel** have been shown to be effective in many situations in

which altered platelet function plays a pathologic role. They are used primarily in combination with **aspirin** in preventing thrombotic events after coronary artery angioplasty and stenting or for other indications as an alternative to **aspirin** in patients intolerant of **aspirin**.

The binding of fibrinogen to activated platelets (Figure 6.2) has been identified as the final step in platelet aggregation. This

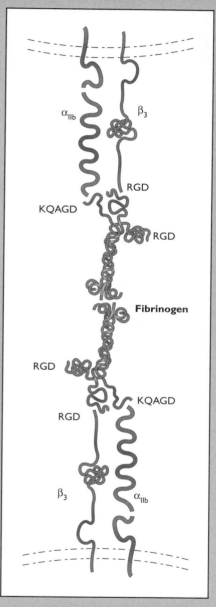

FIGURE 6.2
Glycoprotein IIb/IIIa structure and interactions binding platelets by divalent fibrinogen. (*Adapted from* Colman RW *et al.: Hemostasis and Thrombosis: Basic Principles and Clinical Practice.* Philadelphia: Lippincott; 1994:1638–1660.)

binding can be inhibited by the GP IIb/IIIa integrin receptor antagonists. These drugs prevent thrombosis resulting from vessel damage or atherosclerotic plaque rupture, regardless of the extent of platelet activation.

All three currently available GP IIb/IIIa receptor antagonists are administered parenterally. **Abciximab** is used in high-risk PCI, but is not recommended for patients with non–ST-segment elevation acute coronary syndromes in whom PCI is not planned. **Eptifibatide** and **tirofiban** are recommended for use in patients with unstable angina or non–ST-elevation MI and have also shown benefit in patients undergoing elective PCI. Oral GP IIb/IIIa receptor antagonists have been studied, but clinical trials have thus far demonstrated unacceptably high rates of bleeding with these agents.

MODES OF ACTION

Aspirin affects platelet function by acetylating the cyclooxygenase enzyme, thereby preventing formation of thromboxane A_2, a potent stimulant of platelet aggregation. The effect of **aspirin** is irreversible and lasts the lifetime of the affected platelets (about 7–10 days). Its effect on endothelial cell–derived prostacyclin is dose dependent and less prolonged.

The mechanisms of action of **dipyridamole** and **cilostazol** are uncertain but are believed to involve an increase in platelet cyclic adenosine monophosphate (cAMP). cAMP inhibits the release of calcium from the dense tubular reticulum, reduces the secretion of serotonin and ADP, and thereby increases the resistance of the platelet to activation. **Ticlopidine** and **clopidogrel**, thienopyridine compounds, are prodrugs that require in

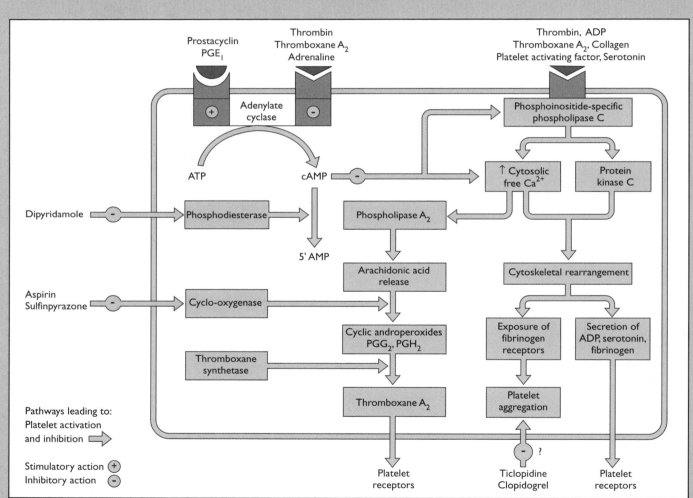

FIGURE 6.3 Sites of action of some of the antiplatelet drugs and the associated mechanisms of platelet activation. Platelet activation results from mobilization of calcium, which in turn results from agonist binding to the platelet receptor. ADP—adenosine diphosphate; AMP—adenosine monophosphate; ATP—adenosine triphosphate; cAMP— cyclic AMP; PGE_1—prostaglandin E_1; PGG_2—prostaglandin G_2; PGH_2—prostaglandin H_2. (*Adapted from* Saltiel E, Ward A: Ticlopidine: a review of its pharmacodynamic and pharmacokinetic properties, and therapeutic efficacy in platelet-dependent disease states. *Drugs* 1987, 34:222–262.)

vivo conversion to the active moieties for antiplatelet effects. These drugs act by blocking ADP receptors within the platelet membrane (Figure 6.3) and act independently of arachidonic acid pathways. The drugs produce a thromboasthenia-like state, resulting in a reduction in platelet aggregation, a prolongation of the bleeding time, a decrease in platelet degranulation, and a reduction in platelet and fibrin deposition on artificial surfaces.

As mentioned earlier, the GP IIb/IIIa receptor antagonists inhibit platelet aggregation by binding to the GP IIb/IIIa receptors of activated platelets and preventing fibrinogen cross-linking between platelets.

INDICATIONS

	Aspirin	Dipyridamole	Ticlopidine	Clopidogrel	GP IIb/IIIa receptor antagonists
Prevention (long-term) of thrombotic complications in patients with previous MI	+	–	–	+	–
Prevention (long-term) of thrombotic complications in patients with unstable angina	+	–	–	(+)*	–
Treatment of acute coronary syndrome	(+)	–	–	+	+
Prevention of thrombotic complications in patients without CAD, but with risk factors for CAD	(+)	–	–	–	–
Secondary prevention of stroke	(+)	+*	+*	+	–
Secondary prevention of cerebrovascular events in patients with TIA	+	+*	+*	(+)	–
Prevention of thrombotic complications in patients with atrial fibrillation	(+)	–	–	–	–
Peripheral vascular disease	–	(+)*	–	+	–
Intermittent claudication	(+)	–	–	(+)	–

*Approved only for limited indications.

+—FDA approved; – —not FDA approved; (+)—clinical uses, not FDA approved; CAD—coronary artery disease; GP—glycoprotein; MI—myocardial infarction; TIA—transient ischemic attacks.

The information here is provided as guidance only. Prescribers should always consult the manufacturer's current prescribing information.

119

ASPIRIN

Aspirin irreversibly binds platelet cyclooxygenase, producing an antiplatelet effect that lasts the life of the platelet (7–10 days). Doses as low as 30 mg have shown antiplatelet effects, although clinically, 81 mg daily is the lowest recommended dosage in the United States. Aspirin has been shown to be effective in both primary and secondary prevention of vascular events in patients with a wide variety of atherosclerotic disease and is recommended for all patients with CAD who do not have a contraindication to therapy. Secondary prevention trials using 300 to 1200 mg daily have consistently demonstrated a decreased incidence of TIA, strokes, and death with aspirin therapy. Aspirin also reduces progression of unstable angina to MI or death and appears to work synergistically with fibrinolytic drugs to improve outcomes.

The ISIS-2 study examined the short-term (5-week) outcome in patients with suspected acute MI randomized to intravenous streptokinase, 162.5 mg enteric-coated aspirin daily, both, or neither. Aspirin was initiated within 24 hours of initial symptoms and continued daily for 5 weeks. The study showed that aspirin substantially decreased nonfatal reinfarction, stroke, and vascular mortality. Streptokinase alone also decreased vascular mortality, and the combination of aspirin and streptokinase decreased vascular mortality more than either drug individually (Figure 6.4).

Studies investigating the effect of aspirin for the treatment of acute ischemic stroke demonstrated a reduction in both stroke recurrence and mortality with aspirin therapy in patients treated within 48 hours of stroke onset.

Aspirin, in dosages of 75 to 325 mg daily, has been shown to be effective for primary prevention of first MI. The Physicians' Health Study, a primary prevention study of 22,071 healthy male physicians, demonstrated a 44% reduction in MI with aspirin therapy (325 mg once every other day; Figure 6.5). However, this was not associated with a reduction in cardiovascular mortality. This finding, coupled with the fact that long-term aspirin therapy is not without risk (ie, GI side effects, hemorrhagic stroke), indicates that primary prevention with aspirin is perhaps not for everybody but may be best reserved for individuals with risk factors for the development of heart disease. There is also evidence that some patients are resistant to the antiplatelet effects of aspirin in therapeutic doses.

Aspirin is a first-line agent for preventing embolic stroke in patients with atrial fibrillation. It is also effective in preventing coronary artery graft reocclusion in patients undergoing coronary bypass surgery and is used in conjunction with a thienopyridine (usually clopidogrel) to prevent ischemic complications following coronary stent placement.

IN BRIEF

INDICATIONS
Only cardiovascular indications are listed (not all indications are FDA approved)
Prevention of thrombotic complications in patients with:
TIA (secondary prevention)
Acute ischemic stroke
MI (acute or previous)
Unstable angina/CAD
Atrial fibrillation
Prosthetic heart valves (with warfarin)
Arteriovenous shunt for hemodialysis
Microcirculatory thrombosis seen in thrombocytosis
Peripheral vascular reconstructive surgery
PCI
Aortocoronary-artery bypass
Other uses: Kawasaki syndrome, diabetic retinopathy, acute pericarditis

CONTRAINDICATIONS
Known hypersensitivity to salicylates or NSAIDs; those with a history of asthma, nasal polyps, or chronic urticaria have a higher prevalence of aspirin hypersensitivity
Active internal bleeding or bleeding diathesis
Hemophilia

DRUG INTERACTIONS
(less problematic with low doses of aspirin)
Urine acidifiers, such as ascorbic acid (vitamin C)[1,5]
Urine alkalinizers, such as antacids[2,5]

Alcohol[1,3]	Probenecid[4]
Angiotensin-converting enzyme inhibitors[4,5]	Valproate[3]
	Carbonic anhydrase inhibitors[1,3,5]
Beta-blockers[4,5]	Anticoagulants[1,3]
Diuretics[4,5]	Other antiplatelet drugs[1,3]
Corticosteroids[2,5]	NSAIDs[1,3]
Methotrexate[3]	Fibrinolytics[1,3]

1 Effect/toxicity of aspirin may increase.
2 Effect of aspirin may decrease.
3 Aspirin may increase the effect/toxicity of this drug.
4 Aspirin may decrease the effect of this drug.
5 For cardiovascular uses, the clinical significance of this interaction is unclear.

ADVERSE EFFECTS
Blood: prolonged bleeding time, blood dyscrasias
GI: nausea, dyspepsia, discomfort, ulceration, bleeding, occult blood loss, liver dysfunction
CNS: tinnitus
Kidney: progressive renal dysfunction, especially in patients with chronic renal insufficiency (rare)
Other: anaphylaxis, bronchospasm, angioedema, hives, rashes, Reye's syndrome

PHARMACOKINETICS AND PHARMACODYNAMICS
Duration of action: platelets are inhibited for 7–10 d, but are also regenerating during this time; the effective duration of antiplatelet action is usually 1–3 d. The analgesic and antipyretic effects last 4–6 h
Onset of action: typically <1 h, but may be 3–4 h for enteric-coated preparations; chewing enteric-coated preparations results in a quicker onset of effect
Peak effect: 1–6 h
Bioavailability: 40%–50%; lower with enteric-coated formulations
Effect of food: decreases the rate/extent of absorption
Protein binding: 33%–90%; concentration dependent (lower doses have more protein binding)
Volume of distribution: 0.15–2.0 L/kg

ASPIRIN (continued)

SPECIAL GROUPS

Race: no differences in response

Children: not recommended in children with acute febrile illness because of the risk for Reye's syndrome

Elderly: no dosage adjustment is required

Renal impairment: use with caution in patients with chronic renal insufficiency because renal function may transiently decrease and aspirin may (rarely) aggravate chronic kidney disease; this effect is more pronounced with higher (analgesic) dosages

Hepatic impairment: use high doses with caution because of the potential for hepatotoxicity

Pregnancy: category D; avoid use in the third trimester of pregnancy, and use only if clearly indicated in the first and second trimesters

Breast-feeding: excreted in human milk; use with caution, although adverse effects on platelet function in the nursing infant have not been reported

DOSAGE

Transient ischemic attack: 1300 mg/d in 2–4 divided doses (males); doses as low as 50 mg/d may be effective

Acute coronary syndrome: 160–325 mg chewed for rapid effect

CAD (chronic prophylaxis): 75–325 mg once daily

See Table 6.5 for additional dosages.

TABLE 6.5 MINIMUM EFFECTIVE DAILY DOSAGE OF ASPIRIN FOR VARIOUS INDICATIONS

Daily dosage	Indication(s)
50 mg	TIA and ischemic stroke*
75 mg	Men at high cardiovascular risk
	Hypertension
	Stable angina
	Unstable angina*
	Severe carotid artery stenosis*
160 mg	Acute myocardial infarction
	Acute ischemic stroke*
325 mg	Atrial fibrillation

*Higher doses have not been found to provide greater risk reduction.

TIA—transient ischemic attack.

Data from The Sixth ACCP Consensus Conference on Antithrombotic Therapy: *Quick Reference Guide for Clinicians.* Northbrook, IL: American College of Chest Physicians; 2001.

PHARMACOKINETICS AND PHARMACODYNAMICS (CONTINUED)

Metabolism: initially hydrolyzed to salicylate in the GI mucosa, the remaining unhydrolyzed aspirin is then almost completely hydrolyzed in liver, plasma, erythrocytes, and synovial fluid

Elimination: in the urine mainly as metabolites; 1% is excreted in the urine as unchanged aspirin

Elimination half-life: about 15–20 min for aspirin; 2–3 h for salicylic acid at low doses; over 20 h with higher anti-inflammatory doses

MONITORING

Clinical evidence of active or occult bleeding (especially if used with other agents that may affect hemostasis); GI intolerance.

OVERDOSE

Manifests first as respiratory alkalosis, hemorrhage, tinnitus and hearing loss, vomiting, oliguria, acute renal failure, behavioral changes, central stimulation followed by central depression, acid–base and electrolyte disturbances, dehydration, hyperpyrexia, and hyperglycemia or hypoglycemia. Symptoms may progress rapidly to depression, coma, and respiratory failure. Treatment may include emptying stomach via induction of emesis or gastric lavage; administering activated charcoal; monitoring and supporting vital function; correcting hypothermia and fluid, electrolyte, and acid–base imbalances; correcting ketosis; and adjusting plasma glucose concentrations as needed.

Monitor serum salicylate concentration until it is apparent that concentration is decreasing to nontoxic range. Induce forced alkaline diuresis to increase salicylate excretion; however, bicarbonate should not be administered orally for this purpose because salicylate absorption may be increased. Also, if acetazolamide is used, the increased risk for severe metabolic acidosis and salicylate toxicity must be considered.

Institute exchange transfusion, hemodialysis, peritoneal dialysis, or hemoperfusion as needed in severe overdose. Monitor for pulmonary edema and convulsions, and institute appropriate therapy if required. Administer blood or vitamin K, if necessary, to treat hemorrhage.

PATIENT INFORMATION

May cause GI irritation (take with food or after meals). Enteric-coated preparations and lower dosages (eg, 81 mg) may reduce GI side effects. Tablet forms should always be administered with a full glass of water, with patient remaining upright for 15–30 min after administration. Tablets should not be placed directly on tooth or gum surface because of possible injury to tissues. No chewing before swallowing for at least 7 d following tonsillectomy or oral surgery. Use caution when taking other medications. Do not take within 3 h of ketoconazole, within 3–4 h of oral tetracycline, or within 2 h of cellulose-containing laxatives. Use caution with other medications containing aspirin or other salicylates (including diflunisal) or when significant quantities of sodium are used. If breathing difficulties (rare), changes in hearing function, rashes, dizziness, or other untoward effects (eg, black, tarry stools or blood in urine) occur, contact your health care provider immediately.

Do not take aspirin 5 d prior to any surgery, unless otherwise directed by a physician.

AVAILABILITY

Tablets—81 mg: chewable tablets, enteric-coated tablets, delayed-release tablets

165 mg: enteric coated tablets

227.5 mg: gum tablets

325 mg: tablets, enteric-coated tablets

500 mg: tablets, enteric-coated tablets

650 mg : enteric-coated tablets, extended-release tablets

800 mg: controlled-release tablets

975 mg: enteric-coated tablets

Rectal suppositories—120 mg, 200 mg, 300 mg, 600 mg

The information here is provided as guidance only. Prescribers should always consult the manufacturer's current prescribing information.

121

ASPIRIN (continued)

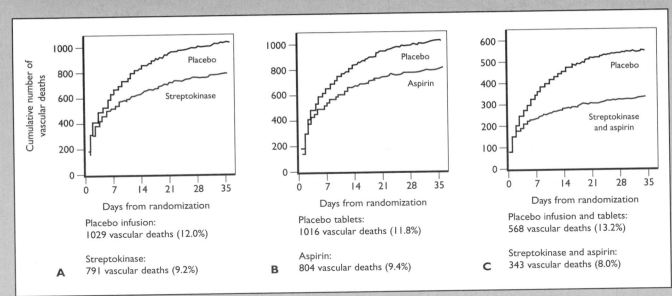

A
Placebo infusion:
1029 vascular deaths (12.0%)

Streptokinase:
791 vascular deaths (9.2%)

B
Placebo tablets:
1016 vascular deaths (11.8%)

Aspirin:
804 vascular deaths (9.4%)

C
Placebo infusion and tablets:
568 vascular deaths (13.2%)

Streptokinase and aspirin:
343 vascular deaths (8.0%)

FIGURE 6.4 Cumulative vascular mortality on days 0 to 35 of the ISIS-2 study. **A**, All patients allocated to receive streptokinase compared with all patients allocated to placebo infusion. **B**, All patients allocated to receive aspirin compared with all patients allocated to placebo tablets. **C**, All patients allocated to both streptok-inase and aspirin regimens compared with all patients allocated to placebo infusion and tablets. (*Adapted from* ISIS 2 Collaborative Group: Randomised trial of intravenous streptokinase, oral aspirin, both or neither among 17,187 cases of suspected acute myocardial infarction. *Lancet* 1988, 2:349–360.)

FIGURE 6.5 Effect of aspirin on primary prevention of myocardial infarction in the US Physicians' Health Study.

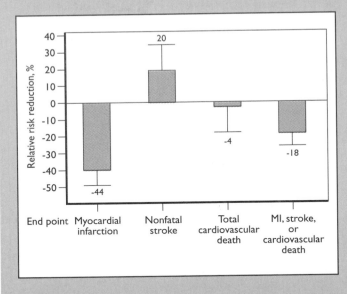

CILOSTAZOL (Pletal®)

Cilostazol, like dipyridamole, is both a vasodilator and an antiplatelet agent. Cilostazol inhibits platelet aggregation by mechanisms that are not completely understood. It is believed that inhibition of phosphodiesterase III (PDE III) is somewhat responsible. PDE III breaks down cAMP, and PDE III inhibition therefore increases cAMP concentrations in platelets and blood vessels, leading to vasodilation and inhibition of platelet aggregation. Cilostazol also may inhibit smooth muscle cell proliferation as well as favorably affect the lipid profile (approximately 10% increase in high-density lipoprotein cholesterol, 15% decrease in triglycerides).

Cilostazol has been shown to improve pain-free and maximal treadmill walking distance and functional status when compared with placebo in patients with intermittent claudication. In these same types of patients, cilostazol has also been shown to be more effective than pentoxifylline in improving walking distance.

Cilostazol is metabolized by hepatic cytochrome P-450 3A4 (CYP3A4), and medications that inhibit CYP3A4 may therefore increase serum cilostazol concentrations. Headache is the most common side effect, occurring in 34% of patients taking 100 mg twice daily (14% incidence with placebo). Cilostazol has been used in combination with aspirin, without a noticeable increase in hemorrhagic events.

Cilostazol carries a black-box warning not to use this medication in patients with heart failure. This is because other PDE III inhibitors (inamrinone and milrinone) that have been studied for the treatment of chronic heart failure have demonstrated increases in mortality in patients with this condition. Cilostazol differs from these medications in that it does not have as much positive inotropic effect, although it shares the vasodilating and antiplatelet properties of the other PDE III inhibitors. Clinical studies involving more than 2000 patients followed for up to 6 months showed cardiovascular death and MI to occur in 0.6% and 1.5% of patients receiving cilostazol and 0.5% and 1.1% of patients receiving placebo, respectively.

SPECIAL GROUPS

Race: no data
Children: safety and effectiveness have not been established
Elderly: safety and efficacy similar to younger patients; no dose adjustment is necessary
Renal impairment: no major pharmacokinetic differences between patients with and without renal insufficiency; no need to reduce dose
Hepatic impairment: no data; dosage adjustment is probably not required
Pregnancy: category C; use only if potential benefit justifies the potential risk to the fetus
Breast-feeding: not recommended; transfer of cilostazol into milk has been shown in rats, but it is unknown whether the drug is excreted in human milk

IN BRIEF

INDICATION
Reduction in symptoms of intermittent claudication

CONTRAINDICATIONS
Known hypersensitivity to any of the product components
CHF of any severity

DRUG INTERACTIONS
Anticoagulants[1,2]
Azole antifungals (ketoconazole, fluconazole, itraconazole, miconazole)[1]
Diltiazem[1]
Erythromycin and other macrolide antibiotics[1]
Fluoxetine[1]
Fluvoxamine[1]
Nefazadone[1]
Omeprazole[1]
Other antiplatelets[1,2]
Sertraline[1]
Fibrinolytics[1,2]

1 Effect/toxicity of cilostazol may increase.
2 Cilostazol may increase the effect/toxicity of this drug.

ADVERSE EFFECTS
CV: palpitation, tachycardia
Pulmonary: increased cough, pharyngitis, rhinitis
CNS: headache, dizziness
GI: abdominal pain, diarrhea, dyspepsia, abnormal stools, flatulence, nausea
Other: back pain, peripheral edema, myalgia

PHARMACOKINETICS AND PHARMACODYNAMICS
Duration of action:	no data
Onset of action:	2–4 wk for symptomatic relief; may take 12 wk in some patients
Peak plasma concentrations:	about 2 h
Bioavailability:	unknown
Effect of food:	high-fat meal increases absorption
Protein binding:	95%–98%, predominantly to albumin
Volume of distribution:	no data
Metabolism:	extensive metabolism by hepatic cytochrome P-450 enzymes, mainly 3A4. Two active metabolites, with one metabolite accounting for at least 50% of the pharmacologic effect of the drug.
Elimination:	eliminated primarily by metabolism and subsequent urinary excretion of metabolites (74% of a 100 mg dose); 20% excreted in the feces
Elimination half-life:	11–13 h

MONITORING
Drug–drug interactions (see above); side effects such as headache and GI distress.

OVERDOSE
Supportive; unlikely to be removed by dialysis.

CILOSTAZOL *(continued)*

DOSAGE

The recommended dose is 100 mg twice daily, taken at least 30 min before or 2 h after breakfast and dinner. Clinical response may be observed after 2-4 wk from initiation of therapy. However, treatment for up to 12 wk may be needed before a beneficial effect is experienced. The dose should be reduced to 50 mg twice daily when cilostazol is coadministered with CYP3A4 or 2C19 inhibitors such as ketoconazole, itraconazole, erythromycin, diltiazem, and omeprazole. Because CYP3A4 is also inhibited by grapefruit juice, this beverage should also be avoided in patients receiving cilostazol.

PATIENT INFORMATION

It typically takes several weeks, and may take up to 3 months, for relief of symptoms. Cilostazol should be taken at least 30 min before or 2 h after eating.

AVAILABILITY

Tablets—50, 100 mg

DIPYRIDAMOLE
(Dipyridamole, Persantine®)

Dipyridamole, like cilostazol, is both a vasodilator and an inhibitor of platelet aggregation. Also similar to cilostazol, the mechanism of action of dipyridamole is largely unknown but is believed to involve inhibition of PDE.

The role of dipyridamole in current clinical practice is somewhat nebulous. When used as monotherapy, dipyridamole does not improve the survival of patients with acute MI, reduce the incidence of postoperative DVT, or produce beneficial effects in patients suffering from TIA. When combined with anticoagulant drugs, there is evidence of added benefit, especially in patients undergoing vascular grafts or those with prosthetic heart valves. When used in combination with other antiplatelet drugs, there is no convincing evidence that dipyridamole has contributed significantly to the benefit derived, except possibly when artificial grafts may have contributed to the risk of thrombosis. The European Stroke Prevention Study 2 (ESPS 2) demonstrated extended-release dipyridamole plus aspirin to be superior to either drug alone in reducing the risk of stroke in patients who had experienced a prior stroke or TIA. The combination reduced stroke risk by 22%, 24%, and 37% compared with aspirin alone, extended-release dipyridamole alone, and placebo, respectively.

The vasodilating properties of dipyridamole are exploited during pharmacologic cardiac stress testing. In this setting, dipyridamole is injected IV to dilate coronary arteries and increase myocardial perfusion.
Special Note: This monograph relates only to oral dipyridamole.

SPECIAL GROUPS
Race: no differences in response
Children: safety and effectiveness have not been established in children under 12 y of age
Elderly: no dose adjustment necessary
Renal impairment: renal elimination is relatively minor; no need to reduce dose
Hepatic impairment: no data; dosage adjustment is probably not required
Pregnancy: category B; should be used only if clearly indicated
Breast-feeding: use with caution; excreted in breast milk

DOSAGE
75–100 mg four times daily (as an adjunct to warfarin therapy)
One capsule (200 mg extended-release dipyridamole + 25 mg aspirin) twice daily (Aggrenox®)

IN BRIEF

INDICATIONS
Prophylaxis of thromboembolism after cardiac valve replacement (as an adjunct to warfarin therapy)
In combination with aspirin to reduce the risk of stroke in patients with a prior history of ischemic stroke or TIA (Aggrenox®)

CONTRAINDICATIONS
Known hypersensitivity to product components

DRUG INTERACTIONS
Adenosine[2]
Anticoagulants[2,4]
Antihypertensives[2]
Antiplatelet drugs[1,2,4]
Cholinesterase inhibitors[3]
Fibrinolytics[2,4]

1 Effect/toxicity of dipyridamole may increase.
2 Dipyridamole may increase the effect/toxicity of this drug.
3 Dipyridamole may decrease the effect of this drug.
4 The clinical significance of this interaction is unclear.

ADVERSE EFFECTS (usually minimal and transient)
CV: hypotension, flushing, angina
CNS: headache, dizziness, syncope
GI: abdominal distress, nausea, vomiting, diarrhea
Skin: rash, pruritus

PHARMACOKINETICS AND PHARMACODYNAMICS
Duration of action: no data
Onset of action: no data
Peak plasma concentrations: 75 min (range, 45–150 min)
Bioavailability: 37%–66%
Effect of food: no data
Protein binding: 91%–99%
Volume of distribution: no data
Metabolism/elimination: metabolized in the liver, excreted in the bile, and eliminated in feces; small amount is eliminated in urine
Elimination half-life: 40–80 min (initial phase); 10–12 h (terminal phase)

MONITORING
Blood pressure (BP), heart rate, and clinical evidence of active or occult bleeding (especially if used with warfarin).

OVERDOSE
Supportive; hypotension is the main concern; fluid and pressor support may be used if necessary; not dialyzable.

PATIENT INFORMATION
Dipyridamole may produce GI discomfort (take with food, preferably before meals). It may also cause dizziness, headache, weakness, or flushing. If chest pain increases, contact your health care provider immediately. Do not chew or crush sustained-release capsules (Aggrenox®).

AVAILABILITY
Tablets—25, 50,75 mg
Combination formulation:
Aggrenox®—extended-release dipyridamole 200 mg/aspirin 25 mg

CLOPIDOGREL BISULFATE
(Plavix®)

Clopidogrel, a thienopyridine derivative, inhibits ADP-induced platelet aggregation. Clopidogrel is a prodrug with no direct antiplatelet activity in vitro. It is believed to be metabolized by hepatic cytochromes P-450 3A4 and 3A5 to its active form. Although chemically similar to ticlopidine, clopidogrel causes less neutropenia (<1200 neutrophils/µL) or agranulocytosis.

Clopidogrel has shown clinical benefits in patients with atherosclerotic vascular disease, patients with non–ST-segment elevation acute coronary syndromes, and patients who have just undergone PCI. The Clopidogrel Versus Aspirin in Patients at Risk of Ischemic Events (CAPRIE) trial demonstrated that clopidogrel was more effective than aspirin in reducing the combined end point of ischemic stroke, MI, or vascular death in 19,185 patients with a history of either MI, ischemic stroke, or peripheral arterial disease. In this study, clopidogrel showed an overall risk reduction of 8.7% compared with aspirin for the primary end point, although the majority of this benefit was in patients with peripheral arterial disease. Subgroup analyses of the patients with stroke and MI did not demonstrate any significant benefit of clopidogrel over aspirin for the primary end point. Because of this, aspirin remains the antiplatelet agent of choice for preventing thrombotic complications in patients with CAD. Clopidogrel is preferred in patients with known histories of aspirin allergy or intolerance and in those who experience recurrent ischemic events while being maintained on aspirin therapy.

The Clopidogrel in Unstable Angina to Prevent Recurrent Ischemic Events (CURE) trial showed a 20% relative risk reduction with clopidogrel plus aspirin compared with placebo plus aspirin for the primary end point of cardiovascular death, MI, or stroke in 12,562 patients hospitalized with a non–ST-segment elevation acute coronary syndrome. Because the majority of patients in the CURE trial did not undergo PCI or receive a GP IIb/IIIa receptor antagonist, less is known about the use of clopidogrel in this setting.

Because clopidogrel does not affect the cyclooxygenase pathway, it may act synergistically with aspirin to inhibit platelet aggregation. The combination of clopidogrel and aspirin has been found to be effective in preventing coronary stent thrombosis and seems to be more effective than aspirin alone in reducing ischemic events when given for up to 1 year following the procedure. This combination has been shown to be as effective as ticlopidine and aspirin, but with fewer adverse effects.

SPECIAL GROUPS

Race: no differences in response
Children: safety and effectiveness have not been established
Elderly: no dosage adjustment is required
Renal impairment: no dosage adjustment is required, but data are limited; use with caution
Hepatic impairment: no dosage adjustment is required, but data are limited; use with caution
Pregnancy: category B; should be used only if clearly indicated
Breast-feeding: not known if the drug is excreted in human milk; however, use is not recommended because of the potential for harm to nursing infants

IN BRIEF

INDICATIONS
Prevention of thrombotic events in patients with recent MI, recent stroke, or peripheral arterial disease
Prevention of thrombotic events in patients with an acute coronary syndrome (unstable angina or non–Q-wave MI)
Prevention of thrombotic events (in combination with aspirin) following coronary stent implantation (not FDA approved)

CONTRAINDICATIONS
Hypersensitivity to product components
Active pathologic bleeding

DRUG INTERACTIONS
Anticoagulants[1,3]
Antiplatelet drugs[1,3]
HMG-CoA reductase inhibitors metabolized by CYP3A4 (atorvastatin, lovastatin, simvastatin)[2,4]
NSAIDs[1,3]
Fibrinolytics[1,3]

1 Effect/toxicity of clopidogrel may increase.
2 Effect of clopidogrel may decrease.
3 Clopidogrel may increase the effect/toxicity of this drug.
4 The clinical significance of this interaction is unclear.

ADVERSE EFFECTS
Blood: bleeding, intracranial hemorrhage, thrombocytopenia (rare)
Cardiac: chest pain
CNS: headache, dizziness
GI: diarrhea, indigestion, nausea, vomiting
Endocrine: abnormal liver function
Skin: rash, pruritus
Other: hypersensitivity
Side effects that were more common vs aspirin include rash, diarrhea, purpura, and pruritus.

PHARMACOKINETICS AND PHARMACODYNAMICS
Duration of action: 5 d after treatment is discontinued
Onset of action: 2 h after a single dose
Peak effect: between day 3 and day 7 after repeated doses
Bioavailability: 50%
Effect of food: none
Protein binding: 94%–98%
Volume of distribution: insufficient data
Metabolism: mainly hepatic; by hydrolysis and glucuronidation
Elimination: mainly as metabolites; urine—50%; feces—46%
Elimination half-life: up to 11 d for platelet-bound clopidogrel and 8 h for a major metabolite; neither one has direct antiplatelet effect

MONITORING
Signs/symptoms of bleeding, rash, and GI side effects

OVERDOSE
Supportive; platelet transfusion may be administered to rapidly reverse prolonged bleeding time.

The information here is provided as guidance only. Prescribers should always consult the manufacturer's current prescribing information.

CLOPIDOGREL BISULFATE (continued)

DOSAGE

75 mg once daily (patients with atherosclerotic vascular disease)

300 mg loading dose, followed by 75 mg once daily (non–ST-elevation acute coronary syndromes) in combination with aspirin

PATIENT INFORMATION

Clopidogrel may cause prolonged bleeding; report any unusual bleeding, and inform your health care provider prior to any surgical procedures or starting any new drugs.

AVAILABILITY

Tablets—75 mg

The information here is provided as guidance only. Prescribers should always consult the manufacturer's current prescribing information.

127

TICLOPIDINE HYDROCHLORIDE (Ticlid®)

Ticlopidine, a thienopyridine derivative, inhibits ADP-induced platelet aggregation. Ticlopidine has no direct antiplatelet activity in vitro. Its metabolites are responsible for the pharmacologic effect observed in vivo. Ticlopidine may also interfere with the binding of von Willebrand factor to platelet receptors. With the therapeutic dose of ticlopidine, 60% to 70% platelet inhibition can be achieved. This effect is irreversible for the life of the platelets.

Clinical studies have supported the effectiveness of ticlopidine in stroke prevention. When compared with placebo in 1072 patients for secondary prevention of stroke, ticlopidine treatment resulted in a 30% reduction in the relative risk of stroke, MI, or vascular death. When compared with aspirin in the Ticlopidine Aspirin Stroke Study (TASS), ticlopidine produced a 21% relative risk reduction for stroke compared with aspirin in patients presenting within 3 months of suffering a minor stroke or TIA.

However, the side effect profile of ticlopidine, especially the bone marrow toxicity, precludes its use as a first-line agent. In fact, ticlopidine carries a black-box warning informing prescribers that life-threatening hematologic side effects may occur with this drug and that close monitoring is required. Aspirin remains the preferred agent of choice in patients with a history of TIA or stroke, with clopidogrel being the preferred alternative

Because ticlopidine has no effect on the cyclooxygenase pathway, it may act synergistically with aspirin. The combination of ticlopidine and aspirin has been studied in patients undergoing coronary stent placement, and has demonstrated lower rates of stent thrombosis and cardiovascular complications compared with aspirin alone. However, clopidogrel plus aspirin is as effective as ticlopidine plus aspirin for this indication, with fewer adverse effects. Ticlopidine may also be useful in peripheral arterial obliterative disease, coronary artery bypass graft (CABG), postsaphenous vein bypass grafting, and diabetic retinopathy, as well as in patients with unstable angina.

SPECIAL GROUPS

Race:	no differences in response
Children:	safety and effectiveness have not been established
Elderly:	no dosage adjustment is required
Renal impairment:	use with caution; drug clearance is reduced, although no unexpected problems have been reported thus far; dosage reduction may be required
Hepatic impairment:	experience is limited in this population, and drug metabolism may be reduced; contraindicated with severe liver dysfunction; use cautiously with mild/moderate liver dysfunction
Pregnancy:	category B; should be used only if clearly indicated
Breast-feeding:	not known if the drug is excreted in human milk; however, use is not recommended because of the potential for harm to nursing infants

IN BRIEF

INDICATIONS
Prevention of thrombotic stroke in patients with TIA or a history of completed thrombotic stroke
Used with aspirin to reduce the incidence of subacute stent thrombosis in patients undergoing successful coronary stent implantation

CONTRAINDICATIONS
Hypersensitivity to product components
Active pathologic bleeding or presence of a hemostatic disorder
Neutropenia
Thrombocytopenia
Past history of thrombotic thrombocytopenic purpura (TTP) or aplastic anemia
Severe hepatic dysfunction

DRUG INTERACTIONS
Antacids[2]
Anticoagulants[1,3]
Antiplatelet drugs[1,3]
Cimetidine[1]
Digoxin[4,5]
Fibrinolytics[1,3]
NSAIDs[1,3]
Phenytoin[3]
Theophylline[3]

1 Effect/toxicity of ticlopidine may increase.
2 Effect of ticlopidine may decrease.
3 Ticlopidine may increase the effect/toxicity of this drug.
4 Ticlopidine may decrease the effect of this drug.
5 The clinical significance of this interaction is unclear.

ADVERSE EFFECTS
Hematologic: bone marrow suppression, neutropenia, thrombocytopenia, agranulocytosis, pancytopenia, bleeding
GI: nausea, vomiting, diarrhea, dyspepsia, liver function abnormalities
Skin: rash, pruritus
Severe/rare: neutropenia, agranulocytosis, hypersensitivity such as Stevens-Johnson syndrome, erythema multiforme, and exfoliative dermatitis

PHARMACOKINETICS AND PHARMACODYNAMICS

Duration of action:	bleeding time normalizes within 2 wk for most patients
Onset of action:	within 2–3 d
Peak effect:	8–11 d
Bioavailability:	>80%
Effect of food:	absorption increased 20% when taken after a meal
Protein binding:	98%
Volume of distribution:	insufficient data
Metabolism:	extensive hepatic metabolism
Elimination:	urine—60%, mainly as metabolites; feces—23%, one third as unchanged drug
Elimination half-life:	12.6 h; increases to 4–5 d with chronic dosing

MONITORING
Lab: Hematologic side effects may be observed as early as within a few days of starting therapy. The incidence of TTP peaks about 3–4 wk, neutropenia 4–6 wk, and aplastic anemia 4–8 wk after starting therapy. The incidence declines thereafter, with only a few cases being reported after more than 3 mo of therapy. Patients should be monitored for hematologic side effects at baseline and every 2 wk for the first 3 mo of therapy. More frequent monitoring and monitoring after the first 3 mo may be performed if clinically indicated. If therapy is discontinued during this time, monitoring must still be performed for an additional 2 wk after drug discontinuation. Monitoring should involve, at minimum, CBC with absolute neutrophil count (WBC x % neutrophils), platelet count, and appearance of the peripheral smear. Clinical symptoms include fever, weakness, pallor, petechiae or purpura, dark urine or jaundice, or neurologic changes.

TICLOPIDINE HYDROCHLORIDE (continued)

DOSAGE

250 mg twice daily with food; duration of therapy following coronary stent placement is up to 30 days (taken with aspirin)

OVERDOSE

Supportive; platelet transfusion may be administered to rapidly reverse prolonged bleeding time.

PATIENT INFORMATION

Ticlopidine may cause prolonged bleeding or affect leukocytes or other blood components; laboratory tests will be performed every couple of weeks at the beginning of therapy to help minimize the risk of these side effects. Report any unusual bleeding, fever, chills, or sore throat to your health care provider; inform your health care provider prior to any surgical procedures or starting any new drugs. Take with food to help minimize stomach discomfort.

AVAILABILITY

Tablets—250 mg

The information here is provided as guidance only. Prescribers should always consult the manufacturer's current prescribing information.

129

ABCIXIMAB (ReoPro®)

Abciximab was the first GP IIb/IIIa receptor antagonist approved for use in the United States. It is the Fab fragment of the chimeric human-murine monoclonal antibody 7E3. Abciximab binds to the GP IIb/IIIa receptor of human platelets and inhibits platelet aggregation by preventing the binding of fibrinogen, von Willebrand factor, and other adhesive molecules to activated platelets. Maximal inhibition of platelet aggregation can be achieved when more than 80% of GP IIb/IIIa receptors are blocked by abciximab. This can be achieved after a bolus dose of 0.25 mg/kg of abciximab and maintained by continuous intravenous infusion. Platelet function gradually returns to normal after discontinuation of abciximab infusion. Abciximab also binds to the vitronectin receptor found on platelets, vascular endothelium, and smooth muscle cells. The vitronectin receptor helps to mediate platelet aggregation and may also be involved with vascular endothelial and smooth muscle cell proliferation.

Abciximab was initially used to prevent ischemic complications of PCI in patients at high risk for abrupt vessel closure. In this setting (the EPIC study), abciximab reduced both the short- (30-day) and long-term (3-year) risk of the primary end point of death, MI, or urgent intervention for recurrent ischemia compared with placebo. Other clinical trials (EPILOG, CAPTURE, EPISTENT, ACE) have shown generally similar benefits with abciximab in different patient populations. Commonalities shared by all of these studies are that abciximab was used with both aspirin and heparin and all patients were either undergoing PCI or scheduled to undergo PCI. The role of abciximab in patients with acute coronary syndromes not scheduled for PCI is discouraged in the most current (2002) American College of Cardiology/American Heart Association guidelines for the management of patients with non–ST-elevation acute coronary syndromes. This is primarily because of the lack of benefit in reducing death or MI seen with abciximab compared with placebo in the GUSTO IV–ACS study in patients with non–ST-elevation acute coronary syndromes not scheduled to undergo PCI. In addition, abciximab combined with half-dose reteplase showed no mortality benefit at 1 year compared with full-dose reteplase in patients with acute MI, although reinfarction within 7 days of randomization was less with the combination.

As expected, bleeding is the most common adverse effect with abciximab, although thrombocytopenia may occur in about 2.3% of patients. Abciximab has a longer duration of action (potentially more problematic should bleeding occur) and is less specific for the GP IIb/IIIa receptor compared with tirofiban and eptifibatide. Abciximab was compared with tirofiban in the TARGET study, and showed a 26% relative reduction in the composite primary end point of death, MI, and target vessel revascularization at 30 days in 4809 patients undergoing elective or urgent stent implantation. However, by 6 months, there were no differences between the two treatments with regard to the primary outcome.

IN BRIEF

INDICATIONS
Prevention of cardiac ischemic complications in patients undergoing PCI or in patients with unstable angina failing conventional therapy with planned PCI within 24 h. Abciximab is intended for use with both aspirin and heparin.

CONTRAINDICATIONS
Hypersensitivity to product components or murine proteins
Intracranial pathology
Active internal bleeding or bleeding diathesis
Severe GI or GU bleeding within 6 wk
History of stroke within 2 y or with a significant residual neurologic deficit
Severe uncontrolled hypertension
Thrombocytopenia (<100,000 cells/L)
Major surgery or severe trauma within 6 wk
Vasculitis
Dextran use
Administration of warfarin within 7 d unless PT <1.2 times control
Intracranial neoplasm, arteriovenous malformation, or aneurysm

DRUG INTERACTIONS
Any agent that may affect hemostasis:
Anticoagulants[1,2]
Fibrinolytics[1,2]
Other antiplatelets[1,2]
NSAIDs[1,2]
Dextran[1]

1 Effect/toxicity of abciximab may increase.
2 Abciximab may increase the effect/toxicity of this drug.

ADVERSE EFFECTS
Major: bleeding and clotting disorders, thrombocytopenia
CV: hypotension, bradycardia, chest pain
CNS: headache, intracranial hemorrhage, stroke
GI: bleeding, abdominal discomfort, nausea, vomiting
Severe/rare: hypersensitivity

PHARMACOKINETICS AND PHARMACODYNAMICS
Duration of action: platelet function normalizes in 24–48 h, although low-level GP IIb/IIIa receptor blockade persists for more than 10 d
Onset of action: <10 min
Protein binding: unknown
Volume of distribution: unknown
Metabolism: insufficient data
Elimination: insufficient data
Elimination half-life: initial phase: <10 min; second phase: 30 min

MONITORING
Lab: CBC with platelet count at baseline and during treatment; PT at baseline to rule out hemostatic abnormalities, aPTT, ACT to monitor heparin effect (and rule out hemostatic abnormalities). Monitor for clinical evidence of active or occult bleeding.

OVERDOSE
Supportive—avoid prolonged infusion; platelet transfusion may restore platelet function.

ABCIXIMAB (continued)

SPECIAL GROUPS

Race: no differences in response
Children: safety and effectiveness have not been established
Elderly: no dosage adjustment is required
Renal impairment: no dosage adjustment is required
Hepatic impairment: insufficient data; dosage adjustment is probably not required
Pregnancy: category C; use only if potential benefit justifies the potential risk to the fetus
Breast-feeding: not recommended; not known if the drug is excreted in human milk

DOSAGE*

PCI: 0.25 mg/kg IV bolus administered 10–60 min before PCI, followed by a continuous infusion of 0.125 µg/kg/min (up to 10 µg/min) for 12 h

Unstable angina with PCI planned in 24 h: 0.25 mg/kg IV bolus followed by a continuous infusion of 10 µg/min for 18–24 h, concluding 1 h after the PCI

*Recommended with concurrent heparin and aspirin therapy

PATIENT INFORMATION

Administration of abciximab has been associated with an increased risk of bleeding, including intracranial, retroperitoneal, GI, and genitourinary bleeding. If you notice any unexpected bleeding, notify your health care provider immediately.

AVAILABILITY

Vials—10 mg/5 mL (2 mg/mL)

EPTIFIBATIDE   (Integrilin®)

Eptifibatide, a peptide antagonist of the platelet GP IIb/IIIa receptor, inhibits platelet aggregation in a dose- and concentration-dependent manner. Unlike abciximab, and similar to tirofiban, eptifibatide is a selective, reversible antagonist of the GP IIb/IIIa receptor that has little or no affinity for vitronectin receptors.

More than 90% and 40% to 50% of inhibition of platelet aggregation can be achieved at steady state with the high-dose (PURSUIT) and low-dose (IMPACT II) regimens, respectively.

In patients with a non–ST-segment elevation acute coronary syndrome who were managed medically or underwent early PCI, adjunct eptifibatide therapy reduced the risk of death and MI compared with placebo (PURSUIT study). This benefit was observed at 72 hours and persisted over 6 months of follow-up; however, this benefit diminished over time and was not statistically significant at the end of the 6-month period.

In patients undergoing elective PCI (IMPACT II study), eptifibatide reduced the rate of death, MI, or urgent revascularization compared with placebo. Again, the benefit diminished over time and did not reach statistical significance at the end of the 6-month period. The ESPRIT study demonstrated eptifibatide to be superior to placebo in reducing the combined end point of death, MI, urgent revascularization, or "bailout" use of open-label eptifibatide due to a thrombotic complication in 2064 patients undergoing PCI with intended coronary stent placement. The benefits of eptifibatide in this study were observed at 48 hours and persisted over 1 year of follow-up.

Similar to other GP IIb/IIIa receptor antagonists, concurrent aspirin and heparin therapy is recommended unless otherwise contraindicated. Bleeding is also the most common complication with eptifibatide, although its shorter duration of action gives it an advantage over abciximab in this regard. Thrombocytopenia may also occur, but is also less frequent compared with abciximab.

SPECIAL GROUPS

Race: no data

Children: safety and effectiveness have not been established

Elderly: no dosage adjustment is required; limited data in patients older than 75 years and weighing <50 kg

Renal impairment: drug is renally cleared and may accumulate with renal insufficiency; dosage should be reduced in these patients

Hepatic impairment: no data; dosage adjustment is probably not required

Pregnancy: category B; should be used only if clearly indicated

Breast-feeding: not recommended; not known if the drug is excreted in human milk

IN BRIEF

INDICATIONS
Prevention of thrombotic complications in patients with acute coronary syndromes (unstable angina or non–ST-elevation MI)
Prevention of thrombotic complications in patients undergoing PCI.
Eptifibatide is intended for use with both aspirin and heparin for both indications.

CONTRAINDICATIONS
Known hypersensitivity to product components
Bleeding diathesis or active bleeding within 30 d
Severe hypertension: systolic BP (SBP) >200 mm Hg; diastolic BP (DBP) >110 mm Hg—not adequately controlled on antihypertensive therapy
Major surgery within 6 wk
History of stroke within 30 d or hemorrhagic stroke at any time
Current or planned administration of another GP IIb/IIIa inhibitor
Dependency on renal dialysis

DRUG INTERACTIONS
Anticoagulants[1,2]
Antiplatelet drugs[1,2]
NSAIDs[1,2]
Fibrinolytics[1,2]

1 Effect/toxicity of eptifibatide may increase.
2 Eptifibatide may increase the effect/toxicity of this drug.

ADVERSE EFFECTS
Blood: bleeding and clotting disorders, thrombocytopenia
Cardiovascular: hypotension
CNS: intracranial hemorrhage, stroke
Severe/rare: anaphylaxis/hypersensitivity reactions

PHARMACOKINETICS AND PHARMACODYNAMICS
Duration of action: 4–6 h (dose dependent)
Onset of action: within 15 min
Protein binding: 25%
Volume of distribution: 185–270 mL/kg
Metabolism: renal, urinary bladder, and plasma
Elimination: urine—50%, mainly unchanged
Elimination half-life: 2.5 h

MONITORING
Lab: CBC with platelet count at baseline and during treatment; PT at baseline to rule out hemostatic abnormalities, aPTT, ACT to monitor heparin effect (and rule out hemostatic abnormalities). Monitor for clinical evidence of active or occult bleeding.

OVERDOSE
Supportive; eptifibatide may be removed by dialysis.

EPTIFIBATIDE (continued)

DOSAGE*

Acute coronary syndrome: 180 µg/kg IV bolus over 1–2 min, followed by 2.0 µg/kg/min (1.0 µg/kg/min with creatinine clearance <50 mL/min or serum creatinine >2.0 mg/dL) continuous infusion for 72 h, until hospital discharge, or until the time of CABG, whichever occurs first. If PCI is performed, the infusion should be continued up to hospital discharge or for up to 18–24 h after the procedure, whichever comes first, allowing for up to 96 h of therapy.

PCI: 180 µg/kg IV bolus over 1–2 min, immediately before the procedure, followed by 2.0 µg/kg/min infusion (1.0 µg/kg/min with creatinine clearance <50 mL/min or serum creatinine >2.0 mg/dL) and then a second 180 µg/kg bolus given 10 min after the first. The infusion should be continued until hospital discharge or for up to 18–24 h, whichever comes first. A minimum infusion time of 12 h is recommended.

*Recommended with concurrent heparin and aspirin therapy. Maximum bolus dose is 22.6 mg and maximum infusion rate is 15 mg/h (7.5 mg/h if creatinine clearance <50 mL/min or serum creatinine >2.0 mg/dL).

PATIENT INFORMATION
Administration of eptifibatide has been associated with an increased risk of bleeding, including intracranial, retroperitoneal, GI, and genitourinary bleeding. If you notice any unexpected bleeding, notify your health care provider immediately.

AVAILABILITY
Vials—20 mg/10 mL, 200 mg/100 mL (2 mg/mL); 75 mg/100 mL (0.75 mg/mL)

TIROFIBAN HYDROCHLORIDE (Aggrastat®)

Tirofiban, a reversible nonpeptide antagonist of the platelet GP IIb/IIIa receptor, inhibits platelet aggregation. Unlike abciximab, and similar to eptifibatide, tirofiban is a selective, reversible antagonist of the GP IIb/IIIa receptor that has little or no affinity for vitronectin receptors. Tirofiban exerts dose- and concentration-dependent inhibition of platelet aggregation. With the recommended dosing regimen, more than 90% platelet inhibition is achieved by the end of a 30-minute bolus infusion and is maintained by the continuous infusion.

Tirofiban has been studied in the setting of non–ST-segment elevation acute coronary syndrome, as well as PCI. The PRISM and PRISM-PLUS studies investigated tirofiban in patients with non–ST-segment elevation acute coronary syndromes. The PRISM study demonstrated tirofiban alone to be more efficacious than heparin alone in reducing the composite end point of MI, death, or refractory ischemia after 48 hours, although no significant differences were noted at 7 and 30 days. PRISM-PLUS compared tirofiban plus heparin with heparin alone, using the same primary end point as the PRISM study. A third arm of this study, tirofiban alone, was prematurely stopped when an interim analysis revealed a higher mortality compared with the other two treatment groups. The results showed 32%, 22%, and 19% risk reductions in the primary end point with tirofiban plus heparin compared with heparin alone at 7, 30, and 180 days, respectively.

The RESTORE study compared tirofiban with placebo (both groups receiving aspirin and heparin) in patients with unstable angina or acute MI undergoing PCI (angioplasty or atherectomy). In this study, the composite end point of death, MI, or repeat revascularization was reduced with tirofiban treatment at 2, 7, and 30 days, although statistical significance was achieved only with the 2- and 7-day outcomes.

Tirofiban was compared with abciximab in the TARGET study, which showed a 26% relative reduction in the composite primary end point of death, MI, and target vessel revascularization at 30 days with abciximab in 4809 patients undergoing elective or urgent stent implantation. However, by 6 months, there were no differences between the two treatments with regard to the primary outcome.

Similar to other GP IIb/IIIa receptor antagonists, concurrent aspirin and heparin therapy is recommended unless otherwise contraindicated. Bleeding is also the most common complication with tirofiban, although its shorter duration of action gives it an advantage over abciximab in this regard. Thrombocytopenia may also occur, but is also less frequent compared with abciximab.

IN BRIEF

INDICATIONS
Prevention of thrombotic complications in patients with acute coronary syndromes (unstable angina or non–Q-wave MI). Tirofiban is intended to be used with aspirin and heparin in this situation.

CONTRAINDICATIONS
Hypersensitivity to product components
Active internal bleeding or bleeding diathesis within the previous 30 days
History of intracranial hemorrhage, intracranial neoplasm, arteriovenous malformation, or aneurysm
History of thrombocytopenia with tirofiban
Acute pericarditis
History of stroke within 30 d or hemorrhagic stroke at any time
Severe hypertension (SBP >180 mm Hg; DBP >110 mm Hg)
Major surgery or severe trauma within 30 d
Dissecting aortic aneurysm
Concomitant use of another GP IIb/IIIa antagonist

DRUG INTERACTIONS
Anticoagulants[1,2]
Antiplatelet drugs[1,2]
Fibrinolytics[1,2]
NSAIDs[1,2]
1 Effect/toxicity of tirofiban may increase.
2 Tirofiban may increase the effect/toxicity of this drug.

ADVERSE EFFECTS
Major: bleeding and clotting disorders, thrombocytopenia
CV: bradycardia, coronary artery dissection
CNS: headache, dizziness
GI: nausea
Severe/rare: anaphylaxis/hypersensitivity reactions

PHARMACOKINETICS AND PHARMACODYNAMICS
Duration of action: 4–8 h
Onset of action: 90% platelet inhibition achieved within 30 min
Protein binding: 65%; concentration dependent
Volume of distribution: 22–42 L
Metabolism: mostly renal excretion, minimally metabolized
Elimination: mainly excreted unchanged; urine—65%; feces—25%
Elimination half-life: 2 h

MONITORING
Lab: CBC with platelet count at baseline and during treatment; PT at baseline to rule out hemostatic abnormalities, aPTT, ACT to monitor heparin effect (and rule out hemostatic abnormalities). Monitor for clinical evidence of active or occult bleeding.

OVERDOSE
Supportive; can be removed by dialysis.

TIROFIBAN HYDROCHLORIDE *(continued)*

AVAILABILITY
Vials—12.5 mg/50 mL (250 µg/mL)
Premixed bags—5 mg/100 mL; 12.5 mg/250 mL (50 µg/mL)

SPECIAL GROUPS

Race: no difference in plasma clearance

Children: safety and effectiveness have not been established

Elderly: slower clearance, but no dosage adjustment is required

Renal impairment: renally cleared; therefore, reduce dose by 50% in patients with a creatinine clearance <30 mL/min

Hepatic impairment: no dosage adjustment is required

Pregnancy: category B; should only be used if clearly indicated

Breast-feeding: not recommended; not known if the drug is excreted in human milk

DOSAGE*

0.4 µg/kg/min for 30 min, followed by 0.1 µg/kg/min for 48–108 h. The infusion should be continued through angiography and for 12–24 h after angioplasty or atherectomy.

*Recommended with concurrent heparin and aspirin therapy.

Fibrinolytic therapy (also known as thrombolytic therapy) has played a critical role in cardiovascular medicine as a result of the appreciation that MIs and ischemic strokes are predominantly caused by blood clots. A localized vascular occlusion is initiated by changes at the endothelial surface, possibly involving a plaque fissure or ulceration. The activation, adherence, and aggregation of platelets, along with the release of coagulation proteins, initiate the clotting cascade. This allows the development of a critical concentration of thrombin sufficient to convert fibrinogen into fibrin. After cross-linkage, fibrin forms a clot anchored to the original site of endothelial surface derangement.

A dynamic situation occurs with the fibrinolytic mechanism being activated on the fibrin network as fibrin continues to be formed. The eventual outcome of the vessel depends on the net balance between the clotting and lysing systems. Clinically, this process is manifest as unstable angina (subtotal occlusion), subendocardial infarction (transient occlusion), or transmural infarction (sustained occlusion) (Figure 6.1A).

Fibrinolytic therapy ultimately increases plasmin release locally to break down the clot while minimizing the risk of adverse events, such as bleeding. Although these drugs are commonly called thrombolytic drugs, it is more correct to refer to them as fibrinolytic drugs, because their function is to dissolve fibrin clots. Five fibrinolytic agents are currently available in the United States and may be roughly divided into two categories: direct (**alteplase, reteplase, tenecteplase, urokinase**) and indirect (**streptokinase**) plasminogen activators. **Alteplase,**

reteplase, and **tenecteplase** are all biosynthetic forms of naturally occurring tissue plasminogen activator (tPA), an enzyme naturally secreted by endothelial cells; streptokinase is a nonenzymatic protein derived from beta-hemolytic streptococci, and **urokinase** is a trypsinlike enzyme produced in the kidney (Table 6.6).

EFFICACY AND USE

Fibrinolytic treatment decreases mortality after coronary thrombosis. Although **streptokinase** was first administered to patients with acute MI more than 30 years ago, thrombolysis has only recently become widely used because of the development of recombinant DNA technology, which allows large-scale production of biosynthetic forms of tPA.

The survival benefits of fibrinolytic drugs are such that they are now considered cornerstones of therapy for treating acute ST-segment elevation MI. For maximum benefit, fibrinolytic therapy should be instituted as soon as possible after the onset of clinical symptoms of acute MI, with current guidelines recommending that fibrinolytic therapy be given to patients presenting within 12 hours after the onset of symptoms of cardiac ischemia. The use of fibrinolytics for treating acute coronary syndromes other than ST-segment elevation MI is unclear and not recommended. Aspirin should be administered to inhibit platelet aggregation and reduce the thrombogenic tendency during or following postfibrinolytic therapy. Angioplasty, coronary bypass surgery, or repeat revascularization procedure may be necessary to provide long-lasting protection against reocclusion.

TABLE 6.6 THROMBOLYTIC AGENTS CURRENTLY AVAILABLE

Characteristic	Streptokinase	Urokinase	Alteplase	Reteplase	Tenecteplase
Molecular weight, D	47,000	35,000–55,000	70,000	39,571	70,000
Half-life, min	18–23	12.6	4–8	13–16	20–24
Fibrin specificity	Minimal	Minimal	Moderate	Mild–moderate	High
Plasminogen binding	Indirect	Direct	Direct	Direct	Direct
Potential allergic reaction	Yes	No	No	No	No
Typical dose (acute MI)	1.5 million units	2 million units	100 mg (max)	20 units	30–50 mg, based on weight
Administration	1-h IV infusion	1 million unit IV bolus, then 1 million unit IV over 1 h	15 mg bolus, then 0.75 mg/kg (max 50 mg) over 30 min, then 0.5 mg/kg (max 35 mg) over 60 min	Two 10-unit IV boluses, each over 2 min, and 30 min apart	Single IV bolus over 5 sec
Average wholesale price/dose	$562	No longer used for acute MI	$2974	$2872	$2832

IV—intravenous; MI—myocardial infarction.

Adapted from Forman R, Frishman WH: Thrombolytic agents. In *Cardiovascular Pharmacotherapeutics Manual,* edn 2. Edited by Frishman WH, Sonnenblick EH, Sica DA. New York: McGraw Hill; 2004:308. *Additional data from* Ohman EM, Harrington RA, Cannon CP, *et al.*: Intravenous thrombolysis in acute myocardial infarction. *Chest* 2001, 119(Suppl):253S–277S. *Drug Topics Red Book.* Montvale, NJ: Medical Economics Company, Inc.; 2004.

It is believed that restoration of myocardial blood flow is one of the primary goals of treatment in patients suffering from an acute MI. With this in mind, there has, and continues to be, much debate regarding the best method of achieving this goal, with the top two options being fibrinolytic therapy and PCI performed as soon as possible on presentation (primary PCI). Currently, many institutions with PCI facilities will perform primary PCI if the procedure can be performed within 60 to 90 minutes from when the patient presents, because this is when primary PCI is likely to yield the most benefit compared with fibrinolytic drugs. After this time period, the two treatment modalities seem to result in similar outcomes.

Cardiac rupture may be a risk with late administration of fibrinolytics. The observation that early atenolol treatment in acute MI may reduce deaths from cardiac rupture suggests that fibrinolytic therapy should be combined with beta-blockade. Allergic reactions, including the rare anaphylactic reactions, have been associated almost exclusively with **streptokinase** because of foreign protein components. Transient hypotension associated with **streptokinase** infusion is a frequent finding. Hypotension may also occur at the time of reperfusion with successful thrombolysis and recanalization. Arrhythmias occurring during fibrinolytic therapy have been used as a nonangiographic marker of reperfusion. Ventricular fibrillation has also been reported. The most common complication of fibrinolytic therapy is hemorrhage, and the most devastating complication is intracerebral bleeding, which occurs more often in the elderly. Intracerebral hemorrhage is less frequent with **streptokinase** than **alteplase**.

MODE OF ACTION

Fibrin and fibrinogen are degraded by the enzyme plasmin that is converted from its inactive proenzyme plasminogen (Figure 6.6). Fibrinolytic therapy aims at increasing plasmin formation by means of additional plasminogen activation. The prothrombin time may be prolonged up to 24 h after discontinuing therapy, a result of relative depletion of fibrinogen or other clotting factors.

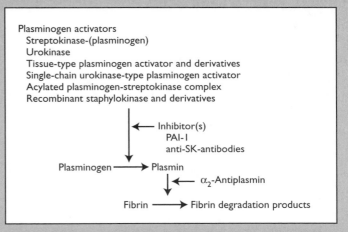

FIGURE 6.6 Schematic representation of the fibrinolytic system. Plasminogen is a proenzyme and is activated by plasminogen activators into the active enzyme plasmin. Plasmin degrades fibrin into degradation products. Fibrinolysis may be inhibited at the level of plasminogen activators by PAI-1 (plasminogen activator inhibitor) and anti-SK (streptokinase) antibodies or the level of plasmin by α_2-antiplasmin. (*From* Forman R, Frishman WH: Thrombolytic agents. In *Cardiovascular Pharmacotherapeutics*, edn 2. Edited by Frishman WH, Sonnenblick EH, Sica DA. New York: McGraw Hill; 2003:302; with permission.)

ALTEPLASE, RECOMBINANT

(Activase®)

Alteplase is a recombinant tPA derived from genetically engineered Chinese hamster ovary cells. At therapeutic concentrations, fibrinolysis is initiated by binding of tPA to fibrin in the thrombus and converting the entrapped plasminogen to plasmin. This localized fibrinolytic activity theoretically may reduce the systemic proteolysis and the risk of bleeding, although clinical trials have not supported this theory.

Alteplase has been shown to result in greater patency of the infarct-related artery at 90 minutes compared with streptokinase. The GUSTO-1 study subsequently demonstrated alteplase therapy to result in lower 30-day mortality compared with streptokinase, although intracranial hemorrhaging was greater with alteplase.

The newer fibrinolytic drugs, reteplase and tenecteplase, share structural and pharmacologic similarities to alteplase, but with the advantage of easier administration (bolus vs infusion) and the potential for fewer medication errors.

Alteplase has been compared with reteplase, which demonstrated greater reperfusion rates at 90 minutes compared with alteplase. However, a follow-up study (GUSTO III) designed to detect the superiority of reteplase over alteplase in terms of overall mortality showed that reteplase (7.47% mortality) was not superior to alteplase (7.24% mortality) in this regard, with similar rates of stroke and hemorrhaging as well.

The Assessment of the Safety and Efficacy of a New Thrombolytic (ASSENT-2) study compared alteplase (rapid infusion) with tenecteplase in 16,949 patients with acute MI. All-cause mortality at 30 days was similar between treatments (6.18% for tenecteplase, 6.15% for alteplase), as was intracranial hemorrhage (0.93% for tenecteplase, 0.94% for alteplase). However, tenecteplase treatment resulted in fewer noncerebral bleeds and blood transfusions.

In patients with acute ischemic stroke, early thrombolysis with alteplase has been shown to improve neurologic recovery and reduce the incidence of disability. These benefits were observed when the treatment was initiated within 3 hours of symptom onset. The potential benefits of administering alteplase to stroke patients should always be assessed against the risk of intracranial hemorrhage. The risk is increased especially in patients presenting with severe neurologic deficit or advanced age.

In patients with pulmonary embolism who are hemodynamically unstable, fibrinolytic therapy may be beneficial. Improvement in pulmonary perfusion scan and embolism-induced pulmonary hypertension has been observed with alteplase therapy when used appropriately.

Alteplase has also been used successfully in restoring patency to occluded intravenous catheters.

IN BRIEF

INDICATIONS
Acute MI
Acute ischemic stroke (administered within 3 h after the onset of symptoms, and after ruling out intracranial hemorrhage)
Acute massive PE

CONTRAINDICATIONS
Active internal bleeding
Known bleeding diathesis
History of cerebrovascular accident
Recent (within 3 months) intracranial or intraspinal surgery or trauma
Intracranial neoplasm, arteriovenous malformation or aneurysm
Severe uncontrolled hypertension (SBP >185 mm Hg or DBP >110 mm Hg)
Evidence of intracranial or subarachnoid hemorrhage
History of recent stroke or intracranial hemorrhage
Seizure at stroke onset (if being considered for stroke treatment)

DRUG INTERACTIONS
Anticoagulants[1,2]
Antiplatelet drugs[1,2]
Fibrinolytics[1,2]
NSAIDs[1,2]

1 Effect/toxicity of alteplase may increase.
2 Alteplase may increase the effect/toxicity of this drug.

ADVERSE EFFECTS
Bleeding: intracranial, retroperitoneal, GI, genitourinary, or respiratory; venous/arterial catheter sites; ecchymosis
CV: cholesterol embolization, cardiogenic shock, arrhythmias, hypotension, bradycardia
GI: nausea, vomiting
Rare: allergic or anaphylactoid reaction, laryngeal edema, rash, and urticaria

PHARMACOKINETICS AND PHARMACODYNAMICS
Duration of action: no data
Onset of action: rapid
Peak effect: thrombolysis occurs within 60–90 min
Bioavailability: 100%
Protein binding: no data
Volume of distribution: 27–53 L
Metabolism: hepatic
Elimination: renal
Elimination half-life: 4–8 min

MONITORING
No specific monitoring required other than monitoring for clinical evidence of active or occult bleeding. Routine monitoring should be performed for other drugs (eg, heparin) and for complications of MI.

OVERDOSE
Supportive; no data.

ALTEPLASE, RECOMBINANT (continued)

AVAILABILITY
Vials—50 mg and 100 mg (potency: 580,000 IU/mg)

SPECIAL GROUPS

Race: no differences in response

Children: safety and effectiveness have not been established

Elderly: elderly patients are more sensitive to bleeding with alteplase, although no specific dosage adjustment is required; adjust dosage based on weight

Renal impairment: no data; use with caution because severe kidney disease may be associated with hemostatic defects

Hepatic impairment: no data; use with caution because severe liver disease may be associated with hemostatic defects

Pregnancy: category C; use only if potential benefit justifies the potential risk to the fetus

Breast-feeding: not recommended; not clear if the drug is excreted in human milk

DOSAGE

Acute MI: The following two regimens should be used with concurrent administration of heparin and aspirin. Treatment should be initiated as soon as possible, preferably within 12 h after the onset of chest pain:

1. Accelerated infusion (preferred because it results in greater reperfusion)—15 mg IV bolus, followed by 0.75 mg/kg (up to 50 mg) infused over 30 min, and then 0.5 mg/kg (up to 35 mg) infused over 60 min. A maximum total dose is 100 mg for patients weighing more than 67 kg.

2. Three-hour infusion—60 mg infused over 60 min (with 6–10 mg administered as a bolus first), followed by 20 mg/h infusion for 2 h to deliver a total dose of 100 mg. For patients weighing less than 65 kg, a total dose of 1.25 mg/kg is recommended.

Acute ischemic stroke: 0.9 mg/kg (up to 90 mg) administered IV over 60 min, with 10% of the total dose administered as a bolus over the first minute. Treatment should be initiated within 3 h after the onset of stroke symptoms. Avoid aspirin and heparin use during the first 24 h.

PE: 100 mg IV over 2 h. Heparin therapy should be initiated near the end or following the alteplase infusion when partial thromboplastin time or thrombin time returns to twice normal or less.

RETEPLASE, RECOMBINANT (Retavase®)

Reteplase is a recombinant plasminogen activator derived from *Escherichia coli*. It catalyzes the cleavage of endogenous plasminogen to generate plasmin, which in turn degrades the fibrin matrix of the thrombus, producing thrombolysis.

Three clinical studies, INJECT, RAPID 1, and RAPID 2 have supported the efficacy of reteplase in restoring coronary artery flow when administered within 6 or 12 hours after the onset of acute MI. With few exceptions, patients were also treated with aspirin and heparin. In the INJECT study, double-bolus reteplase (10 U and 10 U) was compared to streptokinase (1.5 MU over 60 min). Mortality rates were similar between treatments at 35 days and 6 months. Although fewer patients developed CHF and cardiogenic shock, more patients had hemorrhagic strokes in the reteplase group. In RAPID 1 and RAPID 2, reteplase was compared with two different alteplase regimens in patients after acute MI. More patients achieved complete restoration of coronary blood flow with reteplase at 60 and 90 minutes after the initiation of therapy. The reocclusion rates and the incidence of bleeding complications were similar for reteplase and alteplase therapy.

Reteplase was compared with alteplase in the GUSTO III study, which was designed to detect the superiority of reteplase over alteplase in terms of overall mortality. The results showed that reteplase (7.47% mortality) was not superior to alteplase (7.24% mortality) in this regard, with similar rates of stroke and hemorrhaging as well.

The GUSTO V study showed no mortality benefit at 1 year with abciximab combined with half-dose reteplase compared with full-dose reteplase in patients with acute MI, although reinfarction within 7 days of randomization was less with the combination.

With its efficacy in restoring coronary artery blood flow and convenient dosing and administration, reteplase may be useful in treating patients with acute MI before they reach the hospital. This implies earlier thrombolysis, which may further improve the outcome of these patients.

SPECIAL GROUPS

Race: no data

Children: safety and effectiveness have not been established

Elderly: no dosage adjustment is required

Renal impairment: no data; use with caution because severe kidney disease may be associated with hemostatic defects

Hepatic impairment: no data; use with caution because severe liver disease may be associated with hemostatic defects

Pregnancy: category C; use only if potential benefit justifies the potential risk to the fetus

Breast-feeding: not recommended; not clear if the drug is excreted in human milk

IN BRIEF

INDICATIONS
Thrombolysis in patients with acute MI to improve ventricular function, reduce the incidence of heart failure, and reduce mortality

CONTRAINDICATIONS
Active internal bleeding
History of cerebrovascular accident
Recent intracranial or intraspinal surgery or trauma
Intracranial neoplasm, arteriovenous malformation or aneurysm
Known bleeding diathesis
Severe, uncontrolled hypertension
Known hypersensitivity to product components

DRUG INTERACTIONS
Anticoagulants[1,2]
Antiplatelet drugs[1,2]
Fibrinolytics[1,2]
NSAIDs[1,2]

[1] Effect/toxicity of reteplase may increase.
[2] Reteplase may increase the effect/toxicity of this drug.

ADVERSE EFFECTS
Bleeding: intracranial, retroperitoneal, gastrointestinal, genitourinary or respiratory, injection sites, venous/arterial catheter sites
CV: cholesterol embolization, arrhythmias, hypotension, cardiogenic shock
GI: nausea, vomiting
Rare: allergic or anaphylactoid reaction

PHARMACOKINETICS AND PHARMACODYNAMICS
(based on fibrinolytic activity measured)
Duration of action: up to 48 h
Onset of action: rapid
Peak effect: lysis occurs within 60–90 min
Protein binding: insufficient data
Volume of distribution: insufficient data
Metabolism: liver
Elimination: kidney
Elimination half-life: 13–16 min

MONITORING
No specific monitoring required other than monitoring for clinical evidence of active or occult bleeding. Routine monitoring should be performed for other drugs (eg, heparin) and for complications of MI.

OVERDOSE
Supportive; no data.

RETEPLASE, RECOMBINANT (continued)

DOSAGE

Two 10 U bolus injections; each bolus is given IV over 2 min, with the second bolus given 30 min after initiation of the first bolus. Treatment should be initiated as soon as possible, preferably within 12 h after the onset of chest pain. Patients should also receive adjunctive therapy with heparin and aspirin. Reteplase and heparin are incompatible in solution and should not be given through the same IV line.

PATIENT INFORMATION

Reteplase may cause excessive bleeding. If you notice any unexpected bleeding, notify your health care provider immediately.

AVAILABILITY

Kit—reteplase 18.1 mg (10.4 U)/vial, in 1- or 2-vial kits that also contain 10 mL sterile water for injection, reconstitution vials, syringes, dispensing pins, needles, and alcohol swabs

STREPTOKINASE
(Kabikinase®, Streptase®)

Streptokinase, obtained from beta-hemolytic streptococci, is an indirect plasminogen activator that must form an "activator complex" with plasminogen or plasmin in order to convert residual plasminogen to plasmin The formed plasmin acts on fibrinogen and fibrin to yield degradation products. The activator complex is inactivated, in part, by existing antistreptococcal antibodies. The amount of circulating antistreptococcal antibodies varies from person to person, but systemic doses of 250,000 U induce a systemic fibrinolytic state in more than 90% of patients. Generally, a dose of 1.5 MU is used for patients with evolving MI.

Major trials have demonstrated the efficacy of streptokinase in the treatment of acute MI. Streptokinase reduced in-hospital mortality by 18% compared with standard therapy in the GISSI-1 trial, with this benefit being maintained for over 1 year. The ISIS-2 study demonstrated a 25% reduction in 35-day vascular mortality compared with placebo in 17,187 patients with suspected MI (Figure 6.4). Most of the benefit with streptokinase was seen in the patients treated within 12 hours of symptoms.

Compared with alteplase, patency of the infarct-related artery at 90 minutes is greater with alteplase than with streptokinase. The GUSTO-1 study demonstrated alteplase therapy to result in lower 30-day mortality compared with streptokinase, although intracranial hemorrhaging was greater with alteplase.

In the INJECT study, streptokinase (1.5 MU over 60 minutes) was compared with double-bolus reteplase (10 U and 10 U). Mortality rates were similar between treatments at 35 days and 6 months. Although fewer patients developed CHF and cardiogenic shock, more patients had hemorrhagic strokes in the reteplase group.

Streptokinase has been used successfully to lyse PE and DVT. Streptokinase is indicated to clear occluded arteriovenous cannulae, but should not be used to restore patency to occluded IV catheters.

Rapid infusion of large doses of streptokinase (>500 U/min) can induce hypotension, but the relative reduction in BP can reduce myocardial work and may have an oxygen-sparing effect. The production of systemic fibrinolysis also may result in decreased blood viscosity. Both effects may be beneficial.

SPECIAL GROUPS

Race: no differences in response
Children: safety and effectiveness have not been established, although streptokinase has been used safely in patients ranging in age from <1 month to 16 years.
Elderly: no dosage adjustment is required
Renal impairment: no dosage adjustment is required; use with caution because severe kidney disease may be associated with hemostatic defects
Hepatic impairment: no dosage adjustment is required; use with caution because severe liver disease may be associated with hemostatic defects
Pregnancy: category C; avoid use during first 18 wk of pregnancy; otherwise, use only if potential benefit justifies the potential risk to the fetus
Breast-feeding: not recommended; not known if the drug is excreted in human milk

IN BRIEF

INDICATIONS
Acute MI
Acute DVT
Acute arterial thrombosis or embolism
PE
Occlusion of arteriovenous cannulae

CONTRAINDICATIONS
Active internal bleeding
Known bleeding diathesis
Known hypersensitivity reaction to streptokinase
Recent cerebrovascular accident (<2 mo)
Recent intracranial or intraspinal surgery (<2 mo)
Intracranial neoplasm, arteriovenous malformation or aneurysm
Severe uncontrolled hypertension

DRUG INTERACTIONS
Anticoagulants[1,2]
Antiplatelet drugs[1,2]
Fibrinolytics[1,2]
NSAIDs[1,2]
1 Effect/toxicity of streptokinase may increase.
2 Streptokinase may increase the effect/toxicity of this drug.

ADVERSE EFFECTS
Bleeding: intracranial, retroperitoneal, gastrointestinal, genitourinary, or respiratory; venous/arterial catheter sites; ecchymosis
CV: arrhythmias, hypotension, cholesterol embolization, cardiogenic shock
GI: nausea, vomiting
Other: fever, chills, urticaria, pruritus, anaphylactic or anaphylactoid reactions, angioedema, polyneuropathy, noncardiogenic pulmonary edema, elevated serum transaminases

PHARMACOKINETICS AND PHARMACODYNAMICS
Duration of action: 12–24 h; fibrinolytic activity lasts for only a few hours
Onset of action: rapid
Peak effect: rapid
Bioavailability: 100%
Protein binding: insufficient data
Volume of distribution: insufficient data
Elimination: cleared by circulating antibodies and the reticuloendothelial system
Elimination half-life: 18–23 min

MONITORING
No specific monitoring required other than monitoring for clinical evidence of active or occult bleeding. Routine monitoring should be performed for other drugs (eg, heparin) and for complications of acute MI.

OVERDOSE
Supportive; no data.

STREPTOKINASE (continued)

DOSAGE

Acute MI: Although therapeutic benefits have been reported in patients up to 24 h after the onset of symptoms, treatment should be initiated as soon as possible for maximum benefit.
IV—1.5 million IU infused over 60 min
Intracoronary—20,000 IU bolus, followed by 2000 IU/min infusion for 60 min (a total of 140,000 IU).

PE, DVT, arterial thrombosis, or embolism: 250,000 IU bolus infused over 30 min, followed by 100,000 IU/h continuous infusion for up to 24 h for PE, 72 h for DVT, and 24–72 h for arterial thromboembolism. Treatment should be initiated as soon as possible, preferably within 7 d after onset of the symptoms.

Arteriovenous cannulae occlusion: Instill 250,000 IU streptokinase in 2 mL solution into occluded cannula, clamp the cannula for 2 h, then aspirate the contents and flush with saline.

PATIENT INFORMATION
Streptokinase may cause excessive bleeding. If you notice any unexpected bleeding, notify your health care provider immediately.

AVAILABILITY
Vials—250,000, 750,000, 1.5 million IU in 6 mL vials

TENECTEPLASE (TNKase®)

Tenecteplase is a recombinant tPA produced from Chinese hamster ovary cells. It is similar to wild-type tPA but has amino acid substitutions at three sites, which confer increased fibrin specificity; a prolonged half-life; and increased resistance to plasminogen activator inhibitor-1 compared with natural tPA. Tenecteplase has the highest fibrin specificity of all the currently available fibrinolytic drugs and coupled with a relatively long half-life (20–24 minutes), may be given as a single-bolus dose.

The Assessment of the Safety and Efficacy of a New Thrombolytic Agent (ASSENT-2) study compared tenecteplase with alteplase (rapid infusion) in 16,949 patients with acute MI. All-cause mortality at 30 days was similar between treatments (6.18% for tenecteplase, 6.15% for alteplase), as was intracranial hemorrhage (0.93% for tenecteplase, 0.94% for alteplase). However, tenecteplase treatment resulted in fewer noncerebral bleeds and blood transfusions.

The ASSENT-3 study evaluated full-dose tenecteplase in combination with either enoxaparin or heparin or half-dose tenecteplase in combination with abciximab and heparin in 6095 patients with acute MI. The primary composite end point of 30-day mortality, in-hospital reinfarction, or in-hospital refractory ischemia was significantly reduced in the groups receiving tenecteplase with either enoxaparin or abciximab/heparin (15.4% relative risk reductions) compared with the group receiving tenecteplase with only heparin.

SPECIAL GROUPS

Race: no data
Children: safety and effectiveness have not been established
Elderly: more sensitive to bleeding; therefore, use cautiously. No specific dosage adjustment is required.
Renal impairment: no data; use with caution because severe kidney disease may be associated with hemostatic defects
Hepatic impairment: no data; use with caution because severe liver disease may be associated with hemostatic defects
Pregnancy: category C; use only if potential benefit justifies the potential risk to the fetus
Breast-feeding: not recommended; not clear if the drug is excreted in human milk

DOSAGE

Single bolus administered over 5 sec, administered as soon as possible after the onset of acute MI symptoms:

Patient weight, kg	Dose, mg
<60	30
≥60–<70	35
≥70–<80	40
≥80–<90	45
≥90	50

Tenecteplase is intended to be used with aspirin and heparin.

IN BRIEF

INDICATIONS
Reduction of mortality in patients with acute MI; initiate treatment as soon as possible after the onset of acute MI symptoms

CONTRAINDICATIONS
Active internal bleeding
History of cerebrovascular accident
Intracranial or intraspinal surgery or trauma within 2 mo
Intracranial neoplasm, arteriovenous malformation or aneurysm
Known bleeding diathesis
Severe, uncontrolled hypertension

DRUG INTERACTIONS
Anticoagulants[1,2]
Antiplatelet drugs[1,2]
Fibrinolytics[1,2]
NSAIDs[1,2]

1 Effect/toxicity of tenecteplase may increase.
2 Tenecteplase may increase the effect/toxicity of this drug.

ADVERSE EFFECTS
Bleeding: intracranial, retroperitoneal, gastrointestinal, genitourinary or respiratory; injection sites, venous/arterial catheter sites
CV: cholesterol embolization, arrhythmias, hypotension, cardiogenic shock
GI: nausea, vomiting
Rare: allergic or anaphylactoid reaction

PHARMACOKINETICS AND PHARMACODYNAMICS
Duration of action: insufficient data
Onset of action: rapid
Peak effect: lysis occurs within 60–90 min
Protein binding: insufficient data
Volume of distribution: weight related; approximates plasma volume
Metabolism: liver
Elimination: not fully defined
Elimination half-life: 20–24 min (initial phase); 90–130 min (terminal phase)

MONITORING
No specific monitoring required other than monitoring for clinical evidence of active or occult bleeding. Routine monitoring should be performed for other drugs (eg, heparin) and for complications of MI.

OVERDOSE
Supportive; no data.

PATIENT INFORMATION
Tenecteplase may cause excessive bleeding. If you notice any unexpected bleeding, notify your health care provider immediately.

AVAILABILITY
Vial—50 mg, packed with reconstitution kit: 10 mL vial of sterile water for injection, 10 mL syringe with dual cannula device, 3 alcohol prep pads

UROKINASE
(Abbokinase®)

Urokinase, an enzyme produced by the kidney and found in the urine, is a direct plasminogen activator. There are two forms of urokinase with different molecular weights but similar activity. Abbokinase, the commercially available product of urokinase, contains primarily the low molecular weight form. Urokinase, unlike streptokinase, is a direct (vs indirect) plasminogen activator. Urokinase has low antigenicity and low binding affinity for fibrin.

Despite being one of the first fibrinolytics tested in humans, it has little clinical trial data to support its use. Angiographic trials conducted in the 1980s demonstrated arterial patency similar to that achieved with alteplase and generally better than that achieved with streptokinase. In terms of clinical end points, urokinase combined with heparin demonstrated no mortality benefit over heparin alone in patients with acute MI. Intracoronary urokinase administration at a rate of 6000 IU/min up to a maximum dose of 750,000 IU resulted in recanalization in more than 60% of patients suffering from MI. In the TIMI-5 study, IV administration of urokinase, tPA, or a combination of both, achieved 62%, 71%, and 76% coronary patency rates, respectively. The difference was not statistically significant. In aggregate, these data do not support the use of urokinase for treating acute MI.

In the National Institutes of Health (NIH)-sponsored Urokinase Streptokinase Pulmonary Embolism Trial, patients with massive PE receiving urokinase (4400 IU/kg/h IV for 24 h) had significantly greater pulmonary reperfusion on lung scanning and greater reduction of pulmonary hypertension than those receiving streptokinase therapy (100,000 IU/h IV for 24 h). In another study, IV urokinase (3 million IU over 2 h) was compared with tPA (100 mg over 2 h) in patients with PE. Although earlier resolution of emboli was observed in the tPA group, no significant difference was observed at 24 h when assessed by lung scanning.

In patients who have received streptokinase within the prior 12 months and have high antibody titers to streptokinase, urokinase can be used safely and effectively.

Urokinase has been used primarily in the recent past for dissolving clots in occluded intravenous catheters. Because of manufacturing problems, the drug was unavailable in the early part of this decade, but it has recently been reintroduced as a treatment for PE.

IN BRIEF

INDICATIONS
Lysis of acute massive PE
Lysis of PE accompanied by unstable hemodynamics

CONTRAINDICATIONS
Active internal bleeding
Known bleeding diathesis
Recent (within 2 mo) cerebrovascular accident
Recent intracranial or intraspinal surgery (<2 mo)
Intracranial neoplasm, arteriovenous malformation, or aneurysm
Severe, uncontrolled arterial hypertension
Recent trauma, including cardiopulmonary resuscitation
Hypersensitivity to product components

DRUG INTERACTIONS
Anticoagulants[1,2]
Antiplatelet drugs[1,2]
Fibrinolytics[1,2]
NSAIDs[1,2]

1 Effect/toxicity of urokinase may increase.
2 Urokinase may increase the effect/toxicity of this drug.

ADVERSE EFFECTS
Bleeding: intracranial, retroperitoneal, gastrointestinal, genitourinary, or respiratory; venous/arterial catheter sites; ecchymosis
CV: hypotension, hypertension, tachycardia
GI: nausea, vomiting
Rare: allergic reaction, bronchospasm, skin rash, fever, chills, rigors

PHARMACOKINETICS AND PHARMACODYNAMICS
Duration of action: 12–24 h; fibrinolytic activity lasts for only a few hours
Onset of action: immediate
Peak effect: rapid
Bioavailability: 100%
Protein binding: no data
Volume of distribution: 11.5 L
Metabolism/elimination: metabolized by liver; only small amounts are eliminated in urine and bile
Elimination half-life: 12.6 min

MONITORING
Lab: CBC, aPTT. Clinical evidence of active or occult bleeding. Following urokinase administration, other anticoagulants should not be started until the aPTT has dropped below 2 times control.

UROKINASE *(continued)*

SPECIAL GROUPS

Race: no differences in response

Children: safety and effectiveness have not been established

Elderly: no dosage adjustment is required; use with caution because this population has not been adequately studied

Renal impairment: no dosage adjustment is required; use with caution because severe kidney disease may be associated with hemostatic defects

Hepatic impairment: use with caution because urokinase clearance may be reduced with moderate to severe cirrhosis

Pregnancy: category B; should be used only if clearly indicated

Breast-feeding: not recommended; not known if the drug is excreted in human milk

DOSAGE

PE: Initiate therapy as soon as possible. Urokinase 4400 IU/kg administered IV over 10 min, followed by continuous infusion of 4400 IU/kg/h for 12 h. Appropriate anticoagulant therapy should be initiated after urokinase therapy once the aPTT is less than 2 times control.

Occluded catheter (not FDA approved): Urokinase 5000 IU/mL is used, and only the amount equal to the internal volume of the catheter should be injected slowly into the catheter. Specific instructions provided by the manufacturer should be followed to ensure aseptic application and proper urokinase indwelling time before each aspiration attempt, and to avoid the risk for air emboli.

Urokinase is not recommended for use in acute MI.

OVERDOSE
Supportive; no data.

PATIENT INFORMATION
Urokinase may cause excessive bleeding. If you notice any unexpected bleeding, notify your health care provider immediately.

AVAILABILITY
Vials—250,000 IU

SELECTED BIBLIOGRAPHY

Albers GW, Bates VE, Clark WM, *et al.*: Intravenous tissue type plasminogen activator for treatment of acute stroke. The Standard Treatment with Alteplase to Reverse Stroke (STARS) study. *JAMA* 2000, 283:1145–1150.

Alexander RW, Pratt CM, Ryan TJ, Roberts R: ST-segment elevation myocardial infarction: clinical presentations, diagnostic evaluation, and medical management. In *Hurst's The Heart,* edn 11. Edited by Fuster V, Alexander RW, O'Rourke RA. New York: McGraw Hill; 2004:1277–1349.

Amiral J, Bridey F, Wolf M, *et al.*: Antibodies to macromolecular platelet factor 4-heparin complexes in heparin-induced thrombocytopenia: a study of 44 cases. *Thromb Haemost* 1995, 73:21–28.

Ansell J, Hirsh J, Dalen J, *et al.*: Managing oral anticoagulant therapy. *Chest* 2001, 119(Suppl):22S–38S.

Antithrombotic Trialists' Collaboration: Collaborative meta-analysis of randomised trials of antiplatelet therapy for prevention of death, myocardial infarction, and stroke in high risk patients. *BMJ* 2002, 324:71–86.

Antman EM, Guigliano RP, Gibson CM, *et al.* for the TIMI 14 Investigators: Abciximab facilitates the rate and extent of thrombolysis: results from the Thrombolysis in Myocardial Infarction (TIMI) 14 Trial. *Circulation* 1999, 99:2720–2732.

Antoniucci D, Rodriguez A, Hempel A, *et al.*: A randomized trial comparing primary infarct artery stenting with or without abciximab in acute myocardial infarction. *J Am Coll Cardiol* 2003, 42:1879–1885.

Armstrong PW: Heparin in acute coronary disease: requiem for a heavyweight [editorial]. *N Engl J Med* 1997, 337:492.

Assessment of the Safety and Efficacy of a New Thrombolytic Regimen (ASSENT)-3 Investigators: Efficacy and safety of tenecteplase in combination with enoxaparin, abciximab, or unfractionated heparin: the ASSENT-3 randomised trial in acute myocardial infarction. *Lancet* 2001, 358:605–613.

Awtry EH, Loscalzo J: Aspirin. *Circulation* 2000, 101:1206–1218.

Bauer KA, Eriksson BI, Lassen MR, Turpie AGG, the Steering Committee of the Pentasaccharide in Major Knee Surgery Study: Fondaparinux compared with enoxaparin for the prevention of venous thromboembolism after elective major knee surgery. *N Engl J Med* 2001, 345:1305–1310.

Bertrand ME, Rupprecht H-J, Urban P, Gershlick AH, for the CLASSICS Investigators: Double-blind study of the safety of clopidogrel with and without a loading dose in combination with aspirin after coronary stenting. The Clopidogrel Aspirin Stent International Cooperative Study (CLASSICS). *Circulation* 2000, 102:624–629.

Bode C, Smalling R, Gunther B, *et al.*: Randomized comparison of coronary thrombolysis achieved with double bolus reteplase (recombinant plasminogen activator) and front-loaded, accelerated alteplase (recombinant tissue plasminogen activator) in patients with acute myocardial infarction. *Circulation* 1996, 94:891–898.

Braunwald E, Antman EM, Beasley JW, *et al.*: ACC/AHA guideline update for the management of patients with unstable angina and non–ST-segment elevation myocardial infarction: summary article of the American College of Cardiology/American Heart Association Task Force on Practice Guidelines (Committee on the Management of Patients With Unstable Angina), 2002. *Circulation* 2002, 106:1893–1900.

Cairns JA, Theroux P, Lewis D Jr, *et al.*: Antithrombotic agents in coronary artery disease. *Chest* 2001, 119(Suppl):228S–252S.

Cannon CP: Aggrastat in the treatment of unstable angina. *Curr Pract Med* 1998, 1:55–58.

Cannon CP, Weintraub WS, Demopoulos LA, *et al.* for the TACTICS-Thrombolysis in Myocardial Infarction 18 Investigators: Comparison of early invasive and conservative strategies in patients with unstable coronary syndromes treated with the glycoprotein IIb/IIIa inhibitor tirofiban. *N Engl J Med* 2001, 344:1879–1887.

CAPRIE Steering Committee: A randomised, blinded trial of clopidogrel versus aspirin in patients at risk of ischaemic events (CAPRIE). *Lancet* 1996, 348:1329–1339.

CAPTURE Investigators: Randomised, placebo-controlled trial of abciximab before, during and after coronary intervention in refractory unstable angina: the CAPTURE study. *Lancet* 1997, 349:1429–1435.

Challapalli R, Lefkovits J, Topol EJ: Clinical trials of recombinant hirudin in acute coronary syndromes. *Coron Artery Dis* 1996, 7:429–437.

Cheer SM, Dunn CJ, Foster R: Tinzaparin sodium. A review of its pharmacology and clinical use in the prophylaxis and treatment of thromboembolic disease. *Drugs* 2004, 64:1479–1502.

Clopidogrel in Unstable Angina to Prevent Recurrent Events Trial Investigators: Effects of clopidogrel in addition to aspirin in patients with acute coronary syndromes without ST-segment elevation. *N Engl J Med* 2001, 345:494–502.

Cohen M, Demers C, Gurfinkel E, *et al.* for the Efficacy and Safety of Subcutaneous Enoxaparin vs Non–Q-Wave Coronary Events Study Group: A comparison of low molecular weight heparin with unfractionated heparin for unstable coronary artery disease. *N Engl J Med* 1997, 337:447–452.

Collen D: Fibrin-selective thrombolytic therapy for acute myocardial infarction. *Circulation* 1996, 93:857–865.

Danhof M, de Boer A, Magnani HN, *et al.*: Pharmacokinetic considerations of orgaran (org 10172) therapy. *Haemostasis* 1992, 22:73–84.

Deitcher SR: Clinical utility of subcutaneous hirudins. *Am J Health Syst Pharm* 2003, 60(Suppl 5):S27–S31.

Diener HC, Cunha L, Forbes C, *et al.* European Stroke Prevention Study: II. Dipyridamole and acetylsalicylic acid in the secondary prevention of stroke. *J Neurol Sci* 1996, 143:1–13.

Duvall WL, Vorchheimer DA, Fuster V: Thrombogenesis and antithrombotic therapy. In *Hurst's The Heart,* edn 11. Edited by Fuster V, Alexander RW, O'Rourke R. New York: McGraw Hill; 2004:1361–1418.

Eberhardt RT, Coffman JD: Drug treatment of peripheral vascular disease. In *Cardiovascular Pharmacotherapeutics,* edn 2. Edited by Frishman WH, Sonnenblick EH, Sica DA. New York: McGraw Hill; 2003:919–934.

Eberhardt RT, Coffman JD: Drug treatment of peripheral vascular disease. In *Cardiovascular Pharmacotherapeutics Manual,* edn 2. Edited by Frishman WH, Sonnenblick EH, Sica DA. New York: McGraw Hill; 2004:466–484.

EPIC Investigators: Use of a monoclonal antibody directed against the platelet glycoprotein IIb/IIIa receptor in high-risk coronary angioplasty. *N Engl J Med* 1994, 330:956–961.

EPILOG Investigators: Platelet glycoprotein IIb/IIIa receptor blockade and low dose heparin during percutaneous coronary revascularization. *N Engl J Med* 1997, 336:1689–1696.

EPISTENT Investigators: Randomised, placebo-controlled and balloon-angioplasty-controlled trial to assess safety of coronary stenting with use of platelet glycoprotein IIb/IIIa blockade. *Lancet* 1998, 352:87–92.

Eriksson BI, Bauer KA, Lassen MR, Turpie AGG, the Steering Committee of the Pentasaccharide in Hip-Fracture Surgery Study: Fondaparinux compared with enoxaparin for the prevention of venous thromboembolism after hip-fracture surgery. *N Engl J Med* 2001, 345:1298–1304.

ESSENCE trial results: Breaking new ground: efficacy and safety of subcutaneous enoxaparin in non–Q-wave coronary events. *Can J Cardiol* 1998, 14(suppl E):15E–19E.

Forman R, Frishman WH: Thrombolytic agents. In *Cardiovascular Pharmacotherapeutics*, edn 2. Edited by Frishman WH, Sonnenblick EH, Sica DA. New York: McGraw Hill; 2003:301–315.

Foster RH, Wiseman LR: Abciximab: an updated review of its use in ischaemic heart disease. *Drugs* 1998, 56:629–665.

Frishman WH, Hanjis C: Aspirin resistance: mechanisms and clinical implications. *Cardiol Rev* 2004, in press.

Frishman WH, Lerner RG, Klein MD, Roganovic M.: Antiplatelet and antithrombotic drugs. In *Cardiovascular Pharmacotherapeutics*, edn 2. Edited by Frishman WH, Sonnenblick EH, Sica DA. New York: McGraw Hill; 2003:259–299.

Gent M, Easton JD, Hachinski VC, *et al.*: The Canadian American Ticlopidine Study (CATS) in thromboembolic stroke. *Lancet* 1989, 1:1215–1220.

GISSI (Gruppo Italiano per lo Studio della Streptochinasi nell'Infarcto Miocardico): Effectiveness of intravenous thrombolytic treatment in acute myocardial infarction. *Lancet* 1986, 1:397–401.

GISSI Group, GISSI 2: A factorial randomised trial of alteplase versus streptokinase and heparin versus no heparin among 12,490 patient with acute myocardial infarction. *Lancet* 1990, 336:65–71.

Goodman SG, Fitchett D, Armstrong PW *et al.* for the INTERACT trial investigators: Randomized evaluation of the safety and efficacy of enoxaparin versus unfractionated heparin in high-risk patients with non-ST-segment elevation acute coronary syndromes receiving the glycoprotein IIb/IIIA inhibitor eptifibatide. *Circulation* 2003, 107:238–244.

Granger CB, Califf RM, Topol EJ: Thrombolytic therapy for acute myocardial infarction. *Drugs* 1992, 44:293–325.

Greinacher A, Amiral J, Dummel V, *et al.*: Laboratory diagnosis of heparin-associated thrombocytopenia and comparison of platelet aggregation test, heparin-induced platelet activation test, and platelet factor 4-heparin enzyme linked immunosorbent assay. *Transfusion* 1994, 34:381–385.

Greinacher A, Lubenow N: Recombinant hirudin in clinical practice. *Circulation* 2001, 103:1479–1484.

Greinacher A, Volpel H, Janssens U, *et al.*: Recombinant hirudin provides safe and effective anticoagulation in patients with heparin-induced thrombocytopenia: a prospective study. *Circulation* 1999, 99:73–80.

Grotta JC, Norris JW, Kamm B: Prevention of stroke with ticlopidine: who benefits the most? TASS baseline and angiographic subgroup. *Neurology* 1992, 42:111–115.

GUSTO Investigators: An international randomized trial comparing four thrombolytic strategies for acute myocardial infarction. *N Engl J Med* 1993, 329:673–682.

GUSTO IV-ACS Investigators. Effect of glycoprotein IIb/IIIa receptor blocker abciximab on outcome in patients with acute coronary syndromes without early coronary revascularisation: the GUSTO IV-ACS randomised trial. *Lancet* 2001, 357:1915–1924.

Hass WK, Easton JD, Adams HP, *et al.*: A randomized trial comparing ticlopidine hydrochloride with aspirin for the prevention of stroke in high risk patients. *N Engl J Med* 1989, 321:501.

Hennekens CH, O'Donnell CJ, Ridker PM, *et al.*: Current issues concerning thrombolytic therapy for acute myocardial infarction. *J Am Coll Cardiol* 1995, 25(Suppl):18s–22s.

Hiatt WR: Drug therapy: medical treatment of peripheral arterial disease and claudication. *N Engl J Med* 2001, 344:1608–1621.

Hirsh J: Low-molecular-weight heparin: a review of the results of recent studies of the treatment of venous thromboembolism and unstable angina. *Circulation* 1998, 98:1575–1582.

Hirsh J, Dalen JE, Anderson DR, *et al.*: Oral anticoagulants: mechanism of action, clinical effectiveness, and optimal therapeutic range. *Chest* 2001, 119(Suppl):8S–21S.

Hirsh J, Fuster V, Ansell J, Halperin JL: American Heart Association/American College of Cardiology Foundation guide to warfarin therapy. *Circulation* 2003, 107:1692–1711.

Hirsh J, Warkentin TE, Shaughnessy SG, *et al.*: Heparin and low-molecular-weight heparin: mechanisms of action, pharmacokinetics, dosing, monitoring, efficacy, and safety. *Chest* 2001, 119(Suppl):64S–94S.

IMPACT II Investigators: Randomised placebo-controlled trial of effect of eptifibatide on complications of percutaneous coronary intervention: IMPACT-II. *Lancet* 1997, 349:1422–1428.

INJECT Study Group: Randomised, double-blind comparison of reteplase double-bolus administration with streptokinase in acute myocardial infarction (INJECT): trial to investigate equivalence. *Lancet* 1995, 346:329–336.

ISIS 2 Collaborative Group: Randomised trial of intravenous streptokinase, oral aspirin, both or neither among 17,187 cases of suspected acute myocardial infarction. *Lancet* 1988, 2:349–360.

ISIS-3: A randomized comparison of streptokinase vs tissue plasminogen activator vs anistreplase and of aspirin plus heparin vs aspirin alone among 41,299 cases of suspected acute myocardial infarction. *Lancet* 1992, 339:753–770.

Jang I-K, Brown DFM, Giugliano RP, *et al.* and the MINT Investigators: A multicenter, randomized study of argatroban versus heparin as adjunct to tissue plasminogen activator (TPA) in acute myocardial infarction: Myocardial Infarction with Novastatin and TPA (MINT) Study. *J Am Coll Cardiol* 1999, 33:1879–1885.

Janz TG: Using thrombolytic therapy for life-threatening pulmonary embolism. *J Crit Illness* 2003, 18:102.

Kearon C, Ginsberg JS, Kovacs MJ *et al.* for the Extended Low-Intensity Anticoagulation for Thrombo-Embolism Investigators: Comparison of low-intensity warfarin therapy with conventional-intensity warfarin therapy for long-term prevention of recurrent venous thromboembolism. *N Engl J Med* 2003, 349:631–639.

Klein W, Buchwald A, Hillis S, *et al.*: Comparison of low molecular weight heparin with unfractionated heparin acutely and with placebo for 6 weeks in the management of unstable coronary artery disease: the Fragmin in Unstable Coronary Artery Disease study (FRIC). *Circulation* 1997, 96:61–68.

Krumholz HM, Pasternak RC, Weinstein MC, *et al.*: Cost effectiveness of thrombolytic therapy with streptokinase in elderly patients with suspected acute myocardial infarction. *N Engl J Med* 1992, 327:7–13.

Kucher N, Tapson VF: Pulmonary embolism. In *Hurst's The Heart*, edn 11. Edited by Fuster V, Alexander RW, O'Rourke R. New York: McGraw Hill; 2004:1593–1616.

Lee AYY, Levine MN, Baker RI *et al.* for the CLOT Investigators: Low-molecular weight heparin versus a coumarin for the prevention of recurrent venous thromboembolism in patients with cancer. *N Engl J Med* 2003, 349:146–153.

Leon MB, Baim DS, Popma JJ, *et al.*: A clinical trial comparing three antithrombotic-drug regimens after coronary-artery stenting. *N Engl J Med* 1998, 339:1665–1671.

Lerner RG, Frishman WH, Mohan KT: Clopidogrel: a new antiplatelet drug. *Heart Dis* 2000, 2:168–173.

Levine M, Gent M, Hirsh J, *et al.*: A comparison of low-molecular-weight heparin administered primarily at home with unfractionated heparin administered in the hospital for proximal deep vein thrombosis. *N Engl J Med* 1996, 334:677–681.

Lincoff AM, Bittl JA, Harrington RA, *et al.*: Bivalirudin and provisional glycoprotein IIb/IIIa blockade compared with heparin and planned glycoprotein IIb/IIIa blockade during percutaneous coronary intervention. REPLACE-2 randomized trial. *JAMA* 2003, 289:853–863.

Lincoff AM, Califf RM, Van de Werf F, *et al.*: Mortality at 1 year with combination platelet glycoprotein IIb/IIIa inhibition and reduced-dose fibrinolytic therapy vs conventional fibrinolytic therapy for acute myocardial infarction. GUSTO V Randomized Trial. *JAMA* 2002, 288:2130–2135.

Matisse Investigators: Subcutaneous fondaparinux versus intravenous unfractionated heparin in the initial treatment of pulmonary embolism. *N Engl J Med* 2003, 349:1695–1702.

McEwen J, Strauch G, Perles P, *et al.*: Clopidogrel bioavailability is unaffected by food or antacids. *J Clin Pharmacol* 1996, 36:856.

McKeage K, Plosker GL: Argatroban. *Drugs* 2001, 61:515–522.

Mehta SR, Yusuf S, Peters RJG, *et al.*: Effects of pretreatment with clopidogrel and aspirin followed by long-term therapy in patients undergoing percutaneous coronary intervention: the PCI-CURE study. *Lancet* 2001, 358:527–533.

Moliterno DJ, Yakubov SJ, DiBattiste PM, *et al.*: Outcomes at 6 months for the direct comparison of tirofiban and abciximab during percutaneous coronary revascularisation with stent placement: the TARGET follow-up study. *Lancet* 2002, 360:355–360.

Monealescot G, Phillippe F, Ankri A, *et al.*: Early increase in von Willebrand factor predicts adverse outcome in unstable coronary artery disease: beneficial effects of enoxaparin. *Circulation* 1998, 98:294–299.

The information here is provided as guidance only. Prescribers should always consult the manufacturer's current prescribing information.

149

Monreal M, Costa J, Salva P: Pharmacological properties of hirudin and its derivatives: potential clinical advantages over heparin. *Drugs Aging* 1996, 8:171–182.

Nawarskas JJ, Anderson JR: Bivalirudin. A new approach to anticoagulation. *Heart Dis* 2001, 3:131–137.

Noble S, Spencer CM: Enoxaparin: a review of its clinical potential in the management of coronary artery disease. *Drugs* 1998, 56:259–272.

Ohman EM, Harrington RA, Cannon CP, et al: Intravenous thrombolysis in acute myocardial infarction. *Chest* 2001, 119(Suppl):253S–277S.

Organisation to Assess Strategies for Ischemic Syndromes (OASIS-2) Investigators: Effects of recombinant hirudin (lepirudin) compared with heparin on death, myocardial infarction, refractory angina, and revascularisation procedures in patients with acute myocardial ischaemia without ST elevation: a randomised trial. *Lancet* 1999, 353:429–438.

O'Rourke RA: Unstable angina and non–ST-segment elevation myocardial infarction: clinical presentation, diagnostic evaluation, and medical management. In *Hurst's The Heart*, edn 11. Edited by Fuster V, Alexander RW, O'Rourke R. New York: McGraw Hill; 2004:1251–1276.

O'Shea JC, Cantor WJ, Buller CE, et al.: Long-term efficacy of platelet glycoprotein IIb/IIIa integrin blockade with eptifibatide in coronary stent intervention. *JAMA* 2002, 287(5):618-621.

Patrono C: Aspirin as an antiplatelet agent. *N Engl J Med* 1994, 329:1287–1294.

Patrono C, Coller B, Dalen JE, et al.: Platelet-active drugs: the relationships among dose, effectiveness, and side effects *Chest* 2001, 119(Suppl):39S–63S.

Phillips DR, Scarborough RM: Clinical pharmacology of eptifibatide. *Am J Cardiol* 1997, 80:11B–20B.

Pineo GF, Hull RD: Unfractionated and low-molecular-weight heparin: comparison and current recommendations. *Med Clin North Am* 1998, 82:587–599.

Popma JJ, Ohman EM, Weitz J, et al.: Antithrombotic therapy in patients undergoing percutaneous coronary intervention. *Chest* 2001, 119(Suppl):321S–336S.

PRISM Study Investigators: A comparison of aspirin plus tirofiban with aspirin plus heparin for unstable angina. *N Engl J Med* 1998, 338:1498–1505.

PRISM-PLUS Study Investigators: Inhibition of platelet glycoprotein IIb/IIIa receptor with tirofiban in unstable angina and non–Q-wave myocardial infarction. *N Engl J Med* 1998, 338:1488–1497.

PURSUIT Trial Investigators: Inhibition of platelet glycoprotein IIb/IIIa with eptifibatide in patients with acute coronary syndromes. *N Engl J Med* 1998, 339:436–443.

RESTORE Investigators: Effects of platelet glycoprotein IIb/IIIa blockade with tirofiban on adverse cardiac events in patients with unstable angina or acute myocardial infarction undergoing coronary angioplasty. *Circulation* 1997, 96:1445–1453.

Reynolds NA, Perry CM, Scott LJ: Fondaparinux sodium. A review of its use in the prevention of venous thromboembolism following major orthopaedic surgery. *Drugs* 2004, 64:1575–1596.

Ryan TJ, Antman EM, Brooks NH, et al.: 1999 update: ACC/AHA guidelines for the management of patients with acute myocardial infarction: executive summary and recommendations: a report of the American College of Cardiology/American Heart Association Task Force on Practice Guidelines (Committee on Management of Acute Myocardial Infarction). *Circulation* 1999, 100:1016–1030.

Saltiel E, Ward A: Ticlopidine: a review of its pharmacodynamic and pharmacokinetic properties, and therapeutic efficacy in platelet-dependent disease states. *Drugs* 1987, 34:222–262.

SCATI (Studio sulla Calciparina nell' Angina e nella Trombosi Ventricolare nell 'Infarcto) Group: Randomized controlled trial of subcutaneous calcium-heparin in acute myocardial infarction. *Lancet* 1989, 2:182–186.

Sharis PJ, Cannon CP, Loscalzo J: The antiplatelet effects of ticlopidine and clopidogrel. *Ann Intern Med* 1998, 129:394–405.

Sinnaeve P, Alexander J, Belmans A, et al.: One-year follow-up of the ASSENT-2 trial: a double-blind, randomized comparison of single-bolus tenecteplase and front-loaded alteplase in 16,949 patients with ST-elevation acute myocardial infarction. *Am Heart J* 2003, 146:27–32.

Sinnaeve PR, Alexander JH, Bogaerts K, et al.: Efficacy of tenecteplase in combination with enoxaparin, abciximab, or unfractionated heparin: one-year follow-up results of the Assessment of the Safety of a New Thrombolytic-3 (ASSENT-3) randomized trial in acute myocardial infarction. *Am Heart J* 2004, 147:993–998.

Sixth ACCP Consensus Conference on Antithrombotic Therapy: *Quick Reference Guide for Clinicians.* Northbrook, IL: American College of Chest Physicians; 2001.

Smalling R, Bode C, Kalbfleisch J, et al.: More rapid, complete, and stable coronary thrombolysis with bolus administration of reteplase compared with alteplase infusion in acute myocardial infarction. *Circulation* 1995, 91:2725–2732.

Smith P, Amesen H, Holme I: The effect of warfarin on mortality and reinfarction after myocardial infarction. *N Engl J Med* 1990, 323:147–152.

Stein B, Fuster V, Israel DH, et al.: Platelet inhibitor agents in cardiovascular disease: an update. *J Am Coll Cardiol* 1989, 14:813–836.

Stienhubl SR, Berger PB, Mann JT 3d, *et al.*: Early and sustained dual antiplatelet therapy following percutaneous coronary intervention. A randomized controlled trial. *JAMA* 2002, 288:2411–2420.

The Dutch TIA Trial Study Group: A comparison of two doses of aspirin (30 mg vs 283 mg a day) in patients after a transient ischemic attack or minor ischemic stroke. *N Engl J Med* 1991, 325:1261–1266.

The ECASS Study Group: Intravenous thrombolysis with recombinant tissue plasminogen activator for acute hemispheric stroke: The European Cooperative Acute Stroke Study (ECASS). *JAMA* 1995, 274:1017–1025.

The European Myocardial Infarction Project Group: Prehospital thrombolytic therapy in patients with suspected acute myocardial infarction. *N Engl J Med* 1993, 329:383–389.

The Global Use of Strategies to Open Occluded Coronary Arteries (GUSTO III) Investigators: A comparison of reteplase with alteplase for acute myocardial infarction. *N Engl J Med* 1997, 337:1118–1123.

The National Institute of Neurological Disorders and Stroke t-PA Stroke Study Group: Tissue plasminogen activator for acute ischemic stroke. *N Engl J Med* 1995, 333:1581–1587.

The Steering Committee of the Physicians' Health Study Research Group: Final report on the aspirin component of the ongoing Physicians' Health Study. *N Engl J Med* 1989, 321:129–135.

Theroux P, Ouimet H, McCars J, *et al.*: Aspirin, heparin or both to treat acute unstable angina. *N Engl J Med* 1988, 319:1105–1111.

TIMI Study Group: Comparison of invasive and conservative strategies after treatment with intravenous tissue plasminogen activator in acute myocardial infarction: result of the thrombolysis in myocardial infarction (TIMI) phase II trial. *N Engl J Med* 1989, 320:618–627.

Topol EJ, Moliterno DJ, Herrmann HC, *et al.*: Comparison of two platelet glycoprotein IIb/IIIa inhibitors, tirofiban and abciximab, for the prevention of ischemic events with percutaneous coronary revascularization. *N Engl J Med* 2001, 344:1888–1894.

Verstraete M, Fuster V: Thrombogenesis and antithrombotic therapy. In *Hurst's The Heart*, edn 9. Edited by Alexander RW, Schlant RC, Fuster V. New York: McGraw Hill; 1998:1501–1551.

von Domburg RT, Boersma E, Simoons ML: A review of the long-term effects of thrombolytic agents. *Drugs* 2000, 60:293–305.

Warkentin TE, Chong BH, Greinacher A: Heparin-induced thrombocytopenia: towards consensus. *Thromb Haemostas* 1998, 79:1–7.

Warkentin TE, Elavathil LJ, Hayward CPM, *et al.*: The pathogenesis of venous limb gangrene associated with heparin-induced thrombocytopenia. *Ann Intern Med* 1997, 127:804–812.

Weitz JI, Hirsh J: New anticoagulant drugs. *Chest* 2001, 119(Suppl):95S–107S.

Wilcox RG, Von der Lippe G, Olsson CG, *et al.*: Trial of tissue plasminogen activator for mortality reduction in acute myocardial infarction (ASSET). *Lancet* 1988, 2:525–530.

Beta-adrenergic blocking agents exert their major effects through the beta-adrenoceptors in the heart and peripheral vasculature. These agents are generally well tolerated and are widely used for various cardiovascular and other clinical conditions. Heart rate, myocardial contractility, and blood pressure (BP) are all reduced with beta-blockade.

Beta-receptors are also found in a wide range of other tissues. The two main types of beta-receptors, beta$_1$ and beta$_2$, frequently coexist in the same tissue. There is now evidence for a beta$_3$-receptor in brown fat, which is associated with thermogenesis. Table 7.1 shows the distribution of beta-receptors in the body.

During the 1950s, J.W. Black conceived the idea that patients with coronary heart disease might benefit if the work of the heart could be reduced through inhibition of the cardiac beta-receptors. Beta-blockade results in a reduction in heart rate, myocardial contractility, and myocardial oxygen consumption. His work led to the synthesis of propranolol, a nonselective beta-blocker that proved effective in treating ischemic heart disease. Its antihypertensive activity came as a surprise. Today, beta-blockers are indicated for the treatment of hypertension, angina pectoris, myocardial infarction (MI), arrhythmias, pheochromocytoma, Fallot's tetralogy, congestive cardiomyopathy, portal hypertension, thyrotoxicosis, anxiety, tremor, migraine, and glaucoma.

The manufacture of **propranolol** was followed by a number of other beta-blockers with differing pharmacology. Examples include those with partial agonist activity (PAA), such as **pindolol** and **penbutolol**, and beta$_1$-selective (cardioselective) agents, such as **atenolol** and **metoprolol**. The term *partial agonist activity*, also referred to as *intrinsic sympathomimetic activity* (ISA), implies the capacity of beta-blockers to stimulate as well as to inhibit adrenergic receptors (Figure 7.1).

The numerous available beta-blockers can be subdivided on the basis of their pharmacologic properties: nonselective drugs without ISA, beta$_1$-selective (or cardioselective) drugs without ISA, nonselective drugs with ISA, beta$_1$-selective drugs with ISA, and agents with additional alpha-blocking activity ("dual-acting") beta-blockers (Table 7.2).

Beta-blockers can also be classified on the basis of their water solubility (hydrophilicity). The hydrophilic agents are minimally metabolized. These agents tend to have a longer duration of action, which makes them suitable for once-daily administration. Moreover, hydrophilic agents penetrate brain tissue less; thus, they are less likely to produce central nervous system side effects.

MODE OF ACTION

The mode of action of a beta-blocker is best described by considering the actions of the sympathetic nervous system.

The sympathetic nervous system prepares the body for "fight or flight" by accelerating heart rate, raising BP, and shifting blood from the skin and splanchnic bed to the skeletal muscles. Many of these effects result from stimulation of the beta-receptors by the catecholamines, epinephrine and norepinephrine. The former is released by the adrenal medulla and the latter by sympathetic nerve endings. An exogenously administered beta-blocker binds preferentially and reversibly to the beta-receptor, thus competitively inhibiting endogenous catecholamines (Figure 7.1). Some beta-blockers, besides inhibiting sympathetic nerve activity when they occupy the receptor, also possess some sympathomimetic activity (*ie*, PAA or ISA) (Figure 7.1).

The BP-lowering mechanism of the beta-blockers is not entirely understood. The initial fall in cardiac output is counterbalanced by increased peripheral sympathetic nerve activity, leading to vasoconstriction and increased total peripheral resistance. Peripheral sympathetic nerve activity subsides eventually and is accompanied by decreases in total peripheral resistance and BP. The fall in BP, then, is a result of decreased cardiac output. The acute and chronic hemodynamic effects of beta-blockers in hypertensive patients are illustrated in Figure 7.2. Some beta-blockers have a direct effect on peripheral resistance via their beta$_2$ ISA (which causes vasodilatation), via alpha-blockade (which prevents vasoconstriction), or via a nonspecific vasodilatory effect. Several other mechanisms have been proposed to explain the antihypertensive effects of beta-blockers: 1) a central action, 2) inhibition of sympathetic nervous action by prejunctional beta$_2$-receptor blockade, 3) renin-blocking activity, 4) reduction in plasma volume, 5) stimulation of vasodilatory prostaglandins and atrial natriuretic factor, and 6) baroreceptor resetting. These mechanisms are discussed in detail by Cruickshank and Prichard, and Frishman, Sonnenblick, and Sica.

In patients with acute or chronic myocardial ischemia, beta-blockers offset the effects of endogenous catecholamines. This results in reduced heart rate, systolic BP, and myocardial contractility, which in turn reduces myocardial oxygen demand. The slowing of heart rate may also prolong diastolic perfusion time. Beta-blockade has been shown to prevent cardiac rupture in patients with MI.

The class II antiarrhythmic properties of beta-blockers arise directly through the following: 1) reversal of the catecholamine-induced increase of diastolic depolarization of automatic pacemaker cells; 2) increase in the conduction time through the atrioventricular (AV) node; 3) shortening of the refractory period of ventricular cells; and 4) indirectly, through modification of factors that predispose a patient to arrhythmias, such as myocardial ischemia or hypokalemia.

TABLE 7.1 DISTRIBUTION AND RESPONSES MEDIATED BY ADRENOCEPTORS

System	Adrenoceptor type	Response to stimulation
Heart	$beta_1$, $beta_2$	Increase in heart rate
	$beta_1$	Increase in conduction velocity
	$beta_1$	Increase in excitability
	$beta_1$	Increase in force of contraction
Blood vessels	alpha	Constriction of arteries and veins
	$beta_1$	Dilation of coronary arteries
	$beta_2$	Dilation of most arteries
Lung	alpha	Bronchoconstriction
	$beta_2$, $beta_1$	Bronchodilatation
Skeletal muscles	$beta_2$	Tremor
	$beta_2$	Stimulation of Na/K pump, resulting in increased contractility and hypokalemia
Bladder detrusor	beta	Relaxatory urgency
Smooth muscles		
Uterine	$beta_2$	Relaxation
Eye	alpha	Mydriasis
Intestinal	$beta_1$	Relaxation
Mast cells	alpha	Augmented releases of mediators of anaphylaxis
	beta	Inhibition of release of mediators of anaphylaxis
Platelets	$alpha_2$, beta	Aggregation promoted
Eye		
Intraocular pressure	$beta_1$	Increase in intraocular pressure
Tear secretion	$beta_2$	Increase in basic secretion
Central nervous system	$beta_1$	Not known
	$alpha_2$	Fall in blood pressure
Metabolism		
Gluconeogenesis	alpha	Promoted
Glycogenolysis	alpha (liver)	Promoted
	$beta_1$ (heart)	Promoted
	$beta_2$ (skeletal muscle; ? liver)	Promoted
Lipolysis (white adipocytes)	$beta_1$, $beta_2$	Promoted
Thermogenesis (brown adipocytes)	$beta_1$, $beta_3$	Promoted
Hormone secretion		
Glucagon	$beta_2$	Promoted
Insulin	alpha	Inhibited
	$beta_2$	Promoted
Parathyroid hormone	$beta_1$	Promoted
Renin	$beta_1$, $beta_2$	Promoted
Neurotransmitter release		Facilitated: skeletal neuromuscular junction
Acetylcholine	alpha	Inhibited: sympathetic ganglia and intestine, with inhibition/relaxation
Noradrenaline	alpha	Inhibited
	beta (? $beta_2$)	Facilitated

Adapted from Cruickshank JM, Prichard BNC: *Beta Blockers in Clinical Practice.* Edinburgh: Churchill Livingstone; 1987.

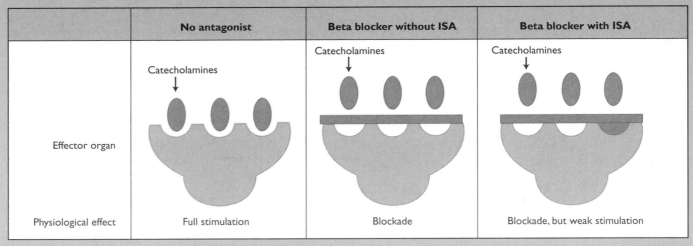

FIGURE 7.1 Nature of beta-adrenoceptor inhibition: effects of intrinsic sympathomimetic activity (ISA) (partial agonist activity) in the presence of high levels of catecholamines. (*Adapted from* Frishman WH, Charlap S, Kostis JB: Clinical significance of ISA in beta-adrenoceptor blocker drugs. In *Beta Blockers in the Treatment of Cardiovascular Disease.* Edited by Kostis JB *et al.* New York: Raven Press; 1984:253–274.)

TABLE 7.2 CLASSIFICATION OF BETA-ADRENERGIC BLOCKERS

Without ISA	With ISA	Dual-acting
Nonselective	Nonselective	
Nadolol	Carteolol	Carvedilol
Propranolol	Penbutolol	Labetalol
Sotalol	Pindolol	
Timolol		
β₁-Selective	β₁-Selective	
Atenolol	Acebutolol	
Betaxolol		
Bisoprolol		
Esmolol		
Metoprolol		

ISA—intrinsic sympathomimetic activity.

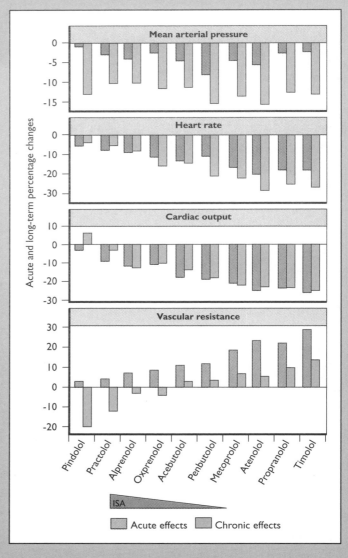

FIGURE 7.2 Acute and chronic hemodynamic effects of 10 beta-adrenoceptor antagonists in hypertensive patients at rest. The degree of intrinsic sympathomimetic activity (ISA) decreases from strong (pindolol) to almost none (penbutolol). Metoprolol, atenolol, propranolol, and timolol lack intrinsic sympathomimetic activity. (*Adapted from* Man In't Veld AJ, van der Meiracker AH: Effects of antihypertensive drugs on cardiovascular haemodynamics. In *Hypertension.* Edited by Laragh JH, Brenner BM. New York: Raven Press; 1990:2117–2130.)

Nonselective beta-blockers competitively inhibit the effects of catecholamines at beta$_1$- and beta$_2$-adrenergic sites. To reverse the effect of beta-blockade, a higher concentration of the agonist is required.

EFFICACY AND USE

Nonselective beta-blockers without ISA are effective in lowering diastolic BP to less than 95 mm Hg in 40% to 50% of patients with mild to moderate hypertension. The BP is lowered in the supine and standing positions and also during exercise. The Medical Research Council trial of mild hypertension showed that in nonsmoking men, **propranolol** decreased the frequency of strokes by 47% and coronary events by 33%. Smoking negated these benefits. Furthermore, **propranolol** significantly reduced the incidence of Q-wave MI (silent and overt); risk for sudden death remained unchanged.

Comparisons among nonselective beta-blockers without ISA (**propranolol, timolol, nadolol**) have found no differences in antihypertensive efficacy. Studies comparing nonselective beta-blockers without ISA (usually **propranolol**) and agents with mild to modest ISA (**carteolol** and **penbutolol**) indicate similar BP-lowering effect. Comparisons of **propranolol** with **pindolol** (which has moderate to high ISA) have shown that they have similar efficacy in lowering daytime BP, but **pindolol** does not significantly lower nocturnal BP. Under conditions of low sympathetic drive, such as sleep, **pindolol** acts as a stimulant to increase the heart rate. Comparisons of nonselective beta-blockers without ISA and beta$_1$-selective blockers without ISA (**atenolol, metoprolol**) indicate similar antihypertensive effects. During strenuous exercise, when catecholamine levels are high, systolic BP is probably better controlled by a beta$_1$-selective than by a nonselective beta-blocker agent.

Diuretics combine well with **propranolol, nadolol**, and **timolol**, producing additive antihypertensive effects. The presence of a beta-blocker mitigates, to some extent, the diuretic-induced hypokalemia. Vasodilators combine well with nonselective beta-blockers, resulting in additive antihypertensive effects. The reflex increase in heart rate associated with vasodilators is diminished by beta-blockade. Calcium antagonists of the dihydropyridine type (eg, **amlodipine, felodipine, nifedipine**) combine well with beta-blockers, adding additional antihypertensive effect. Central-acting antihypertensive agents, such as methyldopa, combine well with beta-blockers such as **propranolol**; they are well tolerated and produce additive antihypertensive effects.

In treating stable angina, **propranolol** has been shown to be superior to long-acting nitrates, and this class of beta-blockers is generally more effective than **nifedipine** in reducing angina symptoms and ischemia. In unstable angina, beta-blockers without ISA are probably more effective than **nifedipine** in providing rapid pain relief, although cardioselective beta-blockers without ISA are often preferred in this situation. Late intervention trials with oral nonselective beta-blockers without ISA (given between days 2 and 28 after MI and continued for up to 3 years) showed a decrease in mortality of about 25%. The incidence of nonfatal reinfarction was also reduced by about 25%. Life-saving benefit has also been achieved in postinfarction patients with coexisting diabetes or congestive heart failure (CHF).

Patients with various arrhythmias may benefit from nonselective beta-blockade. In patients with supraventricular tachycardia, ventricular premature beats, sustained ventricular tachycardia, and ventricular fibrillation associated with ischemia, exercise, or emotion, beta-blockers are often the drugs of choice. **Sotalol**, which is approved for arrhythmias only, is discussed in the antiarrhythmic drug section.

In Fallot's tetralogy, intravenous **propranolol** improves pulmonary artery flow and arterial oxygen saturation. Long-term treatment with oral **propranolol** is highly effective in abolishing syncopal episodes and improving exercise tolerance. Likewise, beta-blockers can benefit patients with hypertrophic obstructive cardiomyopathy, dissecting aneurysms, mitral valve prolapse, mitral stenosis, idiopathic or orthostatic hypotension, and stress-induced cardiac necrosis associated with subarachnoid hemorrhage. Nonselective beta-blockers are also prescribed for a number of noncardiovascular conditions, including portal hypertension, thyrotoxicosis, pheochromocytoma, anxiety, migraine, tremor, and raised intraocular pressure.

MODE OF ACTION

Oral beta-blockers reduce heart rate, systolic BP, and myocardial contractility, thus reducing myocardial oxygen demand. This reduction in myocardial workload is the main mechanism of action in the ischemic patient. Additionally, in acute MI, beta-blockade has been shown to prevent cardiac rupture and life-threatening arrhythmias.

In treating hypertension, both intravenous and oral beta-blockade leads to a reduction in cardiac output by 20% to 25%. This decrease is maintained on chronic oral therapy. Stroke volume is usually unchanged or possibly slightly increased. A fall in heart rate is the main cause of the fall in cardiac output, but left ventricular contractility is also reduced. The fall in cardiac output is counterbalanced by a reflex increase in peripheral resistance magnified by vasoconstriction caused by peripheral beta$_2$-blockade. A nonselective agent may thus produce a lesser fall in diastolic BP than a beta$_1$-selective agent (which preserves beta$_2$-vasodilatation) (Figure 7.2).

Except in the presence of high sympathetic tone or poor left ventricular function, BP does not fall immediately after intravenous beta-blockade. In responders, the reduction in

BP occurs during the first few hours, but maximum reduction may not be achieved after a few months. The fall in coronary blood flow is largely an autoregulatory effect of decreased myocardial oxygen requirement. Autoregulatory processes maintain flow to the brain, whereas less vital tissues, such as skin, muscle, and splanchnic areas, may experience a marked decrease in blood flow.

All the normal hemodynamic responses associated with dynamic exercise or mental stress remain unchanged on nonselective beta-blockade except that heart rate, BP, and cardiac output are 15% to 25% lower. Factors associated with excessive sympathetic activity, such as hypoglycemia and smoking, may be linked to an increase in BP and a reflex decrease in heart rate when nonselective beta-blockers are given.

INDICATIONS

	Nadolol	Propranolol	Sotalol	Timolol
Hypertension	+	+	–	+
Angina	+	+	–	–
Post–myocardial infarction	–	+	–	+
Arrhythmias	–	+	+	–
Hypertrophic subaortic stenosis	–	+	–	–
Essential tremor	–	+	–	–
Migraine headache prophylaxis	–	+	–	+

+ —approved by the FDA; – —not approved by the FDA.

Nadolol, structurally similar to propranolol, is a nonselective beta-adrenergic antagonist. It has no ISA or membrane-stabilizing activity. Nadolol is water soluble, is not metabolized, and has a long duration of action, which offers the advantage of once-a-day dosing. It has been observed that nadolol increases renal blood flow in humans without significant changes in glomerular filtration rate. Its chronic effect on renal hemodynamics remains unclear. Nadolol has also been used for migraine prophylaxis (80–240 mg daily) as well as in the treatment of supraventricular arrhythmias at dosages of 60–160 mg/d (not FDA-approved indications).

SPECIAL GROUPS

Race: black hypertensive patients may be less responsive than white patients

Children: safety and effectiveness have not been established

Elderly: start with low dose, and titrate based on clinical response

Renal impairment: drug clearance is reduced; dosing interval should be increased and adjusted based on clinical response

Hepatic impairment: use with caution, although dosage adjustment is not required

Pregnancy: category C; use only if potential benefit justifies the potential risk to the fetus

Breast-feeding: not recommended; excreted in human milk

DOSAGE*

Hypertension: Usual maintenance dose—40–80 mg daily
Maximum dose—320 mg daily
The dosage is 20–40 mg once daily initially and is increased by 40–80 mg/d every 1–2 wk until desired BP control is achieved.

Angina pectoris: Usual dose—40–80 mg daily
Maximum dose—240 mg daily
The initial dose is 40 mg once daily and is increased by 40–80 mg/d every 3–7 d until adequate control of angina is achieved or there is pronounced slowing of the heart rate.

*Guidelines for dosing intervals in patients with renal impairment.

Creatinine clearance, $mL/min/1.73\ m^2$	Dosing interval
>50	q 24 h
31–50	q 24–36 h
10–30	q 24–48 h
<10	q 40–60 h

IN BRIEF

INDICATIONS
Hypertension   Angina pectoris

CONTRAINDICATIONS
Overt heart failure
Bronchial asthma or related bronchospastic problems
Severe chronic obstructive pulmonary disease
Sinus bradycardia with second- or third-degree AV block
Sick sinus syndrome without a permanent pacemaker in place
Cardiogenic shock
Known hypersensitivity to product components

DRUG INTERACTIONS
Anesthetics, general[1]   Monoamine oxidase (MAO) inhibitors[1]
Antihypertensive agents[1,3]   Neuromuscular blocking agents[3]
Beta-agonists[2,4]   NSAIDs[2]
Calcium channel blockers: Oral hypoglycemic agents[3,4]
  verapamil or diltiazem[1,3]   Reserpine and other
Insulin[3]   catecholamine-depleting drugs[1]

1 Effect/toxicity of nadolol may increase.
2 Effect of nadolol may decrease.
3 Nadolol may increase the effect/toxicity of this drug.
4 Nadolol may decrease the effect of this drug.

ADVERSE EFFECTS
CV: bradycardia, peripheral vascular insufficiency/Raynaud's type, postural hypotension, syncope, hypotension, heart failure, AV block, ventricular arrhythmia, angina
CNS: fatigue, dizziness, drowsiness, paresthesia
Respiratory: dyspnea, bronchospasm, nasal congestion
GI: nausea, vomiting, dyspepsia, constipation
GU: male impotence, ejaculatory failure
Metabolic: hypoglycemia
Other: edema, weight gain, allergic reaction

PHARMACOKINETICS AND PHARMACODYNAMICS
Duration of action:	>24 h
Onset of action:	<2 h
Peak plasma concentration:	2–4 h
Bioavailability:	30%–40%
Effect of food:	no effect
Protein binding:	30%
Volume of distribution:	1.9 L/kg
Metabolism:	not metabolized
Elimination:	urine—24.6%; feces—76.9%
Elimination half-life:	10–24 h (↑ in renal impairment)

MONITORING
BP, heart rate, respiratory status, signs/symptoms of CNS adverse effects.

OVERDOSE
Supportive: For severe bradycardia, atropine 0.25–2.0 mg IV may be administered or a pacemaker should be placed. Isoproterenol may also be used if bradycardia persists. For cardiovascular support, glucagon 50 µg/kg IV bolus may be administered over 1–2 min; up to 10 mg may be needed in some cases. In many cases, this may be followed by 2–5 mg/h (maximum 10 mg/h) continuous infusion. Fluid therapy with vasopressors/inotropic therapy may be added if necessary. Nadolol may be removed by dialysis.

PATIENT INFORMATION
Nadolol therapy should not be discontinued abruptly without consulting your health care provider. Your health care provider should also be consulted for persistent or unusual problems, such as dizziness/faintness, weight gain, worsening edema, or increasing shortness of breath. Sit or lie down if dizziness occurs, and rise slowly from a sitting or lying position. This medication may cause dizziness or drowsiness; use caution if performing activities requiring mental or physical effort.

AVAILABILITY
Tablets—20, 40, 80, 120, 160 mg
Combination formulations with a diuretic:
  Corzide® 40/5 tablets—40 mg nadolol and 5 mg bendroflumethiazide
  Corzide® 80/5 tablets—80 mg nadolol and 5 mg bendroflumethiazide

PROPRANOLOL

(Propranolol, Inderal®, Inderal LA®, InnoPran XL®)

Propranolol has been available for more than 35 years. It is a lipophilic molecule, is extensively metabolized by the liver, and has a short half-life. It also possesses membrane-stabilizing activity, which affects the cardiac action potential. It is administered two to three times daily, except for slow-release formulations, which may be administered once daily.

Propranolol has been shown to be useful for several indications, including hypertension and post-MI. In the large MRC mild hypertension study, propranolol significantly reduced the incidence of fatal and nonfatal stroke (although the benefits were offset by smoking), silent and overt infarctions, and sudden death. In the BHAT postinfarction study, propranolol reduced mortality and the reinfarction rate by about 25%. This benefit was particularly noticeable in diabetic patients and in those with heart failure.

In patients with subarachnoid hemorrhage, propranolol reduced stress-induced myocardial necrosis. In humans, chronic propranolol use may reverse left ventricular hypertrophy. Propranolol is also effective for prophylaxis of migraine headache and for treating essential tremor.

SPECIAL GROUPS

Race: black hypertensive patients may be less responsive than white patients

Children: less extensive data on efficacy and safety in children as in adults, but propranolol has been used safely and effectively in children. The usual antihypertensive dosage is 2–4 mg/kg/d (conventional tablets) in 2 divided doses (max. 16 mg/kg/d). There may be increased bioavailability in children with Down syndrome.

Elderly: start with low dose, and titrate based on clinical response

Renal impairment: use with caution; titrate the dose based on clinical response

Hepatic impairment: use with caution; titrate the dose based on clinical response

Pregnancy: category C; use only if potential benefit justifies the potential risk to the fetus

Breast-feeding: excreted in human milk; use with caution

IN BRIEF

INDICATIONS
Angina pectoris
Cardiac arrhythmias
Essential tremor
Hypertension
Hypertrophic subaortic stenosis
Migraine prophylaxis
MI treatment
Pheochromocytoma

CONTRAINDICATIONS
Bronchial asthma or related bronchospastic problems
Cardiogenic shock
Known hypersensitivity to product components
Second- or third-degree AV block
Severe heart failure
Severe obstructive lung disease
Sick sinus syndrome without a permanent pacemaker in place
Severe bradycardia

DRUG INTERACTIONS
Aluminum hydroxide gel[2]
Antihypertensive drugs[1,3]
Benzodiazepines[3]
Beta-agonists[2,4]
Calcium channel blockers: verapamil or diltiazem[1,3]
Cimetidine[1]
Diuretics (loop)[1]
Insulin[3]
Levodopa[4,5]
Neuromuscular blocking agents[3]
NSAIDs[2]
Oral hypoglycemic agents[3,4]
Phenothiazines[1,3]
Phenytoin[2]
Phenobarbital[2]
Propafenone[1]
Rifampin[2]
Selective serotonin reuptake inhibitors[1]
Theophylline[3]

1 Effect/toxicity of propranolol may increase.
2 Effect of propranolol may decrease.
3 Propranolol may increase the effect/toxicity of this drug.
4 Propranolol may decrease the effect of this drug.
5 The clinical significance of this interaction is unclear.

ADVERSE EFFECTS
CV: bradycardia, peripheral vascular insufficiency/Raynaud's type, postural hypotension, syncope, hypotension, heart failure, AV block, ventricular arrhythmia, angina
CNS: fatigue, dizziness, drowsiness, depression, hallucinations, disorientation, vivid dreams, short-term memory loss, paresthesia
Respiratory: dyspnea, bronchospasm
GI: nausea, vomiting, dyspepsia, constipation
GU: male impotence, ejaculatory failure
Metabolic: hypoglycemia
Other: edema, weight gain, allergic reaction, systemic lupus erythematosus, blood dyscrasias

PHARMACOKINETICS AND PHARMACODYNAMICS

Duration of action:	10–15 min (IV); 6–24 h (po)
Onset of action:	immediate (IV); variable; may occur as soon as 1 h postdose (po)
Peak plasma concentration:	IV—1 min; regular tablets—60–90 min; sustained release—6 h
Bioavailability:	100% (IV); 26% (po; sustained release—9%–18%)
Effect of food:	delayed absorption
Protein binding:	>90%
Volume of distribution:	4.3 L/kg
Metabolism:	mainly metabolized in liver with at least one active metabolite
Elimination:	mainly excreted in urine as metabolites
Elimination half-life:	3.4–6 h

PROPRANOLOL *(continued)*

DOSAGE *(LA—sustained release form)*

Hypertension:* Initial dosage—40 mg twice daily; (LA) 80 mg once daily
Maintenance—120–240 mg/d in 2–3 divided doses; (LA) 120–160 mg once daily
Maximum—640 mg/d in 2–3 divided doses

Angina pectoris:* 80–320 mg/d in 2–4 divided doses; (LA) 80–320 mg once daily

Arrhythmias: 10–30 mg 3 or 4 times daily before meals and at bedtime

Myocardial infarction: 180–240 mg/d in 2–4 divided doses

Migraine prophylaxis:* Dose range: 160–240 mg/d in divided doses starting from 80 mg/d in divided doses and increasing gradually to achieve optimal control; (LA) 80–240 mg once daily

Essential tremor: Usual dose is 120 mg/d in divided doses, starting from 40 mg twice daily and titrating the dose based on the response (maximum dose: 320 mg/d)

Hypertrophic subaortic stenosis:* 20–40 mg 3 or 4 times daily before meals and at bedtime; (LA) 80–160 mg once daily

Pheochromocytoma: 30–60 mg/d in divided doses

Intravenous administration for life-threatening arrhythmias: 1–3 mg, rate ≤1 mg/min; a second dose may be administered after 2 min if indicated

*Patients may also be switched from the regular to sustained-release formulation for once-daily regimen; however, it is not an exact milligram-for-milligram switch. To assure the desired therapeutic effect is maintained, dose should be adjusted based on clinical response.

MONITORING

BP, heart rate, ECG, respiratory status, and appropriate clinical response as per indication; signs/symptoms of CNS adverse effects.

OVERDOSE

Supportive: For severe bradycardia, atropine 0.25–2.0 mg IV may be administered or a pacemaker should be placed. Isoproterenol may also be used if bradycardia persists. For cardiovascular support, glucagon 50 μg/kg IV bolus may be administered over 1–2 min; up to 10 mg may be needed in some cases. In many cases, this may be followed by 2–5 mg/h (maximum 10 mg/h) continuous infusion. Fluid therapy with vasopressors/inotropic therapy may be added if necessary. Propranolol is not readily removed by dialysis.

PATIENT INFORMATION

Propranolol therapy should not be discontinued abruptly without consulting your health care provider. Your health care provider should also be consulted for persistent or unusual problems, such as dizziness/faintness, weight gain, worsening edema, or increasing shortness of breath. Sit or lie down if dizziness occurs, and rise slowly from a sitting or lying position. This medication may cause dizziness or drowsiness; use caution if performing activities requiring mental or physical effort.

AVAILABILITY

Tablets—10, 20, 40, 60, 80, 90 mg
Oral solution—4 mg/mL, 8 mg/mL, 80 mg/mL (concentrate)
Capsules (sustained release)—60, 80, 120, 160 mg
Injectable ampules and vials—1 mg/mL, 1 mL
Combination formulations with a diuretic, HCTZ (hydrochlorothiazide):
  Capsules (sustained release):
    Inderide LA 80/50: propranolol 80 mg/HCTZ 50 mg
    Inderide LA 120/50: propranolol 120 mg/HCTZ 50 mg
    Inderide LA 160/50: propranolol 160 mg/HCTZ 50 mg
  Tablets:
    Inderide 80/25: propranolol 80 mg/HCTZ 25 mg
    Inderide 40/25: propranolol 40 mg/HCTZ 25 mg
    Propranolol/HCTZ (generic): 80/25 mg
    Propranolol/HCTZ (generic): 40/25 mg

SOTALOL

(Betapace®)

Sotalol, a nonselective beta-adrenergic blocking agent without ISA or membrane-stabilizing activity, is water soluble and long acting. Similar to amiodarone, it has class II and III antiarrhythmic actions. The action potential of the myocardial cell is prolonged, resulting in a long QT interval. This property may occasionally predispose a patient to life-threatening arrhythmias, including ventricular fibrillation. Sotalol is indicated for the treatment of documented ventricular arrhythmias, such as sustained ventricular tachycardia, that, in the judgment of the physician, are life threatening. Sotalol is also indicated for the maintenance of normal sinus rhythm in patients with a history of symptomatic atrial fibrillation or flutter who are currently in normal sinus rhythm.

For additional information on sotalol, please refer to the chapter on antiarrhythmic agents.

TIMOLOL

(Timolol, Blocadren®)

Timolol is a nonselective beta-blocker. It has moderate lipophilicity and is metabolized by the liver. It does not have intrinsic sympathomimetic, direct myocardial depressant, or membrane-stabilizing activities. The Norwegian Multicentre Study demonstrated that timolol, begun 7 to 28 days post-MI, reduced overall mortality and reinfarction over 3 years compared with placebo. This benefit was still present at 6-year follow-up. Patients receiving timolol who stopped smoking gained the most benefit.

SPECIAL GROUPS

Race: black hypertensive patients may be less responsive than white patients

Children: safety and effectiveness have not been established

Elderly: start with low dose, and titrate the dose based on clinical response

Renal impairment: use with caution because drug may accumulate; titrate the dose based on clinical response

Hepatic impairment: use with caution because drug may accumulate; titrate the dose based on clinical response

Pregnancy: category C; use only if potential benefit justifies the potential risk to the fetus

Breast-feeding: not recommended; excreted in human milk

IN BRIEF

INDICATIONS
Hypertension
MI
Migraine prophylaxis

CONTRAINDICATIONS
Bronchial asthma or related bronchospastic problems
Cardiogenic shock
Known hypersensitivity to product components
Severe chronic obstructive pulmonary disease
Second- or third-degree AV block
Sick sinus syndrome without a permanent pacemaker in place
Sinus bradycardia
Overt heart failure

DRUG INTERACTIONS
Antihypertensive drugs[1,3]
Beta-agonists[2,4]
Calcium channel blockers:
 verapamil or diltiazem[1,3]
Digoxin[1,3]
Insulin[3]
NSAIDs[2]
Oral hypoglycemic agents[3,4]
Quinidine[1]
Reserpine and other
 catecholamine-depleting drugs[1]

[1] Effect/toxicity of timolol may increase.
[2] Effect of timolol may decrease.
[3] Timolol may increase the effect/toxicity of this drug.
[4] Timolol may decrease the effect of this drug.

ADVERSE EFFECTS
CV: bradycardia, peripheral vascular insufficiency/Raynaud's type, postural hypotension, syncope, hypotension, heart failure, AV block, ventricular arrhythmia, angina
CNS: fatigue, dizziness, drowsiness, depression, hallucinations, disorientation, short-term memory loss, paresthesia
Respiratory: dyspnea, bronchospasm
GI: nausea, vomiting, dyspepsia, constipation
GU: male impotence, ejaculatory failure
Metabolic: hypoglycemia
Other: edema, weight gain, pruritus, rash, fever, allergic reaction, blood dyscrasias

PHARMACOKINETICS AND PHARMACODYNAMICS
Duration of action: 12–24 h
Onset of action: Detectable levels of drug in the bloodstream occur in 30 min
Peak plasma concentration: 1–2 h
Bioavailability: 50%
Effect of food: no effect
Protein binding: 10%–60%
Volume of distribution: 2.1 L/kg
Metabolism: 80% metabolized in the liver
Elimination: excreted in the urine as metabolites
Elimination half-life: 4 h

MONITORING
BP, heart rate, respiratory status, and appropriate clinical response as per indication; signs/symptoms of CNS side effects.

OVERDOSE
Supportive: For severe bradycardia, atropine 0.25–2.0 mg IV may be administered or a pacemaker should be placed. Isoproterenol may also be used if bradycardia persists. For cardiovascular support, glucagon 50 µg/kg IV bolus may be administered over 1–2 min; up to 10 mg may be needed in some cases. In many cases, this may be followed by 2–5 mg/h (maximum 10 mg/h) continuous infusion. Fluid therapy with vasopressors/inotropic therapy may be added if necessary. Timolol is only minimally removed by dialysis.

The information here is provided as guidance only. Prescribers should always consult the manufacturer's current prescribing information.

161

TIMOLOL *(continued)*

DOSAGE

Hypertension: 10 mg twice daily initially, increased no quicker than every 7 d as tolerated to 20–60 mg/d in 2 divided doses

MI: 10 mg twice daily

Migraine prophylaxis: initial dose is 10 mg twice daily. During the maintenance phase, 20 mg once daily may be administered. The dose should be adjusted based on clinical response to a maximum of 30 mg/d in divided doses. If no effect after 6–8 wk of the maximum dose, therapy should be tapered and discontinued.

PATIENT INFORMATION

Timolol therapy should not be discontinued abruptly without consulting your health care provider. Your health care provider should also be consulted for persistent or unusual problems, such as dizziness/faintness, weight gain, worsening edema, or increasing shortness of breath. Sit or lie down if dizziness occurs, and rise slowly from a sitting or lying position. This medication may cause dizziness or drowsiness; use caution if performing activities requiring mental or physical effort.

AVAILABILITY

Tablets—5, 10, 20 mg
Combination formulations:
Timolide® 10–25 tablets—10 mg timolol/25 mg hydrochlorothiazide

BETA₁-SELECTIVE BETA-ADRENERGIC BLOCKERS WITHOUT ISA

Since selective beta₁-antagonism was first described in 1968 with **practolol**, other structures with this property have subsequently been developed. The term *cardioselectivity* was used, indicating that beta₂-receptors in the airway would remain unblocked. The implied safety factor, free from drug-induced bronchospasm in the asthmatic patient, is only relative, as selectivity tends to diminish at higher doses. *Beta₁-selectivity* is a more accurate term than *cardioselectivity* because both beta₁- and beta₂-receptors coexist in human myocardium in a 3:1 ratio.

EFFICACY AND USE

Beta₁-selective blockers may lower diastolic BP more than their nonselective counterparts, a result of their beta₂ vasodilatory-sparing action. The beta₁-selective drugs appear more effective than a thiazide diuretic in lowering BP of young, white hypertensive patients, especially in the presence of sympathetic hyperactivity. They have about the same antihypertensive actions as calcium antagonists and angiotensin-converting enzyme (ACE) inhibitors.

The Heart Attack Primary Prevention in Hypertension (HAPPHY) trial, involving more than 6000 moderately hypertensive middle-aged men, showed that total mortality rates were similar in both diuretic and beta-blocker groups, although death rate from stroke was significantly lower in the beta-blocker group. In the follow-up subgroup analysis, the Metoprolol Atherosclerosis Prevention in Hypertension (MAPHY) trial, selective beta₁-blockade with **metoprolol** significantly reduced MI and sudden death compared with the diuretic in smokers and nonsmokers. Similar to nonselective beta-blockers, beta₁-selective agents are cardioprotective and reverse left ventricular hypertrophy by reducing wall thickness. However, in elderly hypertensives, atenolol has been shown to reduce the frequency of stroke but not MI.

Similar to nonselective beta-blockers, beta₁-selective agents have greater antihypertensive effect in patients with baseline high or normal plasma renin activity (PRA), such as in Asian and white patients. Black patients and the elderly (usually with low PRA) may not respond as well, but this is not a reason to withhold these medications if an indication is present.

Similar to other beta-blockers, beta₁-selective agents work synergistically with antihypertensive agents from other classes. Diuretic-induced hypokalemia may be partially mitigated by the beta₁-blockers, but probably less than by a nonselective agent. **Atenolol** works synergistically with **nifedipine** in lowering BP, especially in patients with eclampsia. The BP response to combination therapy with a beta₁-selective blocker and an ACE inhibitor may be less pronounced because the effects are less than additive.

Beta₁-selective agents are also first-line anti-ischemic agents. Patients with mixed angina who experience frequent silent ischemic episodes may benefit more from beta₁-block-

ade than from nitrates or nifedipine. Patients with angina and mild to moderate aortic stenosis also respond well to beta-blockade.

In unstable angina, beta₁-selective agents were superior to **nifedipine** in preventing cardiac events in the Holland Interuniversity Nifedipine/Metoprolol (HINT) study. Beta₁-selective beta-blockers may be used effectively in combination with nitrates and dihydropyridines. Left ventricular function and AV conduction are not usually suppressed, though hypotension is seen occasionally. The beta₁-selective blockers are currently the preferred antianginal drugs in patients with coronary artery disease without a contraindication to therapy.

Early intervention studies of post-MI patients, such as the First International Study of Infarct Survival (ISIS-1), indicate a 15% reduction in vascular mortality with beta-blockers at 1 week (Figure 7.3). Most of this benefit appears to occur in the first 24 to 36 hours, and prevention of cardiac rupture seems to be the main mechanism of benefit. Bradycardia, hypotension, and heart failure may occur, but rarely require active intervention. Pooled data from 28 randomized trials suggest that the incidence of reinfarction and cardiac arrest is significantly decreased (15%–18%) by early IV beta-blockade. All beta-blockers without ISA, including beta₁-selective drugs, decrease death and recurrent MI by 23% and 32%,

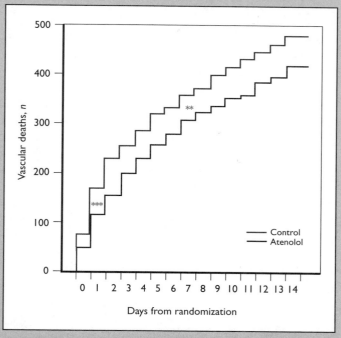

FIGURE 7.3 Mortality reduction in ISIS: comparison of atenolol and usual care (control). **—2P < 0.04; ***—2P < 0.003. (*Adapted from* ISIS-1 Collaborative Group: Randomized trial of intravenous atenolol among 16,027 cases of suspected acute myocardial infarction: ISIS-1. *Lancet* 1986, ii:57–66.)

respectively, with late intervention (beta-blocker begun 1–28 days post-MI).

Beta$_1$-selective drugs also have a role in treating cardiac arrhythmias. Their selectivity for the beta$_1$-receptor means that they are relatively safe and well tolerated in patients with potential airway problems (although they are not recommended if alternative drugs can be given), in insulin-dependent diabetics, and in hypertensives who undergo physical exercise.

The beta$_1$-adrenergic blockers **metoprolol** and **bisoprolol** have also been used as adjunctive therapy in patients with symptomatic CHF who are already receiving conventional therapy with diuretics, ACE inhibitors, and digoxin. The results of placebo-controlled clinical trials demonstrate morbidity and mortality benefits with these drugs in the treatment of systolic heart failure. Currently, sustained-release **metoprolol** (Toprol XL®) is the only beta$_1$-selective antagonist approved by the FDA for the treatment of heart failure.

MODE OF ACTION

Beta$_1$-selective blockade leads to a fall in cardiac output of 20% to 25%. This decrease is maintained on chronic oral therapy. This fall is counterbalanced by a small reflex increase in peripheral resistance. The lack of beta$_2$-blocking effects, however, permits beta$_2$ vasodilatation; thus, peripheral resistance does not increase to the same degree as with nonselective agents (Figure 7.2). As a consequence, beta$_1$-selective agents produce a slightly greater fall in diastolic BP (3–4 mm Hg). Beta$_1$-selective beta-blockers suppress resting heart rate, cardiac output, and exercise-induced increase in heart rate to the same extent as nonselective beta-blockers; however, when the increase in heart rate involves stimulation of beta$_2$- as well as beta$_1$-receptors (*eg*, via isoproterenol or epinephrine), nonselective beta-blockers cause a greater decrease in stimulated heart rate.

Beta$_1$-selective agents decrease coronary flow (mainly a reflection of decreased oxygen requirements) to the same degree as nonselective beta-blockers; however, blood flow to other organs, such as skin, kidney, and liver, is possibly less affected by the beta$_1$-selective agents. A beta$_1$-selective agent may show advantages in terms of lesser impairment of exercise tolerance, probably a result of sparing beta$_2$-blocking effects on muscle glycolytic processes and possibly on blood glucose and potassium levels during exercise. Beta$_1$-selective agents possibly attenuate the hemodynamic changes of isometric exercise to a greater degree than nonselective agents. The hypertensive reaction to nonselective beta-blockers in the presence of excessive sympathetic activity, hypoglycemia, or smoking, is less likely to occur with beta$_1$-selective agents.

INDICATIONS

	Atenolol	Betaxolol	Bisoprolol	Esmolol	Metoprolol
Hypertension	+	+	+	+*	+
Angina pectoris	+	–	–	–	+
Post MI	+	–	–	–	+‡
Arrhythmias	–	–	–	+	–
Heart failure (systolic)	–	–	–	–	+†

Indicated only for treating intraoperative and postoperative hypertension.

†*Sustained-release formulation only (Toprol XL®).*

‡*Immediate-release formulation only.*

MI—myocardial infarction; +—approved by the FDA; – —not approved by the FDA.

ATENOLOL
(Atenolol, Tenormin®)

Atenolol, a beta₁-selective blocker without membrane-stabilizing activity or ISA, is water soluble and long acting. It was the first once-daily beta-blocker in use, and various studies have demonstrated its short- and long-term efficacy and tolerability.

Atenolol has been shown to decrease the risk of MI and stroke (fatal and nonfatal) in hypertensive patients when compared with a control population. Its effect on stroke prevention has been confirmed in elderly hypertensive patients with isolated systolic hypertension. It may be more effective than nifedipine and nitrates in abolishing ischemic episodes in mixed angina, and is beneficial in the treatment of angina with aortic stenosis. It crosses the blood–brain barrier marginally, with fewer CNS side effects than lipid-soluble beta-blockers. It is not recommended in patients with asthma, but its beta₁ selectivity makes it safer than nonselective agents in patients with reactive airways disease, and it does not prolong insulin-induced hypoglycemia in diabetes. It reduces stress-induced cardiac necrosis in patients with head injuries and reverses left ventricular hypertrophy.

The results of four randomized clinical trials demonstrated the efficacy of oral atenolol in relieving ischemia and improving outcomes in patients with documented silent myocardial ischemia. These studies compared atenolol monotherapy with placebo, calcium channel blocker monotherapy, calcium channel blockers plus nitrates, and the combination of atenolol with calcium channel blockers (ie, nifedipine, amlodipine).

The ISIS-1 trial showed atenolol (IV followed by oral therapy) to reduce vascular mortality by 15% within the first week compared with conventional therapy in 16,027 patients with suspected MI.

SPECIAL GROUPS

Race: black hypertensive patients may be less responsive than white patients

Children: safety and effectiveness have not been established

Elderly: because clearance may be reduced, start with a low dose and titrate based on clinical response

Renal impairment: drug clearance is reduced; dosage should be reduced accordingly, based on renal function and clinical response

Hepatic impairment: use with caution, although dosage adjustment is probably not required

Pregnancy: category D; should not be used

Breast-feeding: not recommended; excreted in human milk

IN BRIEF

INDICATIONS
Angina pectoris
Hypertension
Acute MI

CONTRAINDICATIONS
Cardiogenic shock
Known hypersensitivity
Second- or third-degree AV block
Sinus bradycardia
Overt heart failure

DRUG INTERACTIONS
Antihypertensive agents[1,3]
Beta-agonists[2,4]
Calcium channel blockers: verapamil or diltiazem[1,3]
Insulin[3]
NSAIDs[2]
Oral hypoglycemic agents[3,4]
Reserpine and other catecholamine-depleting drugs[1]

1 Effect/toxicity of atenolol may increase.
2 Effect of atenolol may decrease.
3 Atenolol may increase the effect/toxicity of this drug.
4 Atenolol may decrease the effect of this drug.

ADVERSE EFFECTS
CV: bradycardia, peripheral vascular insufficiency/Raynaud's type, postural hypotension, syncope, hypotension, heart failure, AV block, ventricular arrhythmia, angina
CNS: fatigue, dizziness, drowsiness, depression, vertigo, sleep disturbances
Respiratory: dyspnea, bronchospasm, nasal congestion
GI: nausea, diarrhea
GU: male impotence, ejaculatory failure
Metabolic: hypoglycemia
Other: edema, weight gain, allergic reaction, rash, agranulocytosis, lupus syndrome

PHARMACOKINETICS AND PHARMACODYNAMICS
Duration of action: up to 12 h (IV); >24 h (po)
Onset of action: immediate (IV); <1 h (po)
Peak effect: <5 min (IV); 2–4 h (po); 1–2 weeks required for full antihypertensive effect
Bioavailability: 100% (IV); about 50% (po)
Effect of food: ↓ bioavailability
Protein binding: 6%–16%
Volume of distribution: 0.95 L/kg
Metabolism: little or no metabolism
Elimination: mainly renal as unchanged drug
Elimination half-life: 6–7 h (normal renal function)

MONITORING
BP, heart rate, ECG, and respiratory status; signs/symptoms of heart failure; signs/symptoms of CNS side effects

OVERDOSE
Supportive: For severe bradycardia, atropine 0.25–2.0 mg IV may be administered or a pacemaker should be placed. Isoproterenol may also be used if bradycardia persists. For cardiovascular support, glucagon 50 µg/kg IV bolus may be administered over 1–2 min; up to 10 mg may be needed in some cases. In many cases, this may be followed by 2–5 mg/h (maximum 10 mg/h) continuous infusion. Fluid therapy with vasopressors/inotropic therapy may be added if necessary. Atenolol may be removed by dialysis.

ATENOLOL (continued)

DOSAGE*

Hypertension: 50–100 mg once daily

Angina pectoris: 50–200 mg once daily

MI: Treatment should be initiated with intravenous (IV) atenolol 5 mg administered over 5 min, followed by a second IV dose of 5 mg 10 min later. If the patient tolerates the full IV therapy, 50 mg of atenolol should be administered orally 10 min after the last IV dose, followed by a second 50 mg dose 12 h later. Then, the patient can receive atenolol orally either 100 mg once daily or 50 mg twice daily for 6–9 d or until discharge from the hospital. If the patient is unable to receive IV therapy, treatment should begin with the oral regimen (above) and be given for at least 7 days.

*Guidelines for dosing adjustments in patients with renal impairment (including elderly patients)

Creatinine clearance, mL/min/1.73 m²	Maximum dose
15–35	50 mg/d
<15	25 mg/d
On hemodialysis (HD)	25 or 50 mg after HD

PATIENT INFORMATION

Atenolol therapy should not be discontinued abruptly without consulting your health care provider. Your health care provider should also be consulted for persistent or unusual problems, such as dizziness/faintness, weight gain, worsening edema, or increasing shortness of breath. Sit or lie down if dizziness occurs, and rise slowly from a sitting or lying position. This medication may cause dizziness or drowsiness; use caution if performing activities requiring mental or physical effort.

AVAILABILITY

Tablets—25, 50, 100 mg

Ampules—5 mg/10 mL

Combination formulations with a diuretic:
Tenoretic® tablets (also available as generic)—
50 mg atenolol/25 mg chlorthalidone
100 mg atenolol/25 mg chlorthalidone

BETAXOLOL (Kerlone®)

Betaxolol, a beta₁-selective blocker devoid of ISA and membrane-stabilizing activity, is moderately lipid soluble and is extensively metabolized by the liver. It is prescribed once daily for hypertension and is also available in topical form for management of elevated intraocular pressure.

SPECIAL GROUPS

Race: black hypertensive patients may be less responsive than white patients

Children: safety and effectiveness have not been established

Elderly: start with a low dose, and titrate the dose based on clinical response

Renal impairment: use with caution because drug clearance is reduced; start with a lower dose

Hepatic impairment: use with caution, although dosage reduction is usually not necessary

Pregnancy: category C; use only if potential benefit justifies the potential risk to the fetus

Breast-feeding: not recommended; excreted in human milk

DOSAGE

Hypertension: The initial dose is 10 mg once daily (5 mg for elderly patients or patients with impaired renal function). If the desired effect is not achieved, increase the dose by 5 mg/d increments every 1–2 wks to maximum doses of 20–40 mg/d.

IN BRIEF

INDICATIONS
Hypertension

CONTRAINDICATIONS
Cardiogenic shock

Sinus bradycardia

Known hypersensitivity to product components

Overt heart failure

Second- or third-degree AV block

DRUG INTERACTIONS
Antihypertensive agents[1,3]

Beta-agonists[2,4]

Calcium channel blockers: verapamil or diltiazem[1,3]

Insulin[3]

NSAIDs[2]

Oral hypoglycemic agents[3,4]

Reserpine and other catecholamine-depleting drugs[1]

[1] Effect/toxicity of betaxolol may increase.
[2] Effect of betaxolol may decrease.
[3] Betaxolol may increase the effect/toxicity of this drug.
[4] Betaxolol may decrease the effect of this drug.

ADVERSE EFFECTS
CV: bradycardia, peripheral vascular insufficiency/Raynaud's type, postural hypotension, syncope, hypotension, heart failure, AV block, ventricular arrhythmia, angina
CNS: fatigue, dizziness, drowsiness, depression, headache, sleep disturbances
Respiratory: dyspnea, bronchospasm, nasal congestion
GI: dyspepsia, nausea, diarrhea
GU: male impotence, ejaculatory failure
Metabolic: hypoglycemia
Other: edema, weight gain, allergic reaction, rash, blood dyscrasias

PHARMACOKINETICS AND PHARMACODYNAMICS
Duration of action: >24 h
Onset of action: 2–3 h
Peak effect: 3–4 h; 7–14 d may be required for full antihypertensive effect
Bioavailability: 89%
Effect of food: no effect
Protein binding: 50%
Volume of distribution: 4.9–9.8 L/kg
Metabolism: mainly metabolized in the liver
Elimination: 80% via renal excretion (15% as unchanged)
Elimination half-life: 14–22 h

MONITORING
BP, heart rate, respiratory status, and other appropriate clinical response; signs/symptoms of heart failure; signs/symptoms of CNS side effects

OVERDOSE
Supportive: For severe bradycardia, atropine 0.25–2.0 mg IV may be administered or a pacemaker should be placed. Isoproterenol may also be used if bradycardia persists. For cardiovascular support, glucagon 50 µg/kg IV bolus may be administered over 1–2 min; up to 10 mg may be needed in some cases. In many cases, this may be followed by 2–5 mg/h (maximum 10 mg/h) continuous infusion. Fluid therapy with vasopressors/inotropic therapy may be added if necessary. Betaxolol is not successfully removed by dialysis.

PATIENT INFORMATION
Betaxolol therapy should not be discontinued abruptly without consulting your health care provider. Your health care provider should also be consulted for persistent or unusual problems, such as dizziness/faintness, weight gain, worsening edema, or increasing shortness of breath. Sit or lie down if dizziness occurs, and rise slowly from a sitting or lying position. This medication may cause dizziness or drowsiness; use caution if performing activities requiring mental or physical effort.

AVAILABILITY
Tablets—10, 20 mg

The information here is provided as guidance only. Prescribers should always consult the manufacturer's current prescribing information.

167

BISOPROLOL

(Bisoprolol fumarate, Zebeta®)

Bisoprolol, a beta$_1$-selective adrenergic blocking agent, is structurally similar to acebutolol, atenolol, and metoprolol. Bisoprolol does not exhibit ISA or membrane-stabilizing activity. It is not lipid soluble. At high doses (20 mg or higher), bisoprolol loses its cardioselectivity and inhibits both beta$_1$- and beta$_2$-adrenergic receptors. In controlled clinical trials, bisoprolol monotherapy has been shown to produce significant dose-related BP reduction with a 47% to 70% clinical response rate observed in patients with hypertension.

The CIBIS-II study, involving 2647 patients with symptomatic systolic heart failure receiving standard therapy with diuretics and ACE inhibitors, was prematurely terminated once it was revealed that bisoprolol therapy significantly reduced all-cause mortality (34% relative reduction) compared with placebo. To date, however, this drug is FDA approved only for the treatment of hypertension.

SPECIAL GROUPS

Race:	black hypertensive patients may be less responsive than white patients
Children:	safety and effectiveness have not been established
Elderly:	no dosage adjustment is necessary unless underlying renal or hepatic insufficiency is present
Renal impairment:	use with caution; start with a lower dose, and titrate the dose based on clinical response
Hepatic impairment:	use with caution; start with a lower dose, and titrate the dose based on clinical response
Pregnancy:	category C; use only if potential benefit justifies the potential risk to the fetus
Breast-feeding:	not recommended; not known if the drug is excreted in human milk

DOSAGE

Hypertension: 2.5–20 mg once daily
The initial dose should be 2.5–5 mg once daily and increased gradually based on BP response

IN BRIEF

INDICATIONS
Hypertension

CONTRAINDICATIONS
Cardiogenic shock
Known hypersensitivity to product components

Second- or third-degree AV block
Marked sinus bradycardia
Overt heart failure

DRUG INTERACTIONS
Antihypertensive agents[1,3]
Beta-agonists[2,4]
Calcium channel blockers: verapamil or diltiazem[1,3]
Insulin[3]

NSAIDs[2]
Oral hypoglycemic agents[3,4]
Reserpine and other catecholamine-depleting drugs[1]
Rifampin[2,5]

1 Effect/toxicity of bisoprolol may increase.
2 Effect of bisoprolol may decrease.
3 Bisoprolol may increase the effect/toxicity of this drug.
4 Bisoprolol may decrease the effect of this drug.
5 The clinical significance of this interaction is unclear.

ADVERSE EFFECTS
CV: bradycardia, peripheral vascular insufficiency/Raynaud's type, postural hypotension, syncope, hypotension, heart failure, AV block, ventricular arrhythmia, angina
CNS: fatigue, dizziness, drowsiness, depression, vertigo, sleep disturbances
Respiratory: dyspnea, bronchospasm, nasal congestion
GI: nausea, diarrhea
GU: male impotence, ejaculatory failure
Metabolic: hypoglycemia, hyperuricemia
Other: edema, weight gain, allergic reaction, rash, purpura

PHARMACOKINETICS AND PHARMACODYNAMICS
Duration of action:	>24 h
Onset of action:	1–2 h
Peak effect:	2–4 h
Bioavailability:	80%
Effect of food:	no effect
Protein binding:	30%
Volume of distribution:	3.2 L/kg
Metabolism:	50% metabolized by the liver
Elimination:	mainly renal (50% as unchanged); <2% in feces
Elimination half-life:	9–12 h

MONITORING
BP, heart rate, respiratory status, ECG for PR prolongation, and other appropriate clinical markers as indicated (eg, blood glucose if diabetic); also monitor for signs/symptoms of heart failure and signs/symptoms of CNS side effects.

OVERDOSE
Supportive: For severe bradycardia, atropine 0.25–2.0 mg IV may be administered or a pacemaker should be placed. Isoproterenol may also be used if bradycardia persists. For cardiovascular support, glucagon 50 µg/kg IV bolus may be administered over 1–2 min; up to 10 mg may be needed in some cases. In many cases, this may be followed by 2–5 mg/h (maximum 10 mg/h) continuous infusion. Fluid therapy with vasopressors/inotropic therapy may be added if necessary. Bisoprolol is not removed by dialysis.

PATIENT INFORMATION
Bisoprolol therapy should not be discontinued abruptly without consulting your health care provider. Your health care provider should also be consulted for persistent or unusual problems, such as dizziness/faintness, weight gain, worsening edema, or increasing shortness of breath. Sit or lie down if dizziness occurs, and rise slowly from a sitting or lying position. This medication may cause dizziness or drowsiness; use caution if performing activities requiring mental or physical effort.

AVAILABILITY
Tablets—5, 10 mg
Combination formulations with a diuretic:
Ziac® tablets—
    2.5 mg bisoprolol/6.25 mg hydrochlorothiazide
    5 mg bisoprolol/6.25 mg hydrochlorothiazide
    10 mg bisoprolol/6.25 mg hydrochlorothiazide

ESMOLOL

(Brevibloc®)

Esmolol, a beta₁-selective blocker with no significant ISA or membrane-stabilizing activity, is available only in the IV form. It is not lipid soluble and has an elimination half-life of about 9 minutes because of rapid and extensive metabolism. Esmolol has a very rapid onset and a very short duration of action. After termination of infusion, substantial recovery from beta-blockade is observed in 10 to 20 minutes. Esmolol is indicated for the rapid control of ventricular rate in patients with atrial fibrillation or atrial flutter in perioperative, postoperative, or other emergencies in which short-term control of ventricular rate with a short-acting beta-adrenergic agent is desirable. Esmolol is also used in patients with noncompensatory sinus tachycardia when rapid heart rate control is indicated. In addition to its antiarrhythmic activity, esmolol is indicated for the treatment of tachycardia and hypertension that occurs intraoperatively or postoperatively. Esmolol may also be useful in managing patients with unstable angina or dissecting aorta.

SPECIAL GROUPS

Race: black hypertensive patients may be less responsive than white patients

Children: safety and effectiveness have not been established

Elderly: no dosage adjustment necessary

Renal impairment: acid metabolite may accumulate with renal dysfunction; use cautiously

Hepatic impairment: no dosage adjustment necessary

Pregnancy: category C; use only if potential benefit justifies the potential risk to the fetus

Breast-feeding: not recommended; not known if the drug is excreted in human milk

DOSAGE

Supraventricular tachycardia: Treatment should be initiated with a loading infusion of 0.5 mg/kg over 1 min, followed by 50 µg/kg/min infusion. If an adequate response is not achieved after 5 min, the infusion rate may be increased by 50 µg/kg/min every 4 min as needed to a maximum rate of 200 µg/kg/min. An alternative is to repeat the same loading dose over 1 min and increase the rate of infusion to 100 µg/kg/min. This titration process may be repeated in 4 min with a final 0.5 mg/kg bolus followed by an increase in the infusion rate to 150 µg/kg/min. The infusion rate may then be increased after another 4 min to a maximum rate of 200 µg/kg/min if desired. Then, the maintenance infusion may be decreased or increased based on the desired end point. Most patients respond within the range of 25–200 µg/kg/min. Alternative antiarrhythmic agents, such as a longer-acting beta-blocker, verapamil, or digoxin, should also be considered for long-term patient management if indicated.

Intraoperative and postoperative tachycardia and hypertension:
Rapid intraoperative control—Administer an 80 mg (1 mg/kg) IV bolus dose over 30 sec, followed by a 150 µg/kg/min infusion if necessary, and titrate the dose to maintain desired heart rate or BP (up to 300 µg/kg/min).
Gradual postoperative control—Dose titration schedule is the same as the treatment in supraventricular tachycardia; however, higher dosages, up to 250–300 µg/kg/min, may be required for adequate BP control.

IN BRIEF

INDICATIONS
Supraventricular tachycardia

Intraoperative and postoperative tachycardia and/or hypertension

CONTRAINDICATIONS
Cardiogenic shock

Known hypersensitivity to product components

Second- or third-degree AV block

Sinus bradycardia

Overt heart failure

DRUG INTERACTIONS
Antihypertensive agents[1,3]

Beta-agonists[2,4]

Calcium channel blockers: verapamil or diltiazem[1,3]

Digoxin[3,5]

Morphine[1]

Neuromuscular blockers[3]

NSAIDs[2]

Reserpine and other catecholamine-depleting drugs[1]

1 Effect/toxicity of esmolol may increase.
2 Effect of esmolol may decrease.
3 Esmolol may increase the effect/toxicity of this drug.
4 Esmolol may decrease the effect of this drug.
5 The clinical significance of this interaction is unclear.

ADVERSE EFFECTS
CV: bradycardia, hypotension, peripheral vascular insufficiency/Raynaud's type, syncope, heart failure, AV block, ventricular arrhythmia, angina
CNS: fatigue, dizziness, drowsiness, confusion, headache, depression, paresthesia
Respiratory: dyspnea, bronchospasm, nasal congestion
GI: nausea, vomiting
GU: urinary retention
Other: infusion site reactions, edema, weight gain, allergic reaction, rash, purpura

PHARMACOKINETICS AND PHARMACODYNAMICS
Duration of action: 10–20 min
Onset of action: within minutes
Peak effect: <5 min (with bolus); 30 min (without bolus)
Bioavailability: 100%
Effect of food: not applicable
Protein binding: 55%
Volume of distribution: 1.9 L/kg
Metabolism: rapidly metabolized by esterases in the blood
Elimination: (renal) 73%–88%; mainly as metabolites
Elimination half-life: 2 min (distribution); 9 min (elimination)

MONITORING
BP, heart rate, respiratory status.

OVERDOSE
Supportive: Esmolol is a short-acting agent. For severe bradycardia, atropine 0.25–2.0 mg IV may be administered or a pacemaker should be placed. Isoproterenol may also be used if bradycardia persists. For cardiovascular support, glucagon 50 µg/kg IV bolus may be administered over 1–2 min; up to 10 mg may be needed in some cases. In many cases, this may be followed by 2–5 mg/h (maximum 10 mg/h) continuous infusion. Fluid therapy with vasopressors/inotropic therapy may be added if necessary. Esmolol is not removed by dialysis.

PATIENT INFORMATION
Esmolol is used for adequate BP or heart rate control.

AVAILABILITY
Ampules—2500 mg/10 mL (250 mg/mL), not for direct IV injection
Vials—100 mg/10 mL (10 mg/mL); 100 mg/5 mL (20 mg/mL)
Premixed injection bags—2500 mg/250 mL (10 mg/mL); 2000 mg /100 mL (20 mg/mL)

The information here is provided as guidance only. Prescribers should always consult the manufacturer's current prescribing information.

169

METOPROLOL SUCCINATE
(Toprol XL®)
METOPROLOL TARTRATE
(Metoprolol Tartrate, Lopressor®)

SELECTIVE BETA$_1$-ADRENERGIC ANTAGONISTS WITHOUT ISA

Metoprolol is a beta$_1$-antagonist without ISA. It has moderate lipid solubility, and its beta$_1$ selectivity is less than that of atenolol. Metoprolol also lacks membrane-stabilizing activity within the usual therapeutic range.

In addition to its antihypertensive and anti-ischemic effects, metoprolol has been shown to reduce both morbidity and mortality in patients with acute MI. Metoprolol is also effective in controlling ventricular response in patients with atrial fibrillation or flutter.

Metoprolol succinate also has shown long-term benefits in reducing mortality and morbidity in patients with mild to moderate congestive cardiomyopathy in the MERIT-HF trial. When metoprolol tartrate was compared with carvedilol in the COMET study in 1511 patients with chronic heart failure, carvedilol therapy resulted in a 17% relative risk reduction in all-cause mortality ($P = 0.0017$) after a mean follow-up of 58 months. The composite end point of mortality or all-cause admission, however, was not statistically different between treatments.

An equivalent maximal beta-blockade of metoprolol is achieved with oral and intravenous doses in the ratio of approximately 2.5:1. Metoprolol succinate (Toprol XL®) is about two-thirds as potent as metoprolol tartrate (ie, 100 mg succinate ≈ 67 mg tartrate) in patients with heart failure due to lower systemic bioavailability. However, when switching from one salt form to another, the same total daily dosage may be used.

SPECIAL GROUPS

Race: black hypertensive patients may be less responsive than white patients

Children: safety and effectiveness have not been established

Elderly: start with a low dose, and titrate the dose based on clinical response

Renal impairment: no dose reduction is required; titrate the dose based on clinical response

Hepatic impairment: because the drug is hepatically metabolized, use caution; titrate the dose based on clinical response

Pregnancy: category C; use only if potential benefit justifies the potential risk to the fetus

Breast-feeding: not recommended; excreted in human milk in small quantities

IN BRIEF

INDICATIONS
Angina pectoris
Hypertension
MI (tartrate)
Heart failure (succinate)

CONTRAINDICATIONS
Cardiogenic shock
Known hypersensitivity to product components
Second- or third-degree AV block
Severe bradycardia
Severe decompensated heart failure
Sick sinus syndrome without a permanent pacemaker in place
Treatment of MI with heart rate <45 bpm or systolic BP <100 mm Hg

DRUG INTERACTIONS
Antihypertensive agents[1,3]
Beta-agonists[2,4]
Calcium channel blockers: verapamil or diltiazem[1,3]
Cimetidine[1]
Insulin[3]
MAO inhibitors[1]
NSAIDs[2]
Oral hypoglycemic agents[3,4]
Propafenone[1]
Quinidine[1]
Reserpine and other catecholamine-depleting drugs[1]
Selective serotonin reuptake inhibitors[1]

1 Effect/toxicity of metoprolol may increase.
2 Effect of metoprolol may decrease.
3 Metoprolol may increase the effect/toxicity of this drug.
4 Metoprolol may decrease the effect of this drug.

ADVERSE EFFECTS
CV: bradycardia, hypotension, peripheral vascular insufficiency/Raynaud's type, syncope, cold extremities, heart failure, AV block, ventricular arrhythmia, angina
CNS: fatigue, dizziness, drowsiness, confusion, headache, depression, sleep disturbance
Respiratory: dyspnea, bronchospasm, nasal congestion
GI: nausea, vomiting
GU: male impotence, ejaculatory failure
Metabolic: hypoglycemia
Other: edema, weight gain, allergic reaction, rash

PHARMACOKINETICS AND PHARMACODYNAMICS
Duration of action (dose dependent): (IV) 5–8 h; (po) 12–24 h; >24 h for succinate salt
Onset of action: (IV) within minutes; (po) 15 min
Peak effect: (IV) 20 min; (po) 1–2 h; >7 h for slow release; maximum antihypertensive effect occurs in about 1 wk
Bioavailability: (IV) 100%; (po) 50%; 40% for succinate salt
Effect of food: (tartrate salt) increased absorption; (succinate salt) no effect
Protein binding: 12%
Volume of distribution: 4.2 L/kg
Metabolism: metabolized in the liver primarily by cytochrome P-450 (CYP)2D6
Elimination: renal (5%–10% as unchanged)
Elimination half-life: 3–7 h

MONITORING
BP, heart rate, respiratory status, ECG for PR prolongation, and other appropriate clinical markers as indicated (eg, blood glucose if diabetic); also monitor for signs/symptoms of heart failure and signs/symptoms of CNS side effects.

The information here is provided as guidance only. Prescribers should always consult the manufacturer's current prescribing information.

METOPROLOL SUCCINATE
METOPROLOL TARTRATE
(continued)

DOSAGE

Hypertension: Tartrate salt—100–450 mg/d. The initial dose is 100 mg/d in single or divided doses. The dose should be adjusted at weekly (or longer) intervals until the desired BP control is achieved. Lower dosages may not maintain effective 24-h BP control, and twice-daily dosing should be considered.
Succinate salt—50–400 mg once daily. Begin with 50–100 mg/d and titrate at weekly (or longer) intervals to desired effect.

Angina pectoris: Tartrate salt—100–400 mg/d in two divided doses. Same dose titration as recommended in the management of hypertension.
Succinate salt—100 mg once daily initially, titrate dosage weekly to desired effect.

MI (tartrate salt): Treatment should be initiated as soon as the patient's hemodynamic status has stabilized; three 5 mg IV bolus injections of metoprolol should be administered at 2 min intervals. If the full 15 mg dose is tolerated by the patient, 50 mg of oral metoprolol (or 25 mg for those who cannot tolerate the full dose) every 6 h should be initiated 15 min after the last IV dose and continued for 48 h. Then, the dose may be adjusted to 100 mg twice daily. If the full IV dose is not tolerated, give 25–50 mg orally every 6 h either 15 min after the last IV dose or as soon as the clinical condition allows. If IV treatment is not given, institute oral therapy as soon as possible at a dosage of 100 mg twice daily.

Heart failure (succinate salt): 25 mg once daily initially for New York Heart Association (NYHA) class II heart failure (12.5 mg with more severe heart failure). This dosage should be doubled every 2 wk to the maximum dosage tolerated or 200 mg once daily, whichever is less. Do not initiate or up-titrate treatment if the patient is unstable.

OVERDOSE

Supportive: For severe bradycardia, atropine 0.25–2.0 mg IV may be administered or a pacemaker should be placed. Isoproterenol may also be used if bradycardia persists. For cardiovascular support, glucagon 50 µg/kg IV bolus may be administered over 1–2 min; up to 10 mg may be needed in some cases. In many cases, this may be followed by 2–5 mg/h (maximum 10 mg/h) continuous infusion. Fluid therapy with vasopressors/inotropic therapy may be added if necessary. Metoprolol is not removed by dialysis.

PATIENT INFORMATION

Metoprolol therapy should not be discontinued abruptly without consulting your health care provider. Your health care provider should also be consulted for persistent or unusual problems, such as dizziness/faintness, weight gain, worsening edema, or increasing shortness of breath. Sit or lie down if dizziness occurs, and rise slowly from a sitting or lying position. This medication may cause dizziness or drowsiness; use caution if performing activities requiring mental or physical effort.

AVAILABILITY

Tablets—50, 100 mg (Lopressor, generic); 25, 50, 100, 200 mg (Toprol XL)
Ampules—5 mg/5 mL
Combination formulations with a diuretic:
Lopressor HCT tablets:
50/25: 50 mg metoprolol/25 mg hydrochlorothiazide
100/25: 100 mg metoprolol/25 mg hydrochlorothiazide
100/50: 100 mg metoprolol/50 mg hydrochlorothiazide

Some beta-blockers, in addition to inhibiting the effects of sympathetic activity, possess some stimulant activity of their own, termed PAA or ISA. The partial agonist effect, however, differs from that of epinephrine or isoproterenol in that the maximal response of the tissue is lower (Figure 7.4). ISA may be competitively inhibited by a beta-blocker with no such property, such as **propranolol**. The degree of ISA in some of the available beta-blockers has been quantified (Figure 7.5).

EFFICACY AND USE

Beta-blockers with ISA cause a decrease in resting heart rate to a lesser degree than beta-blockers without ISA. Indeed, a beta-blocker with moderate to high ISA can increase resting heart rate if sympathetic tone is low. During exercise or stress, when sympathetic drive is high, beta-blockers with ISA act more like full antagonists, although the maximum heart rate reduction is usually less than that achieved with beta-blockers without ISA. Under resting conditions, cardiac output is minimally depressed by beta-blockers with high ISA. Under conditions of high sympathetic drive, the fall in cardiac output approximates that observed with beta-blockers without ISA. In patients with chronically impaired left ventricular function (dependent on increased sympathetic drive) given beta-blockers with a moderate degree of ISA, such as **pindolol**, the reduction in cardiac output may cause heart failure. Newer investigational agents with a high degree of ISA (45%–50%) may benefit patients with milder forms of heart failure.

The International Prospective Primary Prevention Study in Hypertension (IPPPSH), involving more than 6000 moderately hypertensive patients, suggested that a beta-blocker with ISA could reduce coronary events in nonsmoking men.

Beta-blockers with ISA possess antianginal properties similar to their counterparts without ISA but tend to be less effective (particularly at night, when an increase in heart rate can prolong ischemic episodes). Beta-blockers with ISA are also less effective after infarction, achieving only about a 10% decrease in mortality compared with 25% to 30%

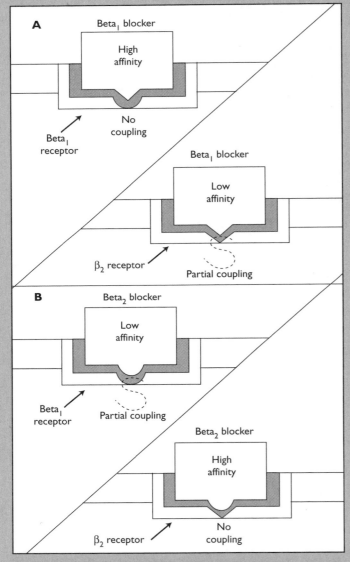

FIGURE 7.4 Examples of receptor affinity/coupling characteristics of a beta$_1$-selective blocker with beta$_2$-selective intrinsic sympathomimetic activity (ISA) (**A**) and a beta$_2$-selective blocker with beta$_1$-selective ISA (**B**). (*Adapted from* Cruickshank JM: Measurement and cardiovascular relevance of partial agonist activity (PAA) involving beta$_1$- and beta$_2$- adrenoceptors. *Pharmacol Ther* 1990, 46:199–242.)

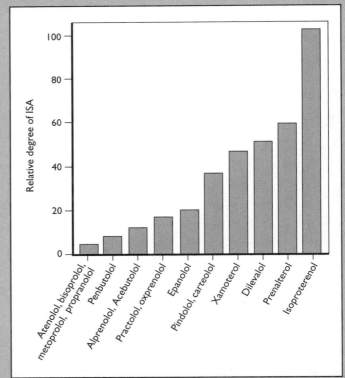

FIGURE 7.5 Relative degree of intrinsic sympathomimetic activity (ISA) of various beta-blockers.

achieved with beta-blockers without ISA. However, **acebutolol** (with only 10% beta$_1$ ISA) was found to be effective in high-risk postinfarction patients. Although speculative, beta-blockers with ISA are probably as effective as non-ISA beta-blockers in reducing the rate of reinfarction.

Under experimental conditions, beta-blockers with moderate ISA tend to affect the cardiac conduction system to a lesser extent than agents without ISA, except under conditions of high sympathetic tone. **Pindolol** has antiarrhythmic activity, but may also increase ventricular ectopic beats.

Nonselective agents with ISA, such as **pindolol**, can still cause marked bronchoconstriction in patients with asthma and hyperreactive airway problems. They also competitively inhibit the bronchodilatory action of beta$_2$-agonists. Although adverse reactions, such as cold peripheries and fatigue, tend to be less common with beta-blockers with ISA, increased incidence of tremor and muscle cramps has been reported.

MODE OF ACTION

ISA is best expressed in humans when baseline sympathetic activity is minimal. For example, at night, **pindolol** acts as a stimulant to increase resting heart rate. During exercise, however, the beta antagonism of **pindolol** predominates and inhibits maximum heart rate acceleration.

Although data are limited, it is probable that the ISA contained within a beta$_1$-selective beta-blocker will express itself only through the beta$_1$-receptor, and the ISA of a nonselective beta-blocker acts on both beta$_1$- and beta$_2$-receptors. A nonselective agent, however, may possess predominantly beta$_2$-selective ISA. Beta-blockers with significant beta$_2$-ISA lower BP mainly by reducing peripheral resistance (beta$_2$ vasodilatation, Figure 7.2). Possession of significant beta$_1$ ISA results in little peripheral action and minimal effect on cardiac output so that resting BP is lowered to a lesser degree or even increased. Resting BP is lowered by a nonselective beta-blocker with moderate nonselective ISA or beta$_2$-selective ISA more by a reduction in peripheral resistance than a fall in cardiac output. Beta$_1$-selective ISA is associated with a diminution or abolition of antihypertensive efficacy.

INDICATIONS

	Nonselective agents			Beta$_1$-selective agent
	Carteolol	**Penbutolol**	**Pindolol**	**Acebutolol**
Hypertension	+	+	+	+
Arrhythmias	–	–	–	+
Angina pectoris	–	–	–	–
Heart failure	–	–	–	–

+—approved by the FDA; – —not approved by the FDA.

ACEBUTOLOL (Acebutolol, Sectral®)

Acebutolol is a selective beta$_1$-adrenergic antagonist with mild ISA within the usual therapeutic range. Its relative potency on beta$_1$-blockade is only 10% to 30% of that of propranolol. At high doses (>800 mg daily), the beta$_1$ selectivity of acebutolol diminishes and it inhibits both beta$_1$- and beta$_2$-receptors competitively. Both acebutolol and its active metabolite, diacetolol, are responsible for the therapeutic effect observed clinically. It has been shown that serum diacetolol levels have been consistently higher than acebutolol secondary to its long half-life. Diacetolol has beta-blockade activity similar to acebutolol and also possesses weak ISA activity. Diacetolol may contribute substantially to the therapeutic effect of acebutolol. Because diacetolol is primarily cleared by the kidney and may accumulate in patients with renal dysfunction, lower maintenance doses are recommended.

Acebutolol has been shown to reduce mortality in post-MI patients compared with placebo. However, most clinicians perceive ISA to be an unfavorable property for treating ischemic heart disease, and this class of drugs is therefore not typically used in this situation. Acebutolol is indicated for hypertension and for treating ventricular premature depolarizations (VPDs). In clinical practice, it is primarily used for its effects on cardiac conduction.

SPECIAL GROUPS

Race: black hypertensive patients may be less responsive than white patients

Children: safety and effectiveness have not been established

Elderly: twofold increase in bioavailability; start with low dose, and titrate the dose based on clinical response. Dosages greater than 800 mg daily should be avoided.

Renal impairment: use with caution; dose reduction is required because diacetolol may accumulate

Hepatic impairment: use with caution, although dosage adjustment is probably not required

Pregnancy: category B; should only be used if clearly indicated

Breast-feeding: not recommended; excreted in human milk

DOSAGE*

Hypertension: 200–1200 mg/d. The initial dose is 200–400 mg administered as a single dose or twice daily. The dose may be gradually increased based on clinical response up to 600 mg twice daily. Most patients require 400–800 mg/d.

VPDs: 400–1200 mg/d in 2 divided doses

*Reduce dosages by 50% when creatinine clearance is <50 mL/min; reduce by 75% when creatinine clearance is <25 mL/min

IN BRIEF

INDICATIONS
Hypertension   Ventricular arrhythmias (management of VPDs)

CONTRAINDICATIONS
Cardiogenic shock
Known hypersensitivity to product components
Second- or third-degree AV block
Sick sinus syndrome without a permanent pacemaker in place
Persistently severe bradycardia
Severe decompensated heart failure

DRUG INTERACTIONS
Antihypertensive agents[1,3]   NSAIDs[2]
Beta-agonists[2,4]   Oral hypoglycemic agents[3,4]
Calcium channel blockers: Reserpine and other
  verapamil or diltiazem[1,3]   catecholamine-depleting drugs[1]
Insulin[3]

1 Effect/toxicity of acebutolol may increase.
2 Effect of acebutolol may decrease.
3 Acebutolol may increase the effect/toxicity of this drug.
4 Acebutolol may decrease the effect of this drug.

ADVERSE EFFECTS
CV: bradycardia, peripheral vascular insufficiency/Raynaud's type, postural hypotension, syncope, hypotension, heart failure, AV block, ventricular arrhythmia, angina
CNS: fatigue, dizziness, drowsiness, depression, headache, sleep disturbances
Respiratory: dyspnea, bronchospasm, nasal congestion
GI: constipation, dyspepsia, nausea, diarrhea, liver function abnormality
GU: male impotence, ejaculatory failure, urinary frequency
Metabolic: hypoglycemia
Other: edema, weight gain, allergic reaction, rash, pruritus, lupuslike syndrome, positive antinuclear antibody (ANA) titer

PHARMACOKINETICS AND PHARMACODYNAMICS
Duration of action: >24 h
Onset of action: 1–2 h
Peak effect: 3–8 h
Bioavailability: 35%–50%
Protein binding: 26%
Volume of distribution: 1.6–3.0 L/kg
Effect of food: slower absorption and lower peak concentration, but similar extent of absorption
Metabolism: mainly metabolized in the liver, diacetolol is the active metabolite
Elimination: 30%–40% in urine; 50%–60% in stool
Elimination half-life: 3–4 h; 8–13 h (diacetolol)

MONITORING
BP, heart rate, respiratory status, ECG for PR prolongation, and other appropriate clinical markers as indicated (eg, blood glucose if diabetic); also monitor for signs/symptoms of heart failure and signs/symptoms of CNS side effects.

OVERDOSE
Supportive: For severe bradycardia, atropine 0.25–2.0 mg IV may be administered or a pacemaker should be placed. Isoproterenol may also be used if bradycardia persists. For cardiovascular support, glucagon 50 µg/kg IV bolus may be administered over 1–2 min; up to 10 mg may be needed in some cases. In many cases, this may be followed by 2–5 mg/h (maximum 10 mg/h) continuous infusion. Fluid therapy with vasopressors/inotropic therapy may be added if necessary. Acebutolol is removed by dialysis.

PATIENT INFORMATION
Acebutolol therapy should not be discontinued abruptly without consulting your health care provider. Your health care provider should also be consulted for persistent or unusual problems, such as dizziness/faintness, weight gain, worsening edema, or increasing shortness of breath. Sit or lie down if dizziness occurs, and rise slowly from a sitting or lying position. This medication may cause dizziness or drowsiness; use caution if performing activities requiring mental or physical effort.

AVAILABILITY
Capsules—200, 400 mg

CARTEOLOL (Cartrol®)

Carteolol is a long-acting, nonselective beta-adrenergic receptor antagonist with ISA and without significant membrane-stabilizing activity. Because of its partial beta-agonist activity, carteolol does not reduce resting heart rate as much as other beta-blockers without ISA. It does not have clinically significant antiarrhythmic activity. Carteolol is used either alone or in combination with other agents for the management of hypertension. It is also available as an ophthalmic solution for open-angle glaucoma.

SPECIAL GROUPS

Race: black hypertensive patients may be less responsive than white patients

Children: safety and effectiveness have not been established

Elderly: start with low dose, and adjust dosing intervals based on renal function

Renal impairment: renally eliminated, therefore use with caution; dosage should be reduced

Hepatic impairment: use with caution; dosage adjustment is probably not required

Pregnancy: category C; use only if potential benefit justifies the potential risk to the fetus

Breast-feeding: not recommended; not known if the drug is excreted in human milk

DOSAGE

2.5–10 mg once daily (usual maintenance dose is 2.5 or 5 mg once daily) Guidelines for dosing intervals in patients with renal impairment (including elderly patients):

Creatinine clearance, mL/min	Dosing interval, h
>60	24
20–60	48
<20	72

IN BRIEF

INDICATIONS
Hypertension

CONTRAINDICATIONS
Bronchial asthma or related bronchospastic problems

Cardiogenic shock

Known hypersensitivity to product components

Second- or third-degree AV block

Severe persistent bradycardia

Overt heart failure

Severe obstructive pulmonary disease

Sick sinus syndrome without a permanent pacemaker in place

DRUG INTERACTIONS
Antihypertensive agents[1,3]

Beta-agonists[2,4]

Calcium channel blockers: verapamil or diltiazem[1,3]

Insulin[3]

NSAIDs[2]

Oral hypoglycemic agents[3,4]

Reserpine and other catecholamine-depleting drugs[1]

1 Effect/toxicity of carteolol may increase.
2 Effect of carteolol may decrease.
3 Carteolol may increase the effect/toxicity of this drug.
4 Carteolol may decrease the effect of this drug.

ADVERSE EFFECTS
CV: bradycardia, peripheral vascular insufficiency/Raynaud's type, postural hypotension, syncope, hypotension, heart failure, AV block, ventricular arrhythmia, angina
CNS: fatigue, dizziness, drowsiness, depression, headache, sleep disturbances, paresthesia
Respiratory: dyspnea, bronchospasm, nasal congestion
GI: nausea, diarrhea
GU: male impotence, ejaculatory failure, urinary frequency
Other: edema, weight gain, allergic reaction, rash

PHARMACOKINETICS AND PHARMACODYNAMICS
Duration of action: >24 h
Onset of action: 1–3 h
Peak effect: 6 h
Bioavailability: 85%
Effect of food: slower absorption but no effect on the extent of absorption
Protein binding: 23%–30%
Volume of distribution: insufficient data
Metabolism: partially metabolized with an active metabolite, 8-hydroxycarteolol
Elimination: mainly in urine (50%–70% unchanged; 5% as 8-hydroxycarteolol)
Elimination half-life: 6 h in normal renal function; 8–12 h (8-hydroxycarteolol, active)

MONITORING
BP, heart rate, respiratory status, ECG for PR prolongation, and other appropriate clinical markers as indicated (eg, blood glucose if diabetic); also monitor for signs/symptoms of heart failure and signs/symptoms of CNS side effects.

OVERDOSE
Supportive: For severe bradycardia, atropine 0.25–2.0 mg IV may be administered or a pacemaker should be placed. Isoproterenol may also be used if bradycardia persists. For cardiovascular support, glucagon 50 µg/kg IV bolus may be administered over 1–2 min; up to 10 mg may be needed in some cases. In many cases, this may be followed by 2–5 mg/h (maximum 10 mg/h) continuous infusion. Fluid therapy with vasopressors/inotropic therapy may be added if necessary. Carteolol is not removed by dialysis.

PATIENT INFORMATION
Carteolol therapy should not be discontinued abruptly without consulting your health care provider. Your health care provider should also be consulted for persistent or unusual problems, such as dizziness/faintness, weight gain, worsening edema, or increasing shortness of breath. Sit or lie down if dizziness occurs, and rise slowly from a sitting or lying position. This medication may cause dizziness or drowsiness; use caution if performing activities requiring mental or physical effort.

AVAILABILITY
Tablets—2.5, 5 mg

PENBUTOLOL (Levatol®)

Penbutolol is a long-acting, nonselective beta-adrenergic receptor antagonist with mild ISA. It is not clear if the ISA activity offers additional advantages in a clinical setting. The beta-blocking potency of penbutolol is approximately four times that of propranolol. Maximum beta antagonism occurs with doses of 10 to 20 mg. Penbutolol may be used alone or in combination with other agents in the management of hypertension.

SPECIAL GROUPS

Race:	black hypertensive patients may be less responsive than white patients
Children:	safety and effectiveness have not been established
Elderly:	start with low dose, and adjust the dose based on clinical response
Renal impairment:	use with caution; dosage adjustment is probably not required
Hepatic impairment:	conjugate accumulation may occur with hepatic insufficiency; use with caution; adjust the dose based on clinical response
Pregnancy:	category C; use only if potential benefit justifies the potential risk to the fetus
Breast-feeding:	not recommended; not known if the drug is excreted in human milk

DOSAGE

20–80 mg once daily (usual maintenance dose is 20 mg once daily)

IN BRIEF

INDICATIONS
Hypertension

CONTRAINDICATIONS
Bronchial asthma or related bronchospastic problems

Cardiogenic shock

Known hypersensitivity to product components

Second- or third-degree AV block

Sinus bradycardia

Overt heart failure

Severe obstructive pulmonary disease

Sick sinus syndrome without a permanent pacemaker in place

DRUG INTERACTIONS
Antihypertensive agents[1,3]

Beta-agonists[2,4]

Calcium channel blockers: verapamil or diltiazem[1,3]

Insulin[3]

NSAIDs[2]

Oral hypoglycemic agents[3,4]

Reserpine and other catecholamine-depleting drugs[1]

1 Effect/toxicity of penbutolol may increase.
2 Effect of penbutolol may decrease.
3 Penbutolol may increase the effect/toxicity of this drug.
4 Penbutolol may decrease the effect of this drug.

ADVERSE EFFECTS
CV: bradycardia, peripheral vascular insufficiency/Raynaud's type, postural hypotension, syncope, hypotension, heart failure, AV block, ventricular arrhythmia, angina
CNS: fatigue, dizziness, drowsiness, depression, headache, sleep disturbances
Respiratory: dyspnea, bronchospasm, nasal congestion
GI: dyspepsia, nausea, diarrhea
GU: male impotence, ejaculatory failure
Metabolic: hypoglycemia
Other: edema, weight gain, allergic reaction

PHARMACOKINETICS AND PHARMACODYNAMICS

Duration of action:	>20 h
Onset of action:	<1 h
Peak effect:	2–3 h
Bioavailability:	100%
Effect of food:	little effect
Protein binding:	80%–98%
Volume of distribution:	insufficient data
Metabolism:	extensively metabolized in the liver by conjugation and oxidation
Elimination:	90% in urine, mainly as metabolites (5% unchanged)
Elimination half-life:	5 h

MONITORING
BP, heart rate, respiratory status, ECG for PR prolongation, and other appropriate clinical markers as indicated (eg, blood glucose if diabetic); also monitor for signs/symptoms of heart failure and signs/symptoms of CNS side effects.

OVERDOSE
Supportive: For severe bradycardia, atropine 0.25–2.0 mg IV may be administered or a pacemaker should be placed. Isoproterenol may also be used if bradycardia persists. For cardiovascular support, glucagon 50 µg/kg IV bolus may be administered over 1–2 min; up to 10 mg may be needed in some cases. In many cases, this may be followed by 2–5 mg/h (maximum 10 mg/h) continuous infusion. Fluid therapy with vasopressors/inotropic therapy may be added if necessary. Penbutolol is not removed by dialysis.

PATIENT INFORMATION
Penbutolol therapy should not be discontinued abruptly without consulting your health care provider. Your health care provider should also be consulted for persistent or unusual problems, such as dizziness/faintness, weight gain, worsening edema, or increasing shortness of breath. Sit or lie down if dizziness occurs, and rise slowly from a sitting or lying position. This medication may cause dizziness or drowsiness; use caution if performing activities requiring mental or physical effort.

AVAILABILITY
Tablets—20 mg

PINDOLOL
(Pindolol, Visken®)

Pindolol is a nonselective beta-adrenergic receptor antagonist with ISA. It is not clear if the ISA activity offers additional advantages in a clinical setting. It also exhibits membrane-stabilizing activity (quinidine-like), although this occurs only at supratherapeutic plasma concentrations. Pindolol has less effect on reducing the heart rate and cardiac output at rest, although its effect on blocking stress- or exercise-induced tachycardia is similar to other beta-blockers without ISA. Pindolol may be used alone or in combination with other agents in the management of hypertension. It may also be useful in the management of stress- or exercise-induced angina (not an indication approved by the FDA), especially in those patients with resting bradycardia and CHF.

SPECIAL GROUPS

Race: black hypertensive patients may be less responsive than white patients

Children: safety and effectiveness have not been established

Elderly: clearance may be reduced; start with low dose, and adjust the dose based on clinical response

Renal impairment: use with caution because clearance may be reduced; initial dosage adjustment is not necessary, but adjust dosage based on clinical response

Hepatic impairment: clearance is reduced with hepatic insufficiency; use with caution; start with a low dosage, and adjust based on clinical response

Pregnancy: category B; should only be used if clearly indicated

Breast-feeding: not recommended; excreted in human milk

IN BRIEF

INDICATIONS
Hypertension

CONTRAINDICATIONS
Bronchial asthma or related bronchospastic problems
Cardiogenic shock
Concomitant thioridazine use
Known hypersensitivity to product components
Second- or third-degree AV block
Sinus bradycardia
Overt heart failure
Severe obstructive pulmonary disease
Sick sinus syndrome without a permanent pacemaker in place

DRUG INTERACTIONS
Antihypertensive agents[1,3]
Beta-agonists[2,4]
Calcium channel blockers: verapamil or diltiazem[1,3]
Digoxin[4,5]
Insulin[3]
NSAIDs[2]
Oral hypoglycemic agents[3,4]
Reserpine and other catecholamine-depleting drugs[1]
Thioridazine[1,3]

1 Effect/toxicity of pindolol may increase.
2 Effect of pindolol may decrease.
3 Pindolol may increase the effect/toxicity of this drug.
4 Pindolol may decrease the effect of this drug.
5 The clinical significance of this interaction is unclear.

ADVERSE EFFECTS
CV: bradycardia, peripheral vascular insufficiency/Raynaud's type, postural hypotension, syncope, hypotension, heart failure, AV block, ventricular arrhythmia, angina
CNS: fatigue, dizziness, drowsiness, depression, headache, sleep disturbances
Respiratory: dyspnea, bronchospasm, nasal congestion
GI: nausea, abdominal discomfort, diarrhea, elevated liver enzymes
GU: male impotence, ejaculatory failure
Metabolic: hypoglycemia
Other: edema, weight gain, allergic reaction

PHARMACOKINETICS AND PHARMACODYNAMICS
Duration of action: 24 h
Onset of action: <3 h
Peak plasma concentration: 1–2 h; 2 wk or longer may be required for maximal antihypertensive effect
Bioavailability: 50%–95%
Effect of food: increases the rate of absorption
Protein binding: 40%–60%
Volume of distribution: 1.2–2 L/kg
Metabolism: 60%–65% metabolized in liver to hydroxylated metabolites
Elimination: 35%–50% excreted in urine unchanged
Elimination half-life: 3–4 h (↑ in elderly, renal dysfunction, and hepatic cirrhosis)

MONITORING
BP, heart rate, respiratory status, ECG for PR prolongation, and other appropriate clinical markers as indicated (eg, blood glucose if diabetic); also monitor for signs/symptoms of heart failure and signs/symptoms of CNS side effects.

The information here is provided as guidance only. Prescribers should always consult the manufacturer's current prescribing information.

177

PINDOLOL (continued)

DOSAGE

Initial dosage is 5 mg twice daily; maintenance dosage is 10–60 mg/d in 2 divided doses (usual maintenance dose is 10–40 mg/d in 2 divided doses). Allow 3–4 wk between dosage increases. Once-daily dosing may be possible in some patients.

OVERDOSE

Supportive: For severe bradycardia, atropine 0.25–2.0 mg IV may be administered or a pacemaker should be placed. Isoproterenol may also be used if bradycardia persists. For cardiovascular support, glucagon 50 µg/kg IV bolus may be administered over 1–2 min; up to 10 mg may be needed in some cases. In many cases, this may be followed by 2–5 mg/h (maximum 10 mg/h) continuous infusion. Fluid therapy with vasopressors/inotropic therapy may be added if necessary. Pindolol is not removed by dialysis.

PATIENT INFORMATION

Pindolol therapy should not be discontinued abruptly without consulting your health care provider. Your health care provider should also be consulted for persistent or unusual problems, such as dizziness/faintness, weight gain, worsening edema, or increasing shortness of breath. Sit or lie down if dizziness occurs, and rise slowly from a sitting or lying position. This medication may cause dizziness or drowsiness; use caution if performing activities requiring mental or physical effort.

AVAILABILITY

Tablets—5, 10 mg

DUAL-ACTING BETA-BLOCKERS

Some beta-blockers, such as **labetalol** and **carvedilol**, have dual beta- and alpha-blocking properties. These agents improve arterial compliance through alpha-blockade, and therefore may be particularly effective in lowering BP and reversing left ventricular hypertrophy. **Carvedilol** was the first beta-blocker approved for use in CHF.

EFFICACY AND USE

Dual-acting agents are effective in lowering BP in patients with hypertension. **Labetalol** produces a fall in supine BP of the same order as pure beta-blockers but is more effective in reducing BP in the upright position. The BP is lowered maximally within 1–2 h, and once controlled, the antihypertensive effect is maintained on chronic therapy. The relatively quick onset of effect of **labetalol** makes it one of the first-line agents for the treatment of hypertensive crises. Severe hypertension often requires a higher dosage. IV **labetalol** has been used effectively in hypertension associated with pregnancy.

Labetalol appears to be as effective as a thiazide diuretic in lowering supine and standing BP. It is more effective than **hydralazine**, although probably less effective than **minoxidil**. It has similar efficacy to **methyldopa** and **clonidine**, and is more effective than the sympatholytic agents, such as **guanethidine**, **bethanidine**, and **debrisoquine**.

INDICATIONS

	Labetalol	Carvedilol
Hypertension	+	+
Hypertensive emergencies	+	–
CHF	–	+

CHF—congestive heart failure; +—approved by the FDA; – —not approved by the FDA.

The combination of **labetalol** with a diuretic is an effective treatment for hypertension, with the fall in BP on the combination being greater than either agent alone. **Labetalol** has been combined with vasodilators, such as **minoxidil**, and calcium antagonists, to manage resistant hypertension.

Carvedilol is approved for use in hypertension, but it is primarily used as an adjunctive therapy in patients with systolic heart failure. **Carvedilol** has been shown to reduce morbidity and mortality in patients with heart failure and is now considered a primary agent for the treatment of this disease.

Vasodilatory side effects relating to alpha-blockade are seen, particularly at higher doses. Postural hypotension, scalp tingling, and genitourinary problems may be troublesome in certain patients. Classic adverse reactions to beta-blockers, such as fatigue and cold peripheries associated with reduced cardiac output, are less common with this class of agents. Coronary risk factors, such as low plasma high-density lipoprotein (HDL) concentrations and high fibrinogen concentrations, are improved. The clinical relevance of these changes has yet to be established. These drugs tend to be lipid neutral, although the clinical significance of this is not yet clear.

MODE OF ACTION

Dual-acting beta-blockers have only a moderate effect on resting cardiac output and, therefore, they lower BP primarily through a reduction in total peripheral resistance via alpha-blockade or direct nonspecific vasodilatory properties. The afterload reduction may be beneficial when left ventricular function is impaired.

The exact mechanism for **carvedilol**'s benefit in patients with heart failure is not clear. Various mechanisms have been postulated (Table 7.3). There is no clinical experience using **labetalol** in patients with heart failure.

TABLE 7.3 POSSIBLE MECHANISMS BY WHICH BETA-ADRENERGIC BLOCKERS IMPROVE VENTRICULAR FUNCTION IN CHRONIC CONGESTIVE HEART FAILURE

Up-regulation of beta-receptors	Restoration of abnormal baroreflex function
Direct myocardial protective action against catecholamine toxicity	Prevention of ventricular muscle hypertrophy and vascular remodeling
Improved ability of noradrenergic sympathetic nerves to synthesize norepinephrine	Antioxidant effects (carvedilol?)
Decreased release of norepinephrine from sympathetic nerve endings	Shift from free fatty acid to carbohydrate metabolism (improved metabolic efficiency)
Decreased stimulation of other vasoconstrictive systems, including renin-angiotensin-aldosterone, vasopressin, and endothelin	Vasodilatation (eg, carvedilol)
	Antiapoptosis effect allowing myocardial cell regeneration to occur
Potentiation of kallikrein-kinin system and natural vasodilatation (increase in bradykinin)	Modulation of postreceptor inhibitory G-proteins
Antiarrhythmic effects raising ventricular fibrillation threshold	Improved left atrial contribution to left ventricular filling
Protection against catecholamine-induced hypokalemia	Normalization of myocyte Ca^{++} regulatory proteins and improved Ca^{++} handling
Increase in coronary blood flow by reducing heart rate and improving diastolic perfusion time; possible coronary dilatation with vasodilator beta-blocker	Increasing natriuretic peptide production
	Attenuation of inflammatory cytokines
	Restoring cardiac calcium release channel (ryanodine receptor)

Adapted from Frishman WH: Alpha- and beta-adrenergic blocking drugs. In *Cardiovascular Pharmacotherapeutics*, edn 2. Edited by Frishman WH, Sonnenblick EH, Sica DA. New York: McGraw Hill; 2003:83.

CARVEDILOL (Coreg®)

Similar to labetalol, carvedilol is a nonselective beta-adrenergic blocking agent with selective alpha$_1$-blocking activity. It has moderate membrane-stabilizing activity, but no ISA.

In general, beta-blockers, in addition to their antihypertensive and cardiac protective effects, may provide long-term clinical benefits in patients with heart failure by blocking the deleterious effects of the overacting sympathetic nervous system. Clinical studies have shown that bisoprolol, carvedilol, and metoprolol, when added to conventional therapy, may slow disease progression and reduce mortality and the frequency of hospitalization in patients with heart failure.

Although carvedilol is the first beta-blocker approved in the United States as an add-on therapy in patients with heart failure, it is still not clear if its dual alpha- and beta-adrenergic blocking activity offers additional advantage over other beta-blockers. When carvedilol was compared to metoprolol tartrate in the COMET study in 1511 patients with chronic heart failure, carvedilol therapy resulted in a 17% relative risk reduction in all-cause mortality ($P = 0.0017$) after a mean follow-up of 58 months. The composite end point of mortality or all-cause admission, however, was not statistically different between treatments. While this study suggests that carvedilol is more effective than metoprolol tartrate in the treatment of heart failure, the study itself has been criticized for not comparing carvedilol to metoprolol succinate, which is currently the only formulation of metoprolol approved for the treatment of heart failure in the United States, and may just be different enough than the tartrate salt to perhaps produce a different outcome when compared to carvedilol.

Because beta-blockers may initially exacerbate heart failure, carvedilol therapy should be initiated with low doses (3.125 mg twice daily). Close patient monitoring for hypotension, bradycardia, and worsening of heart failure is recommended, especially during the first 2–4 wk of therapy and after each dose increase. Doses should be increased gradually or reduced based on patient tolerance and clinical response. A 1–3 mo trial period is required to determine the full benefits of carvedilol therapy.

SPECIAL GROUPS

Race: black hypertensive patients may be less responsive than white patients

Children: safety and effectiveness have not been established

Elderly: drug clearance is reduced, therefore use cautiously; no specific dosage adjustment is required

Renal impairment: drug clearance is reduced, therefore use cautiously; no specific dosage adjustment is required

Hepatic impairment: contraindicated with active liver disease; drug clearance is reduced, therefore use cautiously, although no specific dosage adjustment is required

Pregnancy: category C; use only if potential benefit justifies the potential risk to the fetus

Breast-feeding: not recommended; not known if the drug is excreted in human milk

IN BRIEF

INDICATIONS
CHF
Left ventricular dysfunction following MI
Hypertension

CONTRAINDICATIONS
Bronchial asthma or related bronchospastic problems
Cardiogenic shock
Clinically manifest hepatic impairment
Known hypersensitivity to product components
NYHA class IV decompensated heart failure requiring intravenous inotropic therapy
Second- or third-degree AV block
Severe bradycardia
Sick sinus syndrome without a permanent pacemaker in place

DRUG INTERACTIONS
Antihypertensive agents[1,3]
Beta-agonists[2,4]
Cimetidine[1]
Cyclosporine[3]
Digoxin[3,5]
Diltiazem[1,3]
Fluoxetine[1]
Insulin[3]
Oral hypoglycemics[3]
Paroxetine[1]
Propafenone[1]
Quinidine[1]
Rifampin[2]
Verapamil[1,3]
Catecholamine-depleting agents (such as reserpine, MAO inhibitors)[1]

1 Effect/toxicity of carvedilol may increase.
2 Effect of carvedilol may decrease.
3 Carvedilol may increase the effect/toxicity of this drug.
4 Carvedilol may decrease the effect of this drug.
5 The clinical significance of this interaction is unclear.

ADVERSE EFFECTS
CV: bradycardia, syncope, hypotension, postural hypotension, heart failure exacerbation, AV block, angina
CNS: fatigue, drowsiness, dizziness
Respiratory: dyspnea, bronchospasm, nasal congestion
GI: hepatic injury, nausea, vomiting, diarrhea
GU: male impotence, ejaculatory failure
Metabolic: hyperglycemia, hypoglycemia, dyslipidemia
Other: edema, weight gain, thrombocytopenia, allergic reaction, photosensitivity

PHARMACOKINETICS AND PHARMACODYNAMICS
Duration of action: 12–24 h
Onset of action: <30 min
Peak effect: 1–7 h
Bioavailability: 25%–35%
Effect of food: slower absorption but has no effect on the extent of absorption
Protein binding: 95%–98%
Volume of distribution: 115 L
Metabolism: mainly metabolized in the liver with three active metabolites identified; CYP2D6, CYP2C9, and to a lesser extent, CYP3A4 and other isozymes are involved with the metabolism of carvedilol
Elimination: excreted mainly via the bile into feces and <2% excreted unchanged in urine
Elimination half-life: 7–10 h

CARVEDILOL *(continued)*

DOSAGE

CHF: If the patient is taking ACE inhibitors, diuretics, or digoxin, the dosing of these agents should be stabilized prior to initiation of carvedilol. It is recommended that the patient be euvolemic or have minimal fluid retention upon initiation of therapy and with subsequent dosage increases.

3.125–50 mg twice daily.* The initial dosage is 3.125 mg twice daily for 2 wk. If the dosage is tolerated, then it may be doubled every 2–4 wk to the highest dosage tolerated by the patient (up to 25 mg twice daily in patients weighing less than 85 kg and 50 mg twice daily in patients weighing more than 85 kg).

Left ventricular dysfunction following MI: It is recommended that the patient be euvolemic or have minimal fluid retention upon initiation of therapy and with subsequent dosage increases. The initial dosage is 3.125–6.25 mg twice daily, doubled every 1–2 wk to a target dosage of 25 mg twice daily.*

Hypertension: 6.25–25 mg twice daily.* The initial dose is 6.25 mg twice daily. The dose should be doubled every 1–2 wk based on BP response, up to a maximum dose of 25 mg twice daily.

*The dose should be taken with food to slow down the rate of absorption and reduce the incidence of orthostatic effect. In patients with heart failure, slower titration with temporary dose reduction or withdrawal may be required based on clinical assessment; however, this should not preclude later attempts to reintroduce or increase the dose of carvedilol.

MONITORING

BP, heart rate, weight, fluid status, respiratory status, CBC, liver function and signs/symptoms of liver dysfunction (eg, pruritus, dark urine, jaundice), blood glucose.

OVERDOSE

Supportive: For severe bradycardia, atropine 2 mg IV may be administered or a pacemaker should be placed. For cardiovascular support, glucagon 5–10 mg IV bolus administered over 30 sec, followed by 5 mg/h continuous infusion. Fluid therapy with vasopressors/inotropic therapy added if necessary may also be appropriate.

PATIENT INFORMATION

Carvedilol therapy should not be discontinued abruptly without consulting your health care provider. Your health care provider should also be consulted if you experience dizziness/faintness or signs and symptoms of worsening heart failure, such as unusual weight gain, worsening of edema, or increasing shortness of breath. Sit or lie down if dizziness occurs, and rise slowly from a sitting or lying position. Take with food to minimize side effects. Avoid prolonged exposure to the sun because photosensitivity may occur.

AVAILABILITY

Tablets—3.125, 6.25, 12.5, 25 mg

The information here is provided as guidance only. Prescribers should always consult the manufacturer's current prescribing information.

181

LABETALOL

(Labetalol, Normodyne®, Trandate®)

Labetalol is an adrenergic receptor blocking agent that has both selective alpha$_1$- and nonselective beta-adrenergic receptor blocking actions. In humans, the ratios of alpha- to beta-blockade have been estimated to be approximately 1:2 and 1:7 after oral and IV administration, respectively. Beta$_2$-agonist activity has also been demonstrated, but labetalol does not possess membrane-stabilizing activity. It is effective in lowering BP and alleviating angina pectoris. Vasodilating side effects, such as scalp tingling and postural hypotension, may be a problem for some patients, particularly at higher doses. Several cases of hepatic failure, including deaths, have been reported with labetalol.

Intravenous labetalol, unlike many parenterally administered antihypertensives, has a prompt but gradual antihypertensive effect, with little effect on cardiac output or heart rate. About 80%–90% of patients with severe hypertension will respond adequately to the BP-lowering effects of labetalol, making it one of the preferred agents in this situation. Oral labetalol is also one of the first-line agents for the treatment of hypertensive urgencies.

SPECIAL GROUPS

Race: black hypertensive patients may be less responsive than white patients

Children: safety and effectiveness have not been established

Elderly: more sensitive to the effects of labetalol; start with a lower dosage, and titrate based on response

Renal impairment: no dosage adjustment is necessary unless the patient has severe renal insufficiency, in which case, the dosing interval may be extended (ie, once-daily dosing)

Hepatic impairment: increased bioavailability and slower clearance; titrate the dose based on response

Pregnancy: category C; use only if potential benefit justifies the potential risk to the fetus

Breast-feeding: small amounts excreted in human milk; use with caution

IN BRIEF

INDICATIONS
Hypertension

CONTRAINDICATIONS
Bronchial asthma or related bronchospastic problems
Cardiogenic shock
Severe bradycardia
Second- or third-degree AV block
Overt heart failure
Sick sinus syndrome without a permanent pacemaker in place

DRUG INTERACTIONS
Antihypertensive agents[1,3]
Beta-agonists[2,4]
Calcium channel blockers: verapamil or diltiazem[1,3]
Cimetidine[1]
Glutethimide[2]
Halothane[1,3]
Tricyclic antidepressants[3]
Insulin[3]
Oral hypoglycemic agents[3]

1 Effect/toxicity of labetalol may increase.
2 Effect of labetalol may decrease.
3 Labetalol may increase the effect/toxicity of this drug.
4 Labetalol may decrease the effect of this drug.

ADVERSE EFFECTS
CV: postural hypotension, syncope, hypotension, heart failure exacerbation, bradycardia, AV block, ventricular arrhythmia, angina
CNS: fatigue, drowsiness, headache, paresthesia
Respiratory: dyspnea, bronchospasm, nasal congestion
GI: hepatic injury, jaundice, nausea, vomiting, dyspepsia
GU: male impotence, ejaculatory failure
Other: edema, weight gain, allergic reaction

PHARMACOKINETICS AND PHARMACODYNAMICS
Duration of action: 8–24 h (po); 2–4 h (IV)
Onset of action: 20 min (po); 2–5 min (IV)
Peak effect: 1–4 h (po); 5–15 minutes (IV)
Bioavailability: 26%–36% (po); 100% (IV)
Protein binding: 50%
Volume of distribution: 3.2–15.7 L/kg
Effect of food: delay but increase the extent of absorption
Metabolism: mainly metabolized in the liver and GI mucosa
Elimination: biliary—30%; urine—55%–60% (<5% unchanged)
Elimination half-life: 6–8 h (po), 5.5 h (IV)

MONITORING
BP, heart rate, respiratory status, liver function and signs/symptoms of liver dysfunction (eg, pruritus, dark urine, jaundice).

OVERDOSE
Supportive: For severe bradycardia, atropine 2 mg IV may be administered or a pacemaker should be placed. For cardiovascular support, glucagon 5–10 mg IV bolus administered over 30 sec, followed by 5 mg/h continuous infusion. Fluid therapy with v asopressors/inotropic therapy added if necessary may also be appropriate. Labetalol is not removed by dialysis.

DOSAGE

PO: Initial dose is 100 mg twice daily; dose may be titrated in increments of 100 mg twice daily every 2–3 d based on BP response

Usual maintenance dose: 200–400 mg bid; maximum dose: 1200–2400 mg/d in 2–3 divided doses

Intermittent IV administration: 20 mg (0.25 mg/kg) slow IV over 2 min; additional doses of 20, 40, or 80 mg may be administered every 10 min until a desired supine BP is achieved or a total dose of 300 mg has been injected.

Continuous IV administration: 0.5–2 mg/min

Dose should be titrated based on BP response. The infusion should be continued until an adequate response is achieved or a total dose of 300 mg is infused. The infusion is then discontinued and oral therapy is initiated when supine BP begins to increase. Initial oral dose is 200 mg, followed in 6–12 h by an additional oral dose of 200 or 400 mg, depending on BP response.

PATIENT INFORMATION
Labetalol therapy should not be discontinued abruptly without consulting your health care provider. Your health care provider should also be consulted for persistent or unusual problems, such as dizziness/faintness, weight gain, worsening edema, increasing shortness of breath, anorexia, jaundice, pruritus, dark urine, flulike syndrome, and right upper quadrant tenderness. Sit or lie down if dizziness occurs, and rise slowly from a sitting or lying position.

AVAILABILITY
Tablets—100, 200, 300 mg
Vials—5 mg/mL, in 20 mL and 40 mL multidose vials
Prefilled syringes—5 mg/mL, 4 mL and 8 mL

The information here is provided as guidance only. Prescribers should always consult the manufacturer's current prescribing information.

183

SELECTED BIBLIOGRAPHY

Abrams J, Frishman WH, Bates SM, *et al.*: Pharmacologic options for treatment of ischemic disease. In *Cardiovascular Therapeutics. A Companion to Braunwald's Heart Disease,* edn 2. Edited by Antman EM. Philadelphia: WB Saunders Co.; 2002:97–153.

Auerbach AD, Goldman L: β Blockers and reduction of cardiac events in noncardiac surgery. Clinical applications. *JAMA* 2002, 287:1435–1444.

Australia/New Zealand Heart Failure Research Collaborative Group: Randomised, placebo-controlled trial of carvedilol in patients with congestive heart failure due to ischaemic heart disease. *Lancet* 1997, 349:375–380.

Beta-Blocker Heart Attack Trial Research Group: A randomized trial of propranolol in patients with acute myocardial infarction. *JAMA* 1982, 247:1707–1713.

Black JW: Ahlquist and the development of beta-adrenoceptor antagonists. *Postgrad Med J* 1976, 52(Suppl 4):11–13.

Boissel JP, Leizorovicz A, Picolet H, *et al.*: Secondary prevention after high-risk acute myocardial infarction with low-dose acebutolol. *Am J Cardiol* 1990, 66:251–260.

Carson PE: β-blocker therapy in heart failure: pathophysiology and clinical results. *Curr Prob Card* 1999, 24:421–460.

Cavusoglu E, Frishman WH: Sotalol: a new β-adrenergic blocker for ventricular arrhythmias. *Prog Cardiovasc Dis* 1995, 37:423–440.

Chadda K, Goldstein S, Byington R, Curb JD: Effects of propranolol after acute myocardial infarction in patients with congestive heart failure. *Circulation* 1986, 73:503–510.

CIBIS Investigators and Committees: A randomized trial of b blockade in heart failure: the Cardiac Insufficiency Bisoprolol Study (CIBIS). *Circulation* 1994, 90:1765–1773.

CIBIS II Investigators and Committees: The Cardiac Insufficiency Bisoprolol Study II (CIBIS II): a randomized trial. *Lancet* 1999, 353:9–13.

Coope J, Warrender TS: Randomised trial of treatment of hypertension in elderly patients in primary care. *Br Med J* 1986, 293:1145–1151.

Cruickshank JM: Measurement and cardiovascular relevance of partial agonist activity (PAA) involving beta1- and beta2-adrenoceptors. *Pharmacol Ther* 1990, 46:199–242.

Cruickshank JM, Pennert K, Sorman A, *et al.*: Low mortality from all causes, including myocardial infarction, in well-controlled hypertensives treated with a beta blocker plus other antihypertensives. *J Hypertens* 1987, 5:489–498.

DiBona GF, Sawin LL: Effect of metoprolol administration on renal sodium handling in experimental heart failure. *Circulation* 1999, 100:82–86.

Dwyer N, Walter P, Cruickshank JM, *et al.*: Effect of propranolol and phentolamine on myocardial necrosis after subarachnoid haemorrhage. *Br Med J* 1978, 2:990–992.

Engelmeier RS, O'Connell JB, Walsh R, *et al.*: Improvements in symptoms and exercise tolerance by metoprolol in patients with dilated cardiomyopathy. *Circulation* 1985, 72:536–546.

Frishman WH: Secondary prevention of myocardial infarction: the roles of beta-adrenergic blockers, calcium-channel blockers, angiotensin converting enzyme inhibitors and aspirin. In *Triggering of Acute Coronary Syndromes: Implications for Prevention.* Edited by Willich SN, Muller JE. Dordrecht: Kluwer Academic Publishers; 1995:367–394.

Frishman WH: Carvedilol. *N Engl J Med* 1998, 339:1759–1765.

Frishman WH: Alpha- and beta-adrenergic blocking drugs. In *Cardiovascular Pharmacotherapeutics,* edn 2. Edited by Frishman WH, Sonnenblick EH, Sica DA. New York: McGraw Hill; 2003:67–97.

Frishman WH: Alpha- and beta-adrenergic blocking drugs. In *Cardiovascular Pharmacotherapeutics Manual.* Edited by Frishman WH, Sonnenblick EH, Sica DA. New York: McGraw Hill; 2004:19–57.

Frishman WH, Bryzinski BS, Coulson LR, *et al.*: A multifactorial trial design to assess combination therapy in hypertension: treatment with bisoprolol and hydrochlorothiazide. *Arch Intern Med* 1994, 154:1461–1468.

Frishman WH, Burris FJ, Mroczek WJ, *et al.*: First-line therapy option with low-dose bisoprolol fumarate and low-dose hydrochlorothiazide in patients with stage I and stage II systemic hypertension. *J Clin Pharmacol* 1995, 35:182–188.

Frishman WH, Cheng A: Secondary prevention of myocardial infarction: the role of β-adrenergic blockers and angiotensin converting enzyme inhibitors: based on symposium Agents to Prevent Acute Coronary Disease. *Am Heart J* 1999, 137:S25–S34.

Frishman WH, Christiana J: The current use of beta blockers in cardiovascular disease. In *Cardiology Clinics Annual of Drug Therapy,* vol 2. Edited by Crawford MH. Philadelphia: WB Saunders Co.; 1998:37–59.

Frishman WH, Jorde U: β-Adrenergic blockers. In *Hypertension: A Companion to Brenner & Rector's The Kidney.* Edited by Oparil S, Weber MA. Philadelphia: WB Saunders Co.; 2000:590–595.

Frishman WH, Murthy VS, Strom JA, Hershman D: Ultra-short-acting β-adrenergic blocking drugs. In *Cardiovascular Drug Therapy,* edn 2. Edited by Messerli FH. Philadelphia: WB Saunders Co.; 1996:507–516.

Frishman WH, Opie LH, Sica DA: Adverse cardiovascular drug interactions and complications. In *Hurst's The Heart,* edn 11. Edited by Fuster V, Alexander RW, O'Rourke RA, *et al.* New York: McGraw Hill; 2004:2169–2188.

Frishman WH, Sica DA: β-Adrenergic blockers. In *Hypertension Primer*, edn 3. Edited by Izzo JL Jr, Black HR. Dallas: American Heart Association; 2003:417–421.

Frishman WH, Skolnick AE: Secondary prevention post infarction: the role of β-adrenergic blockers, calcium-channel blockers and aspirin. In *Acute Myocardial Infarction*, edn 2. Edited by Gersh BJ, Rahimtoola SH. New York: Chapman and Hall; 1996:766–796.

Frishman WH, Sonnenblick EH: β-Adrenergic blocking drugs and calcium channel blockers. In *Hurst's The Heart*, edn 9. Edited by Alexander RW, Schlant RC, Fuster V. New York: McGraw Hill; 1998:1583–1618.

Hennekens CH, Albert CM, Godfried SL, *et al.*: Adjunctive drug therapy of acute myocardial infarction—evidence from clinical trials. *N Engl J Med* 1996, 335:1660–1667.

Hjalmarson A, Herlitz J, Holmbert S, *et al.*: The Goteborg Metoprolol Trial: effects on mortality and morbidity in acute myocardial infarction. *Circulation* 1983, 67(Suppl I):I36–I32.

Hohnloser SH, Meinertz T, Klingenheben T, *et al.*: Usefulness of esmolol in unstable angina pectoris. *Am J Cardiol* 1991, 67:1319–1323.

ISIS-1 Collaborative Group: Randomised trial of intravenous atenolol among 16,027 cases of suspected acute myocardial infarction: ISIS-1. *Lancet* 1986, ii:57–66.

Kaplan NM: Treatment of hypertension: drug therapy. In *Kaplan's Clinical Hypertension,* edn 8. Edited by Neal W, Kaplan NM, Lieberman E. Philadelphia: Lippincott Williams & Wilkins; 2002:237–338.

Kjekshus J: Comments: beta blockers and heart rate reduction: a mechanism of benefit. *Eur Heart J* 1985, 6(Suppl A):29–30.

Kjekshus J, Gilpin E, Cali G, *et al.*: Diabetic patients and beta blockers after acute myocardial infarction. *Eur Heart J* 1990, 11:43–50.

LeJemtel TH, Sonnenblick EH, Frishman WH: Diagnosis and medical management of heart failure. In *Hurst's The Heart*, edn 11. Edited by Fuster V, Alexander RW, O'Rourke RA, *et al.* New York: McGraw Hill; 2004:723–762.

Lubsen J, Tijssen JGP, Study Group: Efficacy of nifedipine and metoprolol in the early treatment of unstable angina in the coronary care unit: findings from the Holland Interuniversity Nifedipine/Metoprolol Trial (HINT). *Am J Cardiol* 1987, 60:18A–25A.

Man In't Veld AJ, van den Meiracker AH: Effects of antihypertensive drugs on cardiovascular haemodynamics. In *Hypertension*. Edited by Laragh JH, Brenner BM. New York: Raven Press; 1990:2117–2130.

Mason JW for the Electrophysiologic Study Versus Electrocardiographic Monitoring Investigators (ESVEM): A comparison of seven antiarrhythmic drugs in patients with ventricular tachyarrhythmias. *N Engl J Med* 1993, 329:452–458.

McAinsh H, Cruickshank JM: Beta blockers and the central nervous system side effects. *Pharmacol Ther* 1990, 46:163–197.

MERIT-HF Study Group: Effect of metoprolol CR/XL in chronic heart failure: Metoprolol CR/XL Randomised Intervention Trial in Congestive Heart Failure (MERIT-HF). *Lancet* 1999, 353:2001–2007.

Miall WE, Greenberg D: The Medical Working Party on mild to moderate hypertension: the influence of thiazide and beta-blocker treatment on ECG findings. In *Mild Hypertension: Is There Pressure to Treat? An Account of the MRC Trial*. Cambridge, UK: Cambridge University Press; 1987:78–94; 181–185.

MIAMI Trial Research Group: Metoprolol in Acute Myocardial Infarction (MIAMI): a randomised placebo-controlled international trial. *Eur Heart J* 1985, 6:199–226.

Mohindra SK, Udeani GO: Intravenous esmolol in acute aortic dissection. *Ann Pharmacother* 1991, 25:735–738.

MRC Working Party: MRC Trial of Treatment of Mild Hypertension: principal results. *Br Med J* 1985, 291:97–104.

Norwegian Multicentre Study Group: Timolol-induced reduction in mortality and reinfarction in patients surviving acute myocardial infarction. *N Engl J Med* 1981, 304:801–807.

Opie LH, Sonnenblick EH, Frishman WH, Thadani U: Beta-blocking agents. In *Drugs for the Heart*, edn 4. Edited by Opie LH. Philadelphia: WB Saunders; 1995:1–30.

Packer M, Bristow MR, Cohn JN, *et al.*: The effect of carvedilol on morbidity and mortality in patients with chronic heart failure. *N Engl J Med* 1996, 334:1349–1355.

Pepine CJ, Cohn PF, Deedwania PC, *et al.*: Effects of treatment on outcome in asymptomatic and mildly symptomatic patients with ischemia during daily life: the Atenolol Silent Ischemia Study (ASIST). *Circulation* 1994, 90:762–768.

Poole-Wilson PA, Swedberg K, Cleland JGF, *et al.*: Comparison of carvedilol and metoprolol on clinical outcomes in patients with chronic heart failure in the Carvedilol Or Metoprolol European Trial (COMET): randomised controlled trial. *Lancet* 2003; 362:7–13.

Quyyumi AA, Crake T, Wright CM, *et al.*: Medical treatment of patients with severe exertional and rest angina in a double-bind comparison of beta blocker, calcium antagonist and nitrate. *Br Heart J* 1987, 57:505–511.

Rapaport E: Should beta blockers be given immediately and concomitantly with thrombolytic therapy in acute myocardial infarction? *Circulation* 1991, 83:695–697.

Sandberg A, Blomqvist I, Jonsson UE, Lundborg P: Pharmacokinetic and pharmacodynamic properties of a new controlled-release formulation of metoprolol: a comparison with conventional tablets. *Eur J Clin Pharmacol* 1988, 33(Suppl):S9–S14.

Sharma S, Mitra S, Grover VK, *et al.*: Esmolol blunt the haemodynamic responses to tracheal intubation in treated hypertensive patients. *Can J Anaesth* 1996, 43:778–782.

Sica DA, Frishman WH, Manowitz N: Pharmacokinetics of propranolol after single and multiple dosing with sustained-release propranolol or propranolol CR (Innopran XL), a new chronotherapeutic formulation. *Heart Dis* 2003, 5:176–181.

Smerling A, Gersony WM: Esmolol for severe hypertension following repair of aortic coarctation. *Crit Care Med* 1990, 18:1288–1290.

The SHEP Cooperative Research Group: Prevention of stroke by antihypertensive drug treatment in older persons with isolated systolic hypertension: final results of Systolic Hypertension in the Elderly Program (SHEP). *JAMA* 1991, 265:3255–3264.

Wikstrand J, Warnold I, Olsson G, *et al.*: Primary prevention with metoprolol in patients with hypertension. *JAMA* 1988, 159:1976–1982.

Wilhelmsen L, Berglund G, Elmfeldt D, *et al.*: Beta blockers versus diuretics in hypertensive men: main results from the HAPPHY trial. *J Hypertens* 1987, 5:561–572.

Verapamil, a coronary vasodilator, was reported in 1962 to possess negative inotropic and chronotropic effects that were not seen with other apparently similar vasodilator agents, such as nitroglycerin. The mechanism of action of **verapamil** was initially thought to be a result of coronary vasodilatation and blockade of myocardial beta-adrenergic receptors. Later, however, it was shown that the mechanism of action was not related to beta-receptor blockade but to inhibition of the movement of calcium ions into cells, with resulting inhibition of excitation-contraction coupling. **Verapamil** and the later drugs, **nifedipine** and **diltiazem**, became known as calcium antagonists because they inhibit the flux of calcium through the voltage-dependent "L" channel.

Unlike the beta-blockers, not all calcium antagonists are chemically related (Table 8.1). The prototype calcium antagonist, **verapamil**, is a phenylalkylamine derivative; **nifedipine** is a dihydropyridine derivative; and **diltiazem** is structurally related to the benzothiazepines. The second-generation calcium antagonists are mainly nifedipine-like dihydropyridines. These agents differ in potency, tissue specificity, and possibly even their exact mode of action. Nevertheless, they all have one action in common—that of altering calcium ion homeostasis. **Bepridil**, however, is not chemically related to the other calcium antagonists.

EFFICACY AND USE

In broad terms, the calcium antagonists have found therapeutic use in the treatment of hypertension and angina pectoris. All calcium channel blockers lower arterial pressure by reducing peripheral vascular resistance. They are effective in reducing both systolic and diastolic blood pressure. Their efficacy as antianginal agents is a result of their effects on myocardial oxygen supply and demand. Calcium channel blockers improve myocardial oxygen supply by vasodilating the coronary arteries. Moreover, nondihydropyridines reduce heart rate and myocardial contractility, thus decreasing oxygen demand. In stable angina pectoris, numerous studies have shown that **nifedipine**, **verapamil**, **diltiazem**, **nicardipine**, **bepridil**, and **amlodipine** are effective

antianginal agents. **Verapamil's** antianginal efficacy is similar to that of **diltiazem**, and both are more potent than the dihydropyridines, particularly **nifedipine**. Aggravation of anginal symptoms has, however, been noted with calcium antagonists. This may occur in up to 10% of patients taking **nifedipine** and may be caused by coronary steal or increased sympathetic tone secondary to peripheral vasodilatation. This effect is less apparent with **verapamil** and **diltiazem**, possibly because of the absence of reflex tachycardia.

In comparable studies, beta-blockers and **diltiazem** have had similar efficacy. Although early data suggested that calcium antagonists were beneficial in the treatment of the total ischemic burden (silent and painful episodes), more recent results have suggested otherwise, at least with **nifedipine** and **diltiazem**. By comparison, beta-blockers have been shown to be beneficial in treating the total ischemic burden.

Combined therapy of a dihydropyridine calcium antagonist and a beta-blocker has been found to be effective in the treatment of stable angina, but may be best used when left ventricular function is good. Combination therapy, particularly with **verapamil** or **diltiazem**, should not be used in patients with conduction system disease or moderate to severe left ventricular dysfunction.

Because of their negative chronotropic and dromotropic properties, nondihydropyridines such as **verapamil** and **diltiazem** have been used successfully in the treatment of supraventricular tachycardia. **Verapamil** and **diltiazem** are also very useful for immediate reduction of the ventricular response to atrial fibrillation or atrial flutter.

Nifedipine has produced subjective improvement in Raynaud's disease in more than 60% of patients. High doses of **nifedipine** (and **diltiazem**) appear to improve survival of patients with primary pulmonary hypertension. **Verapamil** was found to improve coronary vasomotor response to physical stress in patients with hypertrophic obstructive cardiomyopathy.

Bepridil hydrochloride is unique among the calcium antagonists. It is a calcium channel blocker and antianginal agent with type I antiarrhythmic and minimal antihypertensive properties. **Bepridil** has inhibitory effects on both the slow calcium and fast sodium inward currents in both myocardial and vascular smooth muscle.

The most common side effects of calcium antagonists are secondary to their vasodilating properties and include headache, flushing, sweating, dizziness, edema, and ankle swelling. In combination with beta-blockers, some of their vasodilatory side effects are reduced. With **diltiazem**, hypotension and depression of atrioventricular (AV) nodal conduction may occur, and constipation has also been noted (the most common side effect of **verapamil**).

An important controversy associated with calcium channel blockers is whether these agents increase the risk of cardiovascular events. Moreover, concerns regarding the use of calcium channel blockers in patients with heart failure have been raised. To address these issues, several large clinical tri-

TABLE 8.1 CURRENTLY AVAILABLE CALCIUM ANTAGONISTS	
Phenylalkylamine	Verapamil
Dihydropyridines	Amlodipine
	Felodipine
	Isradipine
	Nicardipine
	Nifedipine
	Nisoldipine
	Nimodipine
Benzothiazepines	Diltiazem
Miscellaneous	Bepridil

The information here is provided as guidance only. Prescribers should always consult the manufacturer's current prescribing information.

187

als were performed, and their results were helpful in clarifying the role of calcium channel blockers in various patient populations. The Antihypertensive and Lipid-Lowering Treatment to Prevent Heart Attack Trial (ALLHAT) recruited 33,357 subjects aged 55 years or older who had hypertension and at least one other risk factor for coronary heart disease (CHD). Participants were randomized to receive chlorthalidone, **amlodipine**, or lisinopril for a planned follow-up period of approximately 4 to 8 years. At a mean follow-up of 4.9 years, the primary outcome of combined fatal CHD or nonfatal myocardial infarction (MI) was similar in all treatment groups. However, one of the secondary outcomes, which consists of a 6-year rate of heart failure, was significantly higher in the **amlodipine** group compared with the chlorthalidone group (10.2% vs 7.7%). Results from ALLHAT demonstrated that thiazide-type diuretics are preferred as first-line antihypertensive therapy. Dihydropyridines such as **amlodipine** have been recommended as second-line agents in patients who cannot tolerate diuretics, although consideration should be given to the long-term effects of these agents on the occurrence of heart failure. Because more than one agent is often needed to manage hypertension in clinical practice, calcium channel blockers may be used safely when given concurrently with a thiazide diuretic.

More recently, the International Verapamil Slow-Release/Trandolapril Study (INVEST) examined the effects of slow-release **verapamil** in 22,576 patients with hypertension and coronary artery disease. Patients were assigned to treatment with either slow-release **verapamil** or atenolol. Dosage of each drug was increased or a second drug was added (trandolapril in the **verapamil** group and hydrochlorothiazide in the atenolol group) if blood pressure control was not achieved with monotherapy. A third drug was added (hydrochlorothiazide in the **verapamil** group and trandolapril in the atenolol group) if further reduction in blood pressure was needed. At a mean follow-up of 2.7 years, no difference was observed between the slow-release **verapamil** and atenolol arms with regard to overall death, cardiovascular death, and nonfatal MI. Thus, the study investigators concluded that treatment initiation in hypertensive patients with coronary artery disease with a nondihydropyridine (slow-release **verapamil**) or beta-blocker (atenolol) results in similar clinical outcomes.

In the Controlled Onset Verapamil Investigation of Cardiovascular End Points (CONVINCE) trial, a total of 16,602 participants who had hypertension and at least one additional risk factor for cardiovascular disease were randomized to receive initial therapy with controlled-onset extended-release (COER) **verapamil** or the investigator's choice of atenolol or hydrochlorothiazide. Other drugs, such as diuretics, beta-blockers, or angiotensin-converting enzyme (ACE) inhibitors, were added in specified sequence if needed. After a mean follow-up period of 3 years, there was no significant difference in the primary composite outcome of fatal or nonfatal MI, fatal or nonfatal stroke, or cardiovascular disease–related death

between the two treatment arms. Despite this result, the investigators concluded that COER **verapamil** is not equivalent to atenolol or hydrochlorothiazide in preventing cardiovascular disease–related events. This is because the upper bound of the 95% confidence interval for the primary end point exceeded the prespecified boundary for equivalence of COER **verapamil** and atenolol or hydrochlorothiazide. In addition, this study was terminated by the sponsor after a mean follow-up of 3 years, during which less than a third of the planned number of events occurred, which limited the ability to draw long-term conclusions from the trial. Of note, hospitalization for heart failure, a component of the secondary cardiovascular disease end point, was 30% higher with the COER verapamil arm compared with the atenolol or hydrochlorothiazide arm.

Although clinical trials such as ALLHAT and CONVINCE have demonstrated an increased risk of heart failure with the use of calcium channel blockers, other trials have demonstrated a neutral effect, or even a beneficial effect (especially in the context of nonischemic cardiomyopathy), associated with the use of calcium channel blockers in patients with heart failure. The Prospective Randomized Amlodipine Survival Evaluation (PRAISE) studies compared **amlodipine** with placebo in patients with severe heart failure. In PRAISE I, 1153 patients with severe heart failure were randomized to treatment with either placebo or **amlodipine** in addition to their usual therapy for 6 to 33 months. The primary end points were death from any cause and hospitalization for major cardiovascular events. Among patients with ischemic heart disease, there was no difference between the **amlodipine** and placebo groups in the occurrence of either end point. However, among patients with nonischemic cardiomyopathy, **amlodipine** significantly reduced the combined risk of fatal and nonfatal events by 31% and decreased the risk of death by 46%. This mortality

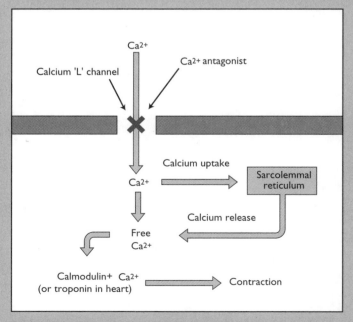

FIGURE 8.1 Mode of action of calcium antagonists.

benefit associated with **amlodipine** was unexpected. Therefore, the subsequent PRAISE II study was initiated to further examine the potential of **amlodipine** in reducing mortality in patients without ischemic heart disease. This study randomized 1652 patients with New York Heart Association (NYHA) class IIIb or IV symptoms of heart failure to either placebo or **amlodipine**. There was no significant difference in all-cause or cardiac mortality and cardiac event rates between the two groups, with trends in favor of placebo. The investigators thus concluded that **amlodipine** can be safely used to treat angina or hypertension in patients with chronic heart failure but is not specifically a treatment to improve symptoms or outcome in chronic heart failure.

Overall, results from the clinical trials described above show that long-acting calcium channel blockers may be safely used in the management of hypertension and angina. However, as a class, these agents are not as protective as other antihypertensive agents against heart failure.

Mode of Action

Definitive evidence shows that depolarization in atrial tissue is mediated by two inwardly directed ionic currents. When a cardiac cell potential reaches threshold, the membrane permeability for sodium increases (Fig. 8.1). The *fast channel* is responsible for this influx of sodium. The time required for the second inward current to reach maximal values is much longer. This current is largely caused by the movement of calcium ions into the cell through a membrane pore termed the *slow channel*. A derivative of **verapamil** was subsequently shown to block the movement of calcium through the slow channel and thereby alter the plateau phase of the cardiac action potential. Although the agents are called *calcium antagonists*, they do not directly antagonize the effects of calcium, but they inhibit the entry of calcium into cells or its mobilization from intracellular stores. For this reason they are also called *calcium channel blockers*. Their vasodilatory activity is not specific to the coronary vasculature but is widespread, reflecting their general ability to modulate calcium transport.

The increase in the cytosolic concentration of calcium by electromechanical or pharmacochemical coupling results in enhanced binding of calcium to calmodulin and to troponin (in the heart). This complex promotes the contraction of smooth muscle. As a consequence, intravenous **nifedipine**, for example, increases forearm blood flow, but the decrease in arterial pressure elicits sympathetic reflexes with resultant tachycardia. Thus, blood pressure (BP) is lowered, and heart rate, as well as cardiac output, is increased (Table 8.2). After oral administration, peripheral blood flow increases because of arterial dilatation. The increase in cardiac output is the result of a decrease in arteriolar resistance coupled with the increase in heart rate that results from the sympathetic reflexes. However, the increases in heart rate, plasma renin activity, and catecholamine release may lead to a reduction in the efficacy of the dihydropyridine calcium antagonists.

By increasing the supply of oxygen to the potentially ischemic myocardium by coronary dilatation or by decreasing the demand secondary to a decrease in BP, calcium antagonists clearly benefit the ischemic patient.

Verapamil and **diltiazem** slow the spontaneous firing of pacemaker cells in the sinus node, leading to a slowing of heart rate that is partially nullified by increased sympathetic activity due to arterial vasodilatation. Nevertheless, unlike the dihydropyridines, **verapamil** and **diltiazem** produce a net 10% to 15% decrease in heart rate. Furthermore, they decrease conduction velocity through the AV node and significantly increase the functional refractory period. The effect on AV nodal conduction is presumably a direct result of calcium channel blockade. However, this effect is not prominent at clinically achieved concentrations of other calcium antagonists, such as the dihydropyridines. For these reasons, **verapamil** and **diltiazem**, unlike **nifedipine**, are useful in the treatment of certain arrhythmias.

The antianginal agent **bepridil** inhibits slow calcium as well as fast sodium channels by interfering with calcium binding to calmodulin and blocking both voltage and receptor-operated calcium channels.

TABLE 8.2 COMPARATIVE HEMODYNAMICS OF FOUR CALCIUM ANTAGONISTS				
	Amlodipine	**Diltiazem**	**Nifedipine**	**Verapamil**
Blood pressure	↓	↓	↓	↓
Heart rate	0/↑	↓	0/↑	↓
Atrioventricular node conduction	0	↓	0	↓
Cardiac output	↑	0/↑	↑	±
Myocardial contractility	0/↓	↓	0/↓	↓↓
Neurohormonal activation	0/↑	↑	↑	↑
Vascular dilatation	↑↑	↑	↑↑	↑
Coronary blood flow	↑	↑	↑	↑
↓—decrease; ↑—increase; 0—no change; ± —minimal but variable effect.				

	Amlodipine	Bepridil	Diltiazem	Diltiazem SR	Diltiazem ER	Diltiazem IV	Felodipine	Isradipine	Nicardipine	Nicardipine SR	Nicardipine IV	Nifedipine	Nifedipine ER	Nimodipine	Nisoldipine	Verapamil	Verapamil SR	Verapamil ER	Verapamil IV
Angina pectoris																			
Vasospastic	+		+		+							+	+†			+		+‡	
Chronic stable	+	+	+		+				+			+	+†			+		+‡	
Unstable																+		+‡	
Atrial fibrillation/flutter						+													+
Hypertension	+			+	+		+	+	+	+	+		+		+	+	+	+	
Hypertrophic cardiomyopathy																(+)			
Paroxysmal supraventricular tachycardia						+										+§			+
Pulmonary hypertension	(+)		(+)				(+)					(+)							
Raynaud's phenomenon	(+)		(+)				(+)	(+)				(+)							
Subarachnoid hemorrhage														+					

*Refer to individual drug monographs for more detailed information.

†Except Adalat CC.

‡Covera-HS only.

§For prophylaxis of repetitive paroxysmal supraventricular tachycardia.

+—FDA approved indication; (+)—clinical use, not FDA approved; ER—extended release; IV—intravenous; SR—sustained release.

AMLODIPINE
(Norvasc®)

Amlodipine is a calcium antagonist of the dihydropyridine group. Because of its long elimination half-life, it is suitable for once-daily administration in hypertension and angina. In contrast to other dihydropyridines, its pharmacodynamic effects are gradual in onset and offset, giving a smooth vascular effect. The slow onset of action and prolonged effect also minimize or abolish stimulation of cardiovascular reflex mechanisms. It invokes beneficial changes in vascular resistance, stroke volume, and cardiac index. Amlodipine may increase heart rate, noradrenaline, and plasma renin activity to a lesser degree than nifedipine. Its natriuretic properties may contribute to its effect in hypertension, in which it provides smooth 24-hour BP control without postural hypotension. Amlodipine is clearly superior to placebo, produces slightly greater reductions in BP than verapamil, and has similar efficacy to hydrochlorothiazide, atenolol, and captopril. Coadministration with diuretics, beta-blockers, and ACE inhibitors also achieves further reductions in BP. A particularly useful combination is amlodipine with benazepril. When this combination was used, BP was reduced to a greater extent compared with when either agent was used alone. Further, this combination therapy was associated with a lower incidence of adverse effects, especially edema, than amlodipine alone. In angina, amlodipine is more effective than placebo and as effective as diltiazem and nadolol.

The results from the PRAISE study demonstrated that amlodipine did not increase cardiovascular morbidity or mortality in patients with severe heart failure. In fact, amlodipine was shown to reduce the risk of death by 46% in patients with nonischemic cardiomyopathy. In contrast, a significantly higher 6-year rate of heart failure was found in the amlodipine treatment arm compared with the chlorthalidone treatment arm (10.2% vs 7.7%) in ALLHAT. Overall, results from clinical trials have shown that calcium channel blockers are not as protective as other antihypertensive agents against heart failure. Because more than one agent is often needed to manage hypertension in clinical practice, calcium channel blockers such as amlodipine may be used safely when given concurrently with a thiazide diuretic.

SPECIAL GROUPS

Race: no differences in response
Children: safety and effectiveness have not been established
Elderly: initiate at lower dose
Renal impairment: normal dosage recommended; amlodipine is not dialyzable
Hepatic impairment: administer with caution; use lower dose
Pregnancy: category C; use only if potential benefit justifies the potential risk to the fetus
Breast-feeding: not recommended; amlodipine may be excreted in breast milk

IN BRIEF

INDICATIONS
Hypertension
Chronic stable angina
Vasospastic (Prinzmetal's or variant) angina

CONTRAINDICATIONS
Hypersensitivity

DRUG INTERACTIONS
Azole antifungals and other inhibitors of CYP450 3A4[1]
Beta-blockers[1,3]
Cyclosporine[3]
Fentanyl[4]
Rifampin[2]
Sildenafil[4]
Tadalafil[4]
Vardenafil[4]

1 Effect/toxicity of amlodipine may increase.
2 Effect of amlodipine may decrease.
3 Amlodipine may increase the effect/toxicity of this drug.
4 May increase the risk of hypotension.

ADVERSE EFFECTS
Cardiovascular: peripheral edema (1%–15%), palpitations (≤1%–5%)
CNS: dizziness/lightheadedness (1%–4%), headache (7%), somnolence(1%–2%), asthenia (1%–2%), fatigue/lethargy (4%–5%)
GI: nausea (3%), abdominal discomfort (1%–2%)
Dermatologic: rash/dermatitis (1%–2%), pruritus/urticaria (1%–2%)
Others: flushing (≤1%–5%), sexual difficulties (1%–2%), shortness of breath (1%–2%), muscle cramps (1%–2%)

PHARMACOKINETICS AND PHARMACODYNAMICS
Duration of action:	24 h
Onset of action:	30–50 min
Time to peak plasma concentration:	6–12 h
Bioavailability:	64%–90%
Effect of food:	none
Protein binding:	93%
Volume of distribution:	no data
Metabolism:	hepatic, extensive, to inactive metabolites
Elimination:	metabolite and parent drug excreted renally
Half-life:	30–50 h

MONITORING
BP, heart rate, hepatic function.

OVERDOSE
If the patient is seen shortly after oral ingestion, employ lavage, activated charcoal, and cathartics. Treatment is supportive. Suggested treatments of possible acute cardiovascular adverse reactions caused by calcium channel blocker overdosage are listed below. Actual treatment and dosage should depend on the severity of the clinical situation and the judgment and experience of the treating physician.
For symptomatic hypotension, administer fluids intravenously, dopamine or dobutamine intravenously, calcium chloride, isoproterenol, metaraminol, or norepinephrine.
For tachycardia, rapid ventricular rate in patients with antegrade conduction in atrial flutter/fibrillation, and accessory pathway with Wolff-Parkinson-White or Lown-Ganong-Levine syndrome, administer direct-current cardioversion, intravenous lidocaine, or intravenous procainamide. Intravenous fluids should be given by slow drip.
For bradycardia, second- or third-degree AV block, with a few patients progressing to asystole, administer intravenous atropine, isoproterenol, norepinephrine, or calcium chloride, or use electronic cardiac pacemaker. Intravenous fluids should be given by slow drip.

AMLODIPINE (continued)

DOSAGE

Hypertension: Initially, give 5 mg once daily. May be increased to a maximum dose of 10 mg once daily, depending on individual response. In elderly patients or patients with hepatic insufficiency, initiate with 2.5 mg once daily.

Angina: Usual dose is 5–10 mg once daily. Use lower dose for elderly and patients with hepatic insufficiency.

PATIENT INFORMATION

This medication may cause palpitations, headache, flushing, ankle edema, and cramps. Notify physician if persistent side effects occur. Do not discontinue therapy without your physician's advice.

AVAILABILITY

Tablets—2.5 mg, 5 mg, 10 mg
Combination formulations:
Lotrel—amlodipine/benazepril hydrochloride combination capsules
    2.5 mg/10 mg
    5 mg/10 mg
    5 mg/20 mg
    10 mg/20 mg
Caduet—amlodipine/atorvastatin combination tablets
    5 mg/10 mg
    5 mg/20 mg
    5 mg/40 mg
    5 mg/80 mg
    10 mg/10 mg
    10 mg/20 mg
    10 mg/40 mg
    10 mg/80 mg

BEPRIDIL

(Vascor®)

Bepridil hydrochloride is an antianginal agent that inhibits slow calcium as well as fast sodium channels. In addition, bepridil demonstrates electrophysiologic effects such as prolongation of QT and QTc intervals that are characteristic of class I antiarrhythmic agents. Structurally, bepridil is a diarylaminopropylamine derivative that is unrelated to other currently available calcium channel blockers. Its precise mechanism of action as an antianginal agent is not fully known. However, the drug is believed to reduce heart rate and arterial pressure at rest and at a given level of exertion by dilating peripheral arterioles and reducing total peripheral resistance (afterload) against which the heart works. Bepridil may be used alone or with beta-blockers or nitrates. An added effect occurs when it is administered to patients already receiving propranolol. Because of bepridil's arrhythmogenic potential and case reports of agranulocytosis associated with this agent, bepridil generally is reserved for patients who have failed to respond or are intolerant to other antianginal agents.

SPECIAL GROUPS

Race: no differences in response

Children: safety and effectiveness have not been established

Elderly: normal dosing with caution

Renal impairment: administer with caution; specific dosage has not been established. Bepridil is not removable by hemodialysis.

Hepatic impairment: use with caution

Pregnancy: category C; use only if potential benefit justifies the potential risk

Breast-feeding: not recommended; bepridil is excreted in breast milk

IN BRIEF

INDICATIONS
Chronic stable angina

CONTRAINDICATIONS
Hypersensitivity

History of serious ventricular or atrial arrhythmias (especially tachycardia or those associated with accessory conduction pathways)

Hypotension (less than 90 mm Hg systolic)

Uncompensated cardiac insufficiency

Congenital QT interval prolongation

Use with other drugs that prolong QT interval

DRUG INTERACTIONS

Amprenavir[1,4]	Histamine$_2$ (H$_2$)-blockers[1]
Atazanavir[1,4]	Quinidine[2]
Antiarrhythmic agents[3]	Ritonavir[1,4]
Beta-blockers[1,2]	Sildenafil[5]
Carbamazepine[2]	Sparfloxacin[1,4]
Cisapride[1,4]	Tadalafil[5]
Cyclosporine[2]	Theophylline[2]
Digitalis glycosides[2]	Vardenafil[5]
Fentanyl[5]	

1 Effect/toxicity of bepridil may increase.
2 Bepridil may increase the effect/toxicity of this drug.
3 May cause prolongation of the QT interval.
4 Concurrent use with bepridil is contraindicated.
5 May increase the risk of hypotension.

ADVERSE EFFECTS
Cardiovascular: palpitation (≤7%), peripheral edema (≤2%), bradycardia (≤2%), tachycardia (≤2%), prolonged QT interval
CNS: dizziness/lightheadedness (12%–27%), headache (7%–14%), nervousness (7%–12%), asthenia (6%–14%), tremor (≤9%), drowsiness (>7%), tinnitus (0%–7%), insomnia (2%–3%), paresthesia (2%–3%)
GI: nausea (7%–26%), diarrhea (0%–11%), abdominal discomfort (≤7%), dry mouth (3%–4%), constipation (2%–3%)
Dermatologic: rash/dermatitis (≤2%)
Others: nasal or chest congestion (≤2%), shortness of breath (≤9%), respiratory infection (2%–3%), sexual difficulties (≤2%)

PHARMACOKINETICS AND PHARMACODYNAMICS

Duration of action:	24 h
Onset of action:	1 h
Time to peak effect:	8 d
Time to peak plasma concentration:	2–3 h
Bioavailability:	60%
Effect of food:	none
Protein binding:	>99%
Volume of distribution:	no data
Metabolism:	highly metabolized by the liver
Elimination:	renal, 70% (none unchanged); biliary/fecal, 22% (none unchanged)
Half-life:	24 h

MONITORING
BP, electrocardiogram (ECG) and serum electrolytes, hepatic function, signs and symptoms of congestive heart failure. Elderly may need close monitoring because of underlying cardiac and organ system insufficiencies.

BEPRIDIL (continued)

DOSAGE

Adult: Individualize therapy according to clinical judgment and each patient's response. Usual initial dose is 200 mg once daily. Upward adjustment may be made after 10 days depending on patient's response. Usual maintenance dose is 300 mg once daily. Maximum daily dose is 400 mg. Minimum effective dose is 200 mg daily.

Elderly: Same initial dose as above. However, careful monitoring must be done after therapeutic response is demonstrated.

Note: If nausea occurs, administer the drug with meals or at bedtime.

OVERDOSE

If the patient is seen shortly after oral ingestion, employ lavage, activated charcoal, and cathartics. Treatment is supportive. Suggested treatments for possible acute cardiovascular adverse reactions caused by calcium channel blocker overdosage are listed below. Actual treatment and dosage should depend on the severity of the clinical situation and the judgment and experience of the treating physician.

For symptomatic hypotension, administer fluids intravenously, dopamine or dobutamine intravenously, calcium chloride, isoproterenol, metaraminol, or norepinephrine.

For tachycardia, rapid ventricular rate in patients with antegrade conduction in atrial flutter/fibrillation, and accessory pathway with Wolff-Parkinson-White or Lown-Ganong-Levine syndrome, administer direct-current cardioversion, intravenous lidocaine, or intravenous procainamide. Intravenous fluids should be given by slow drip.

For bradycardia, second- or third-degree AV block, with a few patients progressing to asystole, administer intravenous atropine, isoproterenol, norepinephrine, or calcium chloride, or use electronic cardiac pacemaker. Intravenous fluids should be given by slow drip.

PATIENT INFORMATION

This medication may cause cardiac arrhythmias if potassium concentration in body is low; maintain potassium supplementation as directed by physician. Notify physician if persistent side effects occur. Follow-up visits must be taken seriously.

AVAILABILITY

Tablets—200 mg, 300 mg

DILTIAZEM

(Diltiazem, Cardizem®, Cardizem® LA, Cardizem® SR, Cardizem® CD, Cartia™ XT, Dilacor™ XR, Diltia® XT, Tiazac™)

Diltiazem is a benzothiazepine calcium ion influx inhibitor that is extensively metabolized and consequently short acting. When administered orally, diltiazem has been used either alone or in combination with other antihypertensive agents for the management of hypertension. Diltiazem increases exercise capacity and improves all indices of myocardial ischemia in patients with angina; it relieves spasm and vasospastic (Prinzmetal's) angina. It is effective in the treatment of chronic stable angina, with effects equal to those of propranolol, nifedipine, and verapamil, but additional benefit may be obtained by combining the drug with propranolol. Diltiazem is also effective in the treatment of variant angina and unstable angina.

Diltiazem has an inhibitory effect on the cardiac conduction system, acting primarily at the AV node, with some effects at the sinus node. This allows diltiazem to be useful in the management of paroxysmal supraventricular tachycardia and atrial fibrillation. Diltiazem also reduces left ventricular hypertrophy. Diltiazem may protect the myocardium against the effects of ischemia and reduces the damage produced by excessive entry of calcium into the myocardial cell during reperfusion (ie, angioplasty). An overview of postinfarction studies with calcium antagonists showed that diltiazem reduced the incidence of reinfarction but did not reduce mortality. The benefit of reinfarction was only seen in patients with uncompromised left ventricular function, and mainly in patients with non–Q-wave MI.

A greater effect on BP lowering was observed when diltiazem was administered with enalapril, and a combination formulation is available. Concomitant use of diltiazem with beta-blockers or digitalis may result in additive effects on cardiac conduction. The use of diltiazem with a beta-blocker may reduce the frequency of attacks and increase exercise tolerance in patients with chronic stable angina pectoris as suggested by controlled study results; however, additional study is needed to confirm the safety and efficacy of this combination therapy, especially in patients with compromised left ventricular function or cardiac conduction abnormalities. Major side effects of diltiazem include vasodilatory reactions (headache, flushing, hypotension), sinus bradycardia, and AV block, although these side effects are relatively infrequent.

SPECIAL GROUPS

Race: no differences in response
Children: safety and effectiveness have not been established
Elderly: half-life may be increased; more likely to have age-related renal impairment
Renal impairment: use with caution; diltiazem is excreted renally. It is not removed by hemodialysis.
Hepatic impairment: use with caution; diltiazem is extensively metabolized by the liver
Pregnancy: category C; use diltiazem in pregnant women only if potential benefit justifies potential risk to fetus
Breast-feeding: not recommended; diltiazem is excreted in breast milk

IN BRIEF

INDICATIONS
Angina (Cardizem, Cardizem CD, Cartia XT, Dilacor XR, Diltia XT, Tiazac)
Hypertension (Cardizem LA, Cardizem SR, Cardizem CD, Cartia XT, Dilacor XR, Diltia XT, Tiazac)
Arrhythmias
Paroxysmal supraventricular tachycardia (Cardizem injectable)
Atrial fibrillation or flutter (Cardizem injectable)

CONTRAINDICATIONS
Hypersensitivity
Severe hypotension (<90 mm Hg systolic)
Sick sinus syndrome or second- or third-degree AV block, except with a functioning pacemaker
Acute MI
Pulmonary congestion

DRUG INTERACTIONS
Amiodarone[1]
Beta-blockers[1,3]
Buspirone[3]
Carbamazepine[3]
Cisapride[3]
Cyclosporine[3]
Digitalis glycosides[3]
Fentanyl[4]
H2-blockers[1]
3-Hydroxy-3-methylglutaryl coenzyme A (HMG-CoA) reductase inhibitors[3]
Imipramine[3]
Lithium[5]
Methylprednisolone[3]
Midazolam[3]
Moricizine[2,3]
Nifedipine[1,3]
Quinidine[3]
Rifampin[2]
Sildenafil[4]
Sirolimus[3]
Tacrolimus[3]
Tadalafil[4]
Theophylline[3]
Triazolam[3]
Vardenafil[4]

1 Effect/toxicity of diltiazem may increase.
2 Effect of diltiazem may decrease.
3 Diltiazem may increase the effect/toxicity of this drug.
4 May increase the risk of hypotension.
5 Coadministration with diltiazem has caused neurotoxicity.

ADVERSE EFFECTS
Cardiovascular: peripheral edema (2%–9%), AV block (≤1%–8%), bradycardia (1%–6%), abnormal ECG (4%)
CNS: headache (2%–12%), dizziness/lightheadedness (1%–7%), asthenia (2%–5%)
GI: abdominal discomfort (1%–2%), nausea (1%–2%), constipation (1%–2%)
Dermatologic: rash/dermatitis (1%–2%)
Others: flushing (1%–3%), micturition disorder (1%–2%)

PHARMACOKINETICS AND PHARMACODYNAMICS
Duration of action: 4–8 h (short acting); 12–24 h (sustained release)
Onset of action: 30–60 min (short acting)
Time to peak serum concentration: 2–3 h (short acting); 6–11 h (sustained release)
Bioavailability: ≈40%–60%
Effect of food: none
Protein binding: 70%–80%
Volume of distribution: ≈305 L (IV)
Metabolism: extensive, hepatic
Elimination: in urine and bile, mostly as metabolites
Half-life: 4–6 h (short-acting), 5–7 h (sustained-release)

MONITORING
BP, ECG, liver function tests.

DILTIAZEM *(continued)*

DOSAGE

Short acting (Diltiazem, Cardizem): As an antianginal agent, usual initial dose is 30 mg 4 times daily (before meals and at bedtime). Dosage should be increased gradually at 1–2-d intervals. Maximum daily dose is 360 mg.

Extended release (Cardizem LA): For hypertension, start with 180–240 mg once daily. The usual dose range is 180–480 mg/d.

Sustained release (Cardizem SR): As monotherapy for hypertension, start with 60–120 mg twice daily, although some patients may respond well to lower doses. Usual dose range is 240–360 mg/d.

Sustained release (Cardizem CD, Cartia XT): As monotherapy for hypertension, initially, 180–240 mg once daily. The usual dose range in clinical trials was 240–360 mg/d. Individual patients may respond to higher doses of up to 480 mg once daily. For angina, start with 120 or 180 mg once daily. Dose may be titrated upward every 7–14 d up to a maximum of 480 mg once daily if necessary.

Sustained release (Dilacor XR, Diltia XT): For hypertension, start with 180–240 mg once daily. Adjust dose as needed, depending on antihypertensive response. In clinical trials, the therapeutic dose range is 180–540 mg once daily. For angina, start with 120 mg once daily. Dose may be titrated upward every 7–14 d up to a maximum of 480 mg once daily if needed.

Sustained release (Tiazac): For hypertension, the usual starting dose is 120–240 mg once daily. Maximum effect is usually observed after 14 d. In clinical trials, doses up to 540 mg daily were effective. For angina, initiate with 120–180 mg once daily. Dosage may be increased every 7–14 d as needed to a maximum dose of 540 mg once daily.

Injection (Diltiazem I.V., Cardizem I.V.): Direct intravenous single injections (bolus): initial 0.25 mg/kg body weight administered as a bolus over 2 min (20 mg is a reasonable dose for an average patient). If response is inadequate after 15 min, a second bolus dose of 0.35 mg/kg administered over 2 min may be given (25 mg is a reasonable dose for an average patient).

Intravenous infusion: An intravenous infusion may be administered for continued reduction of the heart rate (up to 24 h) in patients with atrial fibrillation or atrial flutter. Start an infusion at a rate of 10 mg/h immediately after bolus administration of 0.25 or 0.35 mg/kg. Some patients may maintain response to an initial rate of 5 mg/h. The infusion rate may be increased in 5 mg/h increments up to 15 mg/h as needed. Infusion duration longer than 24 h and infusion rate >15 mg/h are not recommended (refer to package insert for proper dilution of diltiazem for continuous infusion).

OVERDOSE

If the patient is seen shortly after oral ingestion, employ lavage, activated charcoal, and cathartics. Treatment is supportive. Suggested treatments for possible acute cardiovascular adverse reactions caused by calcium channel blocker overdosage are listed below. Actual treatment and dosage should depend on the severity of the clinical situation and the judgment and experience of the treating physician.

For symptomatic hypotension, administer fluids intravenously, dopamine or dobutamine intravenously, calcium chloride, isoproterenol, metaraminol, or norepinephrine.

For tachycardia, rapid ventricular rate in patients with antegrade conduction in atrial flutter/fibrillation, and accessory pathway with Wolff-Parkinson-White or Lown-Ganong-Levine syndrome, administer direct-current cardioversion, intravenous lidocaine, or intravenous procainamide. Intravenous fluids should be given by slow drip.

For bradycardia, second- or third-degree AV block, with a few patients progressing to asystole, administer intravenous atropine, isoproterenol, norepinephrine, or calcium chloride, or use electronic cardiac pacemaker. Intravenous fluids should be given by slow drip.

PATIENT INFORMATION

The sustained-released capsules should be swallowed whole, without breaking, crushing, or chewing. This medication may cause a slowing of the heart rate, headache, ankle edema, or constipation. Notify physician if persistent side effects occur. Do not discontinue therapy without your physician's advice.

AVAILABILITY

Tablets (Diltiazem, Cardizem)—30 mg, 60 mg, 90 mg, 120 mg
Tablets, extended release (Cardizem LA)—120 mg, 180 mg, 240 mg, 300 mg, 360 mg, 420 mg
Capsules, sustained release (Cardizem SR)—60 mg, 90 mg, 120 mg
Capsules, extended release (Cardizem CD, Cartia XT)—120 mg, 180 mg, 240 mg, 300 mg
Capsules, extended release (Cardizem CD)—360 mg
Capsules, extended release (Dilacor XR, Diltia XT)—120 mg, 180 mg, 240 mg
Capsules, extended release (Tiazac)—120 mg, 180 mg, 240 mg, 300 mg, 360 mg
Injection (as hydrochloride)—5 mg/mL (5 mL, 10 mL)
Injection (Cardizem I.V.)—5 mg/mL (5 mL, 10 mL)
Combination formulations:
Teczem—enalapril maleate/diltiazem malate ER (extended-release) combination tablets—5 mg/ 180 mg

FELODIPINE (Plendil®)

Felodipine is a dihydropyridine calcium antagonist that is extensively metabolized. It is supplied as an extended-release formulation based on the hydrophilic gel principle. This allows once-daily administration with smooth control of BP throughout the 24 hours. Its terminal half-life ranges from 11 to 16 hours in young healthy people to about 20 to 27.5 hours in middle-aged hypertensive patients. It is vascularly selective and reduces BP in mild, moderate, and severe hypertension. It causes a fall in BP similar to or greater than that of other antihypertensive agents as monotherapy. Felodipine is also available in a fixed combination with enalapril. This fixed combination therapy has been shown to reduce BP to a greater extent than with felodipine or enalapril alone.

Adverse effects from felodipine are few, except for a constellation of symptoms related to its vasodilator ability. These effects include palpitations, flushing, fatigue, dizziness, and headaches. Ankle edema, however, is the most frequent observed unwanted effect. This agent may produce less reflex tachycardia and a less significant rise in plasma renin activity than does nifedipine. Felodipine has been evaluated in a large international placebo-controlled clinical outcomes study, HOTS, in patients with systemic hypertension. The results of this study showed that intensive lowering of BP (down to a mean diastolic BP of 82.6 mm Hg) in patients with hypertension was associated with a low rate of cardiovascular events.

SPECIAL GROUPS

Race: no differences in response
Children: safety and effectiveness have not been established
Elderly: initiate at lower dose
Renal impairment: normal dosage recommended
Hepatic impairment: administer with caution; use lower dose
Pregnancy: category C; use only if potential benefit justifies the potential risk to the fetus
Breast-feeding: not recommended; felodipine may be excreted in breast milk

IN BRIEF

INDICATIONS
Hypertension (felodipine may be used alone or concomitantly with other antihypertensives)

CONTRAINDICATIONS
Hypersensitivity

DRUG INTERACTIONS
Azole antifungals (eg, itraconazole)[1]
Barbiturates[2]
Beta-blockers[1,3]
Carbamazepine[2]
Cyclosporine[1,3]
Erythromycin[1]
Fentanyl[5]
Grapefruit juice[1]
H2-blockers[1]
Phenytoin[2]
Rifampin[2]
Sildenafil[5]
Tadalafil[5]
Theophylline[4]
Vardenafil[5]

1 Effect/toxcity of felodipine may increase.
2 Effect of felodipine may decrease.
3 Felodipine may increase the effect/toxicity of this drug.
4 Felodipine may decrease the effect of this drug.
5 May increase the risk of hypotension.

ADVERSE EFFECTS
Cardiovascular: peripheral edema (22%), palpitations (1%–2%), hypotension (≤1.5 %), syncope (≤1.5%), AV block (≤1.5%), arrhythmia (≤1.5%), angina (≤1.5%)
CNS: headache (19%), dizziness/lightheadedness (6%), asthenia (5%), paresthesia (2%–3%), nervousness (≤1.5%), psychiatric disturbances (≤1.5%), insomnia (≤1.5%)
GI: nausea (1%–2%), abdominal discomfort (≤1%–2%), diarrhea (1%–2%), constipation (1%–2%), dry mouth/thirst (≤1.5%)
Dermatologic: rash/dermatitis (1%–2%), pruritus/urticaria (1%–2%)
Others: flushing (6%), cough (3%), respiratory infection (≤5.5%), nasal or chest congestion (≤1.5%), sexual difficulties (1%–2%), shortness of breath (1%–2%), muscle cramps (≤1%–2%), anemia (≤1.5%), micturition disorder (≤1.5%), gingival hyperplasia (rare)

PHARMACOKINETICS AND PHARMACODYNAMICS
Duration of action: 16–24 h
Onset of action: 2–5 h
Time to peak plasma concentration: 2.5–5 h
Bioavailability: 20%
Effect of food: bioavailability increased more than twofold when taken with doubly concentrated grapefruit juice compared with water or orange juice
Protein binding: >99%
Volume of distribution: 10 L/kg
Metabolism: hepatic, extensive, to inactive metabolites
Elimination: renal, 70% (less than 0.5% unchanged); biliary/fecal, 10% (less than 0.5% unchanged)
Half-life: 11–16 h

MONITORING
BP, heart rate, hepatic function.

FELODIPINE (continued)

DOSAGE

Adults: Usual initial dose is 5 mg once daily. Dosage may be increased by 5 mg at 2 wk intervals according to response. Maintenance doses range from 2.5–10 mg once daily.

Elderly: Treatment should be initiated at 2.5 mg once daily because of possible accumulation. Maximum dose is 10 mg once daily. Monitor BP closely.

OVERDOSE

If the patient is seen shortly after oral ingestion, employ lavage, activated charcoal, and cathartics. Treatment is supportive. Suggested treatments for possible acute cardiovascular adverse reactions caused by calcium channel blocker overdosage are listed below. Actual treatment and dosage depend on the severity of the clinical situation and the judgment and experience of the treating physician.

For symptomatic hypotension, administer fluids intravenously, dopamine or dobutamine intravenously, calcium chloride, isoproterenol, metaraminol, or norepinephrine.

For tachycardia, rapid ventricular rate in patients with antegrade conduction in atrial flutter/fibrillation, and accessory pathway with Wolff-Parkinson-White or Lown-Ganong-Levine syndrome, administer direct-current cardioversion, intravenous lidocaine, or intravenous procainamide. Intravenous fluids should be given by slow drip.

For bradycardia, second- or third-degree AV block, with a few patients progressing to asystole, administer intravenous atropine, isoproterenol, norepinephrine, or calcium chloride, or use electronic cardiac pacemaker. Intravenous fluids should be given by slow drip.

PATIENT INFORMATION

Swallow tablet whole; do not crush or chew tablets.

This medication may cause palpitations, headache, flushing, ankle edema, and cramps. Notify physician if persistent side effects occur. Do not discontinue therapy without your physician's advice.

AVAILABILITY

Tablets (extended release)—2.5 mg, 5 mg, 10 mg
Combination formulations:
Lexxel—enalapril maleate/felodipine ER (extended-release) combination tablets
5 mg/2.5 mg
5 mg/5 mg

ISRADIPINE (DynaCirc®, DynaCirc CR®)

Isradipine, a typical dihydropyridine and a highly potent drug (milligram for milligram), is extensively metabolized by the liver and has a relatively short half-life, necessitating twice-daily administration for hypertension. Unlike other dihydropyridines, chronic therapy with isradipine does not increase heart rate. The efficacy of isradipine is similar to that of nifedipine, propranolol, atenolol, prazosin, hydrochlorothiazide, and diltiazem. It can be safely combined with beta-blockers, ACE inhibitors, and diuretics. Adverse effects are secondary to vasodilatation. The antiatherosclerotic effect of isradipine has been evaluated in the MIDAS trial. Over 36 months, no difference in the rate of progression of mean maximum intimal-medial thickness in carotid arteries was observed between patients treated with isradipine and patients treated with hydrochlorothiazide. However, there was a higher incidence of major cardiovascular events in the isradipine group compared with the hydrochlorothiazide group ($P = 0.07$).

SPECIAL GROUPS

Race:	no differences in response
Children:	safety and effectiveness have not been established
Elderly:	bioavailability may be increased
Renal impairment:	bioavailability may be increased
Hepatic impairment:	administer with caution; use lower dose
Pregnancy:	category C; use only if potential benefit justifies the potential risk to the fetus
Breast-feeding:	not recommended; isradipine may be excreted in breast milk

IN BRIEF

INDICATIONS
Hypertension (isradipine may be used alone or concomitantly with thiazide-type diuretics)

CONTRAINDICATIONS
Hypersensitivity

DRUG INTERACTIONS
Azole antifungals (eg, itraconazole)[1]
Beta-blockers[1,3]
Fentanyl[5]
H₂-blockers[1]
Lovastatin[4]
NSAIDs (eg, diclofenac)[2]
Rifampin[2]
Sildenafil[5]
Tadalafil[5]
Vardenafil[5]

1 Effect/toxicity of isradipine may increase.
2 Effect of isradipine may decrease.
3 Isradipine may increase the effect/toxicity of this drug.
4 Isradipine may decrease the effect of this drug.
5 May increase the risk of hypotension.

ADVERSE EFFECTS
Cardiovascular: peripheral edema (7%), palpitations (4%), angina (2%–3%), tachycardia (1%–2%)
CNS: headache (14%), dizziness/lightheadedness (7%), fatigue/lethargy (4%)
GI: nausea (2%), vomiting (1%), abdominal discomfort (1%–2%), diarrhea (1%)
Dermatologic: rash/dermatitis (1%–2%), pruritus/urticaria (≤1%)
Others: flushing (2%–3%), sexual difficulties (≤1%), shortness of breath (1%–2%), pollakiuria (1.5%)

PHARMACOKINETICS AND PHARMACODYNAMICS

Duration of action:	12 h (immediate release); 24 h (controlled release)
Onset of action:	2 h
Time to peak plasma concentration:	1.5 h (immediate release)
Time to peak effect:	multiple doses (2–4 wk)
Bioavailability:	15%–24%
Effect of food:	administration of isradipine (DynaCirc) with food significantly increases the time to peak by about an hour but has no effect on the total bioavailability of the drug. Food has been shown to decrease the extent of bioavailability of DynaCirc CR by up to 25%.
Protein binding:	95%
Volume of distribution:	3 L/kg
Metabolism:	extensive first-pass metabolism by liver
Elimination:	renal 60%–65% (none unchanged); biliary/fecal 25%–30% (none unchanged)
Half-life:	8 h (immediate release)

MONITORING
BP, heart rate, hepatic function.

ISRADIPINE (continued)

DOSAGE

Immediate-release (DynaCirc): Initially, give 2.5 mg twice daily alone or in combination with a thiazide diuretic. If necessary, adjust in increments of 2.5–5 mg/d at 2–4 wk intervals. The maximum daily dose is 20 mg.

Note: Most patients show no further improvement with doses >10 mg/d; adverse reactions are increased in frequency above 10 mg/d.

Controlled-release (DynaCirc CR): Initially, give 5 mg once daily alone or in combination with a thiazide diuretic. If necessary, the dose may be adjusted in increments of 5 mg at 2–4 wk intervals up to a maximum dose of 20 mg/d. Adverse experiences are increased in frequency above 10 mg/d.

OVERDOSE

If the patient is seen shortly after oral ingestion, employ lavage, activated charcoal, and cathartics. Treatment is supportive. Suggested treatments for possible acute cardiovascular adverse reactions caused by calcium channel blocker overdosage are listed below. Actual treatment and dosage depend on the severity of the clinical situation and the judgment and experience of the treating physician.

For symptomatic hypotension, administer fluids intravenously, dopamine or dobutamine intravenously, calcium chloride, isoproterenol, metaraminol, or norepinephrine.

For tachycardia, rapid ventricular rate in patients with antegrade conduction in atrial flutter/fibrillation, and accessory pathway with Wolff-Parkinson-White or Lown-Ganong-Levine syndrome, administer direct-current cardioversion, intravenous lidocaine, or intravenous procainamide. Intravenous fluids should be given by slow drip.

For bradycardia, second- or third-degree AV block, with a few patients progressing to asystole, administer intravenous atropine, isoproterenol, norepinephrine, or calcium chloride, or use electronic cardiac pacemaker. Intravenous fluids should be given by slow drip.

PATIENT INFORMATION

The controlled-release tablets (DynaCirc CR) should be swallowed whole and should not be bitten or divided.

This medication may cause palpitations, headache, flushing, ankle edema, and dizziness. Notify physician if persistent side effects occur. Do not discontinue therapy without your physician's advice.

AVAILABILITY

Capsules (DynaCirc)—2.5 mg, 5 mg
Tablets (DynaCirc CR)—5 mg, 10 mg

NICARDIPINE (Cardene®, Cardene® SR)

Nicardipine is a typical dihydropyridine calcium antagonist that is extensively metabolized and has a short half-life, necessitating three-times-daily administration in the oral form. A sustained-release formulation is available for twice-daily dosing in hypertension. It is useful in the treatment of angina pectoris and hypertension. An intravenous formulation is available for short-term management of hypertension. Although no lifesaving benefits after infarction and during unstable angina have been found with nicardipine, studies with other dihydropyridine calcium antagonists have indicated the possibility of benefit when added to or supplementing treatment with beta-blockers. Nicardipine's potential as an antiatherosclerotic agent has been investigated. However, there is no evidence of a reduction in mortality with nicardipine and other dihydropyridines similarly evaluated in patients with coronary disease or peripheral atherosclerosis. Nicardipine is as effective in the management of chronic stable angina pectoris as either diltiazem or verapamil. In hypertension, it is as effective as nifedipine, but perhaps without the reflex tachycardia at lower doses. It may be successfully combined with atenolol or propranolol. Side effects are typical of those seen with vasodilating drugs. Note must be taken of the relatively large peak-to-trough differences in BP effect. However, this does not pertain to the sustained-release formulation.

SPECIAL GROUPS

Race: no differences in response
Children: safety and effectiveness have not been established
Elderly: no change in half-life or protein binding
Renal impairment: titrate dose carefully
Hepatic impairment: use with caution. Initiate with lower doses; titrate dose carefully
Pregnancy: category C; use only if potential benefit justifies the potential risk to the fetus
Breast-feeding: not recommended; nicardipine may be excreted in breast milk

IN BRIEF

INDICATIONS
Hypertension (Cardene, Cardene SR)
Short-term treatment of hypertension when oral therapy cannot be given (Cardene I.V.)
Angina (Cardene)

CONTRAINDICATIONS
Hypersensitivity
Advanced aortic stenosis
Cardiogenic shock
Severe hypotension
Ventricular tachycardia

DRUG INTERACTIONS
Beta-blockers[1,2]
Cyclosporine[2]
Fentanyl[3]
Grapefruit juice[1]
H$_2$-blockers[1]
Sildenafil[3]
Tadalafil[3]
Vardenafil[3]

1 Effect/toxicity of nicardipine may increase.
2 Nicardipine may increase the effect/toxicity of this drug.
3 May increase the risk of hypotension.

ADVERSE EFFECTS
Cardiovascular: peripheral edema (7%–8%), angina (6%), palpitations (3%–4%), tachycardia (1%–4%)
CNS: headache (6%–8%), dizziness/lightheadedness (4%–7%), asthenia (4%–6%)
GI: abdominal discomfort (1%–2%), nausea (1%–2%), dry mouth/thirst (1%–2%)
Dermatologic: rash/dermatitis (1%)
Others: flushing (5%–10%)

PHARMACOKINETICS AND PHARMACODYNAMICS
Duration of action: 8 h (immediate release); 12 h (sustained release)
Onset of action: 20 min
Time to peak serum concentration: 0.5–2 h (immediate release); 1–4 h (sustained release)
Bioavailability: 35%
Effect of food: the mean maximum concentration and area under the curve (AUC) were 20%–30% lower compared with fasting subjects when nicardipine was given 1–3 h after a high-fat meal
Protein binding: >95%
Volume of distribution: 8.3 L/kg (IV)
Metabolism: hepatic; extensive first-pass metabolism
Elimination: renal, 60% (<1% unchanged); biliary/fecal, 35%
Half-life: 2–4 h (early); 8 h (terminal)

MONITORING
BP, heart rate, liver function tests.

NICARDIPINE (continued)

DOSAGE

Immediate-release (Cardene): As an antianginal or antihypertensive agent, administer 20 mg in capsules three times daily. Usual maintenance dose is 20–40 mg three times daily. Allow at least 3 d between dose increases. For patients with renal impairment, titrate dose beginning with 20 mg three times daily. For patients with hepatic impairment, titrate dose starting with 20 mg twice daily.

Sustained-release (Cardene SR): Initiate treatment with 30 mg twice daily. The effective dose ranges from 30–60 mg twice daily. For patients with renal impairment, carefully titrate dose beginning with 30 mg twice daily. The total daily dose of immediate-release product may not automatically be equivalent to the daily sustained-release dose; use caution in converting.

Injection (Cardene I.V.): Intravenously administered nicardipine injection must be diluted before infusion. Administer (concentration of 0.1 mg/mL) by slow, continuous infusion. BP-lowering effect is seen within minutes. For gradual BP lowering, initiate at 50 mL/h (5 mg/h). Infusion rate may be increased by 25 mL/h (2.5 mg/h) every 15 min to a maximum of 150 mL/h (15 mg/h). For rapid BP reduction, initiate at 50 mL/h. Increase infusion rate by 25 mL/h every 5 min to a maximum of 150 mL/h until desirable BP lowering is reached. Infusion rate must be decreased to 30 mL/h (3 mg/h) when desirable BP is achieved. Conditions requiring infusion adjustment include hypotension and tachycardia. The intravenous infusion rate required to produce an average plasma concentration equivalent to a given oral dose at steady state is as follows:

Oral dose (immediate-release)	Equivalent intravenous infusion rate
20 mg every 8 h	0.5 mg/h
30 mg every 8 h	1.2 mg/h
40 mg every 8 h	2.2 mg/h

Intravenous nicardipine should be transferred to oral medication for prolonged control of BP as soon as the clinical condition permits. If treatment includes transfer to an oral antihypertensive agent other than nicardipine, generally initiate therapy upon discontinuation of the infusion. If oral nicardipine is to be used, administer the first dose of a three-times-daily regimen 1 h before discontinuation of the infusion.

OVERDOSE

If the patient is seen shortly after oral ingestion, employ lavage, activated charcoal, and cathartics. Treatment is supportive. Suggested treatments for possible acute cardiovascular adverse reactions caused by calcium channel blocker overdosage are listed below. Actual treatment and dosage depend on the severity of the clinical situation and the judgment and experience of the treating physician.

For symptomatic hypotension, administer fluids intravenously, dopamine or dobutamine intravenously, calcium chloride, isoproterenol, metaraminol, or norepinephrine.

For tachycardia, rapid ventricular rate in patients with antegrade conduction in atrial flutter/fibrillation, and accessory pathway with Wolff-Parkinson-White or Lown-Ganong-Levine syndrome, administer direct-current cardioversion, intravenous lidocaine, or intravenous procainamide. Intravenous fluids should be given by slow drip.

For bradycardia, second- or third-degree AV block, with a few patients progressing to asystole, administer intravenous atropine, isoproterenol, norepinephrine, or calcium chloride, or use electronic cardiac pacemaker. Intravenous fluids should be given by slow drip.

PATIENT INFORMATION

The sustained-released capsules should be swallowed whole, without breaking, crushing, or chewing. This medication may cause headache, flushing, dizziness, and ankle edema. Discuss exertion limits with physician. Notify physician if persistent side effects occur. Do not discontinue therapy without your physician's advice.

AVAILABILITY

Capsules (Cardene)—20 mg, 30 mg
Capsules, sustained release (Cardene SR)—30 mg, 45 mg, 60 mg
Injection (Cardene I.V.)—2.5 mg/mL, 10 mL ampules

NIFEDIPINE
(Nifedipine, Adalat®, Adalat® CC, Nifedical™ XL, Procardia®, Procardia XL®)

Nifedipine, the benchmark dihydropyridine calcium antagonist, is widely prescribed. It undergoes almost complete hepatic oxidation to three pharmacologically inactive metabolites, and its half-life is thus short, necessitating three-times-daily administration. An extended-release formulation has been developed to allow once- or twice-daily administration. It can be used as a first-, second- or third-line agent in mild to moderate hypertension, with an efficacy similar to that of beta-blockers and diuretics. An added effect is obtained when it is combined with beta-blockers, methyldopa, clonidine, and captopril. Side effects are typical of a peripheral vasodilator and include flushing, headaches, and palpitations. In some trials, ankle edema has proved to be troublesome. Serious adverse cardiovascular effects, such as cerebrovascular ischemia, stroke, and MI, have also been reported for the short-acting formulation of nifedipine. Therefore, short-acting nifedipine is no longer recommended for the management of any form of hypertension, including hypertensive crises. Currently, only extended-release formulations of nifedipine are recommended for the treatment of hypertension.

The antianginal efficacy of nifedipine has been seen during acute and chronic administration, but the effect may be reduced in those who smoke. It is less effective than some beta-blockers, but the combination appears to be more effective than either therapy alone. Nifedipine is particularly beneficial in the treatment of variant (Prinzmetal's) angina. An overview of trials with nifedipine and other dihydropyridines in the treatment of unstable angina and acute and post-MI indicates that the combined end points of mortality and reinfarction may be increased with treatment. A large randomized trial, INSIGHT, was initiated to compare nifedipine GITS (gastrointestinal therapeutic system) with a combination of thiazide (hydrochlorothiazide) and potassium-sparing diuretics (amiloride) in the treatment of hypertensive patients with at least one additional cardiovascular risk factor. The results of this trial showed that similar proportions of patients in each treatment arm experienced the primary composite outcome of cardiovascular death, MI, heart failure, or stroke. There were a significantly higher number of withdrawals (8% excess) from the nifedipine group because of peripheral edema. However, serious adverse events were significantly more frequent in the hydrochlorothiazide plus amiloride group compared with the nifedipine group (28% vs 25%). Thus, the investigators of this study concluded that nifedipine once daily and hydrochlorothiazide plus amiloride were equally effective in preventing overall cardiovascular or cerebrovascular complications. Moreover, the investigators of INSIGHT suggest that the choice of therapy in patients with hypertension and cardiovascular risk factors can be decided by tolerability and BP response rather than long-term safety or efficacy.

IN BRIEF

INDICATIONS
Vasospastic angina (Nifedipine, Adalat, Nifedical XL, Procardia, Procardia XL)
Chronic stable angina (Nifedipine, Adalat, Nifedical XL, Procardia, Procardia XL)
Hypertension (Adalat CC, Nifedical XL, Procardia XL)

CONTRAINDICATIONS
Hypersensitivity
Acute MI (short-acting formulation)

DRUG INTERACTIONS
Azole antifungals (eg, itraconazole)[1]   Phenobarbital[2]
Barbiturates[2]   Quinidine[1,4]
Beta-blockers[1,3]   Quinupristin/dalfopristin[1]
Cisapride[1]   Rifampin[2]
Cyclosporine[1]   Sildenafil[5]
Digitalis glycosides[3]   St. John's wort[2]
Diltiazem[1,3]   Tadalafil[5]
Fentanyl[5]   Theophylline[3]
Grapefruit juice[1]   Tacrolimus[3]
H2-blockers[1]   Vardenafil[5]
Melatonin[2]   Vincristine[3]
Nafcillin[2]

1 Effect/toxicity of nifedipine may increase.
2 Effect of nifedipine may decrease.
3 Nifedipine may increase the effect/toxicity of this drug.
4 Nifedipine may decrease the effect of this drug.
5 May increase the risk of hypotension.

ADVERSE EFFECTS
Cardiovascular: peripheral edema (10%–30%), pulmonary edema (7%), palpitations (≤7%), hypotension (≤5%), MI (4%–7%), congestive heart failure (CHF) (2%–7%)
CNS: headache (19%), dizziness/lightheadedness (4%), nervousness (≤7%), fatigue/asthenia (4%), paresthesia (<3%), somnolence (<3%), insomnia (<3%)
GI: nausea (2%), abdominal discomfort (≤3%), constipation (1%), diarrhea (<3%), dry mouth/thirst (<3%)
Dermatologic: rash/dermatitis (≤3%), pruritus/urticaria (≤3%)
Others: giddiness, flushing/heat sensation (4%), shortness of breath (≤8%), muscle cramps (≤8%), cough (6%), nasal or chest congestion (≤6%), fever, chills (≤3%), micturition disorder (<3%), gingival hyperplasia (≤1%)

PHARMACOKINETICS AND PHARMACODYNAMICS
Duration of action: 8 h (short acting); up to 24 h (extended release)
Onset of action: 20 min
Time to peak serum concentration: 0.5 h (short acting); 6 h (extended release)
Bioavailability: 45%–70% (short acting); 86% (extended release)
Effect of food: food may slow the rate but not the extent of nifedipine absorption
Protein binding: 92%–98%
Volume of distribution: no data
Metabolism: extensively metabolized by the liver to three pharmacologically inactive metabolites
Elimination: renal, 80% (as metabolites); biliary/fecal, 20% (as metabolites)
Half-life: 2–5 h

MONITORING
BP, heart rate, liver function tests, signs and symptoms of CHF, peripheral edema.

NIFEDIPINE (continued)

SPECIAL GROUPS

Race: no differences in response

Children: safety and effectiveness have not been established

Elderly: nifedipine may cause a greater hypotensive effect than that seen in younger patients, probably because of age-related alterations in drug disposition

Renal impairment: dosage adjustment is usually not necessary; it is not removed by hemodialysis

Hepatic impairment: use with caution; nifedipine is extensively metabolized by the liver

Pregnancy: category C; use only if potential benefit justifies the potential risk to the fetus

Breast-feeding: not recommended; nifedipine is excreted in breast milk

DOSAGE

Short-acting (nifedipine, Adalat, Procardia): As an antianginal, initiate capsules at 10 mg three times daily, gradually increasing over 7–14 d as needed. For hospitalized patients under close supervision, dosage may be increased by 10 mg increments over 4–6 h periods until symptoms are controlled. For elderly patients and patients with hepatic impairment, initiate treatment at 10 mg twice daily, with careful monitoring.

Note: Labeling states that the short-acting product should not be used for hypertension, hypertensive crisis, acute MI, and some forms of unstable angina and chronic stable angina.

Extended-release (Adalat CC): Initiate with 30 mg once daily, titrate over a 7–14 d period according to response. Usual maintenance dose is 30–60 mg once daily. Titration to doses >90 mg daily is not recommended.

Extended-release (Nifedical XL, Procardia XL): Initiate with 30 or 60 mg once daily, titrate over a period of 7–14 d according to response. Titration may proceed more rapidly if the patient is frequently assessed. Titration to doses >120 mg daily is not recommended. Angina patients maintained on the short-acting formulation (nifedipine capsule) may be switched to the extended-release tablet at the nearest equivalent total daily dose. Experience with doses >90 mg daily in patients with angina is limited.

OVERDOSE

If the patient is seen shortly after oral ingestion, employ lavage, activated charcoal, and cathartics. Treatment is supportive. Suggested treatments for possible acute cardiovascular adverse reactions caused by calcium channel blocker overdosage are listed below. Actual treatment and dosage depend on the severity of the clinical situation and the judgment and experience of the treating physician.

For symptomatic hypotension, administer fluids intravenously, dopamine or dobutamine intravenously, calcium chloride, isoproterenol, metaraminol, or norepinephrine.

For tachycardia, rapid ventricular rate in patients with antegrade conduction in atrial flutter/fibrillation, and accessory pathway with Wolff-Parkinson-White or Lown-Ganong-Levine syndrome, administer direct-current cardioversion, intravenous lidocaine, or intravenous procainamide. Intravenous fluids should be given by slow drip.

For bradycardia, second- or third-degree AV block, with a few patients progressing to asystole, administer intravenous atropine, isoproterenol, norepinephrine, or calcium chloride, or use electronic cardiac pacemaker. Intravenous fluids should be given by slow drip.

PATIENT INFORMATION

The extended-released tablets should be swallowed whole, without breaking, crushing, or chewing. This medication may cause headache, dizziness, flushing, palpitations, and ankle edema. Discuss exertion limits with physician. Notify physician if persistent side effects occur. Do not discontinue therapy without your physician's advice.

AVAILABILITY

Capsules, liquid-filled (Nifedipine, Adalat, Procardia)—10 mg, 20 mg
Tablets, extended-release (Nifedipine, Adalat CC, Procardia XL)—30 mg, 60 mg, 90 mg
Tablets, extended-release (Nifedical XL)—30 mg, 60 mg

NIMODIPINE (Nimotop®)

Nimodipine is a dihydropyridine calcium antagonist that has been approved for use in patients with acute subarachnoid hemorrhage to improve associated neurologic deficits. Nimodipine is lipophilic and can cross the blood–brain barrier easily. It appears to have a greater effect on the cerebral arteries than arteries elsewhere in the body. The drug may prevent cerebral arterial spasm following subarachnoid hemorrhage, but this mechanism has not been confirmed conclusively. Nimodipine's exact mechanism of action in treating neurologic deficits associated with subarachnoid hemorrhage is not known. Nimodipine has also been used in the management of migraine headache, although this indication has not been approved by the Food and Drug Administration (FDA).

SPECIAL GROUPS

Race:	no differences in response
Children:	safety and effectiveness have not been established
Elderly:	risk of hypotension may be increased; use usual dose with caution
Renal impairment:	normal dosage recommended; nimodipine is not likely to be dialyzable
Hepatic impairment:	administer with caution; use lower doses
Pregnancy:	category C; use only if potential benefit justifies the potential risk to the fetus
Breast-feeding:	not recommended; nimodipine may be excreted in breast milk

IN BRIEF

INDICATIONS
Subarachnoid hemorrhage: nimodipine is indicated for the improvement of neurologic outcome by reducing the incidence and severity of ischemic deficits in patients with subarachnoid hemorrhage from ruptured intracranial berry aneurysms regardless of their postictus neurologic condition (eg, Hunt and Hess grades I–V).

CONTRAINDICATIONS
Hypersensitivity

DRUG INTERACTIONS
Beta-blockers[1,3]
Fentanyl[4]
H$_2$-blockers[1]
Omeprazole[1]
Rifampin[2]
Sildenafil[4]
Tadalafil[4]
Valproic acid[1]
Vardenafil[4]

1 Effect/toxicity of nimodipine may increase.
2 Effect of nimodipine may decrease.
3 Nimodipine may increase the effect/toxicity of this drug.
4 May increase the risk of hypotension.

ADVERSE EFFECTS
Cardiovascular: hypotension (1%–8%), peripheral edema (1%), abnormal ECG (1%), bradycardia (≤1%)
CNS: headache (1%–4%), psychiatric disturbances (1%), dizziness/lightheadedness (<1%)
GI: diarrhea (1%–4%), abdominal discomfort (2%), nausea (1%)
Dermatologic: rash/dermatitis (1%–2%), pruritus/urticaria (<1%)
Others: flushing (1%–2%), shortness of breath (1%–2%), muscle cramps (1%–2%)

PHARMACOKINETICS AND PHARMACODYNAMICS

Duration of action:	4 h
Onset of action:	rapid
Time to peak plasma concentration:	≤1 h
Bioavailability:	13%, increased in patients with hepatic impairment
Effect of food:	administration of nimodipine following a standard breakfast resulted in a 68% lower peak plasma concentration and a 38% lower bioavailability relative to dosing under fasted conditions in a study of 24 healthy male volunteers
Protein binding:	>95%
Volume of distribution:	no data
Metabolism:	hepatic, extensive, to inactive metabolites
Elimination:	renal (<1% unchanged); biliary/fecal
Half-life:	1–2 h (early), 8–9 h (terminal)

MONITORING
BP, heart rate, hepatic function.

NIMODIPINE *(continued)*

DOSAGE

Usual dose is 60 mg every 4 h, beginning within 96 h of subarachnoid hemorrhage and continuing for 21 d. In patients with hepatic cirrhosis, dosage should be reduced to 30 mg every 4 h, with close monitoring of BP and heart rate.

Note: This medication is given preferably not less than 1 h before or 2 h after meals. If the capsule cannot be swallowed (*eg*, time of surgery, unconscious patient), make a hole in both ends of the capsule with an 18-gauge needle and extract the contents into a syringe. Empty the contents into the patient's in situ nasogastric tube and wash down the tube with 30 mL of normal saline.

OVERDOSE

If the patient is seen shortly after oral ingestion, employ lavage, activated charcoal, and cathartics. Treatment is supportive. Suggested treatments for possible acute cardiovascular adverse reactions caused by calcium channel blocker overdosage are listed below. Actual treatment and dosage depend on the severity of the clinical situation and the judgment and experience of the treating physician.

For symptomatic hypotension, administer fluids intravenously, dopamine or dobutamine intravenously, calcium chloride, isoproterenol, metaraminol, or norepinephrine.

For tachycardia, rapid ventricular rate in patients with antegrade conduction in atrial flutter/fibrillation, and accessory pathway with Wolff-Parkinson-White or Lown-Ganong-Levine syndrome, administer direct-current cardioversion, intravenous lidocaine, or intravenous procainamide. Intravenous fluids should be given by slow drip.

For bradycardia, second- or third-degree AV block, with a few patients progressing to asystole, administer intravenous atropine, isoproterenol, norepinephrine, or calcium chloride, or use electronic cardiac pacemaker. Intravenous fluids should be given by slow drip.

PATIENT INFORMATION

Take this medication at least 1 h before or 2 h after meals. This medication may cause dizziness, headache, flushing, ankle edema, and cramps. Notify physician if persistent side effects occur. Do not discontinue therapy without your physician's advice.

AVAILABILITY

Capsules, liquid-filled—30 mg

NISOLDIPINE (Sular®)

Nisoldipine is a dihydropyridine calcium antagonist that is structurally related to nifedipine. Because of its vascular selectivity, nisoldipine is capable of lowering BP without affecting the functioning of the myocardium and skeletal muscle. This drug has been used as monotherapy, or in combination with other classes of antihypertensive agents, in the management of hypertension. Nisoldipine currently is available in the United States only as extended-release tablets, nisoldipine coat core (nisoldipine CC), which consist of an external coat and an internal core. Both coat and core contain nisoldipine: the coat as a slow-release formulation and the core as a fast-release formulation. This allows the drug to be released gradually over 24 hours, minimizing fluctuations in plasma concentration and providing a good trough-to-peak ratio.

Nisoldipine's efficacy in hypertensive patients has been demonstrated to be similar to that of thiazide diuretics, beta-blockers, ACE inhibitors, and other calcium antagonists, without adverse effects on metabolic parameters. Further, nisoldipine was shown to reduce early-morning rise in BP without reflex tachycardia in a large South African multicenter trial. Similar to other calcium antagonists, nisoldipine works equally well as an antihypertensive agent in both black and white patients. Regression of left ventricular hypertrophy was demonstrated in black patients with severe diastolic hypertension in another South African study. Nisoldipine CC was also demonstrated to be safe and had no adverse effect on mortality when given to postinfarction patients with impaired left ventricular function in the DEFIANT-II study. In addition, nisoldipine CC was shown to be well tolerated in all groups of patients. The most frequently reported adverse effects were headache and peripheral edema, which were usually mild and transient.

SPECIAL GROUPS

Race: no differences in response
Children: safety and effectiveness have not been established
Elderly: initiate at lower dose
Renal impairment: normal dosage recommended in patients with mild to moderate renal impairment
Hepatic impairment: administer with caution; use lower initial and maintenance doses
Pregnancy: category C; use only if the potential benefit justifies the potential risk to the fetus
Breast-feeding: not recommended; nisoldipine may be excreted in breast milk

IN BRIEF

INDICATIONS
Hypertension (nisoldipine may be used alone or in combination with other antihypertensive agents)

CONTRAINDICATIONS
Hypersensitivity

DRUG INTERACTIONS
Azole antifungals (ketoconazole)[1]
Beta-blockers[1,3]
Digoxin[3]
Fentanyl[4]
Grapefruit juice[1]
H$_2$-blockers[1]
Omeprazole[1]
Phenytoin[2]
Quinidine[2,3]
Rifampin[2]
Sildenafil[4]
Tadalafil[4]
Vardenafil[4]

1 Effect/toxicity of nisoldipine may increase.
2 Effect of nisoldipine may decrease.
3 Nisoldipine may increase the effect/toxicity of this drug.
4 May increase the risk of hypotension.

ADVERSE EFFECTS
Cardiovascular: peripheral edema (22%), palpitations (3%), chest pain (2%)
CNS: headache (22%), dizziness/lightheadedness (5%)
GI: nausea (2%), abdominal discomfort (≤1%)
Dermatologic: rash/dermatitis (2%)
Others: pharyngitis (5%), vasodilation (4%), sinusitis (3%), sexual difficulties (≤1%), shortness of breath (≤1%)

PHARMACOKINETICS AND PHARMACODYNAMICS
Duration of action: 24 h (extended release)
Onset of action: no data
Time to peak plasma concentration: 6–12 h
Bioavailability: 5%
Effect of food: food with a high fat content has a pronounced effect on the release of nisoldipine from the coat-core formulation and results in a significant increase in peak plasma concentration by up to 300%. Total exposure, however, is decreased about 25%. Grapefruit juice may interfere with nisoldipine metabolism, resulting in a mean increase in peak plasma concentration of about threefold and AUC of almost twofold.
Protein binding: >99%
Volume of distribution: no data
Metabolism: extensive presystemic metabolism in the intestinal wall and the liver; hepatically metabolized to inactive metabolites
Elimination: urinary excretion (60%–80%); only traces of unchanged drug are found in the urine
Half-life: 7–12 hours

MONITORING
BP, heart rate, hepatic function.

NISOLDIPINE (continued)

DOSAGE

Initiate therapy with 20 mg orally once daily, then increase by 10 mg/wk, or longer intervals, to attain adequate response. The usual maintenance dose is 20–40 mg once daily. Doses greater than 60 mg daily are not recommended. For elderly patients and patients with hepatic function impairment, initiate with a dose not exceeding 10 mg daily. Monitor BP closely during any dosage adjustment.

Note: Nisoldipine has been used safely with diuretics, ACE inhibitors, and beta-blockers. Administration of this medication with a high-fat meal may lead to excessive peak drug concentration and should be avoided. In addition, grapefruit products should be avoided before and after dosing.

OVERDOSE

If the patient is seen shortly after oral ingestion, employ lavage, activated charcoal, and cathartics. Treatment is supportive. Suggested treatments for possible acute cardiovascular adverse reactions caused by calcium channel blocker overdosage are listed below. Actual treatment and dosage depend on the severity of the clinical situation and the judgment and experience of the treating physician.

For symptomatic hypotension, administer fluids intravenously, dopamine or dobutamine intravenously, calcium chloride, isoproterenol, metaraminol, or norepinephrine.

For tachycardia, rapid ventricular rate in patients with antegrade conduction in atrial flutter/fibrillation, and accessory pathway with Wolff-Parkinson-White or Lown-Ganong-Levine syndrome, administer direct-current cardioversion, intravenous lidocaine, or intravenous procainamide. Intravenous fluids should be given by slow drip.

For bradycardia, second- or third-degree AV block, with a few patients progressing to asystole, administer intravenous atropine, isoproterenol, norepinephrine, or calcium chloride, or use electronic cardiac pacemaker. Intravenous fluids should be given by slow drip.

PATIENT INFORMATION

Nisoldipine (Sular) is an extended-release formulation; swallow whole, do not bite or divide tablets. Avoid taking this medication with high-fat meals. Grapefruit products should also be avoided before and after dosing. This medication may cause dizziness, palpitations, headache, flushing, and ankle edema. Notify physician if persistent side effects occur. Do not discontinue therapy without your physician's advice.

AVAILABILITY

Tablets (extended-release)—10 mg, 20 mg, 30 mg, 40 mg

VERAPAMIL
(Verapamil, Sustained-release Verapamil, Calan®, Calan® SR, Isoptin®, Isoptin® SR, Verelan®, Verelan® PM, Covera-HS™, Verapamil I.V., Isoptin® I.V.)

Verapamil hydrochloride is a phenylalkylamine calcium antagonist. It exerts its pharmacologic effects by modulating ionic calcium across the cell membrane of the arterial smooth muscle as well as in conductile and contractile myocardial cells. Verapamil lowers peripheral vascular resistance with little or no reflex tachycardia and may, in fact, reduce heart rate. The decrease in systemic and coronary vascular resistance and the sparing effect on intracellular oxygen consumption appear to explain its powerful antianginal properties. In the treatment of angina, verapamil is at least as effective as beta-blockers and probably more so than nifedipine. As monotherapy, it can control BP for 24 hours in patients with uncomplicated hypertension given the sustained-release preparations. Verapamil has been combined with beta-blockers, diuretics, ACE inhibitors, and reserpine successfully. Caution should be exercised when coadministering verapamil with a beta-blocker, particularly in patients with myocardial conduction disease, because heart block may result. A particularly useful fixed combination available commercially is verapamil SR (sustained release) and trandolapril (verapamil SR/trandolapril). This combination has been shown to reduce BP to a greater extent than when verapamil SR or trandolapril is used alone. Verapamil SR/trandolapril was demonstrated to reduce proteinuria to a greater extent than the individual agents in patients with diabetic or nondiabetic proteinuria. In a double-blind, randomized trial involving 100 post–acute MI patients with CHF, cardiac events occurred less frequently after verapamil SR/trandolapril than after monotherapy with trandolapril. Further, verapamil SR/trandolapril does not adversely influence glucose, insulin, or lipid parameters in patients with mild to moderate essential hypertension and type II diabetes mellitus.

Verapamil is very effective in suppressing supraventricular arrhythmias, and it slows the ventricular rate in patients with chronic atrial flutter or atrial fibrillation. However, this drug should not be used when these arrhythmias are associated with an accessory bypass tract (eg, Wolff-Parkinson-White). Verapamil is the only calcium antagonist for which a protective effect has been shown in patients who endured an acute coronary event. Decreased mortality and a lower rate of reinfarction were found in the DAVIT II study among patients treated with verapamil for 12 to 18 months after an MI. However, the mortality rate was only significantly reduced in patients without heart failure who were in the verapamil group. A large, randomized clinical trial, CONVINCE, was initiated to compare COER verapamil with hydrochlorothiazide or atenolol for the management of hypertensive patients who have at least one additional risk factor for cardiovascular disease. After a mean follow-up of 3 years, there was no significant difference in the primary composite outcome of morbidity and mortality between the two treatment arms. However, the ability to draw long-term conclusions from this trial was limited because this study was terminated by the sponsor prematurely at 3 years. Of note, hospitalization for heart failure was 30% higher with the COER verapamil arm compared with the atenolol or hydrochlorothiazide arm. Similar to ALLHAT, results from the CONVINCE trial showed that calcium channel blockers are not as protective as other antihypertensive agents against heart failure.

IN BRIEF

INDICATIONS
Hypertension (all oral formulations)
Angina (all oral immediate-release formulations and Covera-HS)
Arrhythmias (all oral immediate-release formulations)
Supraventricular tachyarrhythmias (intravenous formulations)

CONTRAINDICATIONS
Hypersensitivity
Severe left ventricular dysfunction
Hypotension (systolic pressure less than 90 mm Hg)
Sick sinus syndrome (except in patients with a functioning artificial ventricular pacemaker)
Second- or third-degree AV block (except in patients with a functioning artificial ventricular pacemaker)
Patients with atrial flutter or atrial fibrillation and an accessory bypass tract (eg, Wolff-Parkinson-White, Lown-Ganong-Levine syndromes)
Cardiogenic shock and severe CHF, unless secondary to a supraventricular tachycardia amenable to verapamil therapy
Ventricular tachycardia (the use of intravenous verapamil in patients with wide-complex ventricular tachycardia [QRS ≥0.12 sec] may result in marked hemodynamic deterioration and ventricular fibrillation)

DRUG INTERACTIONS
Amiodarone[1,3]	Grapefruit juice[1]
Antineoplastics[2]	H$_2$-blockers[1]
Astemizole[3,5]	HMG-CoA reductase inhibitors[3]
Barbiturates[2]	Imipramine[3]
Beta-blockers[1,3,6]	Lithium[4]
Buspirone[3]	Nondepolarizing muscle relaxants[3,5]
Calcium salts[2]	Phenytoin[2]
Carbamazepine[3]	Prazosin[3]
Cisapride[3,5]	Quinidine[3]
Cyclosporine[3]	Rifampin[2]
Digitalis glycosides[3]	Sildenafil[8]
Disopyramide[3,5]	Sirolimus[3]
Dofetilide[3,7]	Tacrolimus[3]
Doxorubicin[3]	Tadalafil[8]
Ethanol[3]	Theophylline[3]
Fentanyl[8]	Vardenafil[8]
Flecainide[3]	

1 Effect/toxicity of verapamil may increase.
2 Effect of verapamil may decrease.
3 Verapamil may increase the effect/toxicity of this drug.
4 Verapamil may decrease the effect of this drug.
5 Concurrent use with verapamil is not recommended.
6 IV verapamil and IV beta-adrenergic blocking drugs should not be administered in close proximity to each other (within a few hours) because both may have a depressant effect on myocardial contractility and AV conduction.
7 Concurrent use of dofetilide with verapamil is contraindicated.
8 May increase the risk of hypotension.

ADVERSE EFFECTS
Cardiovascular: peripheral edema (2%), hypotension (2%), CHF (2%), pulmonary edema (2%), AV block (1%), bradycardia (1%–2%)
CNS: dizziness/lightheadedness (3%–4%), headache (2%), asthenia (2%)
GI: constipation (7%), nausea (2%–3%)
Dermatologic: rash/dermatitis (1%–2%)
Others: shortness of breath (1%–2%), flushing (<1%), micturition disorder (<1%), sexual difficulties (<1%), muscle cramps (<1%)

VERAPAMIL (continued)

SPECIAL GROUPS

Race: no differences in response

Children: safety and effectiveness have not been established; however, verapamil has been used in the pediatric population

Elderly: verapamil may cause a greater hypotensive effect compared with that seen in younger patients, probably because of age-related alterations in drug disposition. Lower doses may be required.

Renal impairment: use with caution; lower doses may be required. Verapamil is not removed by hemodialysis.

Hepatic impairment: use with caution; verapamil is extensively metabolized by the liver. Use lower doses.

Pregnancy: category C; use verapamil in pregnant women only if potential benefit justifies potential risk to the fetus

Breast-feeding: not recommended; verapamil is excreted in breast milk

DOSAGE

Immediate-release tablets (verapamil, Calan, Isoptin): Adults—as an antianginal, antiarrhythmic, and antihypertensive, initiate at 80–120 mg three times daily, increase at daily or weekly intervals as needed and tolerated. Limit to 480 mg daily in divided doses.

Elderly or patients with hepatic impairment—Initiate at 40 mg three times daily; adjust as needed.

Sustained-release capsules (Verelan): Adults—as an antihypertensive, initiate at 240 mg once daily in the morning; increase in increments of 120 mg/d at daily or weekly intervals as needed and tolerated.

Note: Initiate dose at 120 mg/d for patients who may have an increased response to verapamil. Usual total daily dose range, 240–480 mg

Sustained-release tablets (verapamil SR, Calan SR, Isoptin SR): Adults—as an antihypertensive, initiate at 120–240 mg once daily in the morning with food; increase in increments of 60–120 mg/d at daily or weekly intervals as needed and as tolerated. Usual total daily dose range is 240–480 mg (total daily dose may be given in two divided doses).

Extended-release tablets, controlled onset (Covera-HS): Adults—initiate with 180 mg dose at bedtime for both hypertension and angina; if response is inadequate, the dose may be titrated upward to 480 mg/d given at bedtime.

Extended-release capsules, controlled onset (Verelan PM): Adults—initiate with 200 mg dose at bedtime for hypertension; if response is inadequate, the dose may be titrated upward to 300 or 400 mg/d given at bedtime.

PHARMACOKINETICS AND PHARMACODYNAMICS

Duration of action: 8 h (immediate release); 24 h (sustained release); 10–20 min (duration of hemodynamic effects after a single intravenous dose)

Onset of action: 30 min (oral); 1–5 min (intravenous)

Time to peak serum concentration: 1–2 h (immediate release); 4–9 h (sustained release)

Bioavailability: 20%–35% (immediate release)

Effect of food: food decreases the rate and extent of absorption of sustained-release verapamil tablets but produces smaller differences between peak and trough plasma concentrations of the drug; food does not appear to substantially affect the absorption of immediate-release tablets, extended-release tablets, or sustained-release capsules

Protein binding: 90%

Volume of distribution: no data

Metabolism: extensive; principle metabolite is norverapamil, which has approximately 20% of the cardiovascular activity of verapamil

Elimination: renal, 70% (3%–4% as unchanged drug); biliary/fecal, 9%–16%

Half-life: single oral dose (3–7 h), repetitive oral dose (4.5–12 h), intravenous (4 min, early; 2–5 h, terminal)

MONITORING

BP, ECG, liver function tests.

OVERDOSE

If the patient is seen shortly after oral ingestion, employ lavage, activated charcoal, and cathartics. Treatment is supportive. Suggested treatments for possible acute cardiovascular adverse reactions caused by calcium channel blocker overdosage are listed below. Actual treatment and dosage depend on the severity of the clinical situation and the judgment and experience of the treating physician.

For symptomatic hypotension, administer fluids intravenously, dopamine or dobutamine intravenously, calcium chloride, isoproterenol, metaraminol, or norepinephrine.

For tachycardia, rapid ventricular rate in patients with antegrade conduction in atrial flutter/fibrillation, and accessory pathway with Wolff-Parkinson-White or Lown-Ganong-Levine syndrome, administer direct-current cardioversion, intravenous lidocaine, or intravenous procainamide. Intravenous fluids should be given by slow drip.

For bradycardia, second- or third-degree AV block, with a few patients progressing to asystole, administer intravenous atropine, isoproterenol, norepinephrine, or calcium chloride, or use electronic cardiac pacemaker. Intravenous fluids should be given by slow drip.

DOSAGE *(continued)*

Injection (Verapamil I.V., Isoptin I.V.): Adults—initiate as 5–10 mg (or 75–150 µg/kg body weight [0.075–0.15 mg/kg]) slowly over at least 2 min with continuous ECG and BP monitoring. If response is inadequate, 10 mg (or 150 µg/kg body weight [0.15 mg/kg]) may be administered 30 min after completion of the initial dose. Elderly—Administer intravenous dose slowly over 3 min to minimize undesired effects.

Note: A small fraction (<1%) of patients may have life-threatening adverse responses (rapid ventricular rate in atrial flutter/fibrillation, and an accessory bypass tract, marked hypotension or extreme bradycardia/asystole) to verapamil injections; monitor initial use of intravenous verapamil and have resuscitation facilities available. See package insert for information on compatibility.

PATIENT INFORMATION

Take sustained-release tablets (verapamil SR, Calan SR, Isoptin SR) with food. The sustained- or extended-release formulation of this medication should be swallowed whole, without breaking, crushing, or chewing. Verapamil may cause a slowing of the heart rate, headache, dizziness, ankle edema, or constipation. Discuss exertion limits with physician. Notify physician if persistent side effects occur. Do not discontinue therapy without your physician's advice.

AVAILABILITY

Tablets, immediate-release (verapamil, Calan, Isoptin)—40 mg, 80 mg, 120 mg
Capsules, sustained-release (Verelan)—120 mg, 180 mg, 240 mg, 360 mg
Tablets, extended-release and controlled-onset (Covera-HS)—180 mg, 240 mg
Capsules, extended-release and controlled-onset (Verelan PM)—100 mg, 200 mg, 300 mg
Tablets, sustained-release (verapamil)—180 mg, 240 mg
Tablets, sustained-release (Calan SR, Isoptin SR)—120 mg, 180 mg, 240 mg
Injection (verapamil I.V., Isoptin I.V.)—5 mg/2 mL (2 and 4 mL ampules and vials; syringes)
Combination formulations:
Tarka—trandolapril/verapamil hydrochloride ER combination tablets
   1 mg/240 mg
   2 mg/180 mg
   2 mg/240 mg
   4 mg/240 mg

The information here is provided as guidance only. Prescribers should always consult the manufacturer's current prescribing information.

211

SELECTED BIBLIOGRAPHY

Antonios TFT, MacGregor GA: Some similarities and differences between verapamil and the dihydropyridines. *J Hypertens* 1998, 16(Suppl 1):S31–S34.

Black HR, Elliott WJ, Grandits G, *et al.* for the CONVINCE research group: Principal results of the controlled onset verapamil investigation of cardiovascular end points (CONVINCE) trial. *JAMA* 2003, 289:2073–2082.

Borhani NO, Mercuri M. Borhani PA, *et al.*: Final outcome results of the Multicenter Isradipine Diuretic Atherosclerosis study (MIDAS). A randomized controlled trial. *JAMA* 1996, 276:785–791.

Brown MJ, Palmer CR, Castaigne A, *et al.*: Morbidity and mortality in patients randomised to double-blind treatment with a long-acting calcium-channel blocker or diuretic in the International Nifedipine GITS study: intervention as a goal in hypertension treatment (INSIGHT). *Lancet* 2000, 356:366–372.

Conlin PR, Williams GH: Use of calcium channel blockers in hypertension. *Adv Intern Med* 1998, 43:533–562.

Dooley M, Goa KL: Fixed combination verapamil SR/trandolapril. *Drugs* 1998, 56:837–844.

Eisenberg MJ, Brox A, Bestawros AN: Calcium channel blockers: an update. *Am J Med* 2004, 116:35–43.

Fodor JG: Nisoldipine CC: efficacy and tolerability in hypertension and ischemic heart disease. *Cardiovasc Drugs Ther* 1997, 10(Suppl 3):873–879.

Freher M, Challapalli S, Pinto JV, *et al.*: Current status of calcium channel blockers in patients with cardiovascular disease. *Curr Probl Cardiol* 1999, 24:229–340.

Frishman WH: Comparative efficacy and concomitant use of bepridil and beta blockers in the management of angina pectoris. *Am J Cardiol* 1992, 69(Suppl):50D–60D.

Frishman WH: Current status of calcium channel blockers. *Curr Probl Cardiol* 1994, 19:637–688.

Frishman WH: Calcium channel blockers. In *Cardiovascular Pharmacotherapeutics*. Edited by Frishman WH, Sonnenblick EH. New York: McGraw Hill; 1997:101–130.

Frishman WH, Hershman D: Amlodipine. In *Cardiovascular Drug Therapy*, edn 2. Edited by Messerli FH. Philadelphia: WB Saunders; 1996:1024–1040.

Frishman WH, Rosenberg A, Katz B: Calcium antagonists in the management of systemic hypertension: the impact of sustained-release drug delivery systems. *Coronary Art Dis* 1994, 5:4–13.

Frishman WH, Sica DA: Calcium channel blockers. In *Cardiovascular Pharmacotherapeutics Manual*. Edited by Frishman WH, Sonnenblick EH, Sica DA. New York: McGraw Hill; 2004:65–95.

Frishman WH, Sonnenblick EH: Cardiovascular uses of calcium antagonists. In *Cardiovascular Drug Therapy*, edn 2. Edited by Messerli FH. Philadelphia: WB Saunders; 1996:891–901.

Frishman WH, Sonnenblick EH: Beta-adrenergic blocking drugs and calcium channel blockers. In *Hurst's The Heart*, edn 9. Edited by Alexander RW, Schlant RC, Fuster V. New York: McGraw Hill; 1998:1583–1618.

Hansson L, Zanchetti A, Carruthers SG, *et al.*: Effects of intensive blood-pressure lowering and low-dose aspirin in patients with hypertension: principal results of the Hypertension Optimal Treatment (HOT) randomised trial. HOT Study Group. *Lancet* 1998, 351:1755–1762.

Lopez LM, Santiago TM: Isradipine—another calcium-channel blocker for the treatment of hypertension and angina. *Ann Pharmacother* 1992; 26:789–799.

Mancia G, Grassi G: The International Nifedipine GITS Study of Intervention as a Goal in Hypertension Treatment (INSIGHT) trial. *Am J Cardiol* 1998; 82:23R–28R.

Messerli FH: What, if anything, is controversial about calcium antagonists? *Am J Hypertens* 1996, 9(12 Pt 2):177S–181S.

Messerli FH, Weiner DA: Are all calcium antagonists equally effective for reducing reinfarction rate? *Am J Cardiol* 1993, 72:818–820.

Opie LH: What does nisoldipine coat core (CC) add to current therapy that is clinically meaningful? *Am J Cardiol* 1997, 79:29–32.

Packer M: Combined beta-adrenergic and calcium-entry blockade in angina pectoris. *N Engl J Med* 1989, 302:709–718.

Packer M: Calcium channel blockers in chronic heart failure. *Circulation* 1990, 82:2254–2256.

Packer M, Frishman WH: *Calcium Channel Antagonists in Cardiovascular Disease*. Norwalk, CT: Appleton Century Crofts, 1984.

Packer M, O'Connor CM, Ghali JK, *et al.* for the Prospective Randomized Amlodipine Survival Evaluation Study Group: Effect of amlodipine on morbidity and mortality in severe chronic heart failure. *N Engl J Med* 1996, 335:1107–1114.

Rich S, Kaufmann E, Levy PS: The effect of high doses of calcium-channel blockers on survival in primary pulmonary hypertension. *N Engl J Med* 1992, 327:76–81.

Thackray S, Witte K, Clark AL, *et al.*: Clinical trials update: OPTIME-CHF, PRAISE-2, ALL-HAT. *Eur J Heart Fail* 2000, 2:209–212.

The ALLHAT Officers and Coordinators for the ALLHAT Collaborative Research Group: Major outcomes in high-risk hypertensive patients randomized to angiotensin-converting enzyme inhibitor or calcium channel blocker vs diuretic. The Antihypertensive and Lipid-Lowering Treatment to Prevent Heart Attack Trial (ALLHAT). *JAMA* 2002, 288:2981–2997.

The DEFIANT-II Research Group: Doppler flow and echocardiography in functional cardiac insufficiency: assessment of nisoldipine therapy. Results of the DEFI-ANT-II Study. *Eur Heart J* 1997, 18:31–40.

The Multicentre Diltiazem Postinfarction Trial Research Group: The effect of diltiazem on mortality and reinfarction after myocardial infarction. *N Engl J Med* 1988, 319:386–392.

Waters D: Calcium channel blockers: an evidence-based review. *Can J Cardiol* 1997, 13:757–766.

Yusuf S, Held P, Furberg C: Update of effects of calcium antagonists in myocardial infarction or angina in light of the second Danish Infarction Trial (DAVIT-II) and other recent studies [editorial]. *Am J Cardiol* 1991, 67:1295–1297.

The information here is provided as guidance only. Prescribers should always consult the manufacturer's current prescribing information.

213

9

DIURETICS

Diuretics have been in widespread use for more than 40 years and have been the mainstay of treatment for hypertension and congestive heart failure (CHF). Despite the advent of newer agents, they continue to enjoy a large clinical demand and remain among the most widely prescribed drugs. Although originally intended for the treatment of edematous conditions, the most common application of diuretics is in the management of hypertension, and their efficacy as antihypertensive agents in mild to moderate hypertension is impressive. They remain the cornerstone of treatment for conditions in which the presence of edema is a feature, notably CHF.

Diuretics are classified into three main categories and are defined by their structures, their sites of action, and their effects on electrolyte excretion. The three main types of diuretics are the thiazides (and related drugs), the loop diuretics, and the potassium-sparing diuretics.

The thiazides (benzothiadiazines) and loop diuretics act predominantly at the luminal face of the distal tubule. Differences in their diuretic potency and electrolyte effects are attributable to their actions at different functional loci in the renal tubular apparatus.

MODE OF ACTION

By definition, diuretics are drugs that increase urine output. Their primary effect, however, is to inhibit tubular electrolyte reabsorption. This inhibition leads to an increase in the osmolar pressure, resulting in depressed fluid reabsorption so that an increase in urine output occurs. The individual segments of the nephron differ in selectivity of ion reabsorption. The main action of the thiazide diuretics is to inhibit sodium-chloride cotransport in the distal tubule. Loop diuretics, which can achieve urine output of about 25% of glomerular filtration rate, inhibit sodium-potassium-chloride cotransport in the medullary portion of the ascending limb of the loop of Henle, although they may also have a minor effect on the proximal tubule. The potassium-sparing diuretics act on a sodium channel in the distal tubule. The result is a reduction of the membrane potential that drives potassium secretion, and the end result is a mild natriuretic action combined with potassium retention (Figure 9.1).

All diuretics increase the excretion of sodium as the main cation and are effective in lowering blood pressure (BP) in hypertensive patients and animals. They are effective antihypertensive agents at doses that are not overtly diuretic. Their initial effect is to reduce the plasma volume, although later this change is largely compensated for and the peripheral vascular resistance falls. There is usually a fall in plasma volume, which in turn may result in increased plasma renin activity; this may or may not be accompanied by a rise in plasma catecholamines. The action of diuretics in stimulating renin responsiveness makes them particularly useful for treating elderly and black patients.

In addition to the three groups of diuretics in common use, organomercurials and carbonic anhydrase inhibitors were once used. Because of the toxicity of the former and the poor efficacy of the latter, neither type of compound is now viewed as useful. (Carbonic anhydrase inhibitors, however, have retained a role in the topical treatment of glaucoma.) Further discussion will therefore be confined to the three types of drugs in current use: the thiazides, the loop diuretics, and the potassium-sparing agents.

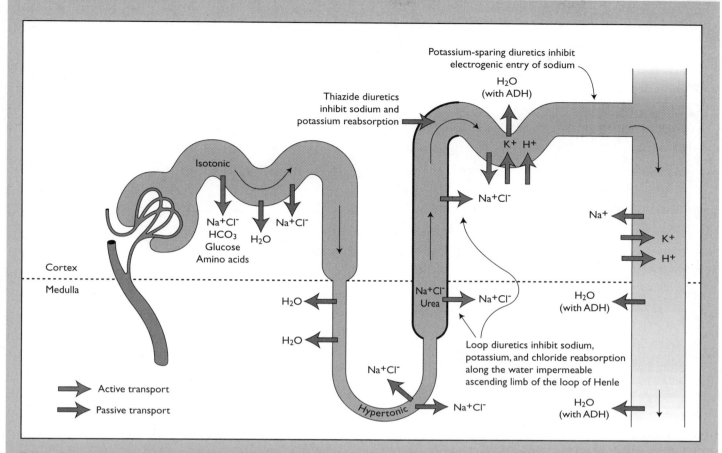

FIGURE 9.1 A simplified schema of the functional divisions of a mammalian nephron. ADH—antidiuretic hormone.

LOOP DIURETICS

Loop diuretics are one of the mainstays in the treatment of CHF and other edematous conditions. The group comprises **furosemide, ethacrynic acid, bumetanide, and torsemide.** All have similar efficacies and modes of action, but differ in their pharmacokinetic profiles.

EFFICACY AND USE

Loop diuretics are of particular value in treating CHF. They not only relieve the symptoms of congestion, but may also increase exercise capacity. Clinical signs, such as edema, are rarely refractory to treatment, except in the terminal stage; apparent resistance may reflect inadequate dosage or failure to combine the actions of drugs that act on different segments of the renal tubule. Intermittent administration has proved more efficacious in promoting fluid loss than has continuous treatment.

Some loop diuretics may have a useful antihypertensive effect, particularly in patients resistant to thiazides or with severe renal impairment. Loop diuretics have an adjunctive place in the treatment of acute pulmonary edema. Intravenous furosemide or ethacrynic acid produces rapid losses of salt and water. A reduction in BP may be apparent before diuresis occurs; this benefit has been attributed to venodilatation and a reduced cardiac filling pressure.

MODE OF ACTION

Loop diuretics exert their main action in the thick ascending limb of the loop of Henle. Although their chemical structures are diverse, they are all actively secreted by the proximal tubule in the lumen; their concentration in the loop of Henle is thus high. This high concentration appears to be a prerequisite for their inhibitory effect on ion reabsorption. They appear to inhibit the sodium-chloride cotransport system at the luminal membrane of the loop of Henle. The excretion of calcium and potassium is also increased.

Loop diuretics are sometimes referred to as high-ceiling diuretics because a good correlation is observed between the diuretic effect and the dose administered. How much of the diuretic response can be attributed solely to direct interference with transport systems at specific membrane sites, and how much can be attributed to secondary effects resulting from the release of intrarenal mediators and the associated redistribution of blood flow in the kidneys remains unclear.

INDICATIONS

	Bumetanide	Ethacrynic Acid	Furosemide	Torsemide
CHF (edema)	+	+	+	+
Edema (hepatic/renal disease)	+	+	+	+
Hypertension	–	–	+	+

+—FDA approved; – —not FDA approved; CHF—congestive heart failure.

BUMETANIDE (Bumetanide, Bumex®)

Bumetanide, similar to furosemide, is a sulfonamide-type loop diuretic. The diuretic potency of bumetanide is approximately 40 times that of furosemide. In addition to the inhibition of sodium reabsorption in the ascending limb of the loop of Henle, bumetanide also acts in the proximal tubule by blocking the reabsorption of phosphate. Bumetanide enhances renal blood flow via renal vascular dilation. However, its effect on glomerular filtration rate is variable. Bumetanide therapy is indicated for the management of excessive fluid overload or edema in various clinical conditions. Bumetanide may be effective in some patients who are unresponsive or refractory to other diuretics. Chronic bumetanide therapy has been associated with increases in plasma renin activity.

SPECIAL GROUPS

Race: no differences in response

Children: safety and effectiveness have not been established

Elderly: use with caution; no dosage adjustment is required

Renal impairment: use with caution; higher doses may be required to enhance diuresis; contraindicated in patients with anuria or progressive oliguric renal failure unresponsive to diuretic therapy

Hepatic impairment: use with caution and use lowest effective dosage possible with careful titration

Pregnancy: category C; use only if potential benefit justifies the potential risk to the fetus

Breast-feeding: not recommended; not known if the drug is excreted in human milk

IN BRIEF

INDICATIONS
Edema associated with CHF or hepatic or renal disease, including the nephrotic syndrome

CONTRAINDICATIONS
Known hypersensitivity to bumetanide, furosemide (has been used safely in patients with furosemide allergy), torsemide, sulfonylureas, or sulfur
Anuria or severe, progressive oliguria unresponsive to diuretic therapy
Hepatic coma
Severe electrolyte depletion

DRUG INTERACTIONS
Antihypertensive agents[1,3]
Cardiac glycosides[3]
Diuretics[1,3]
Lithium[3]
NSAIDs[2]
Non-depolarizing neuromuscular blockers[3]
Ototoxic agents (aminoglycosides, erythromycin, cisplatin)[3]
Potassium-depleting agents (corticosteroids, amphotericin B)[1]
Probenecid[2]
Sulfonylureas[4]

[1] Effect/toxicity of bumetanide may increase.
[2] Effect of bumetanide may decrease.
[3] Bumetanide may increase the effect/toxicity of this drug.
[4] Bumetanide may decrease the effect of this drug.

ADVERSE EFFECTS
CV: hypotension, arrhythmias, chest pain
CNS: dizziness, headache, fatigue, ototoxicity, encephalopathy (in patients with liver disease)
GI: nausea, vomiting, abdominal pain, diarrhea
GU: sexual dysfunction, polyuria
Hematologic: leukopenia, thrombocytopenia
Kidney: volume and electrolyte depletion ($\downarrow$K, $\downarrow$Cl, $\downarrow$Na, $\downarrow$Ca, $\downarrow$Mg, $\uparrow$uric acid), azotemia, $\uparrow$serum creatinine
Liver: elevated liver function tests
Metabolic: metabolic alkalosis, hyperglycemia, dyslipidemia
Skin: pruritus, urticaria, rash
Other: dehydration, muscle cramps

PHARMACOKINETICS AND PHARMACODYNAMICS
Duration of action: (po/IM) 4–6 h; (IV) 2–3 h
Onset of action: (po/IM) 30–60 min; (IV) few min
Peak effect: (po/IM) 1–2 h; (IV) 15–30 min
Bioavailability: (po) 85%–95%; (IV/IM) 100%
Effect of food: insignificant, but may delay the absorption
Volume of distribution: 9.45–19.7 L
Protein binding: 94%–96%
Metabolism: partially metabolized in liver to at least 5 metabolites
Elimination: urine—80% (50% unchanged); feces—10%–20% (<2% unchanged); $\uparrow$nonrenal clearance in renal insufficiency
Elimination half-life: 1–3 h

MONITORING
Clinical: BP, urine output, weight, hearing acuity
Lab: serum electrolytes (especially potassium, but also magnesium, calcium, sodium, and chloride), kidney function (blood urea nitrogen [BUN], serum creatinine), CO_2, CBC for blood dyscrasias

OVERDOSE
Supportive: replace fluid and electrolyte losses.

BUMETANIDE (continued)

DOSAGE

Oral: Usual dose range—0.5–2 mg/d as a single dose*

In patients with edema, if the initial diuresis is inadequate, repeated doses may be administered every 4–5 h until the desired diuretic response or a maximum daily dose of 10 mg is achieved. Intermittent dosing schedule—administer bumetanide on alternate days or daily for 3–4 d with a drug holiday of 1–2 d in between. This schedule, although less convenient than daily administration, is usually more effective.

Intravenous (IV) or intramuscular (IM): Usual dose range—0.5–1 mg*

In patients with edema, if the initial diuresis is inadequate, repeated doses may be administered every 2–3 h until the desired diuretic response or a maximum daily dose of 10 mg is achieved. *Higher dosage (>1–2 mg daily) may be required to achieve the desired therapeutic response in patients with renal insufficiency. In patients with severe renal insufficiency, a continuous IV infusion (12 mg over 12 h) may be safer and more effective than intermittent dosing.

PATIENT INFORMATION

Bumetanide is used to reduce excessive water in the body. Take the medication as instructed. Taking the medication earlier in the day may reduce nighttime awakenings to urinate. Avoid excessive dietary sodium intake while on this therapy. Potassium-rich diet is encouraged to avoid potassium depletion. Notify your health care provider if you develop any unusual muscle cramps, nausea, or dizziness. Sit or lie down if dizziness occurs, and rise slowly from a sitting or lying position.

AVAILABILITY

Tablets—0.5, 1, 2 mg
Ampules—0.25 mg/mL, 2 mL
Vials—0.25 mg/mL, in 2, 4, and 10 mL vials

ETHACRYNIC ACID
ETHACRYNATE SODIUM
(Edecrin®, Sodium Edecrin®)

Ethacrynic acid is a loop diuretic with pharmacologic effects similar to those of furosemide. It is metabolized to a cysteine conjugate, which may contribute to its diuretic effects. Ethacrynic acid enhances the excretion of sodium, chloride, potassium, hydrogen, calcium, and magnesium, but has no effect on urinary phosphate content. The agent has little or no direct effect on glomerular filtration rate or renal blood flow, although these parameters may be reduced with severe intravascular volume depletion associated with aggressive diuresis. Ethacrynic acid is mainly used for the treatment of refractory edema or fluid overload when response to other diuretic therapy is inadequate.

Ethacrynic acid inhibits the resorption of filtered sodium to a greater extent than other available diuretics, making it an attractive option in patients with renal dysfunction. Although ethacrynic acid is effective even in patients with significant renal insufficiency, its use has been limited by ototoxicity. This problem manifests as deafness, tinnitus, and vertigo with a sense of fullness in the ears. Ototoxicity associated with ethacrynic acid therapy may be irreversible and has been reported most frequently in patients with severe renal insufficiency, especially after receiving high IV doses. To alleviate the problem, it is recommended that a single IV dose should not exceed 100 mg and rapid IV administration should be avoided. Ethacrynic acid, structurally free of sulfur, may be used safely in patients with a known allergy to sulfonamides or thiazide diuretics.

IN BRIEF

INDICATIONS
Edema associated with CHF, liver cirrhosis, and renal disease, including the nephrotic syndrome

Ascites (short-term management) associated with malignancy, idiopathic edema, and lymphedema

Hospitalized pediatric patients (short-term management) with congenital heart disease or the nephrotic syndrome (not indicated for infants)

IV for rapid diuresis (eg, acute pulmonary edema) or when oral administration is not feasible

CONTRAINDICATIONS
Known hypersensitivity to product components

Anuria

Increasing electrolyte imbalance, azotemia, and/or oliguria in the setting of severe, progressive renal disease

History of severe, watery diarrhea caused by ethacrynic acid

Infants

DRUG INTERACTIONS
Antihypertensive agents[1,3]
Cardiac glycosides[3]
Diuretics[1,3]
Lithium[3]
NSAIDs[2]
Non-depolarizing neuromuscular blockers[3]
Ototoxic agents (aminoglycosides, erythromycin, cisplatin)[3]
Potassium-depleting agents (corticosteroids, amphotericin B)[1]
Probenecid[2]
Sulfonylureas[4]
Warfarin[3]

1 Effect/toxicity of ethacrynic acid may increase.
2 Effect of ethacrynic acid may decrease.
3 Ethacrynic acid may increase the effect/toxicity of this drug.
4 Ethacrynic acid may decrease the effect of this drug.

ADVERSE EFFECTS
CV: hypotension, orthostatic symptoms, arrhythmias, chest pain
CNS: dizziness, headache, fatigue, ototoxicity, encephalopathy (in patients with liver disease)
Hematologic: agranulocytosis, thrombocytopenia
GI: anorexia, nausea, vomiting, constipation, diarrhea, pancreatitis
GU: sexual dysfunction, polyuria
Kidney: volume and electrolyte depletion ($\downarrow$K, $\downarrow$Cl, $\downarrow$Na, $\downarrow$Ca, $\downarrow$Mg, $\uparrow$uric acid), azotemia, $\uparrow$serum creatinine
Liver: elevated liver enzymes, hepatocellular injury
Metabolic: metabolic alkalosis, hyperglycemia, hypoglycemia (high dose in uremic patients)
Skin: rash
Other: dehydration, muscle cramps, fever, chills

PHARMACOKINETICS AND PHARMACODYNAMICS
Duration of action: (po) 6–8 h or longer; (IV) 2–7 h
Onset of action: (po) <30 min; (IV) <5 min
Peak effect: (po) 2 h; (IV) 15–30 min
Bioavailability: 100%
Effect of food: no data
Protein binding: 90%
Volume of distribution: no data
Metabolism: partially metabolized in liver; with one active metabolite (cysteine conjugate)
Elimination: (IV) 30%–65% in urine (partly unchanged); 35%–40% in bile
Elimination half-life: 1–4 h

MONITORING
Clinical: BP, urine output, weight, hearing acuity
Lab: serum electrolytes (especially potassium, but also magnesium, calcium, sodium, and chloride), kidney function (BUN, serum creatinine), CO_2, CBC for blood dyscrasias

ETHACRYNIC ACID
ETHACRYNATE SODIUM (continued)

SPECIAL GROUPS

Race: no differences in response

Children: Oral doses of 25 mg, with stepwise titration of 25 mg to desired effect, are approved in children. Oral dosing is contraindicated in infants. IV dosing is not recommended by the manufacturer, but doses of 1 mg/kg have been shown to be safe and effective.

Elderly: use with caution; no dosage adjustment is required

Renal impairment: use with caution; higher doses may be required to enhance diuresis; contraindicated in patients with anuria or progressive oliguric renal failure unresponsive to diuretic therapy

Hepatic impairment: use with caution; titrate dose based on clinical assessment

Pregnancy: category B; should be used only if clearly indicated

Breast-feeding: not recommended; not known if the drug is excreted in human milk

DOSAGE

Oral (ethacrynic acid): Usual dose range—50–200 mg/d in 1–2 divided doses taken after a meal

The initial dose is 50 mg* once daily administered after a meal. The dose may be increased in 50 mg* increments daily until the desired diuresis or a maximum dose of 100 mg twice daily is achieved. In patients with severe, refractory edema, a dose of 200 mg twice daily may be required to maintain adequate diuresis.

Intermittent dosing schedule: After an effective diuresis or an ideal dry weight is achieved, ethacrynic acid may be administered on alternate days, or daily for a few days interspersed with a drug holiday of 1–2 d.

*Lower dose (25 mg) is recommended in patients who receive other diuretic therapy concurrently.

IV (ethacrynate sodium): Indicated when a rapid onset of diuresis is desired, such as in acute pulmonary edema, or when oral administration is not practical

Usual dose—50 mg (0.5–1 mg/kg, up to 100 mg) as a single dose infused over a few minutes (or, over 20–30 min), may be repeated once after 2–3 h if the desired diuresis is not achieved.

OVERDOSE
Supportive: replace fluid and electrolyte losses.

PATIENT INFORMATION
Ethacrynic acid is used to reduce excessive water in the body. Take the medication as instructed. Taking the medication earlier in the day may reduce nighttime awakenings to urinate. Avoid excessive dietary sodium intake while on this therapy. Potassium-rich diet is encouraged to avoid potassium depletion. Notify your health care provider if you develop any unusual muscle cramps, nausea, or dizziness. Sit or lie down if dizziness occurs, and rise slowly from a sitting or lying position.

AVAILABILITY
Tablets—25, 50 mg
Vials—50 mg

FUROSEMIDE (Furosemide, Lasix®)

Furosemide is the most widely used loop diuretic. It is useful in the management of edema associated with various cardiac, hepatic, and renal dysfunctions. Furosemide has also been used in the treatment of hypertension, especially in patients with concurrent clinical evidence of fluid overload. Furosemide therapy enhances renal excretion of sodium, chloride, potassium, hydrogen, calcium, magnesium, ammonium, bicarbonate, and possibly phosphate. Its calcium-lowering effect has been utilized, along with normal saline hydration, to increase renal calcium excretion in patients with hypercalcemia.

SPECIAL GROUPS

Race: no differences in response

Children: recommended in infants and children for the management of edema, but not for hypertension

Elderly: use with caution; no dosage adjustment is required

Renal impairment: use with caution; higher doses may be required to enhance diuresis; contraindicated in patients with anuria or progressive oliguric renal failure unresponsive to diuretic therapy

Hepatic impairment: use with caution; titrate dose based on clinical assessment

Pregnancy: category C; use only if potential benefit justifies the potential risk to the fetus

Breast-feeding: not recommended; drug excreted in human milk

IN BRIEF

INDICATIONS
Edema associated with CHF, liver cirrhosis, and renal disease, including the nephrotic syndrome (both adults and children)
Hypertension (adults only)

CONTRAINDICATIONS
Anuria

Increasing electrolyte imbalance, azotemia, and/or oliguria in the setting of severe, progressive renal disease

Known hypersensitivity to furosemide, bumetanide, torsemide, or sulfur

DRUG INTERACTIONS
Antihypertensive agents[1,3]
Cardiac glycosides[3]
Diuretics[1,3]
Lithium[3]
NSAIDs[2]
Non-depolarizing neuromuscular blockers[3,4]
Ototoxic agents (aminoglycosides, erythromycin, cisplatin)[3]
Phenytoin[2]
Potassium-depleting agents (corticosteroids, amphotericin B)[1]
Probenecid[2]
Propranolol[3]
Salicylates[3]
Sucralfate[2]
Sulfonylureas[4]

1 Effect/toxicity of furosemide may increase.
2 Effect of furosemide may decrease.
3 Furosemide may increase the effect/toxicity of this drug.
4 Furosemide may decrease the effect of this drug.

ADVERSE EFFECTS
CV: hypotension, orthostatic symptoms, arrhythmias, chest pain
CNS: dizziness, headache, fatigue, ototoxicity
GI: anorexia, nausea, vomiting, constipation, diarrhea, pancreatitis
GU: sexual dysfunction, polyuria
Hematologic: blood dyscrasias
Kidney: volume and electrolyte depletion ($\downarrow$K, $\downarrow$Cl, $\downarrow$Na, $\downarrow$Ca, $\downarrow$Mg, $\uparrow$uric acid), azotemia, $\uparrow$serum creatinine, interstitial nephritis
Liver: jaundice
Metabolic: metabolic alkalosis, hyperglycemia, dyslipidemia
Skin: rash, pruritus, urticaria, photosensitivity, exfoliative dermatitis, erythema multiforme
Other: dehydration, muscle cramps, fever, vasculitis

PHARMACOKINETICS AND PHARMACODYNAMICS
Duration of action: (po) 6–8 h; (IV) ≥2 h
Onset of action: (po) 30–60 min; (IV) 2–5 min; somewhat later with IM administration
Peak effect: (po) 1–2 h (may take several days for maximal antihypertensive effect); (IV) <30 min
Bioavailability: (po) 60%–70%
Effect of food: may slow down the rate and reduce the amount of absorption
Protein binding: 91%–99%
Volume of distribution: 0.11 L/kg
Metabolism: small amount (10%) metabolized in the liver ($\uparrow$ in renal failure)
Elimination: urine—60%–90% (>50% unchanged); bile/feces—6%–9%
Elimination half-life: 0.5–2 h ($\uparrow$ in renal and/or hepatic dysfunction)

MONITORING
Clinical: BP, urine output, weight, hearing acuity
Lab: serum electrolytes (especially potassium, but also magnesium, calcium, sodium, and chloride), kidney function (BUN, serum creatinine), CO_2, CBC for blood dyscrasias

FUROSEMIDE *(continued)*

DOSAGE (ADULT)

Edema: Oral—The usual initial dose is 20–80 mg given as a single dose. The same dose may be repeated, or increased in 20–40 mg increments every 6–8 h until the desired diuresis is achieved. The effective dose may then be given once or twice daily to maintain adequate fluid balance. For chronic maintenance therapy, furosemide given on alternate days or on 2–4 consecutive days each week is the most effective regimen for fluid mobilization. Up to 600 mg/d has been used in patients with severe fluid overload.

IV/IM—The usual dose is 20–40 mg given as a single injection. The IV route is preferred when rapid diuresis is indicated. The same dose may be repeated, or increased in 20–40 mg increments every 2 h until the desired response is achieved. Each IV dose should be administered over 1–2 min.

Furosemide has been administered as a continuous IV infusion in some patients to maintain adequate urine flow. A bolus of 20–40 mg should be given first, followed by an infusion of 0.25–0.5 mg/min. The rate should be titrated, up to a maximum of 4 mg/min, based on clinical response.

Hypertension: The usual initial dose is 20–40 mg twice daily. Dosage should then be adjusted based on response. The maximum dose is 240 mg/d in 2–3 divided doses.

Higher dosages (480 mg/d in divided doses) may be required for the management of edema or hypertension in patients with renal insufficiency or CHF. These patients should be monitored closely to ensure efficacy and avoid undesired toxicity.

OVERDOSE

Supportive: replace fluid and electrolyte loss. Furosemide is not removed by hemodialysis.

PATIENT INFORMATION

Furosemide is used to reduce excessive water in the body. Take the medication as instructed. Taking the medication earlier in the day may reduce nighttime awakenings to urinate. Avoid excessive dietary sodium intake while on this therapy. Potassium-rich diet is encouraged to avoid potassium depletion. Notify your health care provider if you develop any unusual muscle cramps, nausea, or dizziness. Sit or lie down if dizziness occurs, and rise slowly from a sitting or lying position.

AVAILABILITY

Tablets—20, 40, 80 mg
Ampules/syringes/vials (single dose)—10 mg/mL in 2, 4, 10 mL
Oral solution—8 mg/mL, 10 mg/mL

TORSEMIDE (Demadex®)

Similar to furosemide and bumetanide, torsemide is a sulfonamide-type loop diuretic. It inhibits sodium and chloride reabsorption in the ascending limb of the loop of Henle, which is mainly responsible for its diuretic activity. Torsemide lowers BP via an unknown mechanism of action in low doses (2.5–10 mg/d) that have little diuretic effect. Torsemide is available for oral and IV administration. The absorption is reliable and nearly complete, 80% to 90%, after an oral dose. Oral and IV doses of torsemide are equivalent. After entering the systemic circulation, 80% of torsemide is metabolized in the liver. As a result, there is less drug accumulation in patients with renal failure. This may account for the lower risk of ototoxicity reported with torsemide therapy. It is an effective but relatively more expensive alternative for the management of edema and hypertension.

SPECIAL GROUPS

Race: no differences in response
Children: safety and effectiveness have not been established
Elderly: no dosage adjustment is required
Renal impairment: use with caution; higher doses may be required to enhance diuresis; contraindicated in patients with anuria or progressive oliguric renal failure unresponsive to diuretic therapy
Hepatic impairment: use with caution; titrate dose based on clinical assessment
Pregnancy: category B; should be used only if clearly indicated
Breast-feeding: not recommended; not known if the drug is excreted in human milk

DOSAGE

CHF/chronic renal failure: Usual dose range—10–200 mg/d
The usual initial dose is 10–20 mg once daily via oral or IV administration. If the diuretic response is inadequate, the dose may be doubled until the desired response or the maximum single dose of 200 mg is achieved.

Hepatic cirrhosis: Usual dose range—5–40 mg/d
The usual initial dose is 5–10 mg once daily administered orally or IV along with an aldosterone antagonist or a potassium-sparing diuretic. If the diuretic response is inadequate, the dose may be doubled until the desired response or the maximum single dose of 40 mg is achieved.

Hypertension: Usual dose range—5–10 mg/d
The usual initial dose is 5 mg once daily administered orally. If adequate reduction in BP is not achieved in 4–6 wk, the dose may be increased up to 10 mg once daily. If the response is still inadequate, an additional antihypertensive agent should be added.

IN BRIEF

INDICATIONS
Edema associated with CHF, liver cirrhosis, and renal disease
Hypertension

CONTRAINDICATIONS
Anuria
Increasing electrolyte imbalance, azotemia, and/or oliguria in the setting of severe, progressive renal disease
Known hypersensitivity to torsemide, sulfonylureas, or other sulfur-containing agents

DRUG INTERACTIONS
Antihypertensive agents[1,3]
Cardiac glycosides[3]
Cholestyramine[2]
Diuretics[1,3]
Lithium[3]
NSAIDs[2]
Non-depolarizing neuromuscular blockers[3]
Ototoxic agents (aminoglycosides, erythromycin, cisplatin)[3]
Potassium-depleting agents (corticosteroids, amphotericin B)[1]
Probenecid[2]
Salicylates[3]
Sulfonylureas[4]

1 Effect/toxicity of torsemide may increase.
2 Effect of torsemide may decrease.
3 Torsemide may increase the effect/toxicity of this drug.
4 Torsemide may decrease the effect of this drug.

ADVERSE EFFECTS
CV: hypotension, orthostatic symptoms, arrhythmias, chest pain
CNS: dizziness, headache, fatigue, ototoxicity
GI: anorexia, nausea, vomiting, constipation, diarrhea
GU: sexual dysfunction, polyuria
Kidney: volume and electrolyte depletion ($\downarrow$K, $\downarrow$Cl, $\downarrow$Na, $\downarrow$Ca, $\downarrow$Mg, $\uparrow$uric acid), azotemia, $\uparrow$serum creatinine
Metabolic: metabolic alkalosis, hyperglycemia, dyslipidemia
Skin: rash
Other: dehydration, thirst, arthralgia, angioedema

PHARMACOKINETICS AND PHARMACODYNAMICS
Duration of action: (po/IV) 6–8 h
Onset of action: (po) <1 h; (IV) <10 min
Peak effect: (po) 1–2 h; (IV) <1 h
Bioavailability: 75%–89%
Effect of food: delayed absorption but no effect on bioavailability and diuretic activity
Volume of distribution: 12–15 L
Protein binding: >99%
Metabolism: 80% metabolized in liver
Elimination: renal (20% unchanged)
Elimination half-life: 3.5 h

MONITORING
Clinical: BP, urine output, weight, hearing acuity
Lab: serum electrolytes (especially potassium, but also magnesium, calcium, sodium, and chloride), kidney function (BUN, serum creatinine), CO_2

OVERDOSE
Supportive: replace fluid and electrolyte loss. Torsemide is not removed by hemodialysis.

PATIENT INFORMATION
Torsemide is used to reduce excessive water in the body. Take the medication as instructed. Taking the medication earlier in the day may reduce nighttime awakenings to urinate. Avoid excessive dietary sodium intake while on this therapy. Potassium-rich diet is encouraged to avoid potassium depletion. Notify your health care provider if you develop any unusual muscle cramps, nausea, or dizziness. Sit or lie down if dizziness occurs, and rise slowly from a sitting or lying position.

AVAILABILITY
Tablets—5, 10, 20, 100 mg
Ampules—10 mg/mL in 2 mL and 5 mL

THIAZIDE DIURETICS

Thiazide diuretics remain the most commonly used agents in the initial treatment of essential hypertension and are recognized as the preferred diuretic for this condition. They are very effective in lowering BP in up to 60% of patients with mild-to-moderate essential hypertension. During the first few days after administration, systolic and diastolic pressures are significantly reduced, and this effect is sustained during continued treatment. The longer-acting thiazides and their congeners are distinctly superior to loop diuretics in treating uncomplicated hypertension. In comparative studies, the benzothiazides have been shown to be as effective as other classes of drugs commonly used for the treatment of uncomplicated hypertension. Their effect adds to that of other antihypertensives, especially beta-blockers and angiotensin-converting enzyme (ACE) inhibitors, and to a lesser extent, calcium antagonists.

EFFICACY AND USE

The Medical Research Council (MRC) trial identified several side effects of thiazide diuretics, particularly impotence. The metabolic effects of these drugs (increases in uric acid levels,

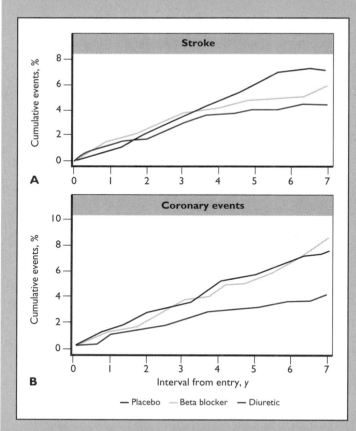

FIGURE 9.2 Cumulative percentage of patients experiencing stroke (**A**) and coronary events (**B**) according to randomized treatment in the Medical Research Council trial of hypertension in older adults. (*Adapted from* Medical Research Council Working Party: MRC trial of treatment of mild hypertension: principal results. *Br Med J* 1985, 291:97–104.)

decreases in serum potassium levels, the appearance of insulin resistance, and changes in the blood lipid profile) are well established. Left ventricular hypertrophy may be reversed, an effect also seen in the Trial of Mild Hypertension Study. The risk of stroke in middle-aged and older patients is significantly reduced (Figure 9.2).

Thiazide diuretics were used as initial therapy in the specially treated group in the Hypertension Detection and Follow-Up Program. Overall death rate fell by 17%, cerebrovascular deaths fell by 45%, and deaths from heart disease fell by 20%, compared with a less aggressively treated group. The Australian Therapeutic Trial in Mild Hypertension demonstrated a significant reduction in cardiovascular events when thiazide diuretics were compared with placebo. In the Oslo Study, however, which compared no active treatment with thiazide diuretic therapy over 10 years, significantly more deaths resulting from myocardial infarction (MI) occurred in the active-treatment group. This finding has led to the suggestion that the metabolic effects of diuretics may reduce the potential benefit derived from the lowering of BP. The MRC showed a beneficial effect with stroke prevention, but failed to detect a benefit with deaths caused by MI (Figure 9.3). In a subsequent analysis, significant increases in MI (Q waves on the ECG, including silent and overt MI) and sudden death were noted in patients treated with diuretics. These findings lend some support to those of the Multiple Risk Factor Intervention Trial.

A study examining the association between thiazide diuretic therapy and the risk of primary cardiac death found a direct correlation between the daily thiazide dose and the risk of primary cardiac arrest in patients with hypertension. Low-dose thiazide treatment and the presence of a potassium-sparing diuretic in the regimen were associated with lower risk as compared with moderate- or high-dose thiazide therapy and the absence of a potassium-sparing component in the regimen.

These findings may partially explain the results of some earlier clinical trials (as mentioned above) in which diuretic therapy was associated with no improvement or an increase in the number of cardiac events.

Any negative findings, however, are often overshadowed by the benefits seen in multiple clinical trials using diuretic therapy for the treatment of hypertension. For example, in the Systolic Hypertension in the Elderly Program of elderly patients with isolated systolic hypertension, treatment with low-dose **chlorthalidone** (12.5–25 mg) was shown to significantly reduce stroke (by 36%), coronary death or MI (by 27%), and CHF (by 55%) at a mean follow-up of 4.5 years compared with placebo.

The Antihypertensive and Lipid-Lowering Treatment to Prevent Heart Attack Trial (ALLHAT) randomized 33,357 patients 55 years of age or older with hypertension and at least one other risk factor for coronary heart disease (CHD) to either **chlorthalidone, amlodipine,** or **lisinopril,** for a

The information here is provided as guidance only. Prescribers should always consult the manufacturer's current prescribing information.

mean follow-up of 4.9 years. The primary outcome of fatal CHD or nonfatal MI was similar among treatment groups, as was all-cause mortality. However, systolic BPs were significantly lower with **chlorthalidone** versus the other two treatments, although diastolic BP was significantly lower with **amlodipine**. Compared with **amlodipine**, **chlorthalidone** therapy resulted in less heart failure, and compared with **lisinopril**, less cardiovascular disease events, stroke, and heart failure. This study further confirmed the role of (thiazide) diuretics as first-line antihypertensive therapy.

The Second Australian National Blood Pressure Study (ANBP2) compared diuretic (mostly **hydrochlorothiazide**) with ACE inhibitor (mostly **enalapril**) therapy in 6083

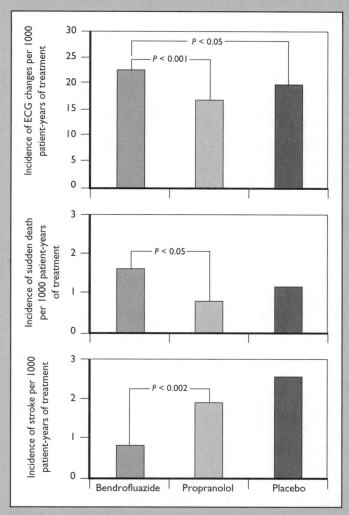

FIGURE 9.3 Close analysis of the Medical Research Council trial showed an increased frequency of infarction, as gauged by abnormalities on the electrocardiogram, after diuretic treatment, and by an increase in the incidence of sudden death compared with beta-blocker treatment. (*Adapted from* Medical Research Council Working Party: MRC trial of treatment of mild hypertension: principal results. *Br Med J* 1985, 291:97–104.)

hypertensive subjects 65 to 84 years of age who were followed for a median of 4.1 years. Despite similar reductions in BP, cardiovascular events or deaths occurred less frequently with ACE inhibitor therapy (11% relative risk reduction; $P = 0.05$). Male patients seemed to derive the most benefit (17% relative risk reduction; $P = 0.02$), whereas event rates in women were similar between groups.

There have been many explanations for the lack of concordance between the ALLHAT and ANBP2 studies; for example, different diuretics and ACE inhibitors were used, add-on antihypertensive therapies used may have confounded the results, and racial demographics were different between studies. The most recent hypertension guidelines (Seventh Report of the Joint National Committee on Prevention, Detection, Evaluation, and Treatment of High Blood Pressure), which included these studies, state that "diuretics have been virtually unsurpassed in preventing the cardiovascular complications of hypertension" and that "thiazide-type diuretics should be used as initial therapy for most patients with hypertension, either alone or in combination with one of the other (drug) classes."

With declining renal function, sodium and water retention become increasingly more difficult to control. In these situations (most clinicians use a creatinine clearance cutoff of <30 mL/min), thiazide diuretics (except **metolazone**) tend to lose their antihypertensive efficacy and the use of a more potent (loop) diuretic is usually required.

MODE OF ACTION

The precise mechanisms that underlie the antihypertensive action of thiazide diuretics have not been defined. As with other diuretics, however, their effect on BP presumably results from their action in producing a negative sodium balance. Thiazide diuretics may have a weak potassium channel–opening action, similar to that of **diazoxide**, and this weak action may cause smooth muscle relaxation and may also explain their diabetogenic effect because of the reverse of the action of glyburide on the pancreatic islet cells. Thiazide diuretics gain access to tubular fluid via the organic secretory pathway in the proximal tubules. During diuresis, in addition to enhanced sodium and chloride excretion, potassium loss is also promoted. Urinary calcium excretion is decreased, in contrast to what is seen with loop diuretics. This decrease may reduce the risk of hip fractures, and thus may benefit elderly patients.

Natriuretic effects of thiazide diuretics last only 3 to 5 days with chronic administration. Sodium concentrations and extracellular fluid volumes remain steady and lower than baseline values thereafter.

The antihypertensive effects of thiazide diuretics may be noted after 3 to 4 days, although up to 3 to 4 weeks may be required for the optimal effect. Antihypertensive effects persist for up to 1 week after therapy withdrawal.

INDICATIONS

	Bendro-flume*	Benz	Chloro	Chlorthal	Hydrochloro	Hydroflum	Indap	Methyclo	Metola	Poly	Quineth	Trichlor
Hypertension	+	+	+	+	+	+	+	+	+	+	+	+
Edema (CHF)	–	+	+	+	+	+	+	+	+	+	+	+
Edema (renal/hepatic disease)	–	+	+	+	+	+	–	+	+†	+	+	+

*No longer available as monotherapy, only available in combination with nadolol.

†Approved only for edema of renal disease.

+—FDA approved; – —not FDA approved; CHF—congestive heart failure; Bendroflume—bendroflumethiazide; Benz—benzthiazide; Chloro—chlorothiazide; Chlorthal—chlorthalidone; Hydrochloro—hydrochlorothiazide; Hydroflum—hydroflumethiazide; Indap—indapamide; Methyclo—methyclothiazide; Metola—metolazone; Poly—polythiazide; Quineth—quinethazone; Trichlor—trichlormethaizide.

BENDROFLUMETHIAZIDE
(Available only in combination with nadolol—Corzide®)

Bendroflumethiazide is a thiazide diuretic. All thiazide diuretics share similar pharmacologic activity and adverse-effect profile when equivalent dosages are employed clinically. In addition to enhancing diuresis, thiazide diuretics are effective antihypertensive agents. Diuresis usually occurs within 2 hours, peaks within 2 to 6 hours, and lasts for 6 to 12 hours or longer. The onset of antihypertensive effect requires several days. Two to 4 weeks are usually required to achieve optimal BP effect for a given dose. The antihypertensive effect persists longer than the diuretic effect after an oral dose, and the effect may last up to 7 days after discontinuing a chronic thiazide diuretic regimen. For more information, please refer to the hydrochlorothiazide monograph.

Bendroflumethiazide alone is no longer available in the United States; it is only available in combination with nadolol (Corzide®) for the treatment of hypertension. The following information pertains only to bendroflumethiazide unless otherwise indicated (eg, under "Dosage"). For more information on nadolol, please refer to the chapter on beta-adrenergic blockers.

SPECIAL GROUPS (BENDROFLUMETHIAZIDE)

Race: no differences in response

Children: safety and effectiveness have not been established

Elderly: use with caution; no dosage adjustment is required

Renal impairment: use with caution; may exacerbate azotemia; contraindicated in anuria. Thiazide diuretics tend to lose efficacy with creatinine clearances <30 mL/min and may be ineffective in severe renal failure.

Hepatic impairment: use with caution; dosage adjustment is probably not required

Pregnancy: category C; use only if potential benefit justifies the potential risk to the fetus

Breast-feeding: use with caution; excreted in human milk in low concentrations

IN BRIEF

INDICATIONS
(Corzide®)
Hypertension

CONTRAINDICATIONS
(Bendroflumethiazide)
Known hypersensitivity to thiazides, other related diuretics, or sulfonamide-derived agents
Anuria or renal decompensation

DRUG INTERACTIONS
(Bendroflumethiazide)
Alcohol[1]
Amphetamines[3]
Antidiabetic agents[4]
Antihypertensive drugs[1,3]
Barbiturates[1]
Cardiac glycosides[3]
Cholestyramine, colestipol[2]
Diuretics[1,3]
Lithium[3]
Narcotics[1]
NSAIDs[2]
Non-depolarizing neuromuscular blockers[3]
Potassium-depleting agents (corticosteroids, amphotericin B)[1]
Quinidine[3]

1 Effect/toxicity of bendroflumethiazide may increase.
2 Effect of bendroflumethiazide may decrease.
3 Bendroflumethiazide may increase the effect/toxicity of this drug.
4 Bendroflumethiazide may decrease the effect of this drug.

ADVERSE EFFECTS
(Bendroflumethiazide)
CV: hypotension, orthostatic symptoms
CNS: dizziness, headache, weakness, vertigo
Hematologic: blood dyscrasias
GI: anorexia, nausea, vomiting, constipation, diarrhea, pancreatitis, cholestatic jaundice, hepatitis
GU: sexual dysfunction, polyuria
Kidney/electrolyte: volume and electrolyte depletion ($\downarrow$K, $\downarrow$Cl, $\downarrow$Na, $\downarrow$Mg, $\uparrow$Ca, $\uparrow$uric acid), dilutional hyponatremia, azotemia, $\uparrow$serum creatinine
Metabolic: metabolic alkalosis, hyperglycemia, hyperuricemia, hypercholesterolemia
Skin: rash, purpura, urticaria, photosensitivity, exfoliative dermatitis
Other: dehydration, muscle cramps, allergic reaction

PHARMACOKINETICS AND PHARMACODYNAMICS
(Bendroflumethiazide)
Duration of action: 6–12 h
Onset of action: 2 h
Peak effect: 4 h
Bioavailability: 100%
Effect of food: not known
Protein binding: not known
Volume of distribution: not known
Metabolism: not metabolized
Elimination: mainly excreted unchanged in the urine
Elimination half-life: 3–4 h

MONITORING
(Bendroflumethiazide)
Clinical: BP, urine output, weight
Lab: serum electrolytes (especially potassium, but also magnesium, calcium, sodium, and chloride), kidney function (BUN, serum creatinine), CO_2

OVERDOSE
Supportive: replace fluid and electrolyte loss. Dialysis is unlikely to be effective.

The information here is provided as guidance only. Prescribers should always consult the manufacturer's current prescribing information.

227

BENDROFLUMETHIAZIDE
(continued)

DOSAGE (CORZIDE®)

Hypertension: Initial dose—5 mg bendroflumethiazide + 40 mg nadolol once daily, eventually increasing to 5 mg/80 mg once daily if desired.

When switching from bendroflumethiazide monotherapy to Corzide®, keep in mind that this represents a 30% increase in bendroflumethiazide dose as a result of increased bioavailability.

Dosing with renal insufficiency:

Creatinine clearance, mL/min/1.73 m^2	Dosing interval
>50	q 24 h
31–50	q 24–36 h
10–30	q 24–48 h
<10	q 40–60 h

PATIENT INFORMATION
(Corzide®)

Corzide® is used to lower blood pressure. Take this medication as instructed. This medication may cause your body to lose potassium. Notify your health care provider if you develop any unusual muscle cramps, nausea, or dizziness. Sit or lie down if dizziness occurs, and rise slowly from a sitting or lying position. Take with food to minimize gastrointestinal side effects. This therapy should not be discontinued abruptly without consulting your health care provider. Your health care provider should also be consulted for persistent or unusual problems, such as dizziness/faintness, weight gain, worsening edema, or increasing shortness of breath. This medication may cause dizziness or drowsiness; use caution if performing activities requiring mental or physical effort.

AVAILABILITY

Combination formulations:
Corzide® 80/5—bendroflumethiazide 5 mg/nadolol 80 mg
Corzide® 40/5—bendroflumethiazide 5 mg/nadolol 40 mg

BENZTHIAZIDE (Exna®)

Note: Benzthiazide is no longer commercially available in the United States. Benzthiazide is a thiazide diuretic. All thiazide diuretics share similar pharmacologic activity and adverse-effect profile when equivalent dosages are employed clinically. In addition to enhancing diuresis, thiazide diuretics are effective antihypertensive agents. Diuresis usually occurs within 2 hours, peaks within 4 to 6 hours, and lasts for 16 to 18 hours or longer. The onset of antihypertensive effect requires several days. Two to 4 weeks are usually required to achieve optimal BP effect for a given dose. The antihypertensive effect persists longer than the diuretic effect after an oral dose, and the effect may last up to 7 days after discontinuing a chronic thiazide diuretic regimen. For more information, please refer to the hydrochlorothiazide monograph.

SPECIAL GROUPS

Race: no differences in response, although blacks tend to have better BP response to diuretic monotherapy compared with ACE inhibitor, angiotensin-receptor blocker or beta-blocker monotherapy

Children: safety and effectiveness have not been established

Elderly: use with caution; no dosage adjustment is required

Renal impairment: use with caution; may exacerbate azotemia; contraindicated in anuria. Thiazide diuretics tend to lose efficacy with creatinine clearances <30 mL/min and may be ineffective in severe renal failure.

Hepatic impairment: use with caution; dosage adjustment is probably not required

Pregnancy: category C; use only if potential benefit justifies the potential risk to the fetus

Breast-feeding: use with caution; excreted in human milk in low concentrations

DOSAGE

Edema: Initial dose—50–200 mg/d administered in 1–2 doses for a few days until the desired diuresis/weight is achieved (for dosages above 100 mg/d, divide and administer in 2 doses after morning and evening meal)

Maintenance—50–150 mg/d; intermittent therapy may be more effective and safer; in this situation, give the dose every other day or on a 3–5 d/wk schedule

Hypertension: Initial dose—25–50 mg twice daily after breakfast and lunch

Maintenance—up to 100 mg twice daily

IN BRIEF

INDICATIONS
Hypertension
Edema

CONTRAINDICATIONS
Known hypersensitivity to thiazides, other related diuretics, sulfonamide-derived agents, or tartrazine
Anuria or renal decompensation

DRUG INTERACTIONS

Alcohol[1]	Lithium[3]
Amphetamines[3]	Narcotics[1]
Antidiabetic agents[4]	NSAIDs[2]
Antihypertensive drugs[1,3]	Non-depolarizing neuromuscular
Barbiturates[1]	blockers[3]
Cardiac glycosides[3]	Potassium-depleting agents
Cholestyramine, colestipol[2]	(corticosteroids, amphotericin B)[1]
Diuretics[1,3]	Quinidine[3]

1 Effect/toxicity of benzthiazide may increase.
2 Effect of benzthiazide may decrease.
3 Benzthiazide may increase the effect/toxicity of this drug.
4 Benzthiazide may decrease the effect of this drug.

ADVERSE EFFECTS
CV: hypotension, orthostatic symptoms
CNS: dizziness, headache, fatigue, weakness
Hematologic: blood dyscrasias
GI: anorexia, nausea, vomiting, constipation, diarrhea, pancreatitis, cholestatic jaundice
GU: sexual dysfunction, polyuria
Kidney/electrolyte: volume and electrolyte depletion ($\downarrow$K, $\downarrow$Cl, $\star$Na, $\downarrow$Mg, $\uparrow$Ca, $\uparrow$uric acid), dilutional hyponatremia, azotemia, $\uparrow$serum creatinine
Metabolic: metabolic alkalosis, hyperglycemia, hyperuricemia, hypercholesterolemia
Skin: rash, purpura, urticaria, photosensitivity
Other: dehydration, muscle cramps, allergic reaction

PHARMACOKINETICS AND PHARMACODYNAMICS
Duration of action: 16–18 h
Onset of action: 2 h
Peak effect: 4–6 h
Bioavailability: 25% or less
Effect of food: not known
Protein binding: not known
Volume of distribution: not known
Metabolism: not fully defined
Elimination: partially cleared renally as unchanged drug
Elimination half-life: not known

MONITORING
Clinical: BP, urine output, weight
Lab: serum electrolytes (especially potassium, but also magnesium, calcium, sodium, and chloride), kidney function (BUN, serum creatinine), CO_2

OVERDOSE
Supportive: replace fluid and electrolyte loss. Dialysis is unlikely to be effective.

PATIENT INFORMATION
Benzthiazide is used to lower blood pressure and reduce excessive water in the body. Take this medication as instructed. This medication may cause your body to lose potassium. Notify your health care provider if you develop any unusual muscle cramps, nausea, or dizziness. Sit or lie down if dizziness occurs, and rise slowly from a sitting or lying position. Take with food to minimize gastrointestinal side effects.

AVAILABILITY
Tablets—50 mg

CHLOROTHIAZIDE
(Chlorothiazide, Diuril®, Diurigen®, various generics)

Chlorothiazide is the only thiazide diuretic available in both oral and IV formulations in the United States. All thiazide diuretics share similar pharmacologic activity and adverse-effect profile when equivalent dosages are employed clinically. In addition to enhancing diuresis, thiazide diuretics are effective antihypertensive agents. Diuresis usually occurs within 2 hours, peaks within 2 to 6 hours, and lasts for 6 to 12 hours or longer. The onset of antihypertensive effect requires several days. Two to 4 weeks are usually required to achieve optimal BP effect for a given dose. The antihypertensive effect persists longer than the diuretic effect after an oral dose, and the effect may last up to 7 days after discontinuing a chronic thiazide diuretic regimen. For more information, please refer to the hydrochlorothiazide monograph.

SPECIAL GROUPS

Race: no differences in response, although blacks tend to have better BP response to diuretic monotherapy compared with ACE inhibitor, angiotensin-receptor blocker or beta-blocker monotherapy

Children: only oral administration is indicated; IV use is not recommended

Elderly: use with caution; no dosage adjustment is required

Renal impairment: use with caution; may exacerbate azotemia; contraindicated in anuria. Thiazide diuretics tend to lose efficacy with creatinine clearances <30 mL/min and may be ineffective in severe renal failure.

Hepatic impairment: use with caution; dosage adjustment is probably not required

Pregnancy: category B; should be used only if clearly indicated

Breast-feeding: use with caution; excreted in human milk in low concentrations

IN BRIEF

INDICATIONS
Hypertension
Edema

CONTRAINDICATIONS
Known hypersensitivity to thiazides, other related diuretics, or sulfonamide-derived agents
Anuria or renal decompensation

DRUG INTERACTIONS
Alcohol[1]
Amphetamines[3]
Antidiabetic agents[4]
Antihypertensive drugs[1,3]
Barbiturates[1]
Cardiac glycosides[3]
Cholestyramine, colestipol[2]
Diuretics[1,3]
Lithium[3]
Narcotics[1]
NSAIDs[2]
Non-depolarizing neuromuscular blockers[3]
Potassium-depleting agents (corticosteroids, amphotericin B)[1]
Quinidine[3]
[1] Effect/toxicity of chlorothiazide may increase.
[2] Effect of chlorothiazide may decrease.
[3] Chlorothiazide may increase the effect/toxicity of this drug.
[4] Chlorothiazide may decrease the effect of this drug.

ADVERSE EFFECTS
CV: hypotension, orthostatic symptoms
CNS: dizziness, headache, fatigue, vertigo
Hematologic: blood dyscrasias
GI: anorexia, nausea, vomiting, constipation, diarrhea, pancreatitis, cholestatic jaundice
GU: sexual dysfunction, polyuria
Kidney/electrolyte: volume and electrolyte depletion ($\downarrow$K, $\downarrow$Cl, $\downarrow$Na, $\downarrow$Mg, $\uparrow$Ca, $\uparrow$uric acid), dilutional hyponatremia, azotemia, $\uparrow$serum creatinine, interstitial nephritis
Metabolic: metabolic alkalosis, hyperglycemia, hyperuricemia, hypercholesterolemia
Skin: rash, purpura, urticaria, photosensitivity, exfoliative dermatitis (IV formulation), erythema multiforme (IV formulation)
Other: dehydration, muscle cramps, allergic reaction

PHARMACOKINETICS AND PHARMACODYNAMICS
Duration of action: 6–12 h
Onset of action: (po) 2 h; (IV) 15 min
Peak effect: (po) 4 h; (IV) 30 min
Bioavailability: 10%–20%
Protein binding: 95%
Volume of distribution: 0.2 L/kg
Effect of food: increases absorption (doubled)
Metabolism: not metabolized; excreted unchanged in the urine
Elimination: mainly cleared renally as unchanged drug (96% after an IV dose; only 10%–15% after an oral dose because of the low bioavailability)
Elimination half-life: 45–120 min

MONITORING
Clinical: BP, urine output, weight
Lab: serum electrolytes (especially potassium, but also magnesium, calcium, sodium, and chloride), kidney function (BUN, serum creatinine), CO_2

OVERDOSE
Supportive: replace fluid and electrolyte loss. Dialysis is unlikely to be effective.

CHLOROTHIAZIDE *(continued)*

DOSAGE

Edema: Adults—500–1000 mg once daily in the morning or twice daily, administered orally or IV (only for patients who are unable to take oral medication or for emergency)

Intermittent therapy may be safer and more effective; in this situation, give the dose every other day or on a 3–5 d/wk schedule.

Hypertension: Adults—500–1000 mg/d in 1–2 divided doses initially, titrated based on response up to 2 g/d in divided doses

CHLORTHALIDONE
(Chlorthalidone, Hygroton®, Thalitone®)

Chlorthalidone is a thiazide diuretic. All thiazide diuretics share similar pharmacologic activity and adverse-effect profile when equivalent dosages are employed clinically. In addition to enhancing diuresis, thiazide diuretics are effective antihypertensive agents. Diuresis usually occurs within 2 hours, peaks within 2 to 6 hours, and lasts for 24 to 72 hours or longer. The onset of antihypertensive effect requires several days. Two to 4 weeks are usually required to achieve optimal BP effect for a given dose. The antihypertensive effect persists longer than the diuretic effect after an oral dose, and the effect may last up to 7 days after discontinuing a chronic thiazide diuretic regimen. For more information, please refer to the hydrochlorothiazide monograph.

The ALLHAT study randomized 33,357 patients 55 years of age or older with hypertension and at least one other risk factor for CHD to either chlorthalidone, amlodipine, or lisinopril, for a mean follow-up of 4.9 years. The primary outcome of fatal CHD or nonfatal MI was similar among treatment groups, as was all-cause mortality. However, systolic BPs were significantly lower with chlorthalidone versus the other two treatments, although diastolic BP was significantly lower with amlodipine. Compared with amlodipine, chlorthalidone therapy resulted in less heart failure, and compared with lisinopril, less cardiovascular disease events, strokes, and heart failure.

SPECIAL GROUPS

Race: no differences in response, although blacks tend to have better BP response to diuretic monotherapy compared with ACE inhibitor, angiotensin-receptor blocker, or beta-blocker monotherapy.

Children: safety and effectiveness have not been established, although chlorthalidone has been used safely and effectively in children.

Elderly: use with caution; no dosage adjustment is required

Renal impairment: use with caution; may exacerbate azotemia; contraindicated in anuria. Thiazide diuretics tend to lose efficacy with creatinine clearances <30 mL/min, and may be ineffective in severe renal failure.

Hepatic impairment: use with caution; dosage adjustment is probably not required

Pregnancy: category B; should only be used if clearly indicated

Breast-feeding: not recommended; excreted in human milk with significant concentrations reported

IN BRIEF

INDICATIONS
Hypertension
Edema

CONTRAINDICATIONS
Known hypersensitivity to thiazides, other related diuretics, or sulfonamide-derived agents
Anuria or renal decompensation

DRUG INTERACTIONS
Alcohol[1]
Amphetamines[3]
Antidiabetic agents[4]
Antihypertensive drugs[1,3]
Barbiturates[1]
Cardiac glycosides[3]
Cholestyramine, colestipol[2]
Diuretics[1,3]
Lithium[3]
Narcotics[1]
NSAIDs[2]
Non-depolarizing neuromuscular blockers[3]
Potassium-depleting agents (corticosteroids, amphotericin B)[1]
Quinidine[3]

1 Effect/toxicity of chlorthalidone may increase.
2 Effect of chlorthalidone may decrease.
3 Chlorthalidone may increase the effect/toxicity of this drug.
4 Chlorthalidone may decrease the effect of this drug.

ADVERSE EFFECTS
CV: hypotension, orthostatic symptoms
CNS: dizziness, headache, fatigue, vertigo
Hematologic: blood dyscrasias
GI: anorexia, nausea, vomiting, constipation, diarrhea, pancreatitis, cholestatic jaundice
GU: sexual dysfunction, polyuria
Kidney/electrolyte: volume and electrolyte depletion ($\downarrow$K, $\downarrow$Cl, $\downarrow$Na, $\downarrow$Mg, $\uparrow$Ca, $\uparrow$uric acid), dilutional hyponatremia, azotemia, $\uparrow$serum creatinine
Metabolic: metabolic alkalosis, hyperglycemia, hyperuricemia, hypercholesterolemia
Skin: rash, purpura, urticaria, photosensitivity, exfoliative dermatitis
Other: dehydration, muscle cramps, allergic reaction

PHARMACOKINETICS AND PHARMACODYNAMICS
Duration of action: up to 72 h
Onset of action: 2–3 h
Peak effect: 2–6 h
Bioavailability: 65% (104%–116% with Thalitone® compared with oral solution)
Effect of food: not known
Protein binding: 75%
Volume of distribution: 0.1 L/kg
Metabolism: hepatic
Elimination: 50%–74% cleared renally as unchanged drug
Elimination half-life: 40–60 h

MONITORING
Clinical: BP, urine output, weight
Lab: serum electrolytes (especially potassium, but also magnesium, calcium, sodium, and chloride), kidney function (BUN, serum creatinine), CO_2

OVERDOSE
Supportive: replace fluid and electrolyte loss. Dialysis is unlikely to be effective.

CHLORTHALIDONE (continued)

DOSAGE

Edema: Usual dose—50–100 mg (30–60 mg Thalitone®)/d administered as a single dose with breakfast; alternatively, 100 mg (60 mg Thalitone®) may be given every other day. Dosage may be gradually increased up to 200 mg (120 mg Thalitone®) once daily if indicated until the desired diuresis/weight is achieved.

Intermittent therapy may be safer and more effective and is performed by giving the dose every other day or 3–5 d/wk.

Hypertension: Usual dose*—25 mg (15 mg Thalitone®) once daily with breakfast; dosage may be gradually increased up to 100 mg (50 mg Thalitone®) once daily if indicated

*Dosages above 25 mg/d are likely to potentiate potassium waste, but provide no further benefit in BP reduction.

PATIENT INFORMATION

Chlorthalidone is used to lower blood pressure and reduce excessive water in the body. Take this medication as instructed. This medication may cause your body to lose potassium. Notify your health care provider if you develop any unusual muscle cramps, nausea, or dizziness. Sit or lie down if dizziness occurs, and rise slowly from a sitting or lying position. Take with food to minimize gastrointestinal side effects.

AVAILABILITY

Tablets (Thalitone®)—15, 25 mg
Tablets (Chlorthalidone, Hygroton®)—25, 50, 100 mg
Combination formulations:
  Combipres® 0.1, 0.2, and 0.3 tablets; various generics—
    Chlorthalidone 15 mg/clonidine 0.1 mg
    Chlorthalidone 15 mg/clonidine 0.2 mg
    Chlorthalidone 15 mg/clonidine 0.3 mg
  Tenoretic® 50 and 100 tablets; various generics—
    Chlorthalidone 25 mg/atenolol 50 mg
    Chlorthalidone 25 mg/atenolol 100 mg
  Regroton® tablets—
    Chlorthalidone 50 mg/reserpine 0.25 mg
  Demi-Regroton® tablets—
    Chlorthalidone 25 mg/reserpine 0.125 mg

HYDROCHLOROTHIAZIDE
(HydroDiuril®; various other brands and generics)

Hydrochlorothiazide (HCTZ) is the most widely used thiazide diuretic in the United States. Thiazide diuretics act primarily by blocking sodium and chloride reabsorption, therefore blocking water reabsorption, in the cortical thick ascending limb of the loop of Henle and the early distal renal tubule. The natriuretic effect of thiazide diuretics is determined by the amount of sodium reaching the distal renal tubule. Sodium delivery to the site is compromised in patients with severe renal dysfunction (ie, with serum creatinine or BUN concentrations greater than about twice normal), CHF, or liver cirrhosis. As a result, thiazide and thiazide-like diuretics (except metolazone) may not be effective in enhancing diuresis in these patients, and a more potent diuretic (ie, loop) may be required. Thiazide diuretics themselves have an antihypertensive effect and work synergistically with other antihypertensive agents as well. Although the exact antihypertensive mechanism is not clear, both direct arteriolar dilation and sodium depletion seem to contribute to the BP-lowering effect.

HCTZ is available alone and in combination with different antihypertensive agents for the management of hypertension. When used alone, BP reduction is usually observed after 3 to 4 days of therapy, which lags behind its diuretic effect. Although the diuretic effect occurs within 2 hours after an oral dose and may last for 6 to 12 hours, the antihypertensive effect may last up to 7 days after discontinuing chronic HCTZ therapy.

SPECIAL GROUPS

Race: no differences in response, although blacks tend to have better BP response to diuretic monotherapy compared with ACE inhibitor, angiotensin-receptor blocker, or beta-blocker monotherapy

Children: HCTZ has been used safely and effectively in infants and children; dose based on weight or body surface area and clinical response

Elderly: use with caution; no dosage adjustment is required

Renal impairment: use with caution; may exacerbate azotemia; contraindicated in anuria. Thiazide diuretics tend to lose efficacy with creatinine clearances <30 mL/min, and may be ineffective in severe renal failure.

Hepatic impairment: use with caution; dosage adjustment is probably not required

Pregnancy: category B; should be used only if clearly indicated

Breast-feeding: use not recommended; excreted in human milk, although in low concentrations

IN BRIEF

INDICATIONS
Hypertension
Edema

CONTRAINDICATIONS
Known hypersensitivity to thiazides, other related diuretics, sulfonamide-derived agents, or sulfites (some products contain sulfites)
Anuria or renal decompensation

DRUG INTERACTIONS
Alcohol[1]
Amphetamines[3]
Antidiabetic agents[4]
Antihypertensive drugs[1,3]
Barbiturates[1]
Cardiac glycosides[3]
Cholestyramine, colestipol[2]
Diuretics[1,3]
Lithium[3]
Narcotics[1]
NSAIDs[2]
Non-depolarizing neuromuscular blockers[3]
Potassium-depleting agents (corticosteroids, amphotericin B)[1]
Quinidine[3]

1 Effect/toxicity of HCTZ may increase.
2 Effect of HCTZ may decrease.
3 HCTZ may increase the effect/toxicity of this drug.
4 HCTZ may decrease the effect of this drug.

ADVERSE EFFECTS
CV: hypotension, orthostatic symptoms
CNS: dizziness, headache, fatigue, vertigo
Hematologic: blood dyscrasias
GI: anorexia, nausea, vomiting, constipation, diarrhea, pancreatitis, cholestatic jaundice
GU: sexual dysfunction, polyuria
Kidney/electrolyte: volume and electrolyte depletion ($\downarrow$K, $\downarrow$Cl, $\downarrow$Na, $\downarrow$Mg, $\uparrow$Ca, $\uparrow$uric acid), dilutional hyponatremia, azotemia, $\uparrow$serum creatinine, interstitial nephritis
Metabolic: metabolic alkalosis, hyperglycemia, hyperuricemia, hypercholesterolemia
Skin: rash, purpura, urticaria, photosensitivity, exfoliative dermatitis, erythema multiforme
Other: dehydration, muscle cramps, allergic reaction

PHARMACOKINETICS AND PHARMACODYNAMICS
Duration of action: 6–12 h (up to a week for hypotensive effect)
Onset of action: 2 h
Peak effect: 4–6 h
Bioavailability: 65%–75%
Effect of food: reduced plasma levels
Protein binding: 58%
Volume of distribution: 0.83 L/kg
Metabolism: not metabolized, eliminated rapidly by the kidney
Elimination: mainly (>95%) in the urine as unchanged drug
Elimination half-life: 6–15 h ($\uparrow$ in heart or renal failure)

MONITORING
Clinical: BP, urine output, weight
Lab: serum electrolytes (especially potassium, but also magnesium, calcium, sodium, and chloride), kidney function (BUN, serum creatinine), CO_2

OVERDOSE
Supportive: replace fluid and electrolyte loss. Dialysis is unlikely to be effective.

HYDROCHLOROTHIAZIDE
(continued)

DOSAGE

Edema: Initial dose—25–200 mg/d administered in 1–3 divided doses for a few days until the desired diuresis/weight is achieved Maintenance—25–100 mg/d in single or divided doses*; intermittent therapy may be more efficacious and safer and is performed by giving the dose every other day or on a 3–5 d/wk schedule

Hypertension: Initial dose—12.5–25 mg once daily in the morning Maintenance*—up to 50 mg once daily in the morning

Use with other antihypertensives: Use lowest effective dose; most patients do not require more than 50 mg/d.

*Higher doses have been used, but the benefits should be assessed carefully against the potential risks of high-dose diuretic therapy.

PATIENT INFORMATION

HCTZ is used to lower BP and reduce excessive water in the body. Take this medication as instructed. This medication may cause your body to lose potassium. Notify your health care provider if you develop any unusual muscle cramps, nausea, or dizziness. Sit or lie down if dizziness occurs, and rise slowly from a sitting or lying position. Take with food to minimize gastrointestinal side effects.

AVAILABILITY

Tablets—25, 50, 100 mg
Solution—50 mg/5 mL
Capsules—12.5 mg
Combination formulations:
  Various generics—
    HCTZ 50 mg/reserpine 0.125 mg tablets
    HCTZ 25 mg/reserpine 0.125 mg tablets
  Hydrap-ES®, Marpres®, Ser-Ap-Es®, Tri-Hydroserpine® tablets—
    HCTZ 15 mg/reserpine 0.1 mg/hydralazine 25 mg
  Apresazide® capsules and various generics—
    HCTZ 50 mg/hydralazine 100 mg
    HCTZ 50 mg/hydralazine 50 mg
    HCTZ 25 mg/hydralazine 25 mg
  Ziac® tablets—
    HCTZ 6.25 mg/bisoprolol 2.5 mg
    HCTZ 6.25 mg/bisoprolol 5 mg
    HCTZ 6.25 mg/bisoprolol 10 mg
  Timolide 10-25® tablets—
    HCTZ 25 mg/timolol 10 mg
  Inderide LA® 160/50, 120/50, and 80/50 capsules—
    HCTZ 50 mg/propranolol 160 mg
    HCTZ 50 mg/propranolol 120 mg
    HCTZ 50 mg/propranolol 80 mg
  Inderide® tablets and various generics—
    HCTZ 25 mg/propranolol 80 mg
    HCTZ 25 mg/propranolol 40 mg
  Aldoril® tablets and various generics—
    HCTZ 50 mg/methyldopa 500 mg
    HCTZ 30 mg/methyldopa 500 mg
    HCTZ 25 mg/methyldopa 250 mg
    HCTZ 15 mg/methyldopa 250 mg
  Lopressor HCT® 100/50, 100/25, and 50/25 tablets—
    HCTZ 50 mg/metoprolol 100 mg
    HCTZ 25 mg/metoprolol 100 mg
    HCTZ 25 mg/metoprolol 50 mg
  Capozide® 50/25, 25/25, 50/15, and 25/15 tablets—
    HCTZ 25 mg/captopril 50 mg
    HCTZ 25 mg/captopril 25 mg
    HCTZ 15 mg/captopril 50 mg
    HCTZ 15 mg/captopril 25 mg
  Lotensin HCT® 20/25, 20/12.5, 10/12.5, and 5/6.25 tablets—
    HCTZ 25 mg/benazepril 20 mg
    HCTZ 12.5 mg/benazepril 20 mg
    HCTZ 12.5 mg/benazepril 10 mg
    HCTZ 6.25 mg/benazepril 5 mg
  Avalide® tablets—
    HCTZ 12.5 mg/irbesartan 150 mg
    HCTZ 12.5 mg/irbesartan 300 mg
  Vaseretic® 10-25, 5-12.5 tablets—
    HCTZ 25 mg/enalapril 10 mg
    HCTZ 12.5 mg/enalapril 5 mg
  Prinzide® and Zestoretic® tablets—
    HCTZ 12.5 mg/lisinopril 10 mg
    HCTZ 25 mg/lisinopril 20 mg
    HCTZ 12.5 mg/lisinopril 20 mg
  Esimil® tablets—
    HCTZ 25 mg/guanethidine 10 mg
  Hyzaar® tablets—
    HCTZ 12.5 mg/losartan 50 mg
    HCTZ 25 mg/losartan 100 mg
  Uniretic® tablets—
    HCTZ 12.5 mg/moexipril 7.5 mg
    HCTZ 25 mg/moexipril 15 mg
  Diovan HCT® tablets—
    HCTZ 12.5 mg/valsartan 80 mg
    HCTZ 12.5 mg/valsartan 160 mg

HYDROFLUMETHIAZIDE
(Hydroflumethiazide, Diucardin®, Saluron®)

Hydroflumethiazide is a thiazide diuretic. All thiazide diuretics share similar pharmacologic activity and adverse-effect profile when equivalent dosages are employed clinically. In addition to enhancing diuresis, thiazide diuretics are effective antihypertensive agents. Diuresis usually occurs within 2 hours, peaks within 2 to 6 hours, and lasts for 6 to 12 hours or longer. The onset of antihypertensive effect requires several days. Two to 4 weeks are usually required to achieve optimal BP effect for a given dose. The antihypertensive effect persists longer than the diuretic effect after an oral dose, and the effect may last up to 7 days after discontinuing a chronic thiazide diuretic regimen. For more information, please refer to the hydrochlorothiazide monograph.

SPECIAL GROUPS

Race: no differences in response, although blacks tend to have better BP response to diuretic monotherapy compared with ACE inhibitor, angiotensin-receptor blocker, or beta-blocker monotherapy.

Children: safety and effectiveness have not been established

Elderly: use with caution; no dosage adjustment is required

Renal impairment: use with caution; may exacerbate azotemia; contraindicated in anuria. Thiazide diuretics tend to lose efficacy with creatinine clearances <30 mL/min and may be ineffective in severe renal failure.

Hepatic impairment: use with caution; dosage adjustment is probably not required

Pregnancy: category C; use only if potential benefit justifies the potential risk to the fetus

Breast-feeding: not recommended; excreted in human milk, although in low concentrations

DOSAGE

Edema: Usual dose range—25–200 mg/d once daily in the morning, or given in two divided doses.
For dosages above 100 mg/d, divide and administer in 2 doses. Intermittent therapy may be safer and more effective, and is performed by giving the dose every other day or on a 3–5 d/wk schedule.

Hypertension: Usual dose range—25–100 mg/d once daily in the morning, or given in 2 divided doses. Do not exceed 200 mg/d.

IN BRIEF

INDICATIONS
Hypertension
Edema

CONTRAINDICATIONS
Known hypersensitivity to thiazides, other related diuretics, or sulfonamide-derived agents
Anuria or renal decompensation

DRUG INTERACTIONS
Alcohol[1]
Amphetamines[3]
Antidiabetic agents[4]
Antihypertensive drugs[1,3]
Barbiturates[1]
Cardiac glycosides[3]
Cholestyramine, colestipol[2]
Diuretics[1,3]
Lithium[3]
Narcotics[1]
NSAIDs[2]
Non-depolarizing neuromuscular blockers[3]
Potassium-depleting agents (corticosteroids, amphotericin B)[1]
Quinidine[3]

1 Effect/toxicity of hydroflumethiazide may increase.
2 Effect of hydroflumethiazide may decrease.
3 Hydroflumethiazide may increase the effect/toxicity of this drug.
4 Hydroflumethiazide may decrease the effect of this drug.

ADVERSE EFFECTS
CV: hypotension, orthostatic symptoms
CNS: dizziness, headache, fatigue, vertigo
Hematologic: blood dyscrasias
GI: anorexia, nausea, vomiting, constipation, diarrhea, pancreatitis, cholestatic jaundice
GU: sexual dysfunction, polyuria
Kidney/electrolyte: volume and electrolyte depletion ($\downarrow$K, $\downarrow$Cl, $\downarrow$Na, $\downarrow$Mg, $\uparrow$Ca, $\uparrow$uric acid), dilutional hyponatremia, azotemia, $\uparrow$serum creatinine
Metabolic: metabolic alkalosis, hyperglycemia, hyperuricemia, hypercholesterolemia
Skin: rash, purpura, urticaria, photosensitivity
Other: dehydration, muscle cramps, allergic reaction

PHARMACOKINETICS AND PHARMACODYNAMICS
Duration of action: 6–12 h
Onset of action: <2 h
Peak effect: 4 h
Bioavailability: 50%
Effect of food: not known
Protein binding: not known
Volume of distribution: not known
Metabolism: not known
Elimination: mainly excreted in the urine
Elimination half-life: 17 h

MONITORING
Clinical: BP, urine output, weight
Lab: serum electrolytes (especially potassium, but also magnesium, calcium, sodium, and chloride), kidney function (BUN, serum creatinine), CO_2

OVERDOSE
Supportive: replace fluid and electrolyte loss. Dialysis is unlikely to be effective.

PATIENT INFORMATION
Hydroflumethiazide is used to lower blood pressure and reduce excessive water in the body. Take this medication as instructed. This medication may cause your body to lose potassium. Notify your health care provider if you develop any unusual muscle cramps, nausea, or dizziness. Sit or lie down if dizziness occurs, and rise slowly from a sitting or lying position. Take with food to minimize gastrointestinal side effects.

AVAILABILITY
Tablets—50 mg
Combination formulations:
Salutensin® tablets—
Hydroflumethiazide 50 mg/reserpine 0.125 mg

INDAPAMIDE (Indapamide, Lozol®)

Indapamide, a methylindoline derivative, is a sulfonamide diuretic. Although structurally different from thiazide diuretics, it has similar pharmacologic activity. Indapamide lowers BP in hypertensive patients via an unclear mechanism. It reduces BP probably by reducing plasma and extracellular fluid volume, by decreasing peripheral vascular resistance, and by causing direct arteriolar dilation. Indapamide acts synergistically with other antihypertensive agents. Similar to thiazide diuretics, the diuretic effect of indapamide diminishes as renal function declines. However, the hypotensive effect remains in patients with an estimated creatinine clearance above 15 mL/min. Different from thiazide diuretics, indapamide has less of an adverse effect on serum levels of triglyceride, total cholesterol, low-density lipoprotein, very low-density lipoprotein, and high-density lipoprotein. The clinical significance of these differences is not known. As a general rule, thiazide-induced mild changes in serum lipid profile can be managed by a diet low in saturated fat and cholesterol. For more information, please refer to the hydrochlorothiazide monograph.

SPECIAL GROUPS

Race: no differences in response, although blacks tend to have better BP response to diuretic monotherapy compared with ACE inhibitor, angiotensin-receptor blocker, or beta-blocker monotherapy.

Children: safety and effectiveness have not been established

Elderly: use with caution; no dosage adjustment is required

Renal impairment: use with caution; may exacerbate azotemia; contraindicated in anuria. Dosage adjustment is not necessary. May be more effective than other thiazides (except metolazone) in patients with renal insufficiency.

Hepatic impairment: use with caution; dosage adjustment may be required

Pregnancy: category B; should be used only if clearly indicated

Breast-feeding: not recommended; not known if the drug is excreted in human milk

DOSAGE

Edema: Usual dose range—2.5–5 mg once daily in the morning

Hypertension: Usual dose range—1.25–5 mg once daily in the morning. Start with 1.25 mg once daily and double as needed every 4 weeks up to 5 mg once daily.

IN BRIEF

INDICATIONS
Hypertension
Edema associated with heart failure

CONTRAINDICATIONS
Known hypersensitivity to thiazides, other related diuretics, or sulfonamide-derived agents
Anuria or renal decompensation

DRUG INTERACTIONS
Alcohol[1]	Lithium[3]
Amphetamines[3]	Narcotics[1]
Antidiabetic agents[4]	NSAIDs[2]
Antihypertensive drugs[1,3]	Non-depolarizing neuromuscular
Barbiturates[1]	blockers[3]
Cardiac glycosides[3]	Potassium-depleting agents
Cholestyramine, colestipol[2]	(corticosteroids, amphotericin B)[1]
Diuretics[1,3]	Quinidine[3]

1 Effect/toxicity of indapamide may increase.
2 Effect of indapamide may decrease.
3 Indapamide may increase the effect/toxicity of this drug.
4 Indapamide may decrease the effect of this drug.

ADVERSE EFFECTS
CV: hypotension, orthostatic symptoms
CNS: dizziness, headache, fatigue, vertigo
GI: anorexia, nausea, vomiting, constipation, diarrhea
GU: sexual dysfunction, polyuria
Kidney/electrolyte: volume and electrolyte depletion ($\downarrow$K, $\downarrow$Cl, $\downarrow$Na, $\downarrow$Mg, $\uparrow$Ca, $\uparrow$uric acid), dilutional hyponatremia, azotemia, $\uparrow$serum creatinine
Metabolic: metabolic alkalosis, hyperglycemia, hyperuricemia
Skin: rash, pruritus
Other: dehydration, muscle cramps, allergic reaction

PHARMACOKINETICS AND PHARMACODYNAMICS
Duration of action: up to 36 h
Onset of action: 1–2 h
Peak effect: <2 h
Bioavailability: 93%
Effect of food: no effect
Protein binding: 75%
Volume of distribution: 25 L
Metabolism: extensively metabolized in liver
Elimination: excreted in urine (mainly as metabolites, 5% as unchanged) and in feces (16%–23%)
Elimination half-life: 14 h or longer

MONITORING
Clinical: BP, urine output, weight
Lab: serum electrolytes (especially potassium, but also magnesium, calcium, sodium, and chloride), kidney function (BUN, serum creatinine), CO_2

OVERDOSE
Supportive: replace fluid and electrolyte loss. Dialysis is unlikely to be effective.

PATIENT INFORMATION
Indapamide is used to lower blood pressure and reduce excessive water in the body. Take this medication as instructed. This medication may cause your body to lose potassium. Notify your health care provider if you develop any unusual muscle cramps, nausea, or dizziness. Sit or lie down if dizziness occurs, and rise slowly from a sitting or lying position. Take with food to minimize gastrointestinal side effects.

AVAILABILITY
Tablets—1.25, 2.5 mg

The information here is provided as guidance only. Prescribers should always consult the manufacturer's current prescribing information.

237

METHYCLOTHIAZIDE

(Aquatensen®, Enduron®)

Methyclothiazide is a thiazide diuretic. All thiazide diuretics share similar pharmacologic activity and adverse-effect profile when equivalent dosages are employed clinically. In addition to enhancing diuresis, thiazide diuretics are effective antihypertensive agents. Diuresis usually occurs within 2 hours, peaks within 2 to 6 hours, and lasts for 24 hours or longer. The onset of antihypertensive effect requires several days. Two to 4 weeks are usually required to achieve optimal BP effect for a given dose. The antihypertensive effect persists longer than the diuretic effect after an oral dose, and the effect may last up to 7 days after discontinuing a chronic thiazide diuretic regimen. For more information, please refer to the hydrochlorothiazide monograph.

SPECIAL GROUPS

Race: no differences in response, although blacks tend to have better BP response to diuretic monotherapy compared with ACE inhibitor, angiotensin-receptor blocker, or beta-blocker monotherapy

Children: safety and effectiveness have not been established

Elderly: use with caution; no dosage adjustment is required

Renal impairment: use with caution; may exacerbate azotemia; contraindicated in anuria. Thiazide diuretics tend to lose efficacy with creatinine clearances <30 mL/min and may be ineffective in severe renal failure.

Hepatic impairment: use with caution; titrate the dose based on clinical response

Pregnancy: category B; should be used only if clearly indicated

Breast-feeding: not recommended; excreted in human milk, although in low concentrations

DOSAGE

Edema: Initial dose—2.5–10 mg/d once daily in the morning
Maintenance—2.5–5 mg once daily in the morning; intermittent therapy may be safer and more effective, and is performed by giving the dose every other day or on a 3–5 d/wk schedule

Hypertension: Usual dose range—2.5–5 mg once daily in the morning

IN BRIEF

INDICATIONS
Hypertension
Edema

CONTRAINDICATIONS
Known hypersensitivity to thiazides, other related diuretics, or sulfonamide-derived agents
Anuria or renal decompensation

DRUG INTERACTIONS
Alcohol[1]
Amphetamines[3]
Antidiabetic agents[4]
Antihypertensive drugs[1,3]
Barbiturates[1]
Cardiac glycosides[3]
Cholestyramine, colestipol[2]
Diuretics[1,3]
Lithium[3]
Narcotics[1]
NSAIDs[2]
Non-depolarizing neuromuscular blockers[3]
Potassium-depleting agents (corticosteroids, amphotericin B)[1]
Quinidine[3]

1 Effect/toxicity of methyclothiazide may increase.
2 Effect of methyclothiazide may decrease.
3 Methyclothiazide may increase the effect/toxicity of this drug.
4 Methyclothiazide may decrease the effect of this drug.

ADVERSE EFFECTS
CV: hypotension, orthostatic symptoms
CNS: dizziness, headache, fatigue, vertigo
Hematologic: blood dyscrasias
GI: anorexia, nausea, vomiting, constipation, diarrhea, pancreatitis, cholestatic jaundice
GU: sexual dysfunction, polyuria
Kidney/electrolyte: volume and electrolyte depletion ($\downarrow$K, $\downarrow$Cl, $\downarrow$Na, $\downarrow$Mg, $\uparrow$Ca, $\uparrow$uric acid), dilutional hyponatremia, azotemia, $\uparrow$serum creatinine
Metabolic: metabolic alkalosis, hyperglycemia, hyperuricemia, hypercholesterolemia
Skin: rash, purpura, urticaria, photosensitivity, erythema multiforme
Other: dehydration, muscle cramps, allergic reaction

PHARMACOKINETICS AND PHARMACODYNAMICS
Duration of action: $\geq$24 h
Onset of action: 2 h
Peak effect: 6 h
Bioavailability: not known
Effect of food: not known
Protein binding: not known
Volume of distribution: not known
Metabolism: not clear
Elimination: mainly excreted unchanged in the urine
Elimination half-life: not known

MONITORING
Clinical: BP, urine output, weight
Lab: serum electrolytes (especially potassium, but also magnesium, calcium, sodium, and chloride), kidney function (BUN, serum creatinine), CO_2

OVERDOSE
Supportive: replace fluid and electrolyte loss. Dialysis is unlikely to be effective.

PATIENT INFORMATION
Methyclothiazide is used to lower blood pressure and reduce excessive water in the body. Take this medication as instructed. This medication may cause your body to lose potassium. Notify your health care provider if you develop any unusual muscle cramps, nausea, or dizziness. Sit or lie down if dizziness occurs, and rise slowly from a sitting or lying position. Take with food to minimize gastrointestinal side effects.

AVAILABILITY
Tablets—2.5, 5 mg
Combination formulations:
Enduronyl® tablets—methyclothiazide 5 mg/deserpidine 0.25 mg
Enduronyl Forte® tablets—methyclothiazide 5 mg/deserpidine 0.5 mg
Diutensen-R® tablets—methyclothiazide 2.5 mg/reserpine 0.1 mg

METOLAZONE (Mykrox®, Zaroxolyn®)

Metolazone is a quinazoline diuretic with structure and pharmacologic activity similar to thiazide diuretics. It acts primarily to inhibit sodium reabsorption at the cortical diluting site and, to a lesser extent, in the proximal convoluted tubule. Its diuretic potency at maximum therapeutic dosage is comparable to thiazide diuretics. However, different from thiazide diuretics, metolazone continues to promote diuresis in patients with glomerular filtration rates below 20 mL/min. Metolazone has been used together with a loop diuretic in the management of edema in patients with impaired renal function who failed to respond to either agent alone. For more information, please refer to the hydrochlorothiazide monograph.

SPECIAL GROUPS

Race: no differences in response, although blacks tend to have better BP response to diuretic monotherapy compared with ACE inhibitor, angiotensin-receptor blocker, or beta-blocker monotherapy

Children: safety and effectiveness have not been established; use is not recommended

Elderly: use with caution; no dosage adjustment is required

Renal impairment: use with caution; may exacerbate azotemia; contraindicated in anuria; more effective than other thiazides in patients with renal insufficiency

Hepatic impairment: use with caution; dosage adjustment is probably not required

Pregnancy: category B/D; should be used only if clearly indicated

Breast-feeding: not recommended; excreted in human milk, although in low concentrations

DOSAGE*

Edema: Initial dose—5–20 mg/day of Zaroxolyn® once daily in the morning; dosages up to 20 mg once daily may be required in patients with renal insufficiency
Maintenance—2.5–10 mg of Zaroxolyn® once daily in the morning; intermittent therapy may be safer and more effective, and is performed by giving the dose every other day or on a 3–5 d/wk schedule

Hypertension: Usual dose range—2.5–5 mg of Zaroxolyn®, or 0.5–1 mg of Mykrox® once daily in the morning

*Note—Because of the difference in formulations, different products have different dosage recommendations and should not be used interchangeably.

IN BRIEF

INDICATIONS
Hypertension (both Zaroxolyn® and Mykrox®)
Edema (Zaroxolyn® only)

CONTRAINDICATIONS
Known hypersensitivity to thiazides, other related diuretics, or sulfonamide-derived agents
Anuria or renal decompensation
Hepatic coma or precoma

DRUG INTERACTIONS
Alcohol[1]
Amphetamines[3]
Antidiabetic agents[4]
Antihypertensive drugs[1,3]
Barbiturates[1]
Cardiac glycosides[3]
Cholestyramine, colestipol[2]
Diuretics[1,3]
Lithium[3]
Narcotics[1]
NSAIDs[2]
Non-depolarizing neuromuscular blockers[3]
Potassium-depleting agents (corticosteroids, amphotericin B)[1]
Quinidine[3]

1 Effect/toxicity of metolazone may increase.
2 Effect of metolazone may decrease.
3 Metolazone may increase the effect/toxicity of this drug.
4 Metolazone may decrease the effect of this drug.

ADVERSE EFFECTS
CV: hypotension, orthostatic symptoms
CNS: dizziness, headache, fatigue, vertigo
Hematologic: blood dyscrasias
GI: anorexia, nausea, vomiting, constipation, diarrhea, pancreatitis, cholestatic jaundice
GU: sexual dysfunction, polyuria
Kidney/electrolyte: volume and electrolyte depletion ($\downarrow$K, $\downarrow$Cl, $\downarrow$Na, $\downarrow$Mg, $\uparrow$Ca, $\uparrow$uric acid), dilutional hyponatremia, azotemia, $\uparrow$serum creatinine
Metabolic: metabolic alkalosis, hyperglycemia, hyperuricemia, hypercholesterolemia
Skin: rash, purpura, urticaria, photosensitivity
Other: dehydration, muscle cramps, allergic reaction

PHARMACOKINETICS AND PHARMACODYNAMICS
Duration of action: 12–24 h or longer
Onset of action: <1 h
Peak effect: 1–2 h
Bioavailability: 40%–65% (higher for Mykrox®, which has bioavailability similar to oral solution)
Effect of food: not known
Protein binding: 95%
Volume of distribution: 113 L
Metabolism: not significantly metabolized
Elimination: 70%–95% is excreted unchanged in urine; the rest is excreted in bile
Elimination half-life: 8–14 h

MONITORING
Clinical: BP, urine output, weight
Lab: serum electrolytes (especially potassium, but also magnesium, calcium, sodium, and chloride), kidney function (BUN, serum creatinine), CO_2

OVERDOSE
Supportive: replace fluid and electrolyte loss. Dialysis is unlikely to be effective.

PATIENT INFORMATION
Metolazone is used to lower blood pressure and reduce excessive water in the body. Take this medication as instructed. This medication may cause your body to lose potassium. Notify your health care provider if you develop any unusual muscle cramps, nausea, or dizziness. Sit or lie down if dizziness occurs, and rise slowly from a sitting or lying position. Take with food to minimize gastrointestinal side effects.

AVAILABILITY
Zaroxolyn® tablets—2.5, 5, 10 mg
Mykrox® tablets— 0.5 mg

POLYTHIAZIDE (Renese®)

Polythiazide is a thiazide diuretic. All thiazide diuretics share similar pharmacologic activity and adverse-effect profile when equivalent dosages are employed clinically. In addition to enhancing diuresis, thiazide diuretics are effective antihypertensive agents. Diuresis usually occurs within 2 hours, peaks within 2 to 6 hours, and lasts for 24 to 48 hours or longer. The onset of antihypertensive effect requires several days. Two to 4 weeks are usually required to achieve optimal BP effect for a given dose. The antihypertensive effect persists longer than the diuretic effect after an oral dose and the effect may last up to 7 days after discontinuing a chronic thiazide diuretic regimen. For more information, please refer to the hydrochlorothiazide monograph.

SPECIAL GROUPS

Race: no differences in response, although blacks tend to have better BP response to diuretic monotherapy compared with ACE inhibitor, angiotensin-receptor blocker, or beta-blocker monotherapy

Children: safety and effectiveness have not been established

Elderly: use with caution; no dosage adjustment is required

Renal impairment: use with caution; may exacerbate azotemia; contraindicated in anuria. Thiazide diuretics tend to lose efficacy with creatinine clearances <30 mL/min and may be ineffective in severe renal failure.

Hepatic impairment: use with caution; titrate the dose based on clinical response

Pregnancy: category D; not recommended

Breast-feeding: use with caution; excreted in human milk, although in low concentrations

IN BRIEF

INDICATIONS
Hypertension
Edema

CONTRAINDICATIONS
Known hypersensitivity to thiazides, other related diuretics, or sulfonamide-derived agents
Anuria or renal decompensation

DRUG INTERACTIONS
Alcohol[1]
Amphetamines[3]
Antidiabetic agents[4]
Antihypertensive drugs[1,3]
Barbiturates[1]
Cardiac glycosides[3]
Cholestyramine, colestipol[2]
Diuretics[1,3]
Lithium[3]
Narcotics[1]
NSAIDs[2]
Non-depolarizing neuromuscular blockers[3]
Potassium-depleting agents (corticosteroids, amphotericin B)[1]
Quinidine[3]

1 Effect/toxicity of polythiazide may increase.
2 Effect of polythiazide may decrease.
3 Polythiazide may increase the effect/toxicity of this drug.
4 Polythiazide may decrease the effect of this drug.

ADVERSE EFFECTS
CV: hypotension, orthostatic symptoms
CNS: dizziness, headache, fatigue, vertigo
Hematologic: blood dyscrasias
GI: anorexia, nausea, vomiting, constipation, diarrhea, pancreatitis, cholestatic jaundice
GU: sexual dysfunction, polyuria
Kidney/electrolyte: volume and electrolyte depletion ($\downarrow$K, $\downarrow$Cl, $\downarrow$Na, $\downarrow$Mg, $\uparrow$Ca, $\uparrow$uric acid), dilutional hyponatremia, azotemia, $\uparrow$serum creatinine
Metabolic: metabolic alkalosis, hyperglycemia, hyperuricemia, hypercholesterolemia
Skin: rash, purpura, urticaria, photosensitivity
Other: dehydration, muscle cramps, allergic reaction

PHARMACOKINETICS AND PHARMACODYNAMICS
Duration of action: 24–48 h
Onset of action: <2 h
Peak effect: 6 h
Bioavailability: no data, but absorbed rapidly
Effect of food: not known
Protein binding: not known
Volume of distribution: not known
Metabolism: not clear; about 30% of a dose is metabolized in dogs
Elimination: 25% excreted unchanged in the urine
Elimination half-life: 26 h

MONITORING
Clinical: BP, urine output, weight
Lab: serum electrolytes (especially potassium, but also magnesium, calcium, sodium, and chloride), kidney function (BUN, serum creatinine), CO_2

OVERDOSE
Supportive: replace fluid and electrolyte loss. Dialysis is unlikely to be effective.

PATIENT INFORMATION
Polythiazide is used to lower blood pressure and reduce excessive water in the body. Take this medication as instructed. This medication may cause your body to lose potassium. Notify your health care provider if you develop any unusual muscle cramps, nausea, or dizziness. Sit or lie down if dizziness occurs, and rise slowly from a sitting or lying position. Take with food to minimize gastrointestinal side effects.

POLYTHIAZIDE *(continued)*

DOSAGE

Edema: Usual dose range—1–4 mg once daily in the morning. Intermittent therapy may be safer and more effective, and is performed by giving the dose every other day or on a 3–5 d/wk schedule.

Hypertension: Usual dose range—2–4 mg once daily in the morning

AVAILABILITY

Tablets—1, 2, 4 mg
Combination formulations:
Minizide® capsules—
Polythiazide 0.5 mg/prazosin 1 mg
Polythiazide 0.5 mg/prazosin 2 mg
Polythiazide 0.5 mg/prazosin 5 mg
Renese-R® tablets—
Polythiazide 2 mg/reserpine 0.25 mg

QUINETHAZONE (Hydromox®)

Note: Quinethazone is no longer commercially available in the United States. Quinethazone is a thiazide diuretic. All thiazide diuretics share similar pharmacologic activity and adverse effect profile when equivalent dosages are employed clinically. In addition to enhancing diuresis, thiazide diuretics are effective antihypertensive agents. Diuresis usually occurs within 2 hours, peaks within 2 to 6 hours, and lasts for 18 to 24 hours or longer. The onset of antihypertensive effect requires several days. Two to 4 weeks are usually required to achieve optimal BP effect for a given dose. The antihypertensive effect persists longer than the diuretic effect after an oral dose, and the effect may last up to 7 days after discontinuing a chronic thiazide diuretic regimen. For more information, please refer to the hydrochlorothiazide monograph.

SPECIAL GROUPS

Race: no differences in response, although blacks tend to have better BP response to diuretic monotherapy compared with ACE inhibitor, angiotensin-receptor blocker, or beta-blocker monotherapy

Children: safety and effectiveness have not been established

Elderly: use with caution; no dosage adjustment is required

Renal impairment: use with caution; may exacerbate azotemia; contraindicated in anuria. Thiazide diuretics tend to lose efficacy with creatinine clearances <30 mL/min and may be ineffective in severe renal failure.

Hepatic impairment: use with caution; titrate the dose based on clinical response

Pregnancy: category D; not recommended

Breast-feeding: use with caution; excreted in human milk, although in low concentrations

DOSAGE

Edema: Usual dose range—25–200 mg/d as a single dose in the morning or in 2 divided doses

Intermittent therapy may be safer and more effective and is performed by giving the dose every other day or on a 3–5 d/wk schedule.

Hypertension: Usual dose range—25–100 mg/d as a single dose in the morning or in 2 divided doses

IN BRIEF

INDICATIONS
Hypertension
Edema

CONTRAINDICATIONS
Known hypersensitivity to thiazides, other related diuretics, or sulfonamide-derived agents
Anuria or renal decompensation

DRUG INTERACTIONS
Alcohol[1]
Amphetamines[3]
Antidiabetic agents[4]
Antihypertensive drugs[1,3]
Barbiturates[1]
Cardiac glycosides[3]
Cholestyramine, colestipol[2]
Diuretics[1,3]
Lithium[3]
Narcotics[1]
NSAIDs[2]
Non-depolarizing neuromuscular blockers[3]
Potassium-depleting agents (corticosteroids, amphotericin B)[1]
Quinidine[3]

1 Effect/toxicity of quinethazone may increase.
2 Effect of quinethazone may decrease.
3 Quinethazone may increase the effect/toxicity of this drug.
4 Quinethazone may decrease the effect of this drug.

ADVERSE EFFECTS
CV: hypotension, orthostatic symptoms
CNS: dizziness, headache, fatigue, vertigo
Hematologic: blood dyscrasias
GI: anorexia, nausea, vomiting, constipation, diarrhea, pancreatitis, cholestatic jaundice
GU: sexual dysfunction, polyuria
Kidney/electrolyte: volume and electrolyte depletion ($\downarrow$K, $\downarrow$Cl, $\downarrow$Na, $\downarrow$Mg, $\uparrow$Ca, $\uparrow$uric acid), dilutional hyponatremia, azotemia, $\uparrow$serum creatinine
Metabolic: metabolic alkalosis, hyperglycemia, hyperuricemia, hypercholesterolemia
Skin: rash, purpura, urticaria, photosensitivity
Other: dehydration, muscle cramps, allergic reaction

PHARMACOKINETICS AND PHARMACODYNAMICS
Duration of action: 18–24 h
Onset of action: 2 h
Peak effect: 6 h
Bioavailability: not known
Effect of food: not known
Protein binding: not known
Volume of distribution: not known
Metabolism: not known
Elimination: not known
Elimination half-life: not known

MONITORING
Clinical: BP, urine output, weight
Lab: serum electrolytes (especially potassium, but also magnesium, calcium, sodium, and chloride), kidney function (BUN, serum creatinine), CO_2

OVERDOSE
Supportive: replace fluid and electrolyte loss. Dialysis is unlikely to be effective.

PATIENT INFORMATION
Quinethazone is used to lower blood pressure and reduce excessive water in the body. Take this medication as instructed. This medication may cause your body to lose potassium. Notify your health care provider if you develop any unusual muscle cramps, nausea, or dizziness. Sit or lie down if dizziness occurs, and rise slowly from a sitting or lying position. Take with food to minimize gastrointestinal side effects.

AVAILABILITY
Tablets—50 mg

TRICHLORMETHIAZIDE
(Metahydrin®, Diurese®, Naqua®, various generics)

Note: Trichlormethiazide is no longer commercially available in the United States. Trichlormethiazide is a thiazide diuretic. All thiazide diuretics share similar pharmacologic activity and adverse-effect profile when equivalent dosages are employed clinically. In addition to enhancing diuresis, thiazide diuretics are effective antihypertensive agents. Diuresis usually occurs within 2 hours, peaks within 2 to 6 hours, and lasts for 24 hours or longer. The onset of antihypertensive effect requires several days. Two to 4 weeks are usually required to achieve optimal BP effect for a given dose. The antihypertensive effect persists longer than the diuretic effect after an oral dose, and the effect may last up to 7 days after discontinuing a chronic thiazide diuretic regimen. For more information, please refer to the hydrochlorothiazide monograph.

SPECIAL GROUPS

Race: no differences in response, although blacks tend to have better BP response to diuretic monotherapy compared with ACE inhibitor, angiotensin-receptor blocker, or beta-blocker monotherapy.

Children: safety and effectiveness have not been established

Elderly: use with caution; no dosage adjustment is required

Renal impairment: use with caution; may exacerbate azotemia; contraindicated in anuria. Thiazide diuretics tend to lose efficacy with creatinine clearances <30 mL/min and may be ineffective in severe renal failure.

Hepatic impairment: use with caution; titrate the dose based on clinical response

Pregnancy: category C; should be used only if potential benefit outweighs risk

Breast-feeding: use with caution; excreted in human milk, although in low concentrations

DOSAGE

Edema: Usual dose range—2–4 mg once daily in the morning Intermittent therapy may be safer and more effective, and is performed by giving the dose every other day or on a 3–5 d/wk schedule.

Hypertension: Usual dose range—2–4 mg/d as a single dose in the morning or in 2 divided doses

IN BRIEF

INDICATIONS
Hypertension
Edema

CONTRAINDICATIONS
Known hypersensitivity to thiazides, other related diuretics, sulfonamide-derived agents, or tartrazine (contained in some products)
Anuria or renal decompensation

DRUG INTERACTIONS
Alcohol[1]
Amphetamines[3]
Antidiabetic agents[4]
Antihypertensive drugs[1,3]
Barbiturates[1]
Cardiac glycosides[3]
Cholestyramine, colestipol[2]
Diuretics[1,3]
Lithium[3]
Narcotics[1]
NSAIDs[2]
Non-depolarizing neuromuscular blockers[3]
Potassium-depleting agents (corticosteroids, amphotericin B)[1]
Quinidine[3]

1 Effect/toxicity of trichlormethiazide may increase.
2 Effect of trichlormethiazide may decrease.
3 Trichlormethiazide may increase the effect/toxicity of this drug.
4 Trichlormethiazide may decrease the effect of this drug.

ADVERSE EFFECTS
CV: hypotension, orthostatic symptoms
CNS: dizziness, headache, fatigue, vertigo
Hematologic: blood dyscrasias
GI: anorexia, nausea, vomiting, constipation, diarrhea, pancreatitis, cholestatic jaundice
GU: sexual dysfunction, polyuria
Kidney/electrolyte: volume and electrolyte depletion ($\downarrow$K, $\downarrow$Cl, $\downarrow$Na, $\downarrow$Mg, $\uparrow$Ca, $\uparrow$uric acid), dilutional hyponatremia, azotemia, $\uparrow$serum creatinine
Metabolic: metabolic alkalosis, hyperglycemia, hyperuricemia, hypercholesterolemia
Skin: rash, purpura, urticaria, photosensitivity
Other: dehydration, muscle cramps, allergic reaction

PHARMACOKINETICS AND PHARMACODYNAMICS
Duration of action: 24 h
Onset of action: 1–2 h
Peak effect: 3–6 h
Bioavailability: not clear, but absorbed rapidly
Effect of food: not known
Protein binding: not known
Volume of distribution: not known
Metabolism: not fully defined
Elimination: not clear, but excreted renally and half-life is prolonged in renal impairment
Elimination half-life: 2.5–7.5 h

MONITORING
Clinical: BP, urine output, weight
Lab: serum electrolytes (especially potassium, but also magnesium, calcium, sodium, and chloride), kidney function (BUN, serum creatinine), CO_2

OVERDOSE
Supportive: replace fluid and electrolyte loss. Dialysis is unlikely to be effective.

PATIENT INFORMATION
Trichlormethiazide is used to lower blood pressure and reduce excessive water in the body. Take this medication as instructed. This medication may cause your body to lose potassium. Notify your health care provider if you develop any unusual muscle cramps, nausea, or dizziness. Sit or lie down if dizziness occurs, and rise slowly from a sitting or lying position. Take with food to minimize gastrointestinal side effects.

AVAILABILITY
Tablets—2, 4 mg
Combination formulations:
Metatensin® #4 and #2 tablets—
Trichlormethiazide 4 mg/reserpine 0.1 mg
Trichlormethiazide 2 mg/reserpine 0.1 mg

POTASSIUM-SPARING DIURETICS

Although potassium-sparing diuretics have some diuretic capability, this action is relatively weak. Four drugs are recognized as having a potassium-sparing action: **amiloride**, **spironolactone**, **eplerenone**, and **triamterene**. For diuresis, they are generally used in fixed-ratio combinations with the more powerful diuretics, which tend to cause excessive potassium loss. Nevertheless, **amiloride** is regarded in some countries as a single-entity diuretic agent.

EFFICACY AND USE

Until recently, the main applications of the potassium-sparing diuretics were in the treatment of hypertension and edematous states arising from cardiac, renal, and hepatic failure. They are used in conjunction with a thiazide or a loop diuretic in the management of hypertension or fluid overload to prevent excessive potassium loss associated with the diuresis. Potassium-sparing diuretics may also be used alone to correct hypokalemia from causes other than diuresis. **Spironolactone** blocks the effect of aldosterone, and thus is indicated for the treatment of hyperaldosteronism.

The European Working Part on Hypertension in the Elderly (EWPHE) study demonstrated that the treatment of elderly patients with a combination of **hydrochlorothiazide** and **triamterene** resulted in a significant reduction in fatal cardiac events, but increased nonfatal events, with a trend toward a decrease in the incidence of stroke. The MRC study on older hypertensives compared **amiloride** plus **hydrochlorothiazide**, **atenolol**, and placebo in more than 4000 patients. The diuretic combination, but not the beta-blocker, significantly reduced stroke and MI. A study has also shown that the addition of a potassium-sparing diuretic to thiazide treatment in patients with hypertension was associated with a lower risk of primary cardiac arrest when compared with treatment with a thiazide alone.

This class of drugs, particularly **spironolactone** and **eplerenone**, has experienced a resurgence of late, but for reasons unrelated to diuresis or BP control. Both **spironolactone** and **eplerenone**, but not **triamterene** or **amiloride**, are aldosterone receptor antagonists and, as such, are able to block the deleterious effects of aldosterone (eg, sodium/water retention, ventricular hypertrophy) on the cardiovascular system, which plays a prominent role in the pathophysiology of systolic heart failure. The Randomized Aldactone Evaluation Study (RALES) demonstrated that **spironolactone**, when added to conventional heart failure therapy, produced a 30% reduction in mortality, a 35% reduction in hospitalizations for worsening heart failure, and a significant improvement in New York Heart Association (NYHA) functional class. The Eplerenone Post–Acute Myocardial Infarction Heart Failure Efficacy and Survival Study (EPHESUS) compared **eplerenone** with placebo in 6632 patients with acute MI complicated by left ventricular dysfunction and heart failure. In this study, **eplerenone** reduced all-cause mortality by 15% compared with placebo (P = 0.008) and reduced cardiovascular mortality by 17% (P = 0.005). However, the rate of serious hyperkalemia (5.5%) was significantly higher with eplerenone compared with placebo (3.9%). Based on these studies, these drugs are now accepted as part of standard care for patients with systolic heart failure.

MODE OF ACTION

Both **amiloride** and **triamterene** act directly on the distal renal tubule of the nephron to inhibit sodium–potassium exchange. They induce only a modest natriuresis but decrease the excretion of potassium. Hydrogen secretion is also reduced, rendering the urine alkaline. Magnesium excretion is decreased, possibly as a consequence of the alkalinization.

Spironolactone and **eplerenone** act through competition with the binding sites of aldosterone, a mineralocorticoid. Because these drugs are relatively weak diuretics, their diuretic effectiveness may be potentiated by combining any one of them with a diuretic that acts more proximally in the tubule (ie, loop or thiazide-type diuretic). For the treatment of heart failure, these drugs are typically added onto existing heart failure therapy (eg, ACE inhibitors, loop diuretics, beta-blockers, digoxin) at low dosages that are used for their ability to block the aldosterone receptor rather than promote diuresis or a reduction in BP, although these pharmacologic actions may still manifest.

INDICATIONS

	Amiloride	Eplerenone	Spironolactone	Triamterene
Hypertension	+*	+	+*	+*
Edema	+*	−	+	+
Hyperaldosteronism	−	−	+	−
Hypokalemia (diuretic-induced)	+	−	+	+
Congestive heart failure (reduce mortality)	−	+†	−	−

*Used in combination with other diuretics.

†Post–myocardial infarction.

+—FDA approved; − —not FDA approved.

AMILORIDE (Amiloride, Midamor®)

Amiloride is a weak natriuretic, diuretic, and hypotensive agent. It acts directly on the distal renal tubule of the nephron to inhibit sodium–potassium ion exchange, and its diuretic activity is independent of aldosterone. When amiloride is combined with a more potent natriuretic agent, it has additive effects on urinary sodium excretion and an antagonistic effect on potassium excretion. In patients with hypertension, amiloride therapy lowers systolic pressure by 10 to 20 mm Hg and diastolic pressure by 5 to 10 mm Hg. An additive reduction in BP is observed when amiloride is used in combination with a thiazide diuretic. With its potassium-sparing effect, hyperkalemia may be a problem, especially in elderly patients or those with underlying renal insufficiency or diabetes mellitus. Amiloride is not a direct aldosterone antagonist.

SPECIAL GROUPS

Race: no differences in response
Children: safety and effectiveness have not been established, although the drug has been used safely and effectively in this population
Elderly: use with caution; no dosage adjustment is required
Renal impairment: use with caution; contraindicated in anuria and acute or chronic renal insufficiency
Hepatic impairment: use with caution; dosage adjustment is probably not required
Pregnancy: category B; should be used only if clearly indicated
Breast-feeding: not recommended; not known if the drug is excreted in human milk

DOSAGE

(intended for use with either a thiazide or a loop diuretic)
Usual dose range—5–10 mg once daily.
Although dosages exceeding 10 mg/day are usually not necessary, higher dosages (up to 20 mg) have been used occasionally in some patients with persistent hypokalemia. Some clinicians have reported efficacy with daily dosages as high as 40 mg.

IN BRIEF

INDICATIONS
As adjunctive therapy with thiazide or other kaliuretic diuretics in CHF or hypertension to prevent excessive potassium loss.

CONTRAINDICATIONS
Known hypersensitivity to product components
Hyperkalemia (serum potassium >5.5 mEq/L)
Anuria, acute and chronic renal insufficiency, diabetic nephropathy
Concurrent therapy with other potassium-sparing agents or potassium supplements

DRUG INTERACTIONS
ACE inhibitors/angiotensin receptor blockers[1]
Antihypertensive drugs[1,3]
Cardiac glycosides[3,4,5]
Diuretics[1,3]
Lithium[3]
NSAIDs[2]
Potassium and potassium-sparing agents[1]

[1] Effect/toxicity of amiloride may increase.
[2] Effect of amiloride may decrease.
[3] Amiloride may increase the effect/toxicity of this drug.
[4] Amiloride may decrease the effect of this drug.
[5] The clinical significance of this interaction is unknown.

ADVERSE EFFECTS
CV: hypotension, orthostatic symptoms, arrhythmias, angina
CNS: dizziness, headache, fatigue
GI: anorexia, nausea, vomiting, diarrhea, abdominal discomfort, jaundice, abnormal liver function
GU: sexual dysfunction, polyuria
Hematologic: aplastic anemia, neutropenia
Metabolic: hyperkalemia, metabolic acidosis
Skin: rash, pruritus
Other: dehydration, muscle cramps, allergic reaction, interstitial nephritis, cough, dyspnea

PHARMACOKINETICS AND PHARMACODYNAMICS
Duration of action: 24 h
Onset of action: 2 h
Peak effect: 6–10 h
Bioavailability: 50%
Effect of food: ↓ absorption, 30% absorbed
Protein binding: 23%–40%
Volume of distribution: 350–380 L
Metabolism: not metabolized
Elimination: excreted unchanged in the urine (50%) and in the stools (unabsorbed, 40%)
Elimination half-life: 6–9 h or longer

MONITORING
BP, urine output, weight, serum electrolytes, especially potassium. Monitor BUN/serum creatinine periodically. Monitor for signs of hyperkalemia and/or dehydration: muscle pains, oliguria, thirst, tachycardia, GI upset.

OVERDOSE
Supportive: correct severe, symptomatic hyperkalemia or hypotension.

PATIENT INFORMATION
Amiloride is used to prevent excessive water accumulation, to treat high blood pressure, or to reduce potassium loss from the body. Take this medication as instructed. Notify your health care provider if you develop any unusual muscle cramps, nausea, or dizziness. Sit or lie down if dizziness occurs, and rise slowly from a sitting or lying position. Take with food to minimize gastrointestinal side effects.

AVAILABILITY
Tablets—5 mg
Combination formulations:
Moduretic® tablets and various generics—
Amiloride 5 mg/hydrochlorothiazide 50 mg

EPLERENONE (Inspra®)

Eplerenone is an aldosterone receptor antagonist that is chemically and pharmacologically similar to spironolactone. The main difference between eplerenone and spironolactone is selectivity for the aldosterone receptor. Spironolactone is a nonselective aldosterone receptor antagonist that binds to other steroid receptors, thereby causing sex hormone–related side effects (eg, gynecomastia) in a significant percentage of patients. Eplerenone is a selective aldosterone receptor antagonist that was designed to alleviate this problem. The replacement of the 17α-thioacetyl group on the spironolactone molecule with a carbomethoxy group is believed to impart the aldosterone receptor selectivity of eplerenone. The result is a compound believed to have all of the benefits of spironolactone minus the hormonal side effects.

Eplerenone, in both monotherapy and combination therapy, has been shown to be beneficial in lowering elevated BP in patients with hypertension. Eplerenone has been shown to have antihypertensive efficacy similar to that of other antihypertensive agents and has also demonstrated renoprotective effects in diabetic patients with hypertension.

EPHESUS compared eplerenone with placebo in 6632 patients with acute MI complicated by left ventricular dysfunction and heart failure. In this study, eplerenone reduced all-cause mortality by 15% compared with placebo ($P = 0.008$) and reduced cardiovascular mortality by 17% ($P = 0.005$). However, the rate of serious hyperkalemia (5.5%) was significantly higher with eplerenone compared with placebo (3.9%).

Hyperkalemia seems to be the biggest concern with eplerenone. Eplerenone is metabolized by cytochrome P-450 3A4 (CYP3A4), and administration with potent inhibitors of this enzyme is contraindicated to minimize the risk of hyperkalemia.

SPECIAL GROUPS

Race: lower bioavailability in blacks

Children: safety and efficacy have not been established

Elderly: reduced clearance; use with caution; no dosage adjustment is required

Renal impairment: reduced clearance; use with caution; contraindicated with serum creatinine >2.0 mg/dL (1.8 mg/dL in females) or creatinine clearance <30 mL/min (<50 mL/min with hypertension)

Hepatic impairment: use with caution; no dosage adjustment necessary for mild to moderate hepatic dysfunction; not adequately studied with severe hepatic impairment

Pregnancy: category B; should be used only if clearly indicated

Breast-feeding: not recommended; not known if eplerenone is excreted in human milk

IN BRIEF

INDICATIONS
CHF post-MI
Hypertension

CONTRAINDICATIONS
Serum potassium >5.5 mEq/L at initiation
Creatinine clearance ≤30 mL/min
Concomitant use with the following potent CYP3A4 inhibitors: ketoconazole, itraconazole, nefazodone, troleandomycin, clarithromycin, ritonavir, and nelfinavir, or any other drug that is a potent inhibitor of this enzyme
Eplerenone is also contraindicated for the treatment of hypertension in patients with the following: type 2 diabetes with microalbuminuria, serum creatinine >2.0 mg/dL in males or >1.8 mg/dL in females, creatinine clearance <50 mL/min, concomitant use of potassium supplements or potassium-sparing diuretics (amiloride, spironolactone, or triamterene)

DRUG INTERACTIONS
ACE inhibitors, angiotensin II receptor antagonists[1]
Antihypertensive drugs[1,3]
Lithium[3,4]
NSAIDs[2,4]
Potassium-containing products[1]
Potassium-sparing diuretics[1]
St. John's wort[2]
Strong CYP3A4 inhibitors[1]: (eg, ketoconazole, itraconazole, nefazodone, troleandomycin, clarithromycin, ritonavir, and nelfinavir)

1 Effect/toxicity of eplerenone may increase.
2 Effect of eplerenone may decrease.
3 Eplerenone may increase the effect/toxicity of this drug.
4 The clinical significance of this interaction is unclear.

ADVERSE EFFECTS
CV: angina pectoris, MI
CNS: dizziness, headache, fatigue
GI: diarrhea, abdominal discomfort
GU: albuminuria, mastodynia, abnormal vaginal bleeding, gynecomastia
Kidney: abnormal renal function
Liver: increased liver enzymes
Metabolic: hyperkalemia, hyponatremia, elevated uric acid

PHARMACOKINETICS AND PHARMACODYNAMICS
Duration of action: not fully defined
Onset of action: not fully defined; maximum BP response takes about 4 weeks
Peak effect: peak plasma concentrations occur about 1.5 h after a dose
Bioavailability: unknown
Effect of food: none
Protein binding: about 50%
Volume of distribution: 43–90 L
Metabolism: metabolized by CYP3A4 to inactive metabolites
Elimination: eliminated as inactive metabolites: 32% in the feces, 67% in the urine; <5% excreted unchanged in the urine and feces
Elimination half-life: 4–6 h

MONITORING
BP; serum potassium should be measured at baseline, within the first week, and at 1 month after the start of treatment or dose adjustment. Serum potassium should be assessed periodically thereafter. Also monitor liver enzymes, BUN/creatinine, and uric acid.

OVERDOSE
Supportive: correct severe, symptomatic hyperkalemia or hypotension.

EPLERENONE *(continued)*

DOSAGE

Hypertension: Initial dosage is 50 mg once daily. Maintenance dosage is 50 mg once or twice daily. For patients receiving weak CYP3A4 inhibitors, such as erythromycin, saquinavir, verapamil, or fluconazole, the starting dose should be reduced to 25 mg once daily.

CHF post-MI: Initial dosage is 25 mg once daily, titrated to a maintenance dosage of 50 mg once daily, preferably within 4 wk if tolerated by the patient. Serum potassium should be measured at baseline, within the first week, and at 1 month after the start of treatment or dose adjustment. Serum potassium should be assessed periodically thereafter.

Dosage should be adjusted based on the serum potassium concentration as follows:

Serum potassium, mEq/L	Action	Dosage adjustment
<5.0	Increase	25mg QOD to 25mg QD, or 25mg QD to 50mg QD
5.0–5.4	Maintain	No adjustment
5.5–5.9	Decrease	50mg QD to 25mg QD, or 25mg QD to 25mg QOD, or 25mg QOD to withhold
≥6.0*	Withhold	

*After withholding eplerenone because of serum potassium ≥6.0 mEq/L, eplerenone may be restarted at a dose of 25 mg every other day (QOD) when serum potassium levels have fallen below 5.5 mEq/L.

QD—once a day.

PATIENT INFORMATION

Do not use potassium supplements, salt substitutes containing potassium, or contraindicated drugs without consulting with your health care professional. Sit or lie down if dizziness occurs, and rise slowly from a sitting or lying position.

AVAILABILITY

Tablets—25, 50 mg

SPIRONOLACTONE
(Spironolactone, Aldactone®)

Spironolactone is a synthetic steroid aldosterone antagonist. It competitively inhibits the physiologic effects of aldosterone on the distal renal tubules, which enhances the excretion of sodium, chloride, and water, and reduces excretion of potassium, ammonium, phosphate, and titratable acid. The weak diuretic effect of spironolactone is determined by the presence of aldosterone and is most pronounced in patients with liver cirrhosis or hyperaldosteronism. It is usually used together with a thiazide or loop diuretic to enhance diuresis.

The antihypertensive effect of spironolactone has not been fully elucidated but may be the result of blocking the effect of aldosterone on arterial smooth muscle or of affecting the extracellular–intracellular sodium gradient. The RALES trial indicated that in patients with severe heart failure (NYHA class III–IV), adding spironolactone 25 mg daily to standard treatment led to a reduction in long-term mortality. Spironolactone has antiandrogenic effects, which are responsible for the troublesome adverse effects, such as gynecomastia, sexual dysfunction, and menstrual irregularities, reported in some patients. These side effects may be related to both dosage and duration of the therapy. Spironolactone has been shown to be a tumorigen in chronic toxicity studies in rats at doses much higher than the usual human dose. The long-term effect in patients receiving the drug chronically is not clear.

SPECIAL GROUPS

Race: no differences in response

Children: safety and efficacy have not been established, although it has been used safely and effectively in this population

Elderly: use with caution; no dosage adjustment is required

Renal impairment: use with caution; contraindicated in anuria and acute or chronic renal insufficiency

Hepatic impairment: use with caution; dosage should be titrated based on clinical response

Pregnancy: category C/D; spironolactone and its metabolites may cross the placenta barrier; use only if potential benefit justifies the potential risk to the fetus

Breast-feeding: not recommended; canrenone, a metabolite of spironolactone, is excreted in human milk

IN BRIEF

INDICATIONS
Edema associated with CHF, liver cirrhosis, or nephrotic syndrome
Hypokalemia (treatment and prevention)
Hypertension, usually in combination with other agents
Primary hyperaldosteronism

CONTRAINDICATIONS
Known hypersensitivity to product components
Hyperkalemia
Anuria, acute and chronic renal insufficiency, diabetic nephropathy
Concurrent therapy with other potassium-sparing agents or potassium supplements

DRUG INTERACTIONS
ACE inhibitors/angiotensin receptor blockers[1]
Alcohol[1]
Anticoagulants[4]
Antihypertensive drugs[1,3]
Barbiturates[1]
Cardiac glycosides[3]
Diuretics[1,3]
Lithium[3]
Narcotics[1]
NSAIDs[2]
Non-depolarizing neuromuscular blockers[3]
Potassium and potassium-sparing agents[1]
Salicylates[2]

1 Effect/toxicity of spironolactone may increase.
2 Effect of spironolactone may decrease.
3 Spironolactone may increase the effect/toxicity of this drug.
4 Spironolactone may decrease the effect of this drug.

ADVERSE EFFECTS
CNS: drowsiness, lethargy, headache
GI: anorexia, nausea, vomiting, diarrhea, abdominal discomfort, jaundice, hepatocellular injury
GU: sexual dysfunction, amenorrhea or irregular menses, post-menopausal bleeding, polyuria
Hematologic: agranulocytosis
Endocrine/metabolic: gynecomastia, metabolic acidosis
Skin: rash, urticaria
Other: muscle cramps, drug fever, dehydration, anaphylactic reactions

PHARMACOKINETICS AND PHARMACODYNAMICS
Duration of action: 2–3 d
Onset of action: 1–2 h until peak serum concentrations, but usually 24–48 h until effect
Peak effect: 48–72 h
Bioavailability: >90%
Effect of food: increases bioavailability by almost 100%
Protein binding: >90% (spironolactone/metabolites)
Volume of distribution: 14 L
Metabolism: rapid and extensive, with active sulfur-containing products as the major metabolites
Elimination: mainly excreted in the urine as metabolites, and also in the bile
Elimination half-life: spironolactone—1–2 hrs; canrenone (active metabolite)—13–24 h; 7α-thiomethylspironolactone (active metabolite)—3 h

MONITORING
BP, urine output, weight, serum electrolytes, especially potassium. Monitor BUN/serum creatinine periodically. Monitor for signs of hyperkalemia and/or dehydration: muscle pains, oliguria, thirst, tachycardia, GI upset.

OVERDOSE
Supportive: correct severe, symptomatic hyperkalemia or hypotension.

SPIRONOLACTONE (continued)

DOSAGE

Edema: Usual dose range—25–200 mg daily. The usual initial dose is 100 mg administered as a single dose or in divided doses. If used alone, the treatment should be continued for at least 5 d at the initial dosage. Then, the dosage may be adjusted based on the response, or a more potent diuretic may be added.

Diuretic-induced hypokalemia: Usual dose range—25–100 mg daily

Hypertension: Usual dose range—50–100 mg daily administered as a single dose or in divided doses (usually used in combination with another agent, such as a thiazide diuretic). Allow at least 2 wk between dosage adjustments.

Primary hyperaldosteronism: As a diagnostic test: Long test—Spironolactone 400 mg is administered daily for 3–4 wk. Correction of hypokalemia and hypertension provides presumptive evidence for the diagnosis.

Short test—Spironolactone 400 mg is administered daily for 4 d. If serum potassium levels increase during the therapy but decline after discontinuing the drug, a presumptive diagnosis should be considered.

Treatment: Spironolactone in doses of 100–400 mg daily may be administered in preparation for surgery. For patients who are not surgical candidates, long-term spironolactone therapy may be used, and the dose should be titrated individually at the lowest effective dosage.

PATIENT INFORMATION
Spironolactone is used to prevent excessive water accumulation, to treat high blood pressure or heart failure, or to reduce potassium loss from the body. Take this medication as instructed. Notify your health care provider if you develop any unusual muscle cramps, nausea, or dizziness. Sit or lie down if dizziness occurs, and rise slowly from a sitting or lying position. Take with food to minimize gastrointestinal side effects.

AVAILABILITY
Tablets—25, 50, 100 mg
Combination formulations:
 Aldactazide® tablets and various products—
  Spironolactone 25 mg/HCTZ 25 mg
  Spironolactone 50 mg/HCTZ 50 mg

TRIAMTERENE (Triamterene, Dyrenium®)

Similar to amiloride, triamterene inhibits reabsorption of sodium and excretion of potassium and hydrogen in the distal renal tubule. Unlike spironolactone, its activity is independent of aldosterone concentrations in the body and it is not a direct aldosterone antagonist. Triamterene alone has little antihypertensive effect. It is usually used in combination with other diuretics to enhance diuresis and to prevent excessive diuretic-induced potassium loss.

SPECIAL GROUPS

Race: no differences in response

Children: safety and effectiveness have not been established, although it has been used safely and effectively

Elderly: use with caution; start with a low dosage, and adjust the dosage based on response

Renal impairment: use with caution; contraindicated in anuria and severe or progressive kidney disease

Hepatic impairment: use with caution; start with a low dosage, and adjust the dose based on response; contraindicated with severe liver disease

Pregnancy: category B/D; should be used only if clearly indicated

Breast-feeding: not recommended; not known if the drug is excreted in human milk

DOSAGE

As a single agent: The usual initial dose is 100 mg twice daily after meals. Dosage should not exceed 300 mg daily. Once edema is controlled, most patients can be maintained on 100 mg daily or every other day.

In combination with a kaliuretic diuretic for the treatment of hypertension: The initial dose is 25 mg once daily. The dose should be titrated based on response to a maximum of 100 mg daily. Some patients may benefit from splitting the daily dosage into 2 doses.

In combination with a kaliuretic diuretic for the treatment of edema: Use lower initial dosage and adjust dosage based on response.

IN BRIEF

INDICATIONS
Edema associated with CHF, liver cirrhosis, nephrotic syndrome, steroid use, or secondary hyperaldosteronism
Hypertension, when combined with other diuretics

CONTRAINDICATIONS
Known hypersensitivity to product components
Hyperkalemia
Anuria, severe or progressive kidney disease or dysfunction
Concurrent therapy with other potassium-sparing agents or potassium supplements

DRUG INTERACTIONS
ACE inhibitors/angiotensin receptor blockers[1]	Lithium[3]
Amantadine[3]	Non-depolarizing neuromuscular blockers[3]
Antidiabetic agents[4]	NSAIDs[2]
Antihypertensive drugs[1,3]	Potassium and potassium-sparing agents[1]
Cimetidine[1]	
Diuretics[1,3]	

1 Effect/toxicity of triamterene may increase.
2 Effect of triamterene may decrease.
3 Triamterene may increase the effect/toxicity of this drug.
4 Triamterene may decrease the effect of this drug.

ADVERSE EFFECTS
CNS: dizziness, headache, fatigue, weakness
GI: nausea, vomiting, diarrhea, jaundice, abnormal liver enzymes
GU: sexual dysfunction, polyuria, nephrolithiasis
Hematologic: thrombocytopenia, megaloblastic anemia
Kidney: elevated BUN/serum creatinine, azotemia, interstitial nephritis
Metabolic/electrolyte: hyperkalemia
Skin: rash, photosensitivity
Other: dehydration, muscle cramps, anaphylaxis

PHARMACOKINETICS AND PHARMACODYNAMICS
Duration of action: 7–9 h, may be up to 24 h
Onset of action: 2–4 h
Peak effect: several days of therapy
Bioavailability: 30%–70%; 85% with Dyazide® capsules
Effect of food: not known; high-fat meal increases bioavailability from Dyazide® capsules by about 67%
Protein binding: 55%–67%
Volume of distribution: 13.4 L/kg
Metabolism: 80% metabolized in liver; has an active metabolite
Elimination: excreted in urine as unchanged drug (about 21%) and metabolites
Elimination half-life: 1.5–2.5 h

MONITORING
BP, urine output, weight, serum electrolytes, especially potassium. Monitor BUN/serum creatinine periodically. Monitor for signs of hyperkalemia and/or dehydration: muscle pains, oliguria, thirst, tachycardia, GI upset.

OVERDOSE
Supportive: correct severe, symptomatic hyperkalemia or hypotension.

PATIENT INFORMATION
Triamterene is used to prevent excessive water accumulation, to treat high blood pressure, or to reduce potassium loss from the body. Take this medication as instructed. Notify your health care provider if you develop any unusual muscle cramps, nausea, or dizziness. Sit or lie down if dizziness occurs, and rise slowly from a sitting or lying position. Take with food to minimize gastrointestinal side effects.

AVAILABILITY
Capsules—50, 100 mg
Combination formulations:
  Dyazide® capsules, Maxzide® tablets, and various generics—
    Triamterene 75 mg/HCTZ 50 mg
    Triamterene 50 mg/HCTZ 25 mg
    Triamterene 37.5 mg/HCTZ 25 mg

Amery A, Birkenhager W, Brixko P, *et al.*: Mortality and morbidity results from the European Working Party on High Blood Pressure in the Elderly Trial. *Lancet* 1985, 1:1349–1354.

Bayliss J, Norell M, Canepa-Anson R, *et al.*: Untreated heart failure: clinical and neuroendocrine effects of introducing diuretics. *Br Heart J* 1987, 57:17–22.

Channer KS, McLean KA, Lawson-Matthew P, *et al*: Combination diuretic treatment in severe heart failure: a randomized controlled trial. *Br Heart J* 1994, 71:146–150.

Chobanian AV, Bakris GL, Black HR, for the National High Blood Pressure Education Program Coordinating Committee: The seventh report of the Joint National Committee on Prevention, Detection, Evaluation, and Treatment of High Blood Pressure. The JNC 7 report. *JAMA* 2003, 289:2560–2572.

Coope J, Warrender TS: Randomized trial of treatment of hypertension in elderly patients in primary care. *Br Med J* 1986, 293:1145–1151.

Cutler JA, Neaton JD, Hulley SB, *et al.*: Coronary heart disease and all-cause mortality in the Multiple Risk Factor Intervention Trial: subgroup findings and comparisons with other trials. *Prev Med* 1985, 16:293–311.

Epstein M: Aldosterone blockers and potassium sparing diuretics. In *Hypertension Primer*, edn 3. Edited by Izzo JL Jr, Black HR. Dallas: American Heart Assn; 2003:414–416.

Friedel HA, Buckley MMT: Torsemide. A review of its pharmacological properties and therapeutic potential. *Drugs* 1991, 41:81–103.

Frishman WH: Diagnosis and treatment of systolic heart failure in the elderly. *Am J Geriatr Cardiol* 1998, 7:10–16.

Frishman WH, Bryzinski BS, Coulson LR, *et al.*: A multifactorial trial design to assess combination therapy in hypertension: treatment with bisoprolol and hydrochlorothiazide. *Arch Intern Med* 1994, 154:1461–1468.

Frishman WH, Burris JF, Mroczek WJ, *et al.*: First-line therapy option with low-dose bisoprolol fumarate and low-dose hydrochlorothiazide in patients with stage I and stage II systemic hypertension. *J Clin Pharmacol* 1995, 35:182–188.

Frishman WH, Stier CT Jr: Aldosterone and aldosterone antagonism in hypertension. *Curr Hypertens Rep* 2004, 6:195–200.

Frishman WH, Yesenski G, Iqbal MJ: Systemic hypertension in the elderly. In *Cardiovascular Diseases in the Elderly Patient*, edn 3. Edited by Aronow WS, Fleg JL. New York: Marcel Dekker; 2004:131–151.

Frohlich ED: Treating hypertension—what are we to believe? *N Engl J Med* 2003, 348:639–641.

Gehr TWB, Sica DA, Frishman WH: Diuretic therapy in cardiovascular disease. In *Cardiovascular Pharmacotherapeutics*, edn 2. Edited by Frishman WH, Sonnenblick EH, Sica DA. New York: McGraw Hill; 2003:157–176.

Gehr TWB, Sica DA, Frishman WH: Diuretic therapy in cardiovascular disease. In *Cardiovascular Pharmacotherapeutics Manual*, edn 2. Edited by Frishman WH, Sonnenblick EH, Sica DA. New York: McGraw Hill; 2004:131–154.

Grossman E, Messerli FH, Goldbourt U: Does diuretic therapy increase the risk of renal cell carcinoma? *Am J Cardiol* 1999, 83:1090–1093.

Hachamovitch R, Strom JA, Sonnenblick EH, *et al.*: Left ventricular hypertrophy in hypertension and the effects of antihypertensive drug therapy. *Curr Probl Cardiol* 1988, 13:371–421.

Kaplan NM: Treatment of hypertension: drug therapy. In *Kaplan's Clinical Hypertension*, edn 8. Philadelphia: Lippincott Williams & Wilkins; 2002:237–338.

Kiyingi A, Field MJ, Pawsey CC, *et al.*: Metolazone in treatment of severe refractory congestive cardiac failure. *Lancet* 1990, 335:29–31.

Kramer WG, Smith WB, Ferguson J, *et al.*: Pharmacodynamics of torsemide administered as an intravenous injection and as a continuous infusion to patients with congestive heart failure. *J Clin Pharmacol* 1996, 36:265–270.

LaCroix AZ, Wienpahl J, White LR, *et al.*: Thiazide diuretic agents and the incidence of hip fracture. *N Engl J Med* 1990, 322:286–290.

Lakshman MR, Reda DJ, Materson BJ, *et al.*: Diuretics and β-blockers do not have adverse effect at 1 year on plasma lipid and lipoprotein profiles in men with hypertension. *Arch Intern Med* 1999, 159:551–558.

Lant A: Diuretics: clinical pharmacology and therapeutic use (part I). *Drugs* 1985, 29:57–87.

LeJemtel TH, Sonnenblick EH, Frishman WH: Diagnosis and management of heart failure. In *Hurst's The Heart*, edn 11. Edited by Fuster V, Alexander RW, O'Rourke R. New York: McGraw Hill; 2004:723–762.

Leren P, Helgeland A: Coronary heart disease and treatment of hypertension. Some Oslo study data. *Am J Med* 1986, 80:3–6.

Levine SD: Diuretics. *Med Clin North Am* 1989, 73:271–282.

Medical Research Council Working Party: MRC trial of treatment of mild hypertension: principal results. *Br Med J* 1985, 291:97–104.

Moore TD, Nawarskas JJ, Anderson JR: Eplerenone: a selective aldosterone receptor antagonist for hypertension and heart failure. *Heart Dis* 2003, 5:354–363.

Neaton JD, Grimm RH, Prineas RJ, *et al.*: Treatment of Mild Hypertension Study. Final results. *JAMA* 1993, 270:713–724.

Papademetriou V, Sica DA, Izzo JL Jr: Thiazide and loop diuretics. In *Hypertension Primer*, edn 3. Edited by Izzo JR Jr, Black HR. Dallas: American Heart Assn; 2003:411–414.

Parker JD, Parker AB, Farrell B, *et al.*: Effects of diuretic therapy on the development of tolerance to nitroglycerin and exercise capacity in patients with chronic stable angina. *Circulation* 1996, 93:691–696.

Pitt B, Remme W, Zannad F, *et al.*: Eplerenone, a selective aldosterone blocker, in patients with left ventricular dysfunction after myocardial infarction. *N Engl J Med* 2003, 348:1309–1321.

Pitt B, Zannad F, Remme WJ, *et al.*: The effect of spironolactone on morbidity and mortality in patients with severe heart failure. *N Engl J Med* 1999, 341:709–717.

Puschett JB: Diuretics. In *Hypertension: A Companion to Brenner & Rector's The Kidney*. Edited by Oparil S, Weber MA. Philadelphia: WB Saunders Co.; 2000:584–590.

Reader R, Bauer GE, Doyle AE, *et al.*: The Australian Therapeutic Trial of Mild Hypertension: report by the management committee. *Lancet* 1980, 1:1261–1267.

Schuller D, Lynch JP, Fine D: Protocol-guided diuretic management: comparison of furosemide by continuous infusion and intermittent bolus. *Crit Care Med* 1997, 25:1969–1975.

Shapiro PA: Five year findings of the Hypertension Detection and Follow-up Program: 1. Reduction in mortality of persons with high blood pressure, including mild hypertension. *JAMA* 1979, 242:2562–2571.

SHEP Cooperative Research Group: Prevention of stroke by anti-hypertensive drug treatment in older persons with isolated systolic hypertension. Final results of the Systolic Hypertension in the Elderly Program. *JAMA* 1991, 24:3255–3264.

Siscovick DS, Raghunathan TE, Psaty BM, *et al.*: Diuretic therapy for hypertension and the risk of primary cardiac arrest. *N Engl J Med* 1994, 330:1852–1857.

Stier CT Jr, Koenig S, Lee DY, *et al.*: Aldosterone and aldosterone antagonism in cardiovascular disease: focus on eplerenone (INSPRA®). *Heart Dis* 2003, 5:102–118.

The ALLHAT Officers and Coordinators for the ALLHAT Collaborative Research Group: Major outcomes in high-risk hypertensive patients randomized to angiotensin-converting enzyme inhibitor or calcium channel blocker vs diuretic. The Antihypertensive and Lipid-Lowering Treatment to Prevent Heart Attack Trial (ALLHAT). *JAMA* 2002, 288:2981–2997.

Vasan RS, Evans JC, Larson MG, *et al*: Serum aldosterone and the incidence of hypertension in nonhypertensive persons. *N Engl J Med* 2004, 351:33–41.

Velazquez H: Thiazide diuretics. *Renal Physiol* 1987, 10:184–197.

Weber KT: Aldosterone and spironolactone in heart failure. *N Engl J Med* 1999, 341:753–754.

Weber MA, Neutel JM, Frishman WH: Combination drug therapy. In *Cardiovascular Pharmacotherapeutics*, edn 2. Edited by Frishman WH, Sonnenblick EH, Sica DA. New York: McGraw Hill; 2003:355–368.

Wing LMH, Reid CM, Ryan P, *et al.*: A comparison of outcomes with angiotensin-converting–enzyme inhibitors and diuretics for hypertension in the elderly. *N Engl J Med* 2003, 348:583–592.

10

INOTROPIC AND VASOPRESSOR AGENTS

The major aim of inotropic therapy is to improve ventricular contractility of the depressed heart so as to increase cardiac output as needed and reduce elevated ventricular filling pressures. It may be employed intravenously for acute ventricular failure (*eg*, phosphodiesterase [PDE] III inhibitors or catecholamines) or chronically as oral agents (*eg*, digitalis glycosides).

Traditionally, the treatment of decompensated heart failure has included the use of diuretics, vasodilators, and digitalis. The lack of response to these agents has spurred the development of new inotropic drugs. Inotropic agents currently available can be classified into three groups: the PDE inhibitors (**milrinone, inamrinone**); the adrenergic receptor agonists (**dobutamine, dopamine, epinephrine, norepinephrine**) for acute, short-term intravenous

use; and the inhibitors of sodium-potassium ATPase (the digitalis family) for chronic oral therapy as well as intravenous use (Table 10.1).

Although digitalis has been available for more than 200 years, it has only recently been shown to be an effective inotrope for chronic oral use. Short-term inotropic support with newer agents such as PDE inhibitors has been effective when administered intravenously. These agents increase contractility and relax both venous and arterial vasculature. As a result, cardiac output is increased and ventricular filling pressure is decreased. Long-term use of positive inotropes has not been shown to improve mortality of heart failure. In fact, in clinical trials, chronic oral **milrinone** or **vesnarinone** therapy in patients with ventricular dysfunction has been associated with increased mortality.

TABLE 10.1 RELATIVE HEMODYNAMIC EFFECTS OF INOTROPIC AND VASOPRESSOR AGENTS IN HEART FAILURE

	Ventricular filling pressure	Peripheral vascular resistance	Cardiac output	Blood pressure	Ejection fraction
Inotropic agents					
Digoxin	↓	↓	↑	NC	↑
Dobutamine	↓/NC	↓↓	↑↑	↑/NC	↑↑
Inodilators					
Milrinone	↓↓	↓↓	↑↑	↓	↑
Inamrinone	↓↓	↓↓	↑↑	↓	↑
Vasopressor agents					
Dopamine	↓/NC	↑	↑	↑	↑/NC
Isoproterenol	↓/NC	↓	↑	↓	↑/NC
Epinephrine	↓/NC	↑	↑	↑	↑/NC
Metaraminol	↓/NC	↑↑	↑/NC	↑↑	↑/NC
Methoxamine	↓/NC	↑	↑/NC	↑↑	↑/NC
Midodrine	↓/NC	↑	↑/NC	↑	↑/NC
Norepinephrine	↓/NC	↑↑	↑/NC	↑↑	↑/NC
Phenylephrine	↓/NC	↑	↑/NC	↑↑	↑/NC
Vasopressin	NC	↑	NC	↑↑	NC

↓—decrease; ↑—increase; NC—no change.

In addition to their direct cardiac actions, PDE inhibitors also have vasodilatory properties, a combination that theoretically may make them seem ideal for the treatment of congestive heart failure (CHF). Currently, they are only approved for intravenous use, because prolonged oral use in patients with severe left ventricular dysfunction was associated with increased mortality.

EFFICACY AND USE

Administration of the biperidylphosphodiesterase inhibitors, **milrinone** and **inamrinone**, to patients with CHF results in a marked increase in cardiac index and a substantial reduction in cardiac filling pressures. Systemic blood pressure (BP) only slightly alters. At high doses, a reflexive rise in heart rate and fall in BP may be observed. The increase in cardiac contractility observed early in the development of inamrinone and milrinone was presumed to be the result of their inotropic action, but this is now attributed to their vasodilatory action.

Because of their vasodilating action, both **milrinone** and **inamrinone** are very effective in lowering filling pressures and increasing cardiac output. These effects are synergistic with those of dobutamine or other catecholamines.

Inamrinone was formerly known as **amrinone**, until reports of serious adverse events, including deaths, resulting from medication errors involving confusion between the names *amrinone* and *amiodarone* prompted the United States Pharmacopeia and United States Adopted Name (USAN) Council to change the drug name to *inamrinone*.

Milrinone has largely replaced **inamrinone** as the PDE inhibitor of choice, mostly because of the relatively high incidence of thrombocytopenia observed with **inamrinone**.

MODE OF ACTION

Milrinone and **inamrinone** inhibit the enzyme responsible for the breakdown of cyclic adenosine monophosphate (AMP) in the target cell. More specifically, they selectively inhibit PDE III, the isoenzyme specific for cyclic AMP. The subsequent increase in cyclic AMP leads to enhanced phosphorylation of protein in the sarcoplasmic reticulum and sarcolemma, which in turn promotes improved calcium uptake, storage, and release from the sarcoplasmic reticulum during excitation-contraction coupling. Adenosine receptors have also been implicated in the action of these drugs. **Milrinone** may also increase calcium influx into myocardial cells via the slow calcium channel. In addition to their inotropic effect, **milrinone** and **inamrinone** produce vasodilatation and a decrease in both preload and afterload. These agents have a rapid onset and reach a peak hemodynamic effect within 10 minutes when given intravenously.

INDICATIONS

	Milrinone	Inamrinone
Short-term support in CHF	+	+

+—FDA approved; CHF—congestive heart failure.

INAMRINONE (Inamrinone)

Inamrinone is a PDE inhibitor with positive inotropic and vasodilating activity. Inamrinone has a different chemical structure and mechanism of action from either digitalis glycosides or catecholamines. Inamrinone provides hemodynamic benefits and symptomatic relief in patients not adequately controlled by diuretic, vasodilator, and cardioglycoside therapy.

Thrombocytopenia is a concern with inamrinone therapy. This problem may be related to high doses and prolonged administration or high blood concentrations of a metabolite, N-acetylamrinone. For this reason, milrinone has largely replaced inamrinone as the PDE inhibitor of choice. The bone marrow is not involved and the platelet count is usually normalized after withdrawal of inamrinone. Intravenous inamrinone is only indicated for short-term management in patients with low-output heart failure. Prolonged therapy is generally not recommended. Chronic inotropic therapy, with the exception of digitalis glycosides, may improve symptoms of heart failure transiently but has been associated with an excessive increase in mortality.

SPECIAL GROUPS

Race: no differences in response
Children: safety and effectiveness have not been established
Elderly: dose should be adjusted based on renal function
Renal impairment: dose should be adjusted based on renal function
Hepatic impairment: use with caution; adjust dosage based on response
Pregnancy: category C; use only if potential benefit justifies the potential risk to the fetus
Breast-feeding: not recommended; not known if the drug is excreted in human milk

DOSAGE

An IV bolus dose of 750 µg/kg (0.75 mg/kg) should be administered over 2–3 min, followed by a continuous infusion of 5–10 µg/kg/min and titrated to the maximum hemodynamic effect based on close patient monitoring. A second bolus of 750 µg/kg (0.75 mg/kg) may be administered 30 min after the initial bolus. The total dose should not exceed 10 mg/kg/d. Duration of therapy is determined by the responsiveness of the patient.

IN BRIEF

INDICATIONS
CHF, short-term inotropic support

CONTRAINDICATIONS
Known hypersensitivity to milrinone, inamrinone, or bisulfites

DRUG INTERACTIONS
Not clear; any agents that may affect cardiac or hemodynamic system can potentially interact with inamrinone.

ADVERSE EFFECTS
CV: arrhythmias, angina, hypotension
CNS: headache
GI: hepatotoxicity, nausea, vomiting
Other: thrombocytopenia, hypokalemia, tremor, hypersensitivity reaction, fever

PHARMACOKINETICS AND PHARMACODYNAMICS
Duration of action:	up to 2 h
Onset of action:	2–5 min
Time to peak effect:	within 10 min
Bioavailability:	100%
Effect of food:	not applicable
Protein binding:	10%–49%
Volume of distribution:	1.2 L/kg
Metabolism:	partially metabolized by conjugative pathway
Elimination:	renal (10%–40% as unchanged within 24 h)
Elimination half-life:	5.8 h (3–15 h)

MONITORING
BP, heart rate, electrocardiogram (ECG), platelet count, serum electrolytes, renal function, weight, cardiac index, central venous or pulmonary wedge pressure, and improvement in signs and symptoms of heart failure.

OVERDOSE
Supportive: Fluid therapy and vasopressors may be used in severe hypotension for circulatory support.

PATIENT INFORMATION
Inamrinone is used to treat decompensated heart failure.

AVAILABILITY
Parenteral—100 mg/20 mL (5 mg/mL)

MILRINONE (Milrinone, Primacor®)

Milrinone is a PDE inhibitor with positive inotropic and vasodilating activity. Milrinone has a different mechanism of action from either digitalis glycosides or catecholamines. However, milrinone has rarely been associated with thrombocytopenia, a significant problem reported with inamrinone. Milrinone IV is only indicated for short-term management in patients with low-output heart failure. Prolonged IV maintenance therapy has been associated with increased risk of arrhythmias and sudden death. Actually, when oral milrinone was investigated as a chronic inotropic support in heart failure patients, the study was terminated because an excessive mortality rate was observed.

SPECIAL GROUPS

Race: no differences in response
Children: safety and effectiveness have not been established
Elderly: dose should be adjusted based on renal function
Renal impairment: dose should be lowered and adjusted based on renal function
Hepatic impairment: use with caution; dosage adjustment is probably not required
Pregnancy: category C; use only if potential benefit justifies the potential risk to the fetus
Breast-feeding: not recommended; not known if the drug is excreted in human milk

DOSAGE

A loading dose of 50 µg/kg should be administered IV over 10 min, followed by a continuous infusion of 0.375 µg/kg/min (start with lower infusion rate if patient has renal dysfunction, see table below) and titrated to the maximum hemodynamic effect based on close patient monitoring.* The total dose should not exceed 1.13 mg/kg/d (or, 0.75 µg/kg/min). Duration of therapy is determined by the responsiveness of the patient.

*Recommended infusion rate in patients with renal impairment:

Creatinine clearance, mL/min/1.73 m^2	Starting infusion rate, µg/kg/min
5	0.20
10	0.23
20	0.28
30	0.33
≥40	0.375

IN BRIEF

INDICATIONS
CHF, short-term inotropic support.

CONTRAINDICATIONS
Known hypersensitivity to milrinone or inamrinone

DRUG INTERACTIONS
Not clear; any agents that may affect cardiac and hemodynamic system can potentially interact with milrinone.

ADVERSE EFFECTS
CV: arrhythmias, angina, hypotension
CNS: headache
Other: thrombocytopenia, hypokalemia, tremor, hypersensitivity reaction

PHARMACOKINETICS AND PHARMACODYNAMICS
Duration of action: 3–5 h
Onset of action: immediate
Peak effect: within 5–15 min
Bioavailability: 100%
Protein binding: 70%
Volume of distribution: 0.3–0.4 L/kg
Effect of food: not applicable
Metabolism: 12% converted to O-glucuronide
Elimination: renal (83% unchanged)
Elimination half-life: 2.3 hours (↑ in renal dysfunction)

MONITORING
BP, heart rate, ECG, serum electrolytes, platelet count, renal function, weight, and improvement in signs and symptoms of heart failure, cardiac index, central venous or pulmonary wedge pressure.

OVERDOSE
Supportive: Fluid therapy and vasopressors may be used in severe hypotension for circulatory support.

PATIENT INFORMATION
Milrinone is used to treat decompensated heart failure.

AVAILABILITY
Vials—10 mg/10 mL, 20 mg/20 mL, 50 mg/50 mL
Syringes—5 mg/5 mL
Pre-Mix—20 mg/100 mL D5W, 40 mg/200 mL

INOTROPIC AND VASOPRESSOR AGENTS: ADRENERGIC RECEPTOR AGONISTS

Drugs that belong to the adrenergic receptor agonist group (*eg*, **dobutamine** and **dopamine**) have a common feature: they stimulate cardiac or peripheral tissues at specific adrenergic or dopaminergic receptors to produce a combination of either peripheral vasodilatation or constriction with positive inotropic support to the heart. They differ in their receptor selectivities, and this is reflected in different hemodynamic responses. Because of their pharmacokinetic or pharmacodynamic properties, most are used for short-term hemodynamic support only. An orally active alpha$_1$-adrenergic agonist is approved for use in patients with orthostatic hypotension (*ie*, **midodrine**).

EFFICACY AND USE

These inotropic agents are available for intravenous (IV), and thus, short-term use. Evidence suggests that tachyphylaxis to these drugs may appear with sustained use. To date, there has been no evidence to support their long-term benefit in terms of mortality, and they may even increase the risk of death. Nevertheless, these agents are valuable in providing short-term hemodynamic support.

Because these drugs tend to enhance atrioventricular (AV) conduction, they have proarrhythmic potential in patients with atrial arrhythmias. In these cases, pretreatment with digitalis may be useful. Because their actions are not identical, they may work synergistically, either together or with other vasodilators. This strategy permits the use of low-dose **dopamine** when its vasodilatory effects are apparent, rather than risking unwanted vasoconstriction with too high a dose. These drugs have a relatively weak effect on pulmonary wedge pressure. Therefore, when used in combination with preload reducers, such as nitrates or angiotensin-converting enzyme (ACE) inhibitors, they may produce valuable benefits. Because of the inotropic effects, they may worsen ischemia; it is therefore advisable to use them only with ECG monitoring.

MODE OF ACTION

Dobutamine stimulates beta$_1$-adrenergic receptors and, to a lesser extent, beta$_2$-receptors. It has a very short half-life. When given IV, it raises cardiac output and reduces systemic vascular resistance. Renal blood flow improves, and this may result in an improved urine output.

Dopamine is among the oldest known direct inotropic drugs. As a precursor of the catecholamines, it is capable of interacting with a variety of adrenergic receptors. As a result, its hemodynamic actions are, to some extent, dose dependent. Dopamine receptors are found in the renal, mesenteric, coronary, and cerebrovascular beds. Low doses of dopamine stimulate dopamine receptors to produce vasodilatation in these areas. Higher doses release norepinephrine from storage sites. As a result, indirect beta$_1$-adrenergic stimulation is observed producing hemodynamic effects similar to those of **dobutamine**. At even higher doses, dopamine stimulates alpha-adrenergic receptors, producing vasoconstriction and opposing the dopaminergic vasodilatory action. Hypertension is sometimes observed in this situation. Table 10.2 shows the different pharmacologic actions of these inotropic agents.

Isoproterenol is a stimulant of both beta$_1$- and beta$_2$-adrenergic receptors. The drug must be given IV. It causes vasodilatation accompanied by direct and reflex cardiac stimulation. Cardiac output is increased while mean BP falls. It can cause tachycardia and significant arrhythmogenesis, which has limited its clinical use.

Norepinephrine, a naturally occurring catecholamine, stimulates beta$_1$-, alpha$_1$-, and alpha$_2$-adrenergic receptors, and to a much less extent, beta$_2$-receptors. Its major hemody-

INDICATIONS

	CHF (short-term)	Cardiogenic shock	Hypotension	Bradycardia
Dobutamine	+	+		
Dopamine	+	+	+	
Epinephrine			+	
Isoproterenol	+	+		+
Metaraminol			+	
Methoxamine			+	
Midodrine			+	
Norepinephrine			+	
Phenylephrine			+	
Vasopressin			+*	

*Not an FDA-approved indication.
+—clinically used.

namic effect is to cause vasoconstriction and direct cardiac stimulation, leading to increased systolic and diastolic BP. Reflex bradycardia may occur. It has limited clinical use except as a pressor agent in the treatment of shock with hypotension.

Epinephrine, a naturally occurring catecholamine, stimulates beta-adrenergic receptors, and to a lesser extent, alpha-receptors. It causes cardiac stimulation accompanied by venoconstriction. It causes vasoconstriction in certain vascular beds, but dilation in others (*eg*, skeletal muscle). Cardiac output is increased and systolic BP is elevated, whereas diastolic BP falls, with little change in peripheral vascular resistance. The drug remains an emergency treatment for cardiac arrest, for preserving cerebral blood flow during resuscitation, and for treatment of severe allergic reactions. It is used as an adjunctive vasoconstrictor during local anesthesia.

Metaraminol is an IV pressor agent that indirectly causes alpha$_1$ stimulation by causing the release of neuronal norepinephrine.

Methoxamine and **phenylephrine** are both sympathomimetic amines, which act predominantly on postsynaptic alpha-adrenergic receptors to increase arterial BP. In addition, phenylephrine has an indirect effect to release norepinephrine from its storage sites.

Midodrine is an orally active alpha$_1$-receptor agonist that causes both arterial and venous constriction without tachycardia. It is approved for use in patients with symptomatic orthostatic hypotension. It has limited benefit in the management of vasovagal syncope.

TABLE 10.2 COMPARATIVE AGONIST ACTIVITIES AND ACTIONS OF DOPAMINE AND DOBUTAMINE

Activity	Response to activity	Dopamine	Dobutamine
DA$_1$	Renal and mesenteric vasodilatation; natriuresis, diuresis	+++	NA
DA$_2$	Presynaptic sympathetic inhibition of norepinephrine release; generalized reduction of sympathetic tone (excessive stimulation leads to increased risk of nausea and emesis)	++	NA
Beta$_1$	Positive chronotropy or inotropy. Increased AV conduction (leads to increased risk of arrhythmias)	++	+++
Beta$_2$	Peripheral vasodilatation (afterload reduction)	+	++
Alpha	Peripheral and arteriolar vasoconstriction	++	++
Uptake inhibition	Increase in amount of norepinephrine in sympathetic synaptic cleft	++	+

+—mild; ++—moderate; +++— powerful; Alpha—Alpha-adrenergic receptor; AV—atrioventricular; Beta$_1$ —Beta$_1$-adrenergic receptor; Beta$_2$—Beta$_2$-adrenergic receptor; DA$_1$—dopamine type I receptor; DA$_2$—dopamine type 2 receptor; NA—not active; uptake inhibition—norepinephrine uptake mechanism.

DOBUTAMINE (Dobutamine, Dobutrex®)

Dobutamine is a selective beta$_1$-adrenergic agonist. In therapeutic doses, dobutamine also exhibits mild beta$_2$- and alpha$_1$-adrenergic activities. Dobutamine does not cause release of endogenous norepinephrine and has no effect on dopaminergic receptors. The major effect of dobutamine is beta$_1$-mediated cardiac stimulation, which results in a positive inotropic effect. Dobutamine may reduce peripheral vascular resistance, but BP may remain unchanged or be increased as a result of increased cardiac output. Heart rate is usually minimally affected, whereas increased contractility may enhance coronary perfusion and myocardial oxygen consumption. Dobutamine enhances atrioventricular conduction. Thus, in atrial fibrillation with rapid ventricular response, patients should be digitalized prior to dobutamine therapy. Dobutamine may reduce pulmonary vascular resistance, which may benefit patients with elevated pulmonary artery pressure.

SPECIAL GROUPS

Race: no differences in response
Children: safety and effectiveness have not been established
Elderly: no dosage adjustment is required
Renal impairment: no dosage adjustment is required
Hepatic impairment: no dosage adjustment is required
Pregnancy: category B; should only be used if clearly indicated
Breast-feeding: not recommended; not known if the drug is excreted in human milk

DOSAGE

Usual dose range: 2.5–15 µg/kg/min
The infusion rate and the duration of therapy should be adjusted based on clinical response.

IN BRIEF

INDICATIONS
Short-term inotropic support in patients with cardiac decompensation due to depressed contractility.

CONTRAINDICATIONS
Idiopathic hypertrophic subaortic stenosis
Hypersensitivity

DRUG INTERACTIONS
Any agents that may affect the cardiac/hemodynamic system can potentially interact with dobutamine
Beta-adrenergic antagonists[1,2]

1 Effect of dobutamine may decrease.

2 Dobutamine may decrease the effect of this drug.

ADVERSE EFFECTS
CV: tachycardia, ventricular ectopic beats, hypertension, hypotension, angina
CNS: headache
GI: nausea
Skin: phlebitis, local infiltration/reaction
Other: hypokalemia

PHARMACOKINETICS AND PHARMACODYNAMICS
Duration of action: few minutes
Onset of action: 1–2 min
Peak effect: 10 min
Bioavailability: 100%
Effect of food: not applicable
Protein binding: not known
Volume of distribution: 0.2 L/kg
Elimination: renally excreted as metabolites after methylation and conjugation
Elimination half-life: 2 min

MONITORING
BP, heart rate, ECG, serum electrolytes, urine output, cardiac index, central venous and pulmonary wedge pressure, weight, and improvement in signs and symptoms of heart failure.

OVERDOSE
Supportive: the duration of action is usually short.

PATIENT INFORMATION
Dobutamine is used to increase the contractility of a failing heart.

AVAILABILITY
Vials—250 mg/20 mL (12.5 mg/mL)

DOPAMINE (Dopamine, Intropin®)

Dopamine, an endogenous catecholamine, is the immediate precursor of norepinephrine. Dopamine activates the sympathetic nervous system directly. In addition, dopamine stimulates the release of norepinephrine from storage sites. Dopamine also causes vasodilation by acting on specific dopaminergic receptors in the renal, mesenteric, coronary, and intracerebral vascular beds. The major therapeutic effect of dopamine is dose dependent. In low doses, up to 10 µg/kg/min, cardiac (beta$_1$) stimulation and renal vascular dilatation (dopaminergic) occur, and in higher doses, >10 µg/kg/min, vasoconstriction occurs (alpha-adrenergic stimulation). In clinical practice, dopamine may be used to increase cardiac output, BP, and urine output in the management of persistent circulatory failure after adequate fluid resuscitation. Because dopamine may improve cardiac output and stroke volume, it has been used as a short-term, add-on therapy in patients with severe heart failure. The therapy should only be continued if clinical improvement can be achieved without significant adverse effects such as arrhythmias, cardiac ischemia, and signs and symptoms of peripheral tissue ischemia.

SPECIAL GROUPS

Race: no differences in response
Children: safety and effectiveness have not been established
Elderly: no dosage adjustment is required
Renal impairment: no dosage adjustment is required
Hepatic impairment: no dosage adjustment is required
Pregnancy: category C; use only if potential benefit justifies the potential risk to the fetus
Breast-feeding: not recommended; not known if the drug is excreted in human milk

DOSAGE

Usual dose range: 1–20 µg/kg/min
Infusion should be started at 1–5 µg/kg/min and increased by 1–4 µg/kg/min, every 10–30 min until the desired response is achieved. Then, the dose should be titrated based on clinical assessment. Infusion rates up to 50 µg/kg/min have been used safely. As a general rule, a lower infusion rate (≤1 µg/kg/min) should be initiated in patients with occlusive vascular disease.

IN BRIEF

INDICATIONS
Hemodynamic imbalances, after adequate fluid resuscitation.

CONTRAINDICATIONS
Pheochromocytoma
Ventricular fibrillation
Uncorrected tachyarrhythmias
Known sulfite allergy (some products)

DRUG INTERACTIONS
Any agents that may affect cardiac/hemodynamic system can potentially interact with dopamine
Alpha-adrenergic antagonists[2,3]
Beta-adrenergic antagonists[2,3]
Monoamine oxidase (MAO) inhibitors[1]
Phenytoin[3,4]

1 Effect/toxicity of dopamine may increase.
2 Effect of dopamine may decrease.
3 Dopamine may decrease the effect of this drug.
4 Severe hypotension and bradycardia has been reported with comcomitant therapy.

ADVERSE EFFECTS
CV: tachycardia, ventricular ectopic beats, other dysrhythmias, hypertension, hypotension, angina, polyuria
CNS: headache
GI: nausea, vomiting
Skin: phlebitis, local infiltration/tissue necrosis
Other: peripheral tissue cyanosis/gangrene

PHARMACOKINETICS AND PHARMACODYNAMICS
Duration of action: <10 min
Onset of action: <5 min
Peak effect: 5–10 min
Bioavailability: 100%
Effect of food: not applicable
Protein binding: no data
Volume of distribution: 1.8–2.5 L/kg
Metabolism: metabolized extensively in plasma, liver, and kidney by MAO and catechol-O-methyltransferase to inactive metabolites; about 25% is metabolized to norepinephrine in the adrenergic nerve terminals
Elimination: in urine mainly as metabolites
Elimination half-life: 2 min

MONITORING
BP, heart rate, ECG , serum electrolytes, urine output, cardiac index, central venous and pulmonary wedge pressure, peripheral tissue perfusion, weight.

OVERDOSE
Supportive: the duration of action is usually short.

PATIENT INFORMATION
Dopamine is used to support cardiac function and blood circulation, and maintain tissue oxygenation.

AVAILABILITY
Vials—
40 mg/mL, in 5, 10, 20 mL
80 mg/mL, in 5, 20 mL
160 mg/mL, in 5 mL
Syringes—
40 mg/mL, in 5, 10 mL
80 mg/mL, in 10 mL
160 mg/mL, in 5 mL
Pre-Mix—
0.8 mg/mL, in 250, 500 mL
1.6 mg/mL, in 250, 500 mL
3.2 mg/mL, in 250 mL

ISOPROTERENOL
(Isoproterenol, Isuprel®)

Isoproterenol, a synthetic sympathomimetic agent, acts directly on beta$_1$- and beta$_2$-adrenergic receptors and has negligble effect on alpha-adrenergic receptors. The major therapeutic effects of isoproterenol are bronchodilation, cardiac stimulation, and peripheral vasodilation. Isoproterenol also inhibits antigen-induced release of histamine and the slow-reacting substance of anaphylaxis.

SPECIAL GROUPS

Race: no differences in response
Children: limited data; dosing based on weight
Elderly: use with caution; no dosage adjustment is required
Renal impairment: use with caution; no dosage adjustment is required
Hepatic impairment: use with caution; dosage adjustment is probably not required
Pregnancy: category C; use only if potential benefit justifies the potential risk to the fetus
Breast-feeding: not recommended; not known if the drug is excreted in human milk

DOSAGE

Cardiac arrhythmias (bradycardia/AV block):
 IV—0.02–0.06 mg (1–3 mL of a 1:50,000 dilution); subsequent doses of 0.01–0.2 mg (0.5–10 mL of a 1:50,000 dilution) may be given based on response.
 IV infusion—The initial rate is 5 µg/min (ie, 2.5 mL/min of a 1:500,000 dilution), and the rate is adjusted based on response (usual dose range: 2–20 µg/min).
 IM/SC—0.2 mg (1 mL of a 1:5,000 dilution); subsequent doses of 0.02–1 mg (0.1–5 mL of a 1:5,000 dilution) IM or 0.15–0.2 mg (0.75–1 mL of a 1:5,000 dilution) SC may be given based on response.
 Intracardiac—0.02 mg (0.1 mL of a 1:5,000 dilution)
Shock: Continuous IV infusion (in 1:500,000 dilution, or 2 µg/mL) is initiated at 0.5–5 µg/min and adjusted based on patient's response.
Diagnostic aid: 4 µg/min is administered in the diagnosis of the etiology of mitral valve regurgitation
 1–3 µg/min is administered in the diagnosis of coronary artery disease

IN BRIEF

INDICATIONS
Low cardiac output in hypovolemic and septic shock
Bradycardia in cardiopulmonary resuscitation
Heart block and Adams-Stokes attacks
Diagnostic aid for mitral valve regurgitation and coronary artery disease (not FDA-approved)
Bronchospasm

CONTRAINDICATIONS
Known hypersensitivity to isoproterenol or sulfites
History of cardiac arrhythmias
Angina pectoris
Tachycardia and AV block associated with cardiac glycoside intoxication

DRUG INTERACTIONS
Concurrent beta-adrenergic blocking agents[2,4]
Digitalis[2,3]
Theophylline derivatives[1,4]
Other sympathomimetic agents[1]
1 Effect/toxicity of isoproterenol may increase.
2 Effect of isoproterenol may decrease.
3 Isoproterenol may increase the effect/toxicity of this drug.
4 Isoproterenol may decrease the effect of this drug.

ADVERSE EFFECTS
CV: palpitation, tachycardia, arrhythmias, angina, hypertension/hypotension
CNS: headache, dizziness, nervousness, insomnia, tremor, weakness
GI: nausea, vomiting
Skin: flushing, sweating

PHARMACOKINETICS AND PHARMACODYNAMICS
Duration of action: (IV) a few min; (IM/SQ) 2 h
Onset of action: rapid
Peak effect: 15–30 min for bronchodilation
Bioavailability: 100% (parenteral)
Effect of food: not known
Protein binding: not known
Volume of distribution: not known
Metabolism: metabolized in liver, lungs, GI mucosa and other tissue
Elimination: excreted renally (after IV, 40%–50% as unchanged, the rest as metabolites)
Elimination half-life: not known

MONITORING
BP, heart rate, ECG, respiration, urine output, serum electrolytes, and other appropriate monitoring for adequate tissue perfusion (such as blood lactic acid, pH, pO$_2$, and pCO$_2$ levels, and oxygen saturation)

OVERDOSE
Supportive: a beta-adrenergic blocking agent may be used to treat tachycardia if indicated.

PATIENT INFORMATION
Isoproterenol is used to stimulate the heart and maintain cardiac function (or to relieve bronchospasm).

AVAILABILITY
Ampules/vials—0.2 mg/mL (1:5,000) in 1, 5, 10 mL
Syringes—0.02 mg/mL (1:50,000) in 10 mL

The information here is provided as guidance only. Prescribers should always consult the manufacturer's current prescribing information.

261

EPINEPHRINE
(Epinephrine, Various Sources)

Epinephrine, a sympathomimetic agent, acts directly on alpha- and beta-adrenergic receptors. At usual doses, it acts predominantly on the beta-receptors of the heart, vasculature, and smooth muscle. At higher doses, alpha-adrenergic stimulation predominates. After rapid intravenous injection, such as in cardiopulmonary resuscitation, epinephrine produces a rapid rise in BP and increases in heart rate and contractility while it constricts the arterioles in peripheral and splanchnic circulations. These result in improved myocardial and cerebral blood flow during resuscitation. Epinephrine relaxes bronchial smooth muscle by $beta_1$-adrenergic stimulation and constricts bronchial arterioles by alpha-adrenergic stimulation. It has been used in patients with airway obstruction to relieve bronchospasm, congestion, and edema. Epinephrine also inhibits histamine release and antagonizes its effect on the end organs. It is useful as an adjunct in the management of anaphylaxis to reverse constriction or obstruction of the airway, vasodilation, and edema associated with mediator release.

SPECIAL GROUPS

Race: no differences in response
Children: dosage should be adjusted based on weight
Elderly: use with caution; no dosage adjustment is required
Renal impairment: use with caution; dosage adjustment is probably not required
Hepatic impairment: use with caution; dosage adjustment is probably not required
Pregnancy: category C; use only if potential benefit justifies the potential risk to the fetus
Breast-feeding: not recommended; not known if excreted in human milk

IN BRIEF
(Cardiovascular use mainly)

INDICATIONS
Cardiopulmonary resuscitation/cardiac arrest
Syncope and/or bradycardia resulting from AV block

CONTRAINDICATIONS
Known hypersensitivity to sulfites (some products)
Shock other than anaphylactic shock
Dilated cardiomyopathy and coronary insufficiency
Cerebral arteriosclerosis or organic brain damage
General anesthesia with halogenated hydrocarbons or cyclopropane
Narrow-angle glaucoma
Local use in fingers, toes, ears, nose, or genitalia in combination with local anesthetics

DRUG INTERACTIONS
Concurrent alpha[2]- and beta-adrenergic blocking agents[1,2,4]
Digitalis[1,3]
Ergot alkaloids[1]
Guanethidine[4]
Phenothiazines[2]
Thyroid hormones[1]
Tricyclic antidepressants[1]
Other sympathomimetic agents[1,3]

1 Effect/toxicity of epinephrine may increase.
2 Effect of epinephrine may decrease.
3 Epinephrine may increase the effect/toxicity of this drug.
4 Epinephrine may decrease the effect of this drug.

ADVERSE EFFECTS
CV: hypertension, palpitation, tachycardia, arrhythmias, angina, MI, hypotension (rare)
CNS: headache, dizziness, weakness, syncope, stroke, anxiety, fear, nervousness, tremor, insomnia, disorientation, assaultive behavior, hallucination, psychosis, memory impairment, exacerbation of parkinsonian syndrome
Other: metabolic acidosis, hyperglycemia, ↓ urine output, hepatic or renal ischemia/failure, tissue ischemia, gangrene, or necrosis

PHARMACOKINETICS AND PHARMACODYNAMICS
Duration of action: short, but may persist for a few hours after subcutaneous administration
Onset of action: rapid, within minutes
Peak effect: not known
Bioavailability: (IV) 100%; not known for other routes
Effect of food: not applicable
Protein binding: not known
Volume of distribution: not known
Metabolism: metabolized in sympathetic nerve endings, liver, and peripheral tissues by catechol-O-methyltransferase and monoamine oxidase
Elimination: mainly excreted in urine as metabolites
Elimination half-life: not known

MONITORING
BP, heart rate, ECG, mental status, urine output, serum electrolytes, and other appropriate monitoring for adequate tissue perfusion (such as blood lactic acid, pH, pO_2, and pCO_2 levels, and oxygen saturation).

OVERDOSE
Supportive: an alpha-adrenergic antagonist such as phentolamine may be used for severe hypertension (may be followed by hypotension, which may be treated with a different vasopressor), and a beta-adrenergic antagonist may be used for arrhythmias.

EPINEPHRINE (continued)

DOSAGE

Cardiac arrest, ventricular fibrillation and pulseless ventricular tachycardia, pulseless electrical activity, or asystole in advanced cardiac life support (ACLS):

Intravenous (IV)—The usual dose is 0.5–1 mg (usually as 5–10 mL of a 1:10,000 injection) administered by IV push. This dose may be repeated every 3–5 minutes if needed.

Initial IV administration may be followed by continuous infusion at a rate of 1–4 µg/min.

Endotracheal—1–3 mg diluted in 10 mL of solution before instillation

Symptomatic bradycardia: The usual initial dose is 1 µg/min (1 mg in 500 mL solution) by continuous infusion. The rate is titrated based on clinical response and usually ranges from 2–10 µg/min.

AVAILABILITY
Syringes—1 mg/mL (1:1,000) in 0.3 mL, 1 mL, 2 mL; 0.5 mg/mL (1:2,000) in 0.3 mL; 0.1 mg/mL (1:10,000) in 10 mL
Ampules—5 mg/mL (1:200) in 0.3 mL, suspension; 1 mg/mL (1:1,000) in 1 mL
Vials—5 mg/mL (1:200) in 5 mL, suspension; 1 mg/mL (1:1,000) in 30 mL
Also available as:
  Metered-dose inhalers—160 and 220 µg/spray
  Solutions for nebulization—1%, 2.25%
  Ophthalmic preparations
  In various combinations with a local anesthetic agent

METARAMINOL
(Metaraminol, Aramine®)

Metaraminol, a sympathomimetic amine, has effects similar to norepinephrine, but it has a longer duration of action. Metaraminol acts directly on alpha- and beta$_1$-adrenergic receptors. It also acts indirectly by increasing the release of norepinephrine from the storage sites. The major therapeutic effects of metaraminol are vasoconstriction and cardiac stimulation. Tachyphylaxis may occur after prolonged use of metaraminol secondary to depletion of norepinephrine stores in sympathetic nerve endings. Metaraminol may also act as a weak or false neurotransmitter. It may replace norepinephrine in sympathetic nerve endings, which may result in vasodilation and hypotension on rare occasions.

SPECIAL GROUPS

Race: no differences in response
Children: safety and effectiveness have not been established
Elderly: no dosage adjustment is required
Renal impairment: use with caution; starting with low dose
Hepatic impairment: use with caution; dosage adjustment is probably not required
Pregnancy: category C; use only if potential benefit justifies the potential risk to the fetus
Breast-feeding: not recommended; not known if the drug is excreted in human milk

DOSAGE

Prevention of hypotension:
Usual dose: 2–10 mg IM*. The lowest effective dose should be used for the shortest possible time. At least 10 min should elapse before additional doses are administered.

Severe hypotension or shock:
Usual dose: 0.5–5 mg (direct IV). Direct IV administration may be followed by a continuous infusion (15–100 mg in 500 mL of compatible diluent) if indicated. The rate of infusion should be adjusted to maintain the desired blood pressure.

*Note—Subcutaneous administration of metaraminol has been used. Subcutaneous administration is not recommended because of increased risk of tissue necrosis and abscess formation.

IN BRIEF

INDICATIONS
Hypotension associated with spinal anesthesia (both prevention and treatment)

Hypotension and shock associated with hemorrhage, reactions to medications, surgical complications, and brain damage due to trauma or tumor

CONTRAINDICATIONS
Known hypersensitivity to sulfites
Suspected peripheral or mesenteric vascular thrombosis
Concurrent halothane or cyclopropane anesthesia

DRUG INTERACTIONS
Concurrent alpha- and beta-adrenergic blocking agents[2,4]
Other agents that increase BP[1,3]
Digitalis[1,2]
MAO inhibitors[1,2]
Tricyclic antidepressants[1,2]
Other sympathomimetic agents[1,3]
1 Effect/toxicity of metaraminol may increase.
2 Effect of metaraminol may decrease.
3 Metaraminol may increase the effect/toxicity of this drug.
4 Metaraminol may decrease the effect of this drug.

ADVERSE EFFECTS
CV: hypertension, palpitations, tachycardia, bradycardia, arrhythmias, angina, myocardial infarction, hypotension (rare)
CNS: headache, stroke
Skin: local tissue irritation, abscess, necrosis, and sloughing
Other: metabolic acidosis, ↓ urine output, hepatic or renal ischemia/failure

PHARMACOKINETICS AND PHARMACODYNAMICS
Duration of action: 20–90 min (depends on routes)
Onset of action: (IV) 1–2 min; (IM) <10 min
Peak effect: rapid, < 10 min
Bioavailability: (IV) 100%
Effect of food: not applicable
Protein binding: not known
Volume of distribution: not known
Metabolism: not clear; partially hepatic
Elimination: excreted in urine and stools mainly as metabolites
Elimination half-life: not known

MONITORING
BP, heart rate, ECG, urine output, serum electrolytes, and other appropriate monitoring for adequate tissue perfusion (such as blood lactic acid, pH, pO$_2$, and pCO$_2$ levels, and oxygen saturation).

OVERDOSE
Supportive: a sympatholytic agent, such as phentolamine, may be used for severe hypertension.

PATIENT INFORMATION
Metaraminol is used to maintain BP or prevent hypotension.

AVAILABILITY
Vials—10 mg/mL in 10 mL (1%)

METHOXAMINE
(Methoxamine, Vasoxyl®)

Methoxamine, a synthetic sympathomimetic amine, has pharmacologic activity similar to phenylephrine. It acts primarily on alpha-adrenergic receptors and has negligible effect on $beta_1$- or $beta_2$-adrenergic receptors. Methoxamine administration produces a rapid and sustained rise in BP. It is used to maintain BP during anesthesia. Methoxamine is less arrhythmogenic and may be used safely with cyclopropane or halogenated hydrocarbons during anesthesia. Similar to phenylephrine, methoxamine may cause reflex bradycardia and ventricular ectopic beats. Bradycardia may be prevented by administration of atropine. Methoxamine may be useful in terminating paroxysmal atrial or nodal tachycardia, especially in patients with profound hypotension.

SPECIAL GROUPS

Race: no differences in response
Children: safety and effectiveness have not been established
Elderly: use with caution; no dosage adjustment is required
Renal impairment: use with caution; dosage adjustment is probably not required
Hepatic impairment: use with caution; dosage adjustment is probably not required
Pregnancy: category C; use only if potential benefit justifies the potential risk to the fetus
Breast-feeding: not recommended; not known if the drug is excreted in human milk

DOSAGE

Hypotension: moderate—5–10 mg IM; severe—3–5 mg IV slowly This dose may be repeated after 15 min, or supplemented by IM injection of 10–15 mg to provide more prolonged effect.
Prevention of hypotension during anesthesia—The usual dose is 10–15 mg given IM shortly before or with spinal anesthesia (up to 20 mg may be required at high levels of anesthesia).
Supraventricular tachycardia: 10 mg given IV over 3–5 min, or 10–20 mg given IM; systolic BP should not be raised above 160 mm Hg

IN BRIEF

INDICATIONS
Hypotension associated with anesthesia (both prevention and treatment)
Paroxysmal supraventricular tachycardia associated with hypotension or shock

CONTRAINDICATIONS
Severe hypertension
Known hypersensitivity to methoxamine or sulfites

DRUG INTERACTIONS
Alpha-adrenergic blocking agents and agents with alpha-adrenergic blocking activity (phenothiazines)[2,4]
Atropine[2,4]
Ergot alkaloids[1]
MAO inhibitors[1,3]
Other sympathomimetic agents[1,3]
Tricyclic antidepressants[1]

[1] Effect/toxicity of methoxamine may increase.
[2] Effect of methoxamine may decrease.
[3] Methoxamine may increase the effect/toxicity of this drug.
[4] Methoxamine may decrease the effect of this drug.

ADVERSE EFFECTS
CV: hypertension, reflex bradycardia, heart failure, chest pain, arrhythmias, myocardial infarction
CNS: headache, dizziness, anxiety, nervousness, restlessness, stroke
GI: nausea, vomiting
Skin: cold, piloerection
Other: paresthesia, metabolic acidosis, ↓ urine output, hepatic or renal ischemia/failure

PHARMACOKINETICS AND PHARMACODYNAMICS
Duration of action: (IV) 10–15 min; (IM) 60–90 min
Onset of action: rapid
Peak effect: (IV) 0.5–2 min; (IM) 15–20 min
Bioavailability: (IV) 100%
Effect of food: not applicable
Protein binding: not known
Volume of distribution: not known
Metabolism: not known
Elimination: not known
Elimination half-life: not known

MONITORING
BP, heart rate, ECG, mental status, urine output, serum electrolytes, and other appropriate monitoring for adequate tissue perfusion (such as blood lactic acid, pH, pO_2, and pCO_2 levels, and oxygen saturation).

OVERDOSE
Supportive: an alpha-adrenergic antagonist such as phentolamine may be used for severe hypertension, and atropine may be used for severe bradycardia.

PATIENT INFORMATION
Methoxamine is used to maintain BP (or to treat abnormal cardiac rhythm).

AVAILABILITY
Ampules—20 mg/mL, 1 mL

MIDODRINE HYDROCHLORIDE (ProAmatine®)

Midodrine HCl, an inactive prodrug, is converted to desglymidodrine, a peripheral alpha-agonist, by enzymatic hydrolysis in the body. Desglymidodrine causes vasoconstriction of both arteries and veins. In patients with severe orthostatic hypotension, it can increase both supine and standing BP and help relieve disabling symptoms. Desglymidodrine also acts on alpha-receptors located within the urinary bladder, which accounts for the dysuria problems observed in certain patient groups. Support stockings, used alone or in combination with fludrocortisone, and/or beta-blockers remain the preferred first-line treatment for certain patients with orthostatic hypotension. The patient medication profile should also be evaluated to identify and possibly remove any offending agents that may exacerbate the problem. Midodrine should be reserved in patients who remain symptomatic despite standard clinical care. Midodrine may also have a role in the management of hypotension secondary to hemodialysis, anesthesia, or spinal cord lesions; neurocardiogenic syncope; and stress-induced urinary incontinence in females.

SPECIAL GROUPS

Race: no differences in response
Children: safety and effectiveness have not been established
Elderly: no dosage adjustment is required
Renal impairment: use with caution; starting with 2.5 mg doses
Hepatic impairment: use with caution; dosage adjustment is probably not required
Pregnancy: category C; use only if potential benefit justifies the potential risk to the fetus
Breast-feeding: not recommended; not known if the drug is excreted in human milk

DOSAGE

10 mg orally three times daily at approximately 3–4 h intervals, with first dose administered shortly before or upon arising in the morning; no dose should be administered after dinner or within 3–4 h before bedtime; the dose should be skipped if the patient remains bedbound.

IN BRIEF

INDICATIONS
Symptomatic orthostatic hypotension unresponsive to nonpharmacologic treatment.

CONTRAINDICATIONS
Severe organic heart disease
Urinary retention
Pheochromocytoma
Thyrotoxicosis
Acute renal disease
Supine hypertension, systolic BP >180 mm Hg
Known hypersensitivity to midodrine

DRUG INTERACTIONS
Alpha-adrenergic blocking agents (prazosin, terazosin, etc.)[2,4]
Cardiac glycosides[3]
Mineralocorticoids[1,3]
Vasopressors (phenylephrine, pseudoephedrine, ephedrine, dihydroergotamine)[1,3]

1 Effect/toxicity of midodrine may increase.
2 Effect of midodrine may decrease.
3 Midodrine may increase the effect/toxicity of this drug.
4 Midodrine may decrease the effect of this drug.

ADVERSE EFFECTS
CV: supine and sitting hypertension, bradycardia
GU: urinary retention, frequency, and urgency
Skin: pruritus, piloerection, rash
Other: paresthesia, chills

PHARMACOKINETICS AND PHARMACODYNAMICS
Duration of action: 2–6 h
Onset of action: 45–90 min
Peak effect: 1–2 h
Bioavailability: 93%
Effect of food: no effect
Protein binding: insignificant
Volume of distribution: 4–4.6 L/kg
Metabolism: metabolized in various tissue and liver to desglymidodrine (active)
Elimination: renal; mainly as desglymidodrine
Elimination half-life: 25 min (midodrine); 3–4 h (desglymidodrine)

MONITORING
Supine and standing BP.

OVERDOSE
Supportive: limited data indicate phentolamine may be used to reverse severe hypertension.

PATIENT INFORMATION
To avoid hypertension occurring during sleep, midodrine should not be taken after dinner or within 3–4 h before bedtime. Certain cold remedies and weight control medications may cause hypertension and should be used cautiously with midodrine.

AVAILABILITY
Tablets—2.5 mg, 5 mg, 10 mg

NOREPINEPHRINE
(Norepinephrine, Levophed®)

Norepinephrine, an endogenous catecholamine, acts directly on alpha- and beta$_1$-adrenergic receptors. It does not have beta$_2$-adrenergic activity. The major therapeutic effects of norepinephrine are vasoconstriction and cardiac stimulation. It constricts both arterial and venous blood vessels, resulting in an increase in systolic and diastolic BP. This effect may redirect blood flow from peripheral (such as skin and skeletal muscle) and splanchnic circulations to vital organs (such as brain and myocardium). Renal blood flow and urine output may be reduced initially from constriction of renal blood vessels. However, if adequate intravascular volume is maintained, renal perfusion and urine output will increase as the systemic BP is normalized and cardiac output is increased through the positive inotropic effect on the myocardium. Direct coronary artery constriction is usually overcome by increased systemic BP and enhanced cardiac output.

Norepinephrine may be proarrhythmic, especially at higher doses in patients with cardiovascular diseases, concurrent proarrhythmic medications, or metabolic and electrolyte imbalances. Norepinephrine also causes pulmonary vessel constriction, resulting in an increase in pulmonary arterial pressure. Norepinephrine is administered IV to provide hemodynamic support via vasoconstriction and cardiac stimulation in patients with profound hypotension after adequate intravascular volume replacement. It has also been used in combination with some local anesthetics to enhance and prolong the duration of local anesthesia.

SPECIAL GROUPS

Race: no differences in response
Children: safety and effectiveness have not been established
Elderly: use with caution; no dosage adjustment is required
Renal impairment: use with caution; no dosage adjustment is required
Hepatic impairment: use with caution; no dosage adjustment is required
Pregnancy: category C; use only if potential benefit justifies the potential risk to the fetus
Breast-feeding: not recommended; not known if the drug is excreted in human milk

DOSAGE

Norepinephrine is administered by continuous IV infusion (ie, 4–8 mg in 500–1000 mL solution). The dose should be initiated at a rate of 0.5–1 µg/min and titrated to maintain a desired BP response.

IN BRIEF

INDICATIONS
Hypotensive state
Cardiac arrest (as an adjunct for severe hypotension)

CONTRAINDICATIONS
Known hypersensitivity to sulfites
General anesthesia (halogenated hydrocarbons or cyclopropane)
Suspected peripheral or mesenteric vascular thrombosis
Local use in fingers, toes, ears, nose, or genitalia in combination with local anesthetics

DRUG INTERACTIONS
Atropine[1,3]
Concurrent alpha-adrenergic blocking agents[2,4]
Concurrent beta-adrenergic blocking agents[2,4]
Ergot alkaloids[1]
Guanethidine[1]
MAO inhibitors[1]
Methyldopa[1]
Tricyclic antidepressants[1]
Other sympathomimetic agents[1,3]

[1] Effect/toxicity of norepinephrine may increase.
[2] Effect of norepinephrine may decrease.
[3] Norepinephrine may increase the effect/toxicity of this drug.
[4] Norepinephrine may decrease the effect of this drug.

ADVERSE EFFECTS
CV: hypertension, palpitations, tachycardia, bradycardia, arrhythmias, angina, MI, hypotension (rare)
CNS: headache, dizziness, weakness, syncope, stroke, anxiety, restlessness, tremor, insomnia
Skin: local tissue irritation, extravasation, necrosis, and sloughing
Other: metabolic acidosis, hyperglycemia, ↓ urine output, hepatic or renal ischemia or failure, tissue ischemia, gangrene, or necrosis

PHARMACOKINETICS AND PHARMACODYNAMICS
Duration of action: 1–2 min
Onset of action: rapid
Peak effect: rapid
Bioavailability: (IV) 100%; not absorbed from GI tract
Effect of food: not applicable
Protein binding: not known
Volume of distribution: not known
Metabolism: metabolized in sympathetic nerve endings, liver, and peripheral tissues by catechol-O-methyltransferase and monoamine oxidase
Elimination: mainly excreted in urine as metabolites
Elimination half-life: not known

MONITORING
BP, heart rate, ECG, mental status, urine output, serum electrolytes, and other appropriate monitoring for adequate tissue perfusion (such as blood lactic acid, pH, pO$_2$, and pCO$_2$ levels, and oxygen saturation).

OVERDOSE
Supportive: the effect should subside within a few minutes, and a beta-adrenergic antagonist, such as propranolol, may be used for arrhythmias if indicated.

PATIENT INFORMATION
Norepinephrine is used to maintain BP and prevent severe consequences associated with profound hypotension.

AVAILABILITY
Ampules—1 mg/mL, 4 mL

The information here is provided as guidance only. Prescribers should always consult the manufacturer's current prescribing information.

267

PHENYLEPHRINE
(Phenylephrine, Neo-Synephrine®)

Phenylephrine, a sympathomimetic amine, acts predominantly on postsynaptic alpha-adrenergic receptors, with little effect on the beta$_1$-adrenergic receptors of the heart. It has no effect on the beta$_2$-adrenergic receptors of the bronchi or peripheral blood vessels. Phenylephrine also has an indirect effect by releasing norepinephrine from its storage sites. The major effect of phenylephrine is vasoconstriction. Increased arterial BP may cause an increase in vagal activity and bradycardia. This effect can be blocked by atropine. Phenylephrine is used as an adjunct to provide hemodynamic support in patients with profound hypotension after adequate intravascular volume replacement. Phenylephrine may be used to terminate paroxysmal supraventricular tachycardia, especially in patients with concurrent hypotension or shock. Phenylephrine has also been used in spinal anesthesia to localize and prolong anesthetic activity, as a topical nasal decongestant, and in combination with an inhaled bronchodilator to prolong the effect of bronchodilation while alleviating airway edema and congestion.

SPECIAL GROUPS

Race: no differences in response
Children: dosage should be adjusted based on weight
Elderly: use with caution; no dosage adjustment is required
Renal impairment: use with caution; dosage adjustment is probably not required
Hepatic impairment: use with caution; dosage adjustment is probably not required
Pregnancy: category C; use only if potential benefit justifies the potential risk to the fetus
Breast-feeding: use with caution; not known if the drug is excreted in human milk

IN BRIEF

INDICATIONS
Hypotensive state associated with shock, drug use, or hypersensitivity reactions
Paroxysmal supraventricular tachycardia associated with hypotension or shock
Maintenance of adequate BP during spinal and inhalation anesthesia

CONTRAINDICATIONS
Known hypersensitivity to phenylephrine or sulfites
Severe coronary artery or cardiovascular disease
Pre-existing severe hypertension
Ventricular tachycardia
Hyperthyroidism
Suspected peripheral or mesenteric vascular thrombosis
Local use in fingers, toes, ears, nose, or genitalia in combination with local anesthetics

DRUG INTERACTIONS
Concurrent alpha-adrenergic blocking agents and agents with alpha-adrenergic blocking activity (phenothiazines)[2,4]
Guanethidine[1]
Other sympathomimetic agents[1,3]
MAO inhibitors[1,3]
Tricyclic antidepressants[1]

1 Effect/toxicity of phenylephrine may increase.
2 Effect of phenylephrine may decrease.
3 Phenylephrine may increase the effect/toxicity of this drug.
4 Pheneylephrine may decrease the effect of this drug.

ADVERSE EFFECTS
CV: hypertension, reflex bradycardia, arrhythmias, chest pain, heart failure
CNS: headache, restlessness, excitability, weakness, dizziness, tremor, stroke
Skin: blanching, piloerection, extravasation, necrosis, and sloughing
Other: paresthesia, metabolic acidosis, ↓ urine output, hepatic or renal ischemia or failure

PHARMACOKINETICS AND PHARMACODYNAMICS
Duration of action: (IV) 15–20 min; (IM/SQ) 1–2 hrs
Onset of action: immediate (IV); 10–15 min (IM/SQ)
Peak effect: not completely defined
Bioavailability: (IV) 100%; (po) 38%
Effect of food: not known
Protein binding: not known
Volume of distribution: >40 L
Metabolism: metabolized in liver and intestine by catechol-O-methyltransferase
Elimination: renally excreted, mainly as metabolites
Elimination half-life: 2–3 h

MONITORING
BP, heart rate, ECG, mental status, urine output, serum electrolytes, and other appropriate monitoring for adequate tissue perfusion (such as blood lactic acid, pH, pO$_2$, and pCO$_2$ levels, and oxygen saturation).

OVERDOSE
Supportive: an alpha-adrenergic antagonist, such as phentolamine may be used for severe hypertension, and a beta-adrenergic antagonist, such as propranolol, may be used for arrhythmias if indicated.

PATIENT INFORMATION
Phenylephrine is used to maintain BP (or to treat abnormal cardiac rhythm).

PHENYLEPHRINE (continued)

DOSAGE

Mild or moderate hypotension: The usual dose is 2–5 mg (range: 1–10 mg; max initial dose 5 mg) administered subcutaneously (SQ) or IM, or 0.2 mg (range: 0.1–0.5 mg) administered IV. The dose may be repeated after 10–15 min if indicated.

Severe hypotension: Continuous IV infusion (ie, 10–20 mg in 500 mL solution) at 100–180 µg/min should be initiated and titrated based on the response. Once the BP is stablized, a maintenance rate of 40–60 µg/min is usually sufficient.

Hypotension associated with spinal anesthesia:
Prophylaxis—2–3 mg administered IM or SQ 3–4 min before administration of the anesthetic agent
Treatment—0.2 mg administered IV; any subsequent doses should be given in increments of 0.1–0.2 mg if indicated and should never exceed 0.5 mg in a single dose

Paroxysmal supraventricular tachycardia: up to 0.5 mg may be given IV over 20–30 sec; subsequent doses may be given in increments of 0.1–0.2 mg if indicated and should never exceed 1 mg in a single dose

---

AVAILABILITY
Ampules or syringes—10 mg/mL (1%), 1 mL
Vials—10 mg/mL (1%), 1 mL and 5 mL
Also available (for noncardiovascular indications) as:
  Metered-dose inhalers—240 µg/spray + isoproterenol
  160 µg/spray
Ophthalmic preparations
Otic preparations
Or, in combination with antihistamines, analgesics, antitussives, bronchodilators, decongestants, and expectorants for oral administration (remedies for cold and allergy)

OTHER VASOPRESSORS (VASOPRESSOR AGENT: VASOPRESSIN)

Vasopressin is an antidiuretic hormone and has long been an important treatment for diabetes insipidus. However, vasopressin is also a nonadrenergic vasopressor with significant vasoconstrictive effects that is clinically useful in patients with vasodilatory shock or cardiac arrest.

EFFICACY AND USE

In patients unresponsive to advanced cardiac life support (ACLS) standard treatment, vasopressin increases coronary perfusion pressure and the chance of spontaneous recovery of circulation. In some shock/hypotension situations (*eg*, sepsis), vasopressin may be the more preferable agent, as hemodynamic control can be attained while sparing patients from alpha-adrenergic effects such as increased oxygen consumption or from the reduced efficacy of traditional adrenergic vasopressors due the presence of systemic acidosis. Similarly, vasopressin raises systolic arterial pressure in patients with vasodilatory shock despite catecholamine treatment.

MODE OF ACTION

Vasopressin, or antidiuretic hormone, exerts physiologic and pharmacologic effects via two types of receptors: type 1 (V_1) and type 2 (V_2). Whereas the osmoregulatory role of vasopressin is mediated primarily by V_2 receptors found in the renal collecting duct system, the hemodynamic effects of vasopressin are mediated by V_1 receptors located in vascular smooth muscle. On a molecular level, binding to V_1 receptors activates Gq protein–linked phospholipases (PLs), including PLC, PLD, and PLA_2. This results in the release of calcium from intracellular stores that contribute to the vasoconstriction.

In normotensive patients, the physiologic antidiuretic level of vasopressin does not affect blood pressure. Circulating vasopressin inhibits sympathetic efferents and resets the cardiac baroreflex to a lower pressure via receptors in the medulla oblongata. However, when blood pressure is compromised, vasopressin-induced vasoconstriction of peripheral vessels helps maintain BP. In patients with baroreflex impairment, such as in vasodilatory shock or autonomic insufficiency, the vasoconstrictive effects of vasopressin achieve or exceed those of angiotensin II or norepinephrine and phenylephrine. In addition, as vasodilation in shock states is prolonged, smooth muscle becomes poorly responsive to catecholamines, possibly because of down-regulation of beta-adrenergic receptors. Therefore, exogenous vasopressin helps to maintain arterial pressure and prevents cardiovascular collapse.

INDICATIONS

	Vasopressin
Prevention and treatment of postoperative abdominal distention	+
Use in abdominal roentgenography to dispel interfering gas shadows	+
Diabetes insipidus	+
Control of bleeding esophageal varices	(+)
Vasodilatory shock	(+)
Cardiac arrest (in ACLS)	(+)

+—FDA approved; (+)—not FDA approved, but clinically used; ACLS—advanced cardiac life support.

VASOPRESSIN (Vasopressin, Pitressin®)

Vasopressin is an antidiuretic hormone that enhances reabsorption of water by the renal tubules. Vasopressin can cause contraction of smooth muscle of the gastrointestinal tract and of all parts of the vascular bed, especially the capillaries, small arterioles, and venules, with less effect on the smooth musculature of the large veins. In normotensive patients, physiologic antidiuretic levels of vasopressin do not affect blood pressure. Circulating vasopressin inhibits sympathetic efferents and resets the cardiac baroreflex to a lower pressure via receptors in the medulla oblongata. However, when blood pressure is compromised, vasopressin-induced vasoconstriction of peripheral vessels helps maintain blood pressure. In patients with baroreflex impairment, such as in vasodilatory shock or autonomic insufficiency, the vasoconstrictive effects of vasopressin achieve or exceed those of angiotensin II or norepinephrine and phenylephrine. In addition, as vasodilation in shock states is prolonged, smooth muscle becomes poorly responsive to catecholamines, possibly because of down-regulation of beta-adrenergic receptors. Therefore, exogenous vasopressin helps to maintain arterial pressure and prevents cardiovascular collapse.

SPECIAL GROUPS

Race: unknown

Children: safety and effectiveness have been established; dosage adjustment is recommended based on age and weight

Elderly: dosage should be adjusted based on liver function and desired effect

Renal impairment: Only 5%–10% excreted unchanged renally; dosage adjustment not needed.

Hepatic impairment: use with caution; lower doses may be sufficient

Pregnancy: category C; use only if potential benefit justifies the potential risk to the fetus

Breast-feeding: use with caution; the amount excreted in human milk is low and should have no pharmacologic effect on a nursing infant

DOSAGE

Vasodilatory shock: 0.02–0.1 U/min IV

Ventricular fibrillation (in ACLS): 40 U IV bolus followed by 300–360 J of direct current cardioversion to restore circulation

Abdominal distention: 5 U IM initially; increase to 10 U IM at subsequent injections (at 3–4 h interval) if necessary

Abdominal roentgenography: Two IM or SC injections of 10 U, given 2 h and 0.5 h, respectively, before films are exposed

Diabetes insipidus: If administered by IM or SC, 5 to 10 U repeated two or three times daily as needed. If administered intranasally by spray or on pledgets, the dosage and interval between treatments must be determined for each patient.

Esophageal bleeding: 0.2–0.9 U/min IV infusion

IN BRIEF

INDICATIONS

Prevention and treatment of postoperative abdominal distention
Use in abdominal roentgenography to dispel interfering gas shadows
Diabetes insipidus
Control of bleeding esophageal varices (not FDA approved)
Vasodilatory shock (not FDA approved)
Cardiac arrest (in ACLS; not FDA approved)

CONTRAINDICATIONS

Known hypersensitivity to vasopressin or its components

DRUG INTERACTIONS

Alcohol[2]	Ganglionic-blocking agents[1]
Carbamazepine[1]	Heparin[2]
Chlorpropamide[1]	Lithium[2]
Clofibrate[1]	Norepinephrine[2]
Demeclocycline[2]	Tricyclic antidepressants[1]
Fludrocortisone[1]	

[1] Effect/toxicity of vasopressin may increase.
[2] Effect of vasopressin may decrease.

ADVERSE EFFECTS

CV: arrhythmias, decreased cardiac output, angina, myocardial ischemia, peripheral vasoconstriction, gangrene
GI: abdominal cramps, nausea, vomiting, passage of gas
CNS: tremor, vertigo, pounding in head
Other: bronchial constriction, sweating, cutaneous gangrene

PHARMACOKINETICS AND PHARMACODYNAMICS

Duration of action: 30–60 min (vasopressor effect); 2–8 h (antidiuretic effect)
Onset of action: not known
Peak effect: not known
Bioavailability: 100%
Effect of food: not applicable
Protein binding: not known
Volume of distribution: not known
Metabolism: Rapidly metabolized in liver to inactive metabolites
Elimination: Metabolized in liver; inactive metabolites are eliminated by the kidney
Elimination half-life: 10–20 min

MONITORING

Cardiovascular side effects are the most important to monitor. Vasopressin causes transient, reversible reductions in cardiac output and heart rate. Patients should be monitored for bradycardia, arrhythmia, and myocardial and/or mesenteric ischemia. Vasopressin may exacerbate regional ischemia by reduction of collateral-dependent myocardial perfusion. Currently, there is a lack of data on adverse events after resuscitation in terms of impaired vital organ function. Because of the presence of vasopressin receptors in various tissues, there is the potential for reduced regional blood circulation in pulmonary, coronary, and splanchnic blood vessels. However, vasopressin has not been reported to be associated with ischemic bowel or increased liver insufficiency. Although there is the potential for increase in pulmonary arterial pressure and hypertension, these side effects also have not been observed following vasopressin treatment.

OVERDOSE

Water intoxication may be treated with water restriction and temporary withdrawal of vasopressin until polyuria occurs. Severe water intoxication may require osmotic diuresis with mannitol, hypertonic dextrose, or urea, along with furosemide.

PATIENT INFORMATION

Side effects such as blanching of skin, abdominal cramps, and nausea may be reduced by taking one or two glasses of water at the time of vasopressin administration. These side effects are usually not serious and probably will disappear within a few minutes.

AVAILABILITY

Injection—20 U/mL (1 mL vial or ampule)

INOTROPIC AGENTS: DIGITALIS

Digitalis differs from other inotropic agents in that it has the pedigree of some 200 years' use. It is interesting that despite such a long period of time, the effectiveness of long-term digitalis therapy is repeatedly questioned. However, studies that have compared **digoxin** with other inotropic and vasodilating drugs in heart failure have demonstrated that the efficacy of many of the newer inotropic agents appears no better than that of this well-tried and inexpensive drug.

EFFICACY AND USE

Cardiac glycosides of the digitalis family are effective inotropic agents for most patients with moderate to severe heart failure and sinus rhythm, particularly those with an S_3 gallop. The beneficial effects of digitalis are additive to those of ACE inhibitors and diuretics.

Although cardiogenic shock is a recognized indication for digitalis, the established effectiveness of these drugs is limited to cardiogenic shock with atrial fibrillation or flutter and an increased ventricular rate. In other cases, digitalis benefits only the noninfarcted areas of the ventricle and has little effect on cardiac output. When treating acute atrial fibrillation, the standard digitalizing dose should not be exceeded. Its antiarrhythmic activity is advantageous (see chapter on antiarrhythmic agents) when used in combination with other inotropic agents, such as beta-adrenergic stimulants, that enhance AV conduction. In patients with atrial fibrillation, the use of beta-adrenergic agonists may promote ventricular arrhythmia; correction of atrial function with digi-

talis may promote safer use of these other agents, but not during exercise. Retrospective analyses suggest that the use of digitalis in the setting of cardiac ischemia, such as after MI, may be associated with increased mortality, particularly in patients with ventricular arrhythmias.

Digitalis drugs are also used in the prevention and treatment of recurrent episodes of paroxysmal atrial tachycardia or paroxysmal AV junctional rhythm in conjunction with measures to increase vagal tone.

MODE OF ACTION

It is now generally accepted that the digitalis glycosides act by binding to and inhibiting the cell membrane–bound sodium-potassium ATPase, the enzyme controlling the cellular sodium pump. This inhibition permits sodium to enter the cardiac cell, which is then expelled using a sodium-calcium exchange process. This, in turn, results in a higher level of intracellular calcium and an increased force of myocardial contraction. This increase in intracellular calcium concentration is accompanied by a fall in intracellular pH, further enhancing sodium movement by a sodium-hydrogen exchange, and further enhancing the inotropic response. Cardiac glycosides slow conduction and increase the refractory period (see chapter on antiarrhythmic agents) in specialized cardiac conducting tissue. Characteristically, the dominant effect is an increase in vagal tone, which manifests itself as a reduced ventricular rate due to slowing of conduction, and increased refractoriness of AV nodal and functional tissues.

INDICATIONS

	Digoxin
Supraventricular arrhythmias	+
CHF	+

+—FDA approved; CHF—congestive heart failure.

DIGOXIN (Digoxin, Lanoxicaps®, Lanoxin®)

Digoxin is the most commonly used digitalis glycoside. As a group, digitalis glycosides are the only inotropic agents that have been shown to provide some benefits in the management of chronic heart failure. In patients with heart failure, digoxin increases myocardial contractility and cardiac output, which results in a reflex reduction in sympathetic tone, thus slowing down the heart rate and promoting diuresis in patients with fluid overload. Digoxin also decreases conduction velocity through the AV node and prolongs the effective refractory period of the AV node by increasing vagal activity, by a direct effect on the AV node, and by a sympatholytic effect. These effects are useful in patients with supraventricular tachycardia, such as atrial fibrillation or atrial flutter, to reduce the conduction reaching the ventricles and thus the rate of ventricular contractions.

Serum digoxin concentrations should be monitored during therapy. Serum electrolyte disturbances, such as hypokalemia, hypomagnesemia, and hypercalcemia, may predispose the patients to digoxin toxicity and should be monitored routinely for chronic therapy. Because digoxin is mainly excreted in the kidney unchanged, it is important to monitor renal function during chronic digoxin therapy. In patients with acute renal failure, depending on the severity, the dose of digoxin should be adjusted or even held temporarily.

SPECIAL GROUPS

Race: no differences in response
Children: safety and effectiveness have been established; dosage adjustment is recommended based on age, weight, renal function, and serum levels
Elderly: dosage should be adjusted based on renal function, desired effect, and serum levels
Renal impairment: dosage should be adjusted based on renal function, desired effect, and serum levels
Hepatic impairment: use with caution; dosage adjustment is probably not required
Pregnancy: category C; use only if potential benefit justifies the potential risk to the fetus
Breast-feeding: use with caution; the amount excreted in human milk is low and should have no pharmacologic effect on a nursing infant

IN BRIEF

INDICATIONS
CHF
Atrial fibrillation
Atrial flutter
Paroxysmal atrial tachycardia

CONTRAINDICATIONS
Ventricular fibrillation
Known hypersensitivity to any digitalis glycosides

DRUG INTERACTIONS
Potassium-depleting agents (corticosteroids, diuretics)[1]
Calcium salts[1]
Sympathomimetics[1]
Quinidine[1]
Verapamil[1]
Amiodarone[1]
Erythromycin[1]
Clarithromycin[1]
Itraconazole[1]
Agents that may slow down GI transit (anticholinergics, diphenoxylate, propantheline)[1]
Propafenone[1]
Indomethacin[1]
Beta-blockers[1,3]
Calcium channel blockers[1,3]
Antacids[2]
Kaolin-pectin[2]
Cholestyramine[2]

1 Effect/toxicity of digoxin may increase.
2 Effect of digoxin may decrease.
3 Digoxin may increase the effect/toxicity of this drug.

ADVERSE EFFECTS
CV: arrhythmias (ventricular premature contraction or tachycardia, AV dissociation, accelerated junctional rhythm, atrial tachycardia, and AV block)
GI: anorexia, nausea, vomiting
CNS: visual disturbance, headache, weakness, dizziness, apathy, psychosis
Other: rash, hypersensitivity reaction, gynecomastia

PHARMACOKINETICS AND PHARMACODYNAMICS
Duration of action: 3–4 d or longer
Onset of action: (po) 0.5–2 h; (IV) 5–30 min
Peak effect: (po) 2–6 h; (IV) 1–4 h
Bioavailability: Tablets/elixir—60%–85%
Capsules—90%–100%
IV—100%
Effect of food: slows the rate but not the extent of absorption
Protein binding: 20%–30%
Volume of distribution: 4–7 L/kg
Metabolism: small amounts are metabolized in liver or by bacteria in GI tract
Elimination: mainly in urine as unchanged drug (50%–70% as unchanged after IV)
Elimination half-life: 1.5–2 d, normal renal function ≥4.5 d, anephric patients

MONITORING
BP, heart rate, ECG, serum electrolytes, renal function, serum digoxin levels, and pertinent signs and symptoms for response or toxicity.

DIGOXIN (continued)

DOSAGE
(*see* Note 1)

Rapid digitalization in adult patients who have not received digoxin in previous 2 wk:

8–12 µg/kg in patients with heart failure and normal sinus rhythm (*see* Note 2)

10–15 µg/kg in patients with atrial fibrillation or flutter for adequate control of ventricular rate (*see* Note 2)

This loading dose is usually administered IV in three divided doses, with 50% given as the first dose and two additional doses (25% each) given at 4–8 h intervals after assessing clinical response. The loading dose may also be given orally in similar divided doses every 6–8 h.

Slow digitalization or chronic maintenance therapy in adult patients: Usual dose—100–375 µg/d given orally as a single dose This is the preferred regimen in patients with heart failure, and the dose should be administered orally whenever possible. Dosage requirement for each individual should be adjusted based on clinical response and renal function. It may take 1–3 wk for a patient to reach steady-state serum digoxin concentrations, depending on the renal function (see Notes 3 and 4). In patients with severe renal dysfunction, a maintenance dose administered every 2–3 d may be adequate to maintain desired serum digoxin concentrations.

NOTES

1. The bioavailability of digoxin may vary significantly depending on the products and different dosage forms selected. Although the difference in bioavailability may not be clinically significant for an individual patient, it may be necessary to adjust the dose when switching a patient between different formulations or products.
2. Lower loading doses should be used in patients with severe renal impairment.
3. Serum digoxin levels should be monitored and kept in the range of 0.5–2 ng/mL based on clinical assessment and indication. Sampling of blood should be at least 6–8 h after the dose or, ideally, just before the next dose.
4. The value of obtaining regular serum digoxin levels, especially in patients with stable renal function is unclear. It is probably reasonable to check digoxin levels every 6–12 mo for chronic therapy. More frequent monitoring is recommended if:
   - heart failure worsens or there is new onset of arrhythmias
   - renal function deteriorates
   - new medication(s) is(are) initiated that may affect digoxin levels
   - digoxin toxicity is suspected based on clinical symptoms

OVERDOSE
Supportive: Correction of serum electrolyte and acid-base disturbances is essential. Potassium should not be administered in heart block, unless primarily related to supraventricular tachycardia. In advanced heart block, atropine and/or temporary pacing may be used. Ventricular arrhythmias may be treated with lidocaine, procainamide, propranolol, and phenytoin.

Digoxin is not dialyzable. In life-threatening digoxin overdose, digoxin immune Fab (ovine) may be used at a dose equimolar to digoxin in the body to reverse the toxicity. Please see the following Appendix for digoxin immune Fab (ovine) dosing guidelines.

PATIENT INFORMATION
Digoxin is used to treat heart rhythm problems or heart failure. Many other medications may interact with digoxin. Do not take any new medications, including over-the-counter products, without consulting a physician or a pharmacist. Check pulse rate routinely as directed. Inform the physician if you experience any unusual palpitation, dizziness, gastrointestinal problems or visual disturbances.

AVAILABILITY
Tablets—0.125, 0.25 mg
Capsules—0.05, 0.1, 0.2 mg
Elixir—0.05 mg/mL
Injection—0.1 mg/mL, 0.25 mg/mL

Dosing guidelines for digoxin immune Fab (ovine source, Digibind®, DigiFab®) in life-threatening digoxin overdose

KEY: Each vial of Digibind contains 38 mg and each vial of DigiFab contains 40 mg of digoxin-specific Fab fragments, which can bind approximately 0.5 mg of digoxin.

1. For *acute* overdose with *known* amount ingested: Total body load = amount of digoxin liquid or capsules ingested in mg, or 0.8 x (amount of digoxin tablets ingested in mg)

   Dose (# of vials*) = Total body load (mg) ÷ 0.5 (mg/vial)

2. For *acute* overdose with known steady-state serum digoxin concentrations:
   Dose (# of vials*) = digoxin level (ng/mL) x weight (kg) ÷ 100

3. For *acute* overdose with *unknown* amount ingested, 20 vials of digoxin immune Fab are recommended.

4. For *life-threatening* toxicity during *chronic* therapy, 6 vials of digoxin immune Fab are recommended.

*Dose of digoxin immune Fab (ovine) should be rounded up to the next whole vial in calculations. The total dose should be administered IV (through a 0.22 micron membrane filter for Digibind) over 30 min. If cardiac arrest is imminent, the dose may be given as an IV bolus.

Alousi AA, Johnson DC: Pharmacology of the bipyridines: amrinone and milrinone. *Circulation* 1986, 70(Suppl II):110–123.

Anversa P, Sonnenblick EH: Ischemic cardiomyopathy: pathophysiological mechanisms. *Prog Cardiovasc Dis* 1990, 33:49–70.

Braunwald E, Ross J Jr, Sonnenblick EH: Mechanisms *of Contraction of the Normal and Failing Heart*, edn. 2. Boston: Little, Brown & Co.; 1976.

Captopril-Digoxin Multicenter Research Group: Comparative effects of therapy with captopril and digoxin in patients with mild to moderate heart failure. *JAMA* 1988, 259:539–544.

Cavusoglu E, Frishman WH, Klapholz M: Vesnarinone: a new inotropic agent for treating congestive heart failure. *J Cardiac Fail* 1995, 1:249–257.

Cheng W, Li B, Kajstura J, et al.: Stretch-induced programmed myocyte cell death. *J Clin Invest* 1995, 96:2247–2259.

Cohn JN, Goldstein SO, Greenberg BH, et al.: A dose-dependent increase in mortality with vesnarinone among patients with severe heart failure. *N Engl J Med* 1998, 339:1810–1816.

Dei Cas L, Metra M, Visioli O: Clinical pharmacology of inodilators. *J Cardiovasc Pharmacol* 1989, 14(suppl8):S60–S71.

Garofalo F, Lalanne GM, Nanni G: Midodrine for female incontinence: a preliminary report. *Clin Ther* 1986, 9:44–46.

Gold JA, Cullinane S, Chen J, et al.: Vasopressin as an alternative to norepinephrine in the treatment of milrinone-induced hypotension. *Crit Care Med* 2000, 28:249–252.

Goldberg LI: The role of dopamine receptors in the treatment of congestive heart failure. *J Cardiovasc Pharmacol* 1989, 14:S19–S27.

Goldberg LI, Rajfer SI: Dopamine receptors: applications in clinical cardiology. *Circulation* 1985, 72:245–248.

Grose R, Strain J, Greenberg M, LeJemtel TH: Systemic and coronary effects of intravenous milrinone and dobutamine in congestive heart failure. *J Am Coll Cardiol* 1986, 7:1107–1113.

Grossman W: Diastolic dysfunction in congestive heart failure. *N Engl J Med* 1991, 325:1557–1564.

Haikala H, Linden I: Mechanisms of action of calcium-sensitizing drugs. *J Cardiovasc Pharm* 1995, 26(Suppl 1):S10–S19.

Insel PA: Adrenergic receptors–evolving concepts and clinical implications. *N Engl J Med* 1996, 334:580–585.

Jakovic J, Gilden JL, Hiner BC, et al.: Neurogenic orthostatic hypotension: a double-blind, placebo-controlled study with midodrine. *Am J Med* 1993, 95:38–48.

Kelley RA, Smith TW: Recognition and treatment of digitalis toxicity. *Am J Cardiol* 1992, 69:108G–119G.

Landry DW, Levin HR, Gallant EM, et al.: Vasopressin deficiency contributes to the vasodilation of septic shock. *Circulation* 1997, 95:1122–1125.

LeJemtel TH, Sonnenblick EH, Frishman WH: Diagnosis and management of heart failure. In *Hurst's The Handbook*, edn 11. Edited by Alexander RW, Schlant RC, Fuster V. New York: McGraw Hill, 2004, in press.

Lewis RP: Clinical use of serum digoxin concentrations. *Am J Cardiol* 1992, 69:97G–107G.

Lilleberg J, Sundberg S, Nieminen MS: Dose-range study of a new calcium sensitizer, levosimendan, in patients with left ventricular dysfunction. *J Cardiovasc Pharmacol* 1995, 26(Suppl 1):S63–S69.

Low PA, Gilden JL, Freeman R, et al.: Efficacy of midodrine vs placebo in neurogenic orthostatic hypotension: a randomized, double-blind multicenter study. Midodrine Study Group. *JAMA* 1997, 227:1046–1051.

McTavish D, Goa KL: Midodrine: a review of its pharmacological properties and therapeutic use in orthostatic hypotension and secondary hypotensive disorders. *Drugs* 1989, 38:757–777.

Majerus TC, Dasta JF, Bauman JL, et al.: Dobutamine: ten years later. *Pharmacotherapy* 1989, 9:245–259.

Morales DLS, Madigan J, Cullinane S, et al.: Reversal by vasopressin of intractable hypotension in the late phase of hemorrhagic shock. *Circulation* 1999, 199:226–229.

Newton GE, Tong JH, Schofield AM, et al.: Digoxin reduces cardiac sympathetic activity in severe congestive heart failure. *J Am Coll Cardiol* 1996, 28:155–161.

Packer M: Do positive inotropic agents adversely affect the survival of patients with chronic congestive heart failure? II. Protagonist's viewpoint. *J Am Coll Cardiol* 1988, 12:562–566.

Packer M, Carver JR, Rodeheffer RJ, et al.: Effect of oral milrinone on mortality in severe chronic heart failure. *N Engl J Med* 1991, 325:1468–1475.

Packer M, Gheorghiade M, Young JB, et al.: Withdrawal of digoxin from patients with chronic heart failure treated with angiotensin-converting-enzyme inhibitors. *N Engl J Med* 1993, 329:1–7.

Rahimtoola SH: Digitalis therapy for patients in clinical heart failure. *Circulation* 2004, 109:2942–2946.

Rector TW, Cohn JN: Assessment of patient outcome with the Minnesota Living with Heart Failure questionnaire: reliability and validity during a randomized, double-blind, placebo-controlled trial of pimobendan. *Am Heart J* 1992, 124:1017–1025.

Rozenfeld V, Cheng JW: The role of vasopressin in the treatment of vasodilation in shock states. *Ann Pharmacother* 2000, 34:250–254.

Ruffolo RR Jr: Review: the pharmacology of dobutamine. *Am J Med Sci* 1987, 294:244–248.

Scholz H: Inotropic drugs and their mechanisms of action. *J Am Coll Cardiol* 1984, 4:389–397.

Smith TW: Digitalis: mechanisms of action and clinical use. *N Engl J Med* 1988, 31:358–365.

Sonnenblick EH, Frishman WH, LeJemtel TH: Dobutamine: a new synthetic cardioactive sympathetic amine. *N Engl J Med* 1979, 300:17–22.

Sonnenblick EH, LeJemtel TH: Heart Failure: its progression and its therapy. *Hosp Pract* 1993, 28:121–130.

Sonnenblick EH, LeJemtel TH, Frishman WH: Inotropic agents. In *Cardiovascular Pharmacotherapeutics*, edn 2. Edited by Frishman WH, Sonnenblick EH, Sica DA. New York: McGraw Hill, 2003:191–202.

Tauke J, Goldstein S, Gheorghiade M: Digoxin for chronic heart failure: a review of the randomized controlled trials with special attention to the PROVED and RADIANCE Trials. *Prog Cardiovasc Dis* 1994, 37:49–58.

The Digitalis Investigation Group: The effect of digoxin on mortality and morbidity in patients with heart failure. *N Engl J Med* 1997, 336:525–533.

Tisdale JE, Patel R, Webb CR, *et al.*: Electrophysiologic and proarrhythmic effects of intravenous inotropic agents. *Prog Cardiovasc Dis* 1995, 38:167–180.

Uretsky BF, Young JB, Shahidi FE, *et al.*: Randomized study assessing the effect of digoxin withdrawal in patients with mild to moderate chronic congestive heart failure: results of the PROVED Trial. *J Am Coll Cardiol* 1995, 22:955–962.

Wright RA, Kaufmann HC, Perera R, *et al.*: A double-blind, dose-response study of midodrine in neurogenic orthostatic hypotension. *Neurology* 1998, 51:120–124.

The links between coronary artery disease (CAD), diet, and hyperlipidemia (excess serum cholesterol and/or triglycerides) are well established, and the biologic factors contributing to hyperlipidemia are now fairly well understood. The hyperlipoproteinemias are defined and treated broadly along the lines of the Fredrickson-Levy classification (Table 11.1).

Cholesterol is an important component of cell membranes, but high serum levels are a major risk factor for CAD. Cholesterol is both synthesized in the liver and derived from diet. Dietary cholesterol and triglycerides are carried into the circulation by chylomicrons, the largest and least dense of the lipoproteins. Chylomicrons consist largely of triglycerides (85%), which are hydrolyzed at sites in the body that store or use these lipids. The chylomicron remnants are then removed from the circulation by the liver.

The liver secretes very low-density lipoproteins (VLDLs), which are triglyceride-rich but also carry some cholesterol synthesized by the liver. The VLDLs are degraded by lipoprotein lipase into VLDL remnants (or intermediate-density lipoproteins [IDLs]). The VLDL remnants are either removed from the circulation by the liver, where excess cholesterol is converted into bile acids, or degraded further into low-density lipoprotiens (LDLs), the major cholesterol-carrying lipoproteins in the body, transporting cholesterol to peripheral cells. LDLs, like the VLDL remnants, are removed from the circulation via receptors on the liver cells. Smaller LDL particles tend to penetrate subendothelial tissue and thereby contribute to the development of atherosclerosis more than larger LDL particles. Very small LDL particles surrounded by apolipoprotein (apo) A, a plasmogen-like glycoprotein, are believed to be an independent risk factor for the development of CAD. These small LDL particles are often referred to as lipoprotein (a). High-density lipoproteins (HDLs) appear to have a protective effect by collecting cholesterol from peripheral cells and transferring it back to VLDL and LDL, so that it can then be removed from the circulation. HDL can be further subdivided into HDL2 and HDL3 fractions, both of which are protective components against CAD. Specific apolipoproteins carried on the surface of LDL and HDL can also be measured and are independently associated with CAD. Nonetheless, current data suggest that

quantification of HDL subfractions and apolipoproteins adds no predictive value to more conventional lipoproteins. The LDL-HDL ratio is also a convenient method of assessing the atherogenic potential of an individual's plasma lipoproteins.

Because LDLs are the main cholesterol transporters, pharmacologic manipulation has focused on decreasing the serum levels of LDL (by inhibiting VLDL synthesis or increasing the number of LDL receptors on the liver) as well as on reducing cholesterol synthesis and increasing its excretion as bile acids (Figure 11.1).

Meta-analyses of prospective studies indicate that high plasma triglyceride concentrations are also a risk factor for CAD. The Third Report of the National Cholesterol Education Program Expert Panel on Detection, Evaluation, and Treatment of High Blood Cholesterol in Adults (Adult Treatment Panel III [NCEP ATP III]) acknowledges this and provides a detailed discussion regarding the implications and treatment of elevated triglycerides. Despite the evidence supporting elevated triglyceride concentrations as an independent risk factor for CAD, studies have not yet been performed investigating the impact of lowering triglycerides on clinical outcomes or addressing whether or not lowering plasma triglycerides lowers the risk for CAD. It is, however, believed

TABLE 11.1 CLASSIFICATION OF HYPERLIPOPROTEINEMIAS

Type	Lipoprotein	Elevated lipid level
I (rare)	Chylomicron	Triglyceride ± cholesterol
IIa	LDL	Cholesterol
IIb	LDL + VLDL	Triglyceride + cholesterol
III (rare)	IDL	Triglyceride + cholesterol
IV	VLDL	Triglyceride ± cholesterol
V	VLDL + chylomicron	Triglyceride ± cholesterol

IDL—intermediate-density lipoprotein; LDL—low-density lipoprotein; VLDL—very-low-density lipoprotein.

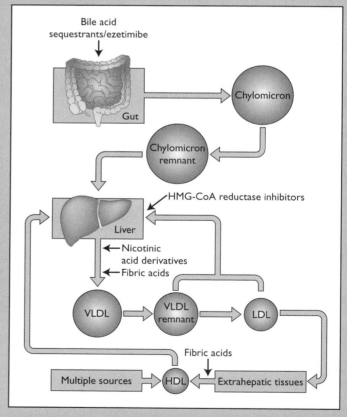

FIGURE 11.1 Interrelationships of the plasma lipoproteins and the sites of action of the lipid-lowering drugs. HDL—high-density lipoprotein; HMG-CoA—hydroxymethylglutaryl coenzyme A; LDL—low-density lipoprotein; VLDL—very-low-density lipoprotein.

that triglyceride-rich remnant lipoproteins (partially degraded VLDL) are atherogenic, making VLDL a potential target of drug therapy. NCEP ATP III establishes LDL+VLDL cholesterol (non-HDL cholesterol) as a secondary therapeutic target in persons with elevated triglycerides. In addition, many individuals with elevated triglyceride concentrations have associated low concentrations of HDL cholesterol or high concentrations of LDL cholesterol, or both, which may further influence decisions about intervention to reduce the risk of CAD.

Drugs currently used for the treatment of dyslipidemias may be classified into four main groups: bile acid sequestrants (BASs)/cholesterol absorption inhibitors, fibric acid derivatives, nicotinic acid, and hydroxymethylglutaryl coenzyme A (HMG-CoA) reductase inhibitors. Because of their varying sites and modes of action, these drugs differ in their effects on lipoprotein fractions (Table 11.2).

The link between successful reduction in total cholesterol or triglyceride levels, or both, and increased HDL cholesterol, as well as morbidity and mortality, has been examined in several drug intervention studies. An overview of diet and drug trials indicates that every 1% decrease in serum cholesterol produces a 2% fall in risk of CAD. It has also been shown that for every 10% lowering of cholesterol, CAD mortality risk decreases by 15% and total mortality risk decreases by 11%. Any additional benefit that might be derived from falls in triglyceride levels and rises in HDL cholesterol remains to be quantified, although there are data from the Helsinki Heart Study and Veterans Administration–HDL Intervention Trial (VA-HIT) to suggest a 3% decrease in cardiac events with each 1% increase in HDL concentration. The benefit of reducing cholesterol appears as a reduction in the incidence of death, providing cholesterol levels are reduced by more than 9% to 10%; reduction of cholesterol seems also to be associated with a reduction in the progression and promotion in the regression of atheromatous lesions.

TABLE 11.2 SUMMARY OF THE EFFECTS OF THE COMMONLY USED GROUPS OF LIPID-LOWERING AGENTS

Group	Primarily lower Cholesterol	Primarily lower Triglycerides	Mechanism of action	Lipoprotein effect VLDL	Lipoprotein effect LDL	Lipoprotein effect HDL
BASs/cholesterol absorption inhibitors	+		BASs increase the excretion of bile acid in stool; biosynthesis of cholesterol is increased slightly and LDL receptors in liver are increased, resulting in increased disposal of circulating LDL cholesterol. Cholesterol absorption inhibitors (ezetimibe) interfere with the absorption of cholesterol in the small intestine.	↓↑0	↓	0 or ↑
FADs		+	Activate lipoprotein lipase; promote lipolysis of VLDL; may also reduce formation of triglycerides	↓	↓↑0	0 or ↑
NA and derivatives	+	+	Inhibit VLDL secretion by liver by decreasing plasma free fatty acids	↓	↓	↑
HMG-CoA reductase inhibitors	+		Inhibit cholesterol synthesis and stimulate suppression of LDL receptors	0 or ↓	↓	0 or ↑

BASs—bile acid sequestrants; FADs—fibric acid derivatives; HDL—high-density lipoprotein; HMG-CoA—hydroxymethylglutaryl coenzyme A; NA—nicotinic acid; LDL—low-density lipoprotein; VLDL—very-low-density lipoprotein; ↑—increase; ↓—decrease; 0—no change.

The Pravastatin or Atorvastatin Evaluation and Infection Therapy–Thrombolysis in Myocardial Infarction 22 (PROVE IT-TIMI 22) study demonstrated that reducing LDL concentrations to a mean of 62 mg/dL with aggressive drug therapy (80 mg **atorvastatin**) resulted in a 16% reduction in risk of death or cardiovascular events compared with a mean LDL of 95 mg/dL achieved with standard drug therapy (40 mg **pravastatin**) in patients recovering from an acute coronary syndrome. This and other studies have led to recent changes in the guidelines regarding what the optimal LDL concentration should be in a given individual to minimize the risk of cardiovascular disease (Table 11.3).

TABLE 11-3 RECOMMENDATIONS FOR MODIFICATIONS TO FOOTNOTE THE ADULT TREATMENT PANEL III TREATMENT ALGORITHM FOR LOW-DENSITY LIPOPROTEIN CHOLESTEROL

TLC remains an essential modality in clinical management. TLC has the potential to reduce cardiovascular risk through several mechanisms beyond LDL lowering.

In high-risk persons, the recommended LDL-C goal is <100 mg/dL.

An LDL-C goal of <70 mg/dL is a therapeutic option on the basis of available clinical trial evidence, especially for patients at very high risk.

If LDL-C is ≥100 mg/dL, an LDL-lowering drug is indicated simultaneously with lifestyle changes.

If baseline LDL-C is <100 mg/dL, institution of an LDL-lowering drug to achieve an LDL-C level <70 mg/dL is a therapeutic option on the basis of available clinical trial evidence.

If a high-risk person has high triglycerides or low HDL-C, consideration can be given to combining a fibrate or nicotinic acid with an LDL-lowering drug. When triglycerides are ≥200 mg/dL, non-HDL-C is a secondary target of therapy, with a goal of 30 mg/dL higher than the identified LDL-C goal.

For moderately high-risk persons (2+ risk factors and 10-year risk 10%–20%), the recommended LDL-C goal is <130 mg/dL; an LDL-C goal <100 mg/dL is a therapeutic option on the basis of available clinical trial evidence. When LDL-C level is 100–129 mg/dL, at baseline or on lifestyle therapy, initiation of an LDL-lowering drug to achieve an LDL-C level <100 mg/dL is a therapeutic option on the basis of available clinical trial evidence.

Any person at high risk or moderately high risk who has lifestyle-related risk factors (eg, obesity, physical inactivity, elevated triglyceride, low HDL-C, or metabolic syndrome) is a candidate for TLC to modify these risk factors regardless of LDL-C level.

When LDL-lowering drug therapy is employed in high-risk or moderately high-risk persons, it is advised that intensity of therapy be sufficient to achieve at least a 30%–40% reduction in LDL-C levels.

For people in lower-risk categories, recent clinical trials do not modify the goals and cutpoints of therapy.

HDL-C—high-density-lipoprotein cholesterol; LDL-C—low-density-lipoprotein cholesterol; TLC—therapeutic lifestyle change.

(*Adapted from* Grundy SM, Cleeman JI, Bairey Merz CN, *et al.*: Implications of recent clinical trials for the National Cholesterol Education Program Adult Treatment Panel III Guidelines. *Circulation* 2004, 110:227–239.)

The information here is provided as guidance only. Prescribers should always consult the manufacturer's current prescribing information.

The BASs, **cholestyramine**, **colestipol**, and **colesevelam**, are safe and effective agents for the treatment of hyperlipidemia. Because they are not absorbed into the circulation, they have the advantages of no systemic drug–drug interactions and few systemic side effects. However, **cholestyramine** and **colestipol** are not well tolerated because of gastrointestinal side effects and poor palatability. **Colesevelam** has better tolerability, albeit at a higher cost. In addition, these drugs are generally less effective than HMG-CoA reductase inhibitors in lowering cholesterol. For these reasons, they are now mainly second-line drugs for treating high cholesterol concentrations. **Ezetimibe** is the first drug in a new class known as selective cholesterol absorption inhibitors. It has efficacy comparable to the BAS and a similar place in therapy. However, gastrointestinal side effects are fewer and palatability is greater compared with the BAS.

EFFICACY AND USE

The cholesterol-lowering effects of 4 g of **cholestyramine** appear to be equivalent to those obtained with 5 g of **colestipol**. Decreases in LDL concentrations of 12% to 20% may be seen with 5 g **colestipol** or 4 g **cholestyramine** twice daily. The response to therapy varies, but daily dosages of **cholestyramine** 16 to 24 g and **colestipol** 15 to 30 g can lower concentrations of LDL by 20% to 25%, making these drugs acceptable first-line agents when modest reductions in LDL cholesterol are desired. Concentrations of HDL may increase from 0% to 8%, and triglycerides may increase (0%–33%). The benefits of dosages exceeding four packets per day (16 g **cholestyramine**, 20 g **colestipol**) are controversial, considering the marginal additional reduction in LDL and the increase in gastrointestinal side effects and poor adherence seen with dosages exceeding this amount.

The newer agents have efficacy similar to **cholestyramine** and **colestipol**. **Colesevelam** has been shown to reduce total LDL cholesterol by about 9% to 20% compared with an average 18% reduction seen with **ezetimibe**. Increases in HDL of about 1% to 5% may be expected with either **colesevelam** or **ezetimibe**. With regard to triglycerides, **colesevelam** behaves like the more traditional BASs, increasing triglycerides by about 10%, whereas **ezetimibe** actually reduces triglycerides by about 7% to 9%. BASs have no place in the treatment of lipid disorders other than the reduction of elevated cholesterol levels. They are generally reserved for the treatment of type II hyperlipidemia. These drugs are commonly used for additive or synergistic effects when given in combination with niacin or an HMG-CoA reductase inhibitor. Studies have shown **colestipol**-niacin combinations to result in 30% to 55% reductions in LDL and 20% to 45% increases in HDL. **Lovastatin** and **colestipol** have also been used in combination, resulting in a 46% reduction in LDL and a 15% increase in HDL concentrations. **Colesevelam** and **ezetimibe** are also used primarily in conjunction with HMG-CoA reductase inhibitors, resulting in additive or synergistic effects in lowering LDL. In patients already stabilized on an HMG-CoA reductase inhibitor, **ezetimibe** has been shown to produce an additional 25% reduction in LDL cholesterol compared with a 4% reduction with placebo (21% absolute reduction). Likewise, 10% to 16% absolute reductions in LDL cholesterol have been observed when **colesevelam** is added to an HMG-CoA reductase inhibitor. The Lipid Research Clinics Coronary Primary Prevention Trial (LRC-CPPT) compared **cholestyramine** (mean daily dose of 16.8 g at 1-year follow-up) to placebo in 3806 men without CAD and with type II hypercholesterolemia receiving a moderate cholesterol-lowering diet. After 7 to10 years of follow-up, total and LDL cholesterol concentrations were reduced by 13.4% and 20.3%, respectively, in patients receiving **cholestyramine**. This corresponded to a 19% reduction in risk of the combined primary end point of definite coronary heart disease (CHD) death (24% reduction) and/or definite nonfatal myocardial infarction (19% reduction) compared with placebo (Figure 11.2). A nonsignificant 7% reduction in all-cause mortality was seen in the **cholestyramine** group, primarily a result of a greater number of violent and accidental deaths in patients taking **cholestyramine**.

Both **cholestyramine** and **colestipol** have been shown to slow the progression of atherosclerosis and promote the regression of atherosclerotic plaques.

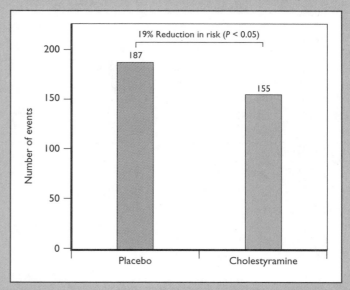

FIGURE 11.2 The effect of cholestyramine treatment on nonfatal myocardial infarction and/or coronary heart disease death in asymptomatic men with type II hyperlipoproteinemia in the LRC-CPPT study. (*Adapted from* Lipid Research Clinics Program: The Lipid Research Clinics Coronary Primary Prevention Trial results. I. Reduction in incidence of coronary heart disease. *JAMA* 1984, 251:351–364.)

Pruritus associated with bile acid retention is believed to be a result of bile acid deposition in the skin. By encouraging the loss of bile acids through the intestine, BASs bring relief of pruritus within 1 to 3 weeks. Diarrhea caused by an excess of fecal bile acids (as in, *eg*, radiation therapy, ileal resection, or Crohn's disease) may also be relieved by bile acid resins. The main problems with these agents, however, are their bulk and gastrointestinal side effects. A report of the 6-year follow-up of the Lipid Research Clinics Program showed that there was an increased incidence of cholecystectomies and gastrointestinal malignancies in subjects receiving **cholestyramine** compared with placebo. Although this association was not statistically significant, it cautions practitioners to pay particular attention to the gastrointestinal complaints of patients receiving bile acid resins.

Cholestyramine and **colestipol** have also been used to treat digoxin toxicity.

Cholestyramine and **colestipol** may interfere with normal fat digestion and absorption and consequently prevent the absorption of fat-soluble vitamins (A, D, E, and K), necessitating supplementation of these vitamins with long-term resin therapy. Malabsorption of vitamin K may lead to hypoprothrombinemia and increased bleeding; folic acid malabsorption may lead to decreased serum or red cell folate concentrations.

MODE OF ACTION

Bile acid sequestrants are anion-exchange resins, which exchange a chloride anion for other anions that have a greater affinity for the resin. The mechanism of drug action is to bind bile acids in the intestinal lumen, thereby preventing their absorption. During normal digestion, bile acids are secreted from the liver and gallbladder into the bile, and are then transported into the intestines. Most of the secreted bile acids are enterohepatically recycled back to the liver through the portal circulation. Bile acids serve to emulsify fats and lipids into a more easily digestible form. BASs, as their name implies, bind bile acids in the intestines to form a complex that is excreted in the feces. Bile acids are therefore removed from enterohepatic recycling.

This process stimulates an increased synthesis of bile acids from endogenous cholesterol, resulting in depletion of the hepatic cholesterol pool. This depletion in turn results in compensatory mechanisms: an increase in the biosynthesis of cholesterol and an increase in the number of specific high-affinity LDL receptors on the liver cell membrane. The increased number of high-affinity LDL receptors expressed on hepatocytes from patients treated with BASs stimulates an enhanced rate of LDL catabolism from plasma and thereby lowers the concentration of this lipoprotein. Despite increased cholesterol production, the net effect of these drugs is a reduction in plasma cholesterol and LDL concentrations in patients with type II hyperlipidemia, possibly because of an increased rate of clearance of LDL from the plasma.

Ezetimibe acts by selectively inhibiting the absorption of cholesterol from the lumen of the small intestine. Through mechanisms that are incompletely defined, **ezetimibe** acts in the brush border of the small intestine at the level of the enterocyte to decrease the absorption of cholesterol through the intestinal wall. About 54% of cholesterol absorption is inhibited by therapeutic doses of **ezetimibe**, with no appreciable effect on plasma concentrations of fat-soluble vitamins.

INDICATIONS

	Cholestyramine	Colestipol	Colesevelam	Ezetimibe
Type I hyperlipoproteinemia	–	–	–	–
Type IIa hyperlipoproteinemia	+	+	+	+
Type IIb hyperlipoproteinemia	+	–	–	–
Type III hyperlipoproteinemia	–	–	–	–
Type IV hyperlipoproteinemia	–	–	–	–
Type V hyperlipoproteinemia	–	–	–	–

+—FDA approved; — —not FDA approved.

CHOLESTYRAMINE

(Cholestyramine, Questran®,
Questran Light®, Prevalite®)

Cholestyramine is an insoluble basic anion-exchange resin containing quaternary ammonium groups that exchange their chloride ions and bind negatively charged bile acids. The complex is then excreted in the feces along with unchanged resin. This excretion results in partial removal of bile acids from the enterohepatic circulation, and these acids are replaced by the oxidation of endogenous cholesterol. Cholestyramine is as effective as the other BASs.

The Lipid Research Clinics Coronary Primary Prevention Trial compared the efficacy of cholestyramine with placebo in reducing the risk of CHD in 3806 men with primary (type II) hypercholesterolemia and no history of heart disease. In addition to reducing total and LDL cholesterol, the cholestyramine group experienced a 19% reduction in risk of the combined primary end point of definite CHD death (24% reduction) and definite nonfatal myocardial infarction (MI) (19% reduction) compared with placebo. A nonsignificant 7% reduction in all-cause mortality was seen in the cholestyramine group. This neutralization of the cardiovascular benefits of cholestyramine was primarily a result of a greater number of violent and accidental deaths in patients taking cholestyramine.

Cholestyramine has been shown to retard the progression of atherosclerosis and promote atherosclerotic plaque regression in patients with CAD. Cholestyramine may also help relieve pruritus due to the deposition of bile acids in dermal tissue in patients with partial biliary obstruction.

SPECIAL GROUPS

Race: not evaluated
Children: optimal dosing has not been established; long-term effects are not known in this population; children are at increased risk for hyperchloremic acidosis
Elderly: no dosage adjustment is required unless constipated (see below); more prone to constipation as a side effect; monitor closely
Renal impairment: the possibility of hyperchloremic acidosis is increased in patients with renal insufficiency; cholestyramine should therefore be used cautiously in this group
Hepatic impairment: contraindicated with total biliary obstruction
Pregnancy: category C; use only if the potential benefit justifies the potential risk to the fetus
Breast-feeding: not evaluated; use cautiously because of the potential malabsorption of fat-soluble vitamins; supplementation may be necessary

IN BRIEF

INDICATIONS
As adjunctive therapy to diet in patients with elevated LDL concentrations (type II hyperlipidemia)
Relief of pruritus associated with partial biliary obstruction

CONTRAINDICATIONS
Complete biliary obstruction
Bowel obstruction
Hypersensitivity to product components

DRUG INTERACTIONS
Note: Because cholestyramine may bind to many medications, it is recommended to give other drugs at least 1 h before or 4–6 h after cholestyramine.
Folic acid[1]
Iron[1]
Phenylbutazone[1]
Warfarin[1]
Thiazide diuretics[1]
Propranolol[1]
Tetracycline[1]
Penicillin G[1]
Phenobarbital[1]
Thyroid and thyroxine preparations[1]
Estrogens and progestins[1]
Digitalis[1]
Drugs that undergo enterohepatic circulation[1]
Fat-soluble vitamins (A, D, E, K)[1]
Spironolactone[2]
Troglitazone[1]

1 Cholestyramine may decrease the effect of this drug.
2 The risk of hyperchloremic acidosis may increase.

ADVERSE EFFECTS
Adverse effects tend to be gastrointestinal and transient in nature. GI: constipation (8%–39%), gas (12%–32%), heartburn (12%–27%), belching/bloating (9%–27%), abdominal pain (7%–15%), diarrhea (4%–10%), nausea (3%–16%), vomiting (2%–6%)

PHARMACOKINETICS AND PHARMACODYNAMICS
Because cholestyramine is not systemically absorbed, many pharmacokinetic parameters are not applicable (9 g of Questran, 5 g of Questran Light, and 5.5 g of Prevalite or generic cholestyramine all contain 4 g of anhydrous cholestyramine resin).
Duration of action: 12–24 h (2–4 wk after stopping therapy)
Onset of action: 24–48 h
Peak effect: within 1 mo
Bioavailability: not applicable
Effect of food: none
Protein binding: not applicable
Metabolism: not applicable
Elimination: 100% fecal
Elimination half-life: not applicable

MONITORING
Plasma lipid profile, bowel function, prothrombin time or International Normalized Ratio (INR).

OVERDOSE
With an overdose of cholestyramine, the primary potential problem would be intestinal obstruction, which is best treated by a specialist in that area.

CHOLESTYRAMINE (continued)

DOSAGE

Usual adult initial dosage is one packet or scoopful once or twice daily. Usual maintenance dosage is two to four packets or scoopfuls (8–16 g of resin) daily divided into two doses. Dosage increases of 4 g should occur at intervals of no less than 4 wk up to a maximum of 24 g of resin (six packets or scoopfuls) daily. Twice-daily dosing is recommended, but may range from one to six doses per day. Pediatric dose is 240 mg/kg/d in two to three divided doses, normally not exceeding 8 g/d. Because cholestyramine may worsen constipation, patients who are constipated should be started on dosages of one packet or scoop once daily for 5–7 d, increasing by one dose per day every month up to a maximum of six doses per day. Consider dosage reductions, combination therapy, or discontinuation or alteration of therapy if triglyceride concentrations increase while on cholestyramine.

PATIENT INFORMATION

Mix each packet or scoopful with 2–6 oz of water or other noncarbonated beverage, soup, or pulpy fruit with a high moisture content (applesauce, crushed pineapple, etc.). Do *not* consume the powder in its dry form. Sipping or retaining the resin in the mouth may cause teeth discoloration or decay. If you miss a dose, take it as soon as you remember. If it is about time for the next dose, take that dose only. Do not take two doses at once. Do not discontinue therapy without your clinician's advice. Take other medications at least 1 h before or 4 h after cholestyramine. Notify your clinician as soon as possible if you become pregnant or intend to become pregnant or breast-feed while taking this medication. Take with plenty of fluid and fiber to minimize constipation. If persistent constipation occurs, notify your clinician. Phenylketonurics: Questran Light and Prevalite contain phenylalanine.

AVAILABILITY

Powder for oral suspension: 4 g resin/9 g powder; 4 g resin/5.7 g powder (light formulation)
Prevalite: 4 g resin/5.5 g powder (contains phenylalanine)
Questran: 4 g resin/9 g powder
Questran Light: 4 g resin/5 g powder (contains phenylalanine)

COLESEVELAM

(WelChol®)

Colesevelam is a new BAS that is effective in lowering total and LDL cholesterol levels. In several short-term, placebo-controlled studies, colesevelam reduced total cholesterol levels by approximately 6% to 10% and LDL cholesterol levels by approximately 9% to 20%. When given in combination with atorvastatin, lovastatin, or simvastatin, LDL cholesterol levels were decreased more than with colesevelam alone. Its unique hydrogel formulation may minimize the potential for gastrointestinal side effects, which are common with other BASs. Further studies and clinical experience are needed to establish the long-term safety and efficacy of this drug.

SPECIAL GROUPS

Race: no information
Children: safety and efficacy have not been established
Elderly: use usual dose
Renal impairment: use usual dose with caution
Hepatic impairment: ineffective in total biliary obstruction
Pregnancy: category B; should be used during pregnancy only if clearly needed
Breast-feeding: exercise caution when administering to a nursing woman; excretion in breast milk unknown

DOSAGE

Monotherapy: The recommended initial dose is 3 tablets taken twice daily with meals (and water or other appropriate fluids) or 6 tablets once daily with a meal. Dose may be increased to 7 tablets daily as needed.

Combination therapy: When colesevelam is administered concurrently with an HMG-CoA reductase inhibitor, the recommended dose is 3 tablets taken twice daily with meals (and water or other appropriate fluids) or 6 tablets taken once daily with a meal. Doses of 4–6 tablets per day are safe and effective when coadministered with an HMG-CoA reductase inhibitor or when the two drugs are dosed apart.

IN BRIEF

INDICATIONS
As adjunctive therapy to diet and exercise, used alone or in combination with an HMG-CoA reductase inhibitor to reduce elevated LDL cholesterol in patients with primary hypercholesterolemia

CONTRAINDICATIONS
Hypersensitivity
Bowel obstruction

DRUG INTERACTIONS
Note: When administering colesevelam with other drugs for which alterations in blood levels could have a clinically significant effect on safety or efficacy, monitoring of drug levels or effects should be considered.
Verapamil (sustained release)[1,2]

1 Colesevelam may decrease the effect of this drug.

2 The clinical significance of this interaction is unclear.

ADVERSE EFFECTS
GI: constipation (11%), dyspepsia (8%)
Neuromuscular and skeletal: weakness (4%), myalgia (2%)
Other: pharyngitis (3%)

PHARMACOKINETICS AND PHARMACODYNAMICS
Time to therapeutic effect: $\approx$ 2 wk
Absorption: insignificant
Elimination: urine (0.05%), after 28 days of chronic dosing

MONITORING
Cholesterol profile, triglyceride levels.

OVERDOSE
Because colesevelam is not absorbed, the risk of systemic toxicity is low. Doses in excess of 4.5 g/d have not been tested.

PATIENT INFORMATION
Colesevelam may be taken once per day with a meal, or taken twice per day in divided doses with meals. This medication should also be taken with water or other appropriate fluids. Follow diet and exercise plan as recommended by physician. Notify physician if persistent side effects occur.

AVAILABILITY
Tablets—625 mg

The information here is provided as guidance only. Prescribers should always consult the manufacturer's current prescribing information.

285

COLESTIPOL (Colestid®, Flavored Colestid®)

Colestipol is an insoluble high molecular weight basic anion-exchange resin containing secondary and tertiary amine groups. The resin forms complexes with bile acids, which are then excreted in the feces. This excretion results in partial removal of bile acids from the enterohepatic circulation; the acids are replaced by the oxidation of endogenous cholesterol. Colestipol is as effective as the other BASs.

Several studies have demonstrated colestipol, in combination with niacin and/or lovastatin, to slow the progression of atherosclerosis and promote atherosclerotic plaque regression in patients with CAD.

SPECIAL GROUPS

Race: not evaluated
Children: not evaluated
Elderly: no dosage adjustment is required unless constipated (see below); more prone to constipation as a side effect; monitor closely
Renal impairment: the possibility of hyperchloremic acidosis is increased in patients with renal insufficiency; colestipol should therefore be used cautiously in this group
Hepatic impairment: ineffective in total biliary obstruction
Pregnancy: not evaluated; use cautiously due to impaired absorption of fat-soluble vitamins
Breast-feeding: not evaluated; the possible lack of proper vitamin absorption may have an effect on nursing infants

DOSAGE

Granules: Usual adult initial dosage is 1 packet or scoopful once or twice daily. Usual maintenance dosage ranges from 1–6 packets or scoopfuls (5–30 g of resin) daily in single or divided doses. Dosage increases of 5 g should occur at intervals of no less than 4 wk up to a maximum of 30 g of colestipol (6 packets or scoopfuls) daily. The prescribed amount of granules must be mixed with a glassful of liquid before administration; it should not be taken dry. Because colestipol may worsen constipation, patients who are constipated should be started on dosages of 1 packet or scoop once daily for 5–7 d, increasing by one dose per day every month up to a maximum of 6 doses/d.

Tablets: Initiate at 2 g once or twice daily; dosage may be increased by 2 g once or twice daily at 1- to 2-mo intervals. The usual daily dose is 2–16 g given once or in divided doses. Tablets should be swallowed whole, one at a time, with plenty of water or other appropriate fluids.

Note: Consider dosage reductions, combination therapy, or discontinuation or alteration of therapy if triglyceride concentrations increase while on colestipol.

IN BRIEF

INDICATIONS
As adjunctive therapy to diet in patients with elevated LDL concentrations (type II hyperlipidemia)

CONTRAINDICATIONS
Hypersensitivity to product components; bowel obstruction.

DRUG INTERACTIONS
Note: Because colestipol may bind to many medications, it is recommended to give other drugs at least 1 h before or 4 h after colestipol administration.

Furosemide[1]	Digitalis[1]
Thiazide diuretics[1]	Oral phosphate supplements[1]
Propranolol[1]	Hydrocortisone[1]
Tetracycline[1]	Drugs that undergo
Penicillin G[1]	enterohepatic circulation[1]
Fat-soluble vitamins (A, D, E, K)[1]	Spironolactone[2]
Gemfibrozil[1]	Warfarin[1]

1 Colestipol may decrease the effect of this drug.
2 The risk of hyperchloremic acidosis may increase.

ADVERSE EFFECTS
Adverse effects tend to be gastrointestinal and transient in nature. The GI effects reported below are event rates with colestipol-niacin combination therapy.
GI: constipation (31%), stomach discomfort (23%), heartburn (20%), sore throat (14%), abdominal pain (15%), nausea (23%), vomiting (6%)
Hepatic: elevated serum transaminases (<1%)

PHARMACOKINETICS AND PHARMACODYNAMICS
Because colestipol is not systemically absorbed, many pharmacokinetic parameters are not applicable.
Duration of action: 12–24 h (2–4 wk after stopping therapy)
Onset of action: 24–48 h
Peak effect: within 1 mo
Bioavailability: not applicable
Effect of food: none
Protein binding: not applicable
Metabolism: not applicable
Elimination: 100% fecal
Elimination half-life: not applicable

MONITORING
Plasma lipid profile, bowel function, prothrombin time or INR, serum transaminases.

OVERDOSE
With an overdose of colestipol, the primary potential problem would be intestinal obstruction, which is best treated by a specialist in that area.

PATIENT INFORMATION
Mix each packet or scoopful of granules with ≥3 oz of water or other noncarbonated beverage, soup, or pulpy fruit with a high moisture content (applesauce, crushed pineapple, etc.). Do not consume the powder in its dry form. Sipping or retaining the resin in the mouth may cause teeth discoloration or decay. If the tablet formulation of colestipol is taken, swallow tablets whole and one at a time. Do not cut, chew, or crush tablets. The tablets should be taken with plenty of water or other appropriate fluids. If you miss a dose, take it as soon as you remember. If it is about time for the next dose, take that dose only. Do not take two doses at once. Do not discontinue therapy without your clinician's advice. Take other medications at least 1 h before or 4 h after colestipol. Notify your clinician as soon as possible if you become pregnant or intend to become pregnant or breast-feed while taking this medication. Take with plenty of fluid and fiber to minimize constipation. If persistent constipation occurs, notify your clinician. Phenylketonurics: Flavored Colestid contains phenylalanine.

AVAILABILITY
Granules, as hydrochloride:
5 g/7.5 g (unflavored)
5 g/7.5 g (orange flavor, contains phenylalanine)
Tablets, as hydrochloride: 1 g

EZETIMIBE (Zetia®)

Ezetimibe is the first agent in a new class of medications known as the selective cholesterol-absorption inhibitors. It has a mechanism of action that differs from those of other classes of cholesterol-lowering agents. Ezetimibe does not inhibit cholesterol synthesis in the liver or increase bile acid excretion. Instead, ezetimibe localizes and appears to act at the brush border of the small intestine and inhibits the absorption of cholesterol, leading to a decrease in the delivery of intestinal cholesterol to the liver. This causes a reduction of hepatic cholesterol stores and an increase in clearance of cholesterol from the blood. Ezetimibe 10 mg daily consistently reduces LDL cholesterol from 15% to 20% and raises HDL cholesterol from 4% to 9% as monotherapy and when combined with a statin or fenofibrate in patients with primary hypercholesterolemia. In contrast to other lipid-lowering medications that act in the gastrointestinal tract, ezetimibe does not appear to worsen hypertriglyceridemia. Ezetimibe has been shown to be useful as monotherapy in patients who need a modest reduction in LDL cholesterol. It can also be used in combination with a statin in patients who are unable to tolerate large doses of statins or need further reductions in LDL cholesterol despite the maximum dose of a statin. The effect of ezetimibe on morbidity and mortality in patients with CAD remains to be established in long-term clinical trials. The combination of ezetimibe and simvastatin has been shown to outperform both atorvastatin and simvastatin monotherapy in reducing LDL cholesterol. The combination of simvastatin and ezetimibe in a single tablet (Vytorin) was recently approved for clinical use in the United States. This combination formulation is well tolerated and has an overall safety profile similar to that of simvastatin monotherapy.

The ongoing Study of Heart and Renal Protection (SHARP) is comparing simvastatin (20 mg daily) + ezetimibe (10 mg daily) with placebo in about 9000 patients with chronic kidney disease (dialysis or predialysis) without a history of MI or coronary revascularization. The study will have a follow-up period of at least 4 years with the primary endpoint being time to a first major vascular event.

SPECIAL GROUPS

Race: no information

Children: treatment with ezetimibe in children <10 years of age is not recommended

Elderly: use usual dose

Renal impairment: use usual dose

Hepatic impairment: not recommended in patients with moderate or severe hepatic impairment

Pregnancy: category C; use ezetimibe during pregnancy only if the potential benefit justifies the potential risk to the fetus

Breast-feeding: not recommended; may be excreted in breast milk

IN BRIEF

INDICATIONS

As monotherapy or in combination with an **HMG-CoA** reductase inhibitor as adjunctive therapy to diet for the reduction of elevated total cholesterol, LDL cholesterol, and apo B in patients with primary (heterozygous familial and nonfamilial) hypercholesterolemia

As adjunctive therapy to diet for the reduction of elevated sitosterol and campesterol levels in patients with homozygous familial sitosterolemia

In combination with atorvastatin or simvastatin for the reduction of elevated total cholesterol and LDL cholesterol levels in patients with homozygous familial hypercholesterolemia as an adjunct to other lipid-lowering treatments (eg, LDL apheresis), or if such treatments are unavailable

CONTRAINDICATIONS/WARNINGS

Hypersensitivity

Active liver disease or unexplained persistent elevations in serum transaminases when used concurrently with a statin

Moderate to severe hepatic impairment

Pregnant and nursing women when used concurrently with a statin

DRUG INTERACTIONS

Antacids[2]

Cholestyramine[2]

Cyclosporine[1]

Fibric acid derivatives (eg, fenofibrate, gemfibrozil)[1,3]

1 Effect/toxicity of ezetimibe may increase.

2 Effect of ezetimibe may decrease.

3 Safety and efficacy of concomitant use with ezetimibe is not established.

ADVERSE EFFECTS

Cardiovascular: chest pain (3%)

CNS: headache (8%), dizziness (3%)

GI: diarrhea (3%–4%), abdominal pain (3%)

Neuromuscular and skeletal: arthralgia (4%)

Respiratory: upper respiratory tract infection (13%, placebo 10.8%), sinusitis (4%–5%), pharyngitis (3%)

PHARMACOKINETICS AND PHARMACODYNAMICS

Time to maximum plasma concentrations:	4–12 h
Bioavailability:	variable
Effect of food:	the maximum concentration of ezetimibe is increased by 38% when it is given with a high-fat meal. Ezetimibe may be administered with or without food.
Protein binding:	>90%
Volume of distribution:	no data
Metabolism:	primarily metabolized in the small intestine and liver via glucuronide conjugation; metabolite ezetimibe-glucuronide is formed; may undergo enterohepatic recycling
Elimination:	feces (78%, 69% as ezetimibe); urine (11%, 9% as metabolite)
Elimination half-life:	22 h (ezetimibe and ezetimibe-glucuronide)

DOSAGE

The usual dose is 10 mg once daily with or without food. Ezetimibe may be administered with an HMG-CoA reductase inhibitor for incremental effect. If a BAS is being used concurrently, dosing of ezetimibe should occur at least 2 h before or at least 4 h after administration of the BAS.

MONITORING

Cholesterol profile, liver function test.

OVERDOSE

Doses of up to 50 mg/d are well tolerated. Treatment should be symptom directed and supportive.

PATIENT INFORMATION

This medication may be taken with or without food. Maintain diet and exercise program as prescribed. Notify physician if persistent side effects occur.

AVAILABILITY

Tablets—10 mg
Combination formulations:
Vytorin—ezetimibe/simvastatin combination tablets
10 mg/10 mg
10 mg/20 mg
10 mg/40 mg
10 mg/80 mg

LIPID-LOWERING DRUGS: FIBRIC ACID DERIVATIVES

The fibric acid derivatives (FADs), **gemfibrozil** and **fenofibrate**, are very effective at reducing triglycerides and as such are primarily used for this purpose. The use of these drugs for treating elevated cholesterol in the absence of elevated triglycerides has not been fully evaluated, and the FADs are therefore not considered first-line agents in these situations. However, the VA-HIT study (*see* below) provides some evidence of benefit for **gemfibrozil** in patients with low HDL concentrations.

EFFICACY AND USE

Gemfibrozil 800 to 1600 mg/d may be expected to reduce triglycerides by about 40% to 60%. **Fenofibrate** has been shown to decrease triglyceride concentrations by 15% to 43% in patients with type IIa hyperlipidemia and by 32% to 53% in patients with type IIb or IV hyperlipidemia. HDL concentrations may be increased anywhere from 1% to 34% with these drugs. LDL concentrations, as mentioned earlier, typically decrease in patients with type II hyperlipidemia (perhaps more so with **fenofibrate**) and may increase in patients with type IV hyperlipidemia. These drugs may also be combined with other antihyperlipidemic agents (*eg*, HMG-CoA reductase inhibitors) for additional triglyceride reduction in the treatment of mixed dyslipidemias. In this case, caution is advised and close monitoring recommended because the risk of rhabdomyolysis is increased when FADs and HMG-CoA reductase inhibitors are used together.

Nonmicronized **fenofibrate** has been shown to reduce total and LDL cholesterol to a greater extent than **gemfibrozil** with comparable decreases in triglycerides in a small study involving patients with type IIb hyperlipidemia.

The Helsinki Heart Study demonstrated a 34% reduction in the risk of developing a serious cardiac event (MI or sudden cardiac death) in patients receiving **gemfibrozil** versus placebo. This was mainly a result of a 37% reduction in the risk of nonfatal MI in patients in the **gemfibrozil** group compared with patients receiving placebo. However, all-cause mortality did not differ between the two groups.

Gemfibrozil has also been shown to retard the progression of coronary and vein graft atherosclerosis and the development of new lesions in post–coronary bypass graft patients and to reduce the need for invasive treatment for milder forms of CAD.

The VA-HIT study investigated the effects of a long-acting gemfibrozil preparation in patients with a history of CAD and a mean HDL, LDL, and triglyceride concentration of 32, 111, and 161 mg/dL, respectively. In this study, **gemfibrozil** reduced the risk of experiencing another cardiac event (MI or cardiac death) by 22% compared with placebo and also reduced the incidence of cerebrovascular disease.

Fibric acid derivatives are generally well tolerated, with most side effects being gastrointestinal in nature. As mentioned earlier, caution should be exercised when combining these drugs with HMG-CoA reductase inhibitors because of the increased risk of rhabdomyolysis. These drugs may also potentiate the anticoagulant effect of **warfarin**, necessitating close monitoring of prothrombin times in patients on concurrent therapy.

MODE OF ACTION

The FADs are believed to increase the activity of the enzyme lipoprotein lipase, thus enhancing the catabolism of triglycerides from VLDL and IDL particles and promoting the transfer of cholesterol to HDL. VLDL production also appears to be decreased. High concentrations of triglyceride-rich VLDL particles may cause a rapid conversion to smaller IDL and LDL particles by lipoprotein lipase, resulting in an increase in LDL concentrations. Patients with normal or only slightly elevated triglyceride concentrations may experience a modest reduction in LDL concentrations.

INDICATIONS

	Fenofibrate	Gemfibrozil
Type I hyperlipoproteinemia	–	–
Type IIa hyperlipoproteinemia	+	–
Type IIb hyperlipoproteinemia	+	+*
Type III hyperlipoproteinemia	–	–
Type IV hyperlipoproteinemia	+	+
Type V hyperlipoproteinemia	+	+

*Limited indication (see drug monograph).
+—FDA approved; − —not FDA approved.

FENOFIBRATE (Lofibra™, TriCor™)

Approved in February 1998, fenofibrate is the latest fibric acid derivative to become available in the United States.

Similar to gemfibrozil, fenofibrate is believed to increase lipoprotein lipase activity and thereby the clearance of triglycerides from the body. Triglyceride concentrations may be decreased by 15% to 43% in patients with type IIa hyperlipidemia and by 32% to 53% in patients with type IIb or IV hyperlipidemia. Studies in patients with type II hyperlipidemia demonstrated fenofibrate 200 mg/d to be generally more effective than 20 mg simvastatin or 20 mg pravastatin daily in reducing triglycerides and increasing HDL, although LDL tended to be reduced more with the HMG-CoA reductase inhibitors. Combination therapy of fenofibrate with an HMG-CoA reductase inhibitor has been shown to be safe and effective in reducing both LDL and triglycerides and increasing HDL concentrations. The effects of fenofibrate on morbidity and mortality from CAD have not been evaluated.

SPECIAL GROUPS

Race: not evaluated
Children: safety and effectiveness have not been established
Elderly: initiate therapy at lowest dose and titrate according to response
Renal impairment: dosage may need to be reduced with creatinine clearance (CrCl) <50 mL/min because of a reduction in clearance of the active metabolite
Hepatic impairment: contraindicated in clinically significant hepatic dysfunction, including primary biliary cirrhosis and in patients with unexplained persistent transaminase elevation
Pregnancy: category C; use only if the potential benefit justifies the potential risk to the fetus
Breast-feeding: nursing mothers should not use fenofibrate because of the potential for tumorigenicity seen in animal studies

DOSAGE

Primary hypercholesterolemia/mixed hyperlipidemia: Initial dose is 160 mg/d in tablet form.
Hypertriglyceridemia: Initial dose ranges from 54 to 160 mg/d in tablet form. Dosage should be individualized according to patient response; adjust if necessary after repeat lipid determinations at 4- to 8-wk intervals. Maximum dose is 160 mg/d.
Renal impairment and the elderly: Initiate treatment at 54 mg/d in tablet form.
Note: The 160 mg tablet is equivalent to the 200 mg capsule (micronized); the 54 mg tablet is equivalent to the 67 mg capsule (micronized).

IN BRIEF

INDICATIONS
As adjunctive therapy to diet for the reduction of LDL cholesterol, total cholesterol, triglycerides, and apo B and to increase HDL cholesterol in patients with primary hypercholesterolemia or mixed dyslipidemia (types IIa and IIb hyperlipidemias)
As adjunctive therapy to diet in adult patients with elevated triglyceride concentrations (types IV and V hyperlipidemia) at risk for pancreatitis

CONTRAINDICATIONS
Hepatic or severe renal dysfunction, including primary biliary cirrhosis, and in patients with unexplained persistent liver function abnormality
Pre-existing gallbladder disease
Hypersensitivity to fenofibrate

DRUG INTERACTIONS
BASs[1]   Rifampin[4]
Cyclosporine[2]   Warfarin[5]
HMG-CoA reductase inhibitors[3]

1 Effect of fenofibrate may decrease if given concurrently; patients should take fenofibrate ≥1 h before or 4–6 h after a bile acid–binding resin.
2 Coadministration may lead to increased risk of nephrotoxicity.
3 Concurrent use may increase the risk of myopathy or rhabdomyolysis.
4 Effect of fenofibrate may decrease.
5 Fenofibrate may increase the effect/toxicity of this drug; monitor prothrombin time/INR.

ADVERSE EFFECTS
CNS: dizziness (2%), decreased libido (2%)
GI: flatulence (3%), nausea/vomiting (4%), constipation (3%), dyspepsia (5%), diarrhea (3%)
Skin: pruritus (3%), rash (6%)
Hepatic: serum transaminases > three times upper limit of normal (8%–10%), hepatitis (<1%)
Pancreatic: pancreatitis (<1%)
Musculoskeletal: rhabdomyolysis (<1%)
Hematologic: decreases in hemoglobin/hematocrit (<1%), thrombocytopenia (<1%)
Other: infections, localized/miscellaneous pain, flu syndrome (2%), headache (3%)

PHARMACOKINETICS AND PHARMACODYNAMICS
Duration of action: not evaluated
Onset of action: 2–5 d
Peak effect: ≥12 wk
Bioavailability: cannot be determined because of the unavailability of a parenteral product for comparison
Effect of food: 35% increase in absorption
Protein binding: 99%
Metabolism: completely hydrolyzed to the active metabolite fenofibric acid
Elimination: mainly renal; 60% recovered in urine, 25% recovered in feces
Elimination half-life: 20 h

MONITORING
Plasma lipid profile, serum transaminases, CBC.

OVERDOSE
Treatment should be symptomatic and supportive. Fenofibrate is not removed by hemodialysis.

PATIENT INFORMATION
Take with food to increase drug absorption. If you miss a dose, take it as soon as you remember. If it is about time for the next dose, take that dose only. Do not take two doses at once. Notify physician if persistent side effects occur. Do not discontinue therapy without your physician's advice.

AVAILABILITY
Capsules, micronized (Lofibra)—67 mg, 134 mg, 200 mg
Tablets (TriCor)—54 mg, 160 mg

GEMFIBROZIL (Gemfibrozil, Lopid®)

Gemfibrozil is currently the most widely used FAD in the United States. Gemfibrozil is most useful in treating patients with elevated triglyceride concentrations (types IV and V hyperlipidemias), with the added ability to increase HDL concentrations. Gemfibrozil generally has only mild effects on decreasing total and LDL cholesterol concentrations and, in fact, may paradoxically increase LDL concentrations in patients with elevated triglycerides and normal cholesterol concentrations.

The Helsinki Heart Study evaluated the effects of gemfibrozil in patients with a non-HDL cholesterol level of ≥200 mg/dL and no history of CAD. Over a 5-year period, patients receiving gemfibrozil experienced a 34% reduction in the risk of developing a serious cardiac event (sudden cardiac death and/or MI) mainly because of a 37% reduction in the risk of developing nonfatal MI compared with patients receiving placebo. However, all-cause mortality did not differ between the two groups. Patients with type IIb hyperlipidemia benefited the most in this particular study. A subgroup of patients excluded from the Helsinki Heart Study because of CHD or electrocardiographic abnormalities demonstrated no benefit of gemfibrozil in reducing cardiac events or cardiac deaths.

The Lopid Coronary Angiography Trial showed gemfibrozil to retard the progression of coronary and vein graft atherosclerosis and the development of new lesions in post–coronary bypass graft patients with a mean total cholesterol, triglyceride, and HDL concentration of 199, 146, and 31 mg/dL, respectively.

The VA-HIT trial studied the effects of a long-acting gemfibrozil preparation (not currently available in the United States) in patients with a history of CAD and a mean HDL, LDL, and triglyceride concentration of 32, 111, and 161 mg/dL, respectively. In this study, gemfibrozil reduced the risk of experiencing a cardiac event (MI or cardiac death) by 22% compared with placebo and also reduced the incidence of cerebrovascular disease. In this trial, the first study demonstrating the benefit of increasing HDL without lowering LDL concentrations, gemfibrozil increased HDL concentrations by 6%, had negligible effects on LDL concentrations, and decreased triglycerides by 31%.

SPECIAL GROUPS

Race: not evaluated
Children: safety and effectiveness have not been established
Elderly: no dosage adjustment is required
Renal impairment: gemfibrozil may worsen renal insufficiency in patients with serum creatinine concentrations >2.0 mg/dL and should therefore be used cautiously in this group
Hepatic impairment: contraindicated in clinically significant hepatic dysfunction, including primary biliary cirrhosis
Pregnancy: category C; use only if the potential benefit justifies the potential risk to the fetus
Breast-feeding: gemfibrozil should not be used in nursing mothers because of the potential for tumorigenicity seen in animal studies

DOSAGE

Usual dosage is 600 mg twice daily 30 min before the morning and evening meal.

IN BRIEF

INDICATIONS
As adjunctive therapy to diet in adult patients with elevated triglyceride concentrations (types IV and V hyperlipidemias) at risk for pancreatitis

Reducing the risk of developing CHD in patients with type IIb hypercholesterolemia with low HDL cholesterol in addition to elevated LDL cholesterol and triglycerides and no history or symptoms of CHD after other treatments have failed

CONTRAINDICATIONS
Hepatic or severe renal dysfunction, including primary biliary cirrhosis
Pre-existing gallbladder disease
Hypersensitivity to gemfibrozil

DRUG INTERACTIONS
Cyclosporine[1]
HMG-CoA reductase inhibitors[2]
Rifampin[3]
Sulfonylureas[4]
Warfarin[4]

1 Gemfibrozil may decrease the effect of this drug.
2 Concurrent use may increase the risk of myopathy or rhabdomyolysis.
3 Effect of gemfibrozil may decrease.
4 Gemfibrozil may increase the effect/toxicity of this drug.

ADVERSE EFFECTS
Cardiac: atrial fibrillation (0.7%)
CNS: paresthesias (1%)
GI: dyspepsia (20%), abdominal pain (10%), acute appendicitis (1%) diarrhea (7%), nausea/vomiting (3%), constipation (1%)
Skin: Eczema (2%), rash (2%), pruritus (1%)
Eyes: blurred vision (1%)
Hepatic: increased serum transaminases (<1%)
Endocrine: gout (1%)
Musculoskeletal: extremity pain (1%), myositis (<1%)
Hematologic: decreases in hemoglobin/hematocrit (<1%), thrombocytopenia, leukopenia (<1%)
Other: dizziness (2%), chest pain (2%), headache (1%), fatigue (4%)

PHARMACOKINETICS AND PHARMACODYNAMICS
Duration of action: 6–8 wk (after stopping therapy)
Onset of action: 2–5 d
Peak effect: 3–4 wk
Bioavailability: 98%
Effect of food: none
Protein binding: >97%
Metabolism: hepatic metabolism partially by CYP3A4
Elimination: mainly renal: 70% recovered in urine, mostly as the glucuronide conjugate; 6% recovered in feces
Elimination half-life: 1.5 h

MONITORING
Plasma lipid profile, serum transaminases, CBC.

OVERDOSE
Treatment should be symptomatic and supportive. Gemfibrozil is not removed by hemodialysis.

PATIENT INFORMATION
If you miss a dose, take it as soon as you remember. If it is about time for the next dose, take that dose only. Do not take two doses at once. If abdominal pain, muscle pain, tenderness, weakness or other persistent side effect occurs, notify your clinician. Do not discontinue therapy without your clinician's advice.

AVAILABILITY
Tablet, scored, film coated—600 mg

The information here is provided as guidance only. Prescribers should always consult the manufacturer's current prescribing information.

291

LIPID-LOWERING DRUGS: NICOTINIC ACID

Nicotinic acid (niacin; vitamin B_3) is a water-soluble vitamin that, at doses much larger than those used as a vitamin supplement, lowers total and LDL cholesterol and triglyceride concentrations and increases HDL concentrations. Unlike other available lipid-lowering drugs, niacin has been shown to lower lipoprotein (a) concentrations by as much as 38%.

EFFICACY AND USE

Nicotinic acid, although an effective and inexpensive agent for treating dyslipidemias, is often overlooked as a first-line drug because of its side effect profile and the availability of the well-tolerated (and more expensive) HMG-CoA reductase inhibitors. Nonetheless, nicotinic acid retains a very prominent role in the treatment of dyslipidemias.

In daily doses of 1.5 to 3 g, nicotinic acid is effective in most patients with a variety of dyslipidemias. A daily dose of 2 g or less may lower LDL cholesterol by 20% to 30% and raise HDL cholesterol by as much as 32%. Compared with placebo, patients receiving 3 g daily of niacin in the Coronary Drug Project experienced an average reduction in triglyceride concentrations of 26%. When used in combination with colestipol, HDL concentrations have been shown to increase and LDL concentrations have been shown to decrease, both by 43%. Adding either an HMG-CoA reductase inhibitor or a BAS to nicotinic acid has yielded greater LDL lowering than niacin alone. The combination of niacin, lovastatin, and colestipol has been shown to produce LDL reductions of almost 70%. Nicotinic acid is effective in the treatment of types II, IV, and V hyperlipidemias.

The Coronary Drug Project studied the effect of nicotinic acid (3 g daily) on reducing total mortality in 1119 men with a previous MI. After 5 years of treatment, there was no difference in total mortality between the nicotinic acid and placebo groups. However, nicotinic acid significantly reduced the incidence of definite nonfatal MI by 27% compared with placebo. At an average follow-up of 15 years (about 9 years after the drug was stopped), mortality in the nicotinic acid group was 11% less than in the placebo group, a statistically significant difference.

Several studies have demonstrated nicotinic acid, in combination with colestipol with or without lovastatin, to slow the progression of atherosclerosis and promote atherosclerotic plaque regression in patients with CAD. Combination nicotinic acid-clofibrate therapy has also been shown to significantly reduce total mortality by 26% and mortality due to ischemic heart disease by 36% in patients with a history of MI. The HDL-Atherosclerosis Treatment Study (HATS) demonstrated simvastatin plus nicotinic acid to cause regression of atherosclerotic arterial plaques in patients with coronary disease, low HDL cholesterol and normal LDL.

As mentioned earlier, the more widespread clinical use of nicotinic acid has been limited by its side-effect profile. The most common side effects are related to the vasodilatory action of the drug: flushing, headache, tingling, itching, and rash. It is believed that slow, gradual upward titration of nicotinic acid helps minimize these adverse effects.

Hepatotoxicity is another worrisome side effect of nicotinic acid, predominantly with the sustained-release preparations. It is incompletely defined as to why the sustained-release preparations have a greater tendency to damage the liver, but it may relate to the difference in metabolic handling between immediate-release (IR) and sustained-release preparations. Some clinicians even advocate avoidance of sustained-release preparations for this reason. A once-daily formulation of nicotinic acid is reported to cause transaminase elevations at an incidence similar to HMG-CoA reductase inhibitors and IR niacin.

MODE OF ACTION

The mechanism of action of nicotinic acid in treating hyperlipidemia remains largely unknown but appears to be independent of its role as a vitamin. Nicotinic acid appears to act, at least in part, by reducing the synthesis of lipoprotein (a) and the hepatic synthesis and secretion of apo B–containing particles, by reducing free fatty acid release from adipose tissue, and by changing the metabolism of HDL particles with a resultant shift in HDL subtype distribution. Nicotinic acid may also increase the rate of removal of chylomicron triglycerides from the plasma secondary to increased lipoprotein lipase activity. Nicotinic acid has no effect on the fecal excretion of fats, sterols, or bile acids.

In addition to its effects on plasma lipid concentrations, nicotinic acid produces peripheral vasodilation, thought to be mediated through prostaglandins. Nicotinic acid reportedly releases histamine, causing increased gastric motility and acid secretion. It also activates the fibrinolytic system. Large doses of nicotinic acid have been reported to decrease uric acid excretion and impair glucose tolerance.

INDICATIONS

	Nicotinic Acid
Type I hyperlipoproteinemia	−
Type IIa hyperlipoproteinemia	+
Type IIb hyperlipoproteinemia	+
Type III hyperlipoproteinemia	−
Type IV hyperlipoproteinemia	+
Type V hyperlipoproteinemia	+

+—FDA approved; − —not FDA approved.

NICOTINIC ACID (NIACIN)

(Nicotinic acid, Niacin extended-release, Niacor®, Slo-Niacin®, Nicotinex®, Niaspan®)

Nicotinic acid (niacin; vitamin B$_3$) is a very effective and inexpensive agent for the treatment of hyperlipidemias. Niacin therapy, however, is usually accompanied by several troublesome side effects, necessitating very slow and deliberate dosage titration. Most side effects are secondary to vasodilation (flushing, headaches, etc.) thought to be induced by prostaglandin release. Sustained-release preparations may blunt these side effects somewhat, but in turn may increase the risk of hepatotoxicity.

Niacin decreases total cholesterol, LDL cholesterol, lipoprotein (a), and triglycerides and, more than any other drug, increases HDL cholesterol. The Coronary Drug Project studied the effect of niacin on reducing total mortality in 1119 men with a previous MI. After 5 years, there was no difference in total mortality between the niacin and placebo groups. However, niacin significantly reduced the incidence of definite nonfatal MI compared with placebo. At an average follow-up of 15 years (about 9 years after the drug was stopped), mortality in the niacin group was 11% less than in the placebo group, a statistically significant difference.

Several studies have demonstrated niacin in combination with an HMG-CoA reductase inhibitor, colestipol, or both to slow the progression of atherosclerosis and promote atherosclerotic plaque regression in patients with CAD. Combination niacin-clofibrate therapy has also been shown to reduce total morbidity and mortality due to ischemic heart disease in patients with a history of MI.

SPECIAL GROUPS

Race: not evaluated

Children: not evaluated

Elderly: no dosage adjustment is required

Renal impairment: not evaluated; use cautiously

Hepatic impairment: not extensively studied; use with caution in patients with a history of liver disease or in patients who consume substantial quantities of alcohol. This drug is contraindicated in patients with active liver disease or unexplained persistent transaminase elevation.

Pregnancy: category C; use only if the potential benefit justifies the potential risk to the fetus

Breast-feeding: not evaluated; breast-feed with caution

IN BRIEF

INDICATIONS

As adjunctive therapy to diet for reducing total cholesterol, LDL cholesterol, apo B, and triglyceride concentrations and to increase HDL cholesterol in patients with primary hypercholesterolemia and mixed dyslipidemia (types IIa and IIb hyperlipidemia)

As adjunctive therapy in adult patients with elevated triglyceride concentrations (types IV and V hyperlipidemias) at risk for pancreatitis

As adjunctive therapy to diet to reduce the risk of recurrent nonfatal MI in patients with a history of MI and hypercholesterolemia (ER niacin, Niaspan)

As combination therapy with a BAS to slow the progression or promote the regression of atherosclerosis in patients with clinical evidence of CHD who have elevated cholesterol concentrations (ER niacin, Niaspan)

CONTRAINDICATIONS

Significant or unexplained hepatic dysfunction

Active peptic ulcer disease

Arterial bleeding

Hypersensitivity to product components

DRUG INTERACTIONS

Adrenergic blocking agents[1]

BASs[2]

Ganglionic-blocking antihypertensives[3]

HMG-CoA reductase inhibitors[5]

Oral hypoglycemic agents[4]

Niacin-containing vitamins[6]

Vasoactive drugs[3]

1 May increase the risk of hypotension because of additive vasodilating effects.

2 Concurrent use may decrease the absorption of niacin; niacin should be given 1 h before or 4–6 h after a BAS.

3 Niacin may increase the effect/toxicity of this drug.

4 Niacin may decrease the effect of this drug.

5 Concurrent use may increase the risk of myopathy or rhabdomyolysis.

6 Effect/toxicity of niacin may increase.

ADVERSE EFFECTS

Where applicable, the first number represents IR niacin, the second, Niaspan

Skin: flushing (92%, 88%), itching of skin (49% with IR), rash (20%, ≤5%)

GI: abdominal pain (14%, ≤5%), diarrhea (5%, ≤11%), nausea (9%, ≤10%), vomiting (2%, ≤8%)

Hepatic: elevated transaminases (5%, 5%, ≤52% with sustained-release preparations)

Endocrine: elevated uric acid concentrations (<1%), reduced phosphorus concentrations (<1%)

Hematologic: decreased platelet count (<1%), elevated prothrombin time (<1%)

Other: headache (4%–11% with Niaspan)

PHARMACOKINETICS AND PHARMACODYNAMICS

Duration of action: 2–6 wk after stopping therapy

Onset of action: 2 wk for cholesterol reduction; several hours for triglyceride reduction

Peak effect: 3–5 wk

Bioavailability: 60%–88%

Effect of food: food may increase bioavailability

Protein binding: <20%

Metabolism: rapid, extensive, and saturable first-pass metabolism via two major pathways to form nicotinamide adenine dinucleotide and nicotinuric acid

Elimination: renal, as unchanged drug and metabolites

Elimination half-life: 20–48 min

NICOTINIC ACID (NIACIN) *(continued)*

DOSAGE

IR preparations: The usual dose of IR niacin (Niacor) is 1–2 g twice daily or three times daily with meals. Initiate with 250 mg/d as a single dose after the evening meal, and increase the frequency of dosing and total daily dose at 4- to 7-d intervals until the desired LDL or triglyceride level is reached or the first-level therapeutic dose of 1.5–2 g/d is reached. If hyperlipidemia is not adequately controlled after 2 mo at this level, dosage may be further increased at 2- to 4-wk intervals to 3 g/d (1 g three times daily). Maximum dose is 6 g/d.

Extended-release (ER) preparations: The usual initial dosage of ER niacin preparation (Niaspan) is 500 mg/d at bedtime. Dosage may be increased by no more than 500 mg daily at 4-wk intervals as needed until the desired response is achieved. Maximum daily dose is 2 g.

Note: IR and ER preparations are not interchangeable. For patients switching from an IR to an ER preparation, therapy should be instituted with the recommended initial dose and gradually titrated upward.

MONITORING

Plasma lipid profile, serum transaminases, blood glucose, uric acid, platelet count, prothrombin time or INR, plasma phosphorus concentrations.

OVERDOSE

Treatment is symptomatic and supportive.

PATIENT INFORMATION

Take with food. Do not crush or chew long-acting preparations. Follow your dosage regimen closely to minimize side effects. Flushing is a common side effect of niacin therapy and usually subsides with repeated dosing. Flushing may last for several hours after dosing and may be minimized by taking aspirin or an NSAID (eg, ibuprofen) about 30–60 min before niacin. Hot beverages or alcohol may worsen flushing. If you miss a dose, take it as soon as you remember. If it is about time for the next dose, take that dose only. Do not take two doses at once. Do not discontinue therapy without your clinician's advice. Notify your clinician as soon as possible if you become pregnant or intend to become pregnant or breast-feed while taking this medication.

AVAILABILITY

Tablets, IR (generic)—50 mg, 100 mg, 250 mg, 500 mg
Tablets, IR (Niacor)—500 mg
Capsules, ER (generic)—125 mg, 250 mg, 400 mg, 500 mg
Tablets, ER (generic)—125 mg, 250 mg
Tablets, ER (Niaspan)—500 mg, 750 mg, 1000 mg
Tablets, controlled release (Slo-Niacin)—250 mg, 500 mg, 750 mg
Elixir (Nicotinex)—50 mg/5 mL
Combination formulations:
  Advicor—niacin ER/lovastatin combination tablets
    500 mg/20 mg
    1000 mg/20 mg

LIPID-LOWERING DRUGS: HMG-CoA REDUCTASE INHIBITORS

Inhibitors of HMG-CoA reductase competitively inhibit the conversion of hydroxymethyl-glutaryl to mevalonic acid, a rate-limiting step in the synthesis of cholesterol in the liver and intestines, the main sites for the production of cholesterol in the body. These drugs are highly effective in reducing LDL cholesterol and are very well tolerated. HMG-CoA reductase inhibitors have repeatedly been shown to reduce cardiovascular mortality and morbidity in patients with and without high cholesterol and/or CAD.

EFFICACY AND USE

The HMG-CoA reductase inhibitors are the most potent drugs available for reducing LDL cholesterol and apo B concentrations. In addition, they reduce triglyceride and increase HDL concentrations. Table 11.4 shows the relative efficacy of each of the drugs in this class. These drugs may also be used in combination with BASs, ezetimibe, or niacin to produce additional decreases in LDL cholesterol, or in combination with a FAD for additional reductions in triglyceride concentrations. Combination therapy with niacin or a FAD should be approached cautiously, however, because of an increase in the risk of rhabdomyolysis.

Six large, randomized, placebo-controlled studies have proven the efficacy of the HMG-CoA reductase inhibitors in reducing cardiovascular morbidity and mortality. These studies are summarized in Table 11.5.

Additional beneficial effects of these drugs are in slowing atherosclerosis progression and in promoting the regression of atherosclerotic plaques and in reducing the incidence of stroke.

HMG-CoA reductase inhibitors are generally the best-tolerated lipid-lowering drugs available. Side effects typically occur in less than 10% of patients and are most commonly abdominal pain, flatulence, headache, constipation, diarrhea, nausea, and vomiting. More serious adverse effects, such as rhabdomyolysis, thrombocytopenia, and liver dysfunction, are rare but necessitate prospective monitoring and withdrawal of drug therapy if necessary. Persistent serum transaminase elevations more than three times the upper limit of normal, severe myalgias, and precipitous drops in platelet counts are all reasons for considering discontinuation of these medications.

MODE OF ACTION

Most of the cholesterol formed in the body is synthesized in the liver. HMG-CoA reductase inhibitors interrupt an early rate-limiting step in cholesterol synthesis: the conversion of HMG-CoA to mevalonic acid. Rates of synthesis of LDL receptors are inversely related to the amount of cholesterol in cells; thus, the action of HMG-CoA reductase inhibitors reduces cholesterol synthesis, reduces cellular concentrations of cholesterol, and increases the expression of LDL receptors in the liver. Because LDL receptors are responsible for clearing two

TABLE 11.4 RELATIVE LIPID EFFECTS OF THE HMG-CoA REDUCTASE INHIBITORS

Drug	Daily dosage, *mg*	Usual total cholesterol reduction, %	Usual LDL reduction, %	Usual HDL increase, %	Usual TG reduction, %
Atorvastatin	10.0	25–29	35–39	6–7	17–23
	80.0	45	60	5	37
Fluvastatin	20.0	16–17	20–25	3–6	12–17
	80.0	22–25	30–35	7–11	19–25
Lovastatin	20.0	17–19	24–28	6–8	7–10
	80.0	29–34	40–42	8–10	19–27
Pravastatin	20.0	19–24	26–32	2–6	11
	40.0	21–25	27–34	5–12	21–24
Rosuvastatin	10.0	36	46–52	14	10–37
	40.0	46	55–63	10	28–43
Simvastatin	20.0	25–28	34–38	6–8	15–19
	80.0	31–36	36–47	8–16	24–34

HDL—high-density lipoprotein; HMG-CoA—hydroxymethylglutaryl coenzyme A; LDL—low-density lipoprotein; TG—triglyceride.

(*Adapted from* Kong SX, Crawford SY, Gandhi SK, *et al.*: Efficacy of 3-hydroxy-3-methylglutaryl coenzyme A reductase inhibitors in the treatment of patients with hypercholesterolemia: a meta-analysis of clinical trials. *Clin Ther* 1997, 19:778–797. Additional information from individual product prescribing information.)

thirds to three fourths of plasma LDL (and the associated cholesterol), HMG-CoA reductase inhibitors may promote the clearance of LDL as well as VLDL and VLDL remnants. They may also, by reducing cholesterol synthesis, interfere with the hepatic formation of lipoproteins. Because cholesterol synthesis peaks at night, the HMG-CoA reductase inhibitors should be given before the patient goes to bed. HMG-CoA reductase inhibitors may also act by inhibiting platelet aggregation, macrophage foam cell formation, and LDL oxidation, major contributors to atherogenesis.

Recent evidence suggests that the beneficial effects of this class of drugs are not limited to their ability to lower cholesterol. These so-called "pleiotropic" effects may involve, but are not limited to, anti-inflammatory effects, enhancement of nitric oxide production in the vasculature and kidney, and improvement in bone mineralization and insulin sensitivity.

INDICATIONS

	Atorvastatin	Fluvastatin	Lovastatin	Pravastatin	Rosuvastatin	Simvastatin
Type I hyperlipoproteinemia	–	–	–	–	–	–
Type IIa hyperlipoproteinemia	+	+	+	+	+	+
Type IIb hyperlipoproteinemia	+	+	+	+	+	+
Type III hyperlipoproteinemia	+	–	–	+	–	+
Type IV hyperlipoproteinemia	+	–	–	+	+	+
Type V hyperlipoproteinemia	–	–	–	–	–	–

+—FDA approved; –—not FDA approved.

TABLE 11.5 LARGE-SCALE PLACEBO-CONTROLLED STUDIES ASSESSING THE EFFECT OF HMG-CoA REDUCTASE INHIBITORS ON CARDIOVASCULAR MORBIDITY AND MORTALITY

Study	Sample size	Mean or median follow-up, y	CAD?	Drug regimen, mg/d	Mean or median baseline total (LDL) cholesterol concentration, mg/dL*	Mean or median post-treatment total (LDL) cholesterol concentration, mg/dL*	Result of primary end point compared with placebo*
4S	4444	5.4	Yes	S 20–40	261 (188)	196 (122)	30% reduction in total mortality
WOSCOPS	6595	4.9	No	P 40	272 (192)	218 (142)	31% reduction in definite nonfatal MI and death from CHD
CARE	4159	5.0	Yes	P 40	209 (139)	NR (97–98)	24% reduction in fatal CHD or nonfatal MI
AFCAPS/TexCAPS	6605	5.2	No	L 20–40	221 (150)[†]	184 (115)[‡]	37% reduction in fatal or nonfatal MI, unstable angina, or sudden cardiac death
LIPID	9014	6.1	Yes	P 40	218 (150)	179 (NR)	24% reduction in death from CHD
HPS	20,536	5.0	Yes (65%), no (35%)	S 40	228 (131)[†]	NR (90)	13% reduction in total mortality

*For the group receiving drug, unless stated otherwise.

[†]For placebo and drug groups combined.

[‡]At 1-year follow up.

4S—Scandinavian Simvastatin Survival Study; AFCAPS/TexCAPS—Air Force Coronary/Texas Atherosclerosis Prevention Study; CAD—coronary artery disease; CARE—Cholesterol and Recurrent Events Trial; CHD—coronary heart disease; HMG-CoA—hydroxymethylglutaryl coenzyme A; HPS—Heart Protection Study; L—lovastatin; LDL—low-density lipoprotein; LIPID—Long-Term Intervention with Pravastatin in Ischaemic Disease; MI—myocardial infarction; NR—not reported; P—pravastatin; S—simvastatin; WOSCOPS—West of Scotland Coronary Prevention Study.

ATORVASTATIN (Lipitor®)

Atorvastatin is a synthetic, reversible HMG-CoA reductase inhibitor indicated for types II, III, and IV hyperlipidemias. Maximum dosages of 80 mg/d have been shown to decrease LDL cholesterol concentrations by 60% in patients with type II hyperlipidemia. Atorvastatin (80 mg/d) has also been shown to decrease triglyceride concentrations by 37% in patients with type II hyperlipidemia, compared with 13% to 35% reductions with other HMG-CoA reductase inhibitors. Reductions in triglyceride concentrations of 26% to 46% have been demonstrated with atorvastatin in patients with hypertriglyceridemia, comparable to the 35% to 44% reductions seen with other HMG-CoA reductase inhibitors. Increases in HDL concentrations produced by atorvastatin range from about 5% to 13%, similar to those seen with other HMG-CoA reductase inhibitors.

The MIRACL (Myocardial Ischemia Reduction with Aggressive Cholesterol Lowering) study demonstrated that aggressive lipid-lowering therapy with 80 mg of atorvastatin, given within 1 to 4 days of hospitalization for unstable angina or acute non–Q-wave MI, reduced the occurrence of death or ischemic events by 16% compared with placebo ($P = 0.048$). In addition, the AVERT (Atorvastatin Versus Revascularization Treatments) study demonstrated atorvastatin to be at least as good as coronary angioplasty in reducing cardiovascular events in patients with CAD.

The PROVE IT-TIMI 22 study demonstrated that reducing LDL concentrations to a mean of 62 mg/dL with aggressive drug therapy (80 mg atorvastatin) resulted in a 16% reduction in risk of death or cardiovascular event compared with a mean LDL of 95 mg/dL achieved with standard drug therapy (40 mg pravastatin) in patients recovering from an acute coronary syndrome. The ongoing Treat to New Targets (TNT) study is investigating the impact of lowering LDL with atorvastatin to target levels of around 75 mg/dL compared with current treatment target levels of 100 mg/dL on cardiovascular end points in patients with CAD.

A substudy of the Anglo-Scandinavian Cardiac Outcomes Trial (ASCOT) assessed the effects of atorvastatin (10 mg) and placebo in hypertensive patients receiving blood pressure–lowering treatment who were not dyslipidemic. There were 100 primary events in the atorvastatin group compared with 154 in the placebo group over a 3-year period, a relative risk reduction of 36%. Surprisingly, there were no significant treatment effects in the diabetic subgroup, although the study was not sufficiently powered to detect this.

SPECIAL GROUPS

Race: not evaluated

Children: safety and efficacy not established in children <10 years of age

Elderly: no dosage adjustment is required

Renal impairment: no dosage adjustment is required

Hepatic impairment: liver disease may increase plasma concentrations of atorvastatin; contraindicated in patients with active liver disease or unexplained persistent transaminase elevation

Pregnancy: category X; if the woman becomes pregnant while on atorvastatin, the drug should be discontinued

Breast-feeding: contraindicated

IN BRIEF

INDICATIONS

As adjunctive therapy to diet for reduction of elevated total cholesterol, LDL cholesterol, apo B, and triglyceride concentrations and to increase HDL cholesterol in patients with primary hypercholesterolemia (heterozygous familial and nonfamilial) and mixed dyslipidemia (types IIa and IIb)

As adjunctive therapy to diet for the management of elevated triglyceride concentrations (type IV hyperlipidemia)

For treatment of patients with primary dysbetalipoproteinemia (type III hyperlipidemia) who do not respond adequately to diet

To reduce total and LDL cholesterol in patients with homozygous familial hypercholesterolemia as an adjunct to other lipid-lowering treatments (eg, LDL apheresis) or if such treatments are unavailable

As adjunctive therapy to diet for reduction of elevated total cholesterol, LDL cholesterol, and apo B levels in boys and postmenarchal girls 10–17 years of age with heterozygous familial hypercholesterolemia if, after an adequate trial of diet therapy, the following findings are present: 1) LDL cholesterol remains ≥190 mg/dL or 2) LDL remains ≥160 mg/dL *and* a) there is a positive family history of premature cardiovascular disease or b) two or more other cardiovascular disease risk factors are present in the pediatric patient

CONTRAINDICATIONS

Active liver disease or persistent elevations of serum transaminases

Pregnancy

Breast-feeding

Hypersensitivity to product components

DRUG INTERACTIONS

Cyclosporine[1,4]

CYP3A4 inhibitors (eg, amiodarone, amprenavir, diltiazem)[1]

FADs[4]

Niacin[4]

Erythromycin[1,4]

Azole antifungals[1,4]

Antacids[2,5]

Colestipol[2,5]

Digoxin[3,5]

Norethindrone[3,5]

Ethinyl estradiol[3,5]

Levothyroxine[3]

1 Effect/toxicity of atorvastatin may increase.

2 Effect of atorvastatin may decrease.

3 Atorvastatin may increase the effect/toxicity of this drug.

4 Concurrent use may increase the risk of myopathy and rhabdomyolysis.

5 The clinical significance of this interaction is unclear.

ADVERSE EFFECTS

CNS: dizziness (≥2%), insomnia (≥2%)

Respiratory: bronchitis (≥2%), rhinitis (≥2%)

GI: diarrhea (3%–5%), nausea (≥2%), constipation (1%–2%)

Skin: rash (1%–4%)

Urogenital: urinary tract infection (≥2%)

Extremities: peripheral edema (≥2%)

Hepatic: serum transaminases >3 times upper limit of normal (0.7%)

Musculoskeletal: myalgia (1%–6%), arthritis (≥2%), rhabdomyolysis (<1%)

Hematologic: thrombocytopenia (<1%)

Other: infections (3%–10%), chest pain (≥2%), abdominal pain (2%–4%), headache (3%–17%)

ATORVASTATIN (continued)

Recently, the Collaborative Atorvastatin Diabetes Study (CARDS) demonstrated that treatment with atorvastatin 10 mg provided early and significant benefits in primary prevention of CAD and stroke in type 2 diabetic patients with relatively low LDL cholesterol levels (mean LDL cholesterol of 118 mg/dL). The treatment benefits were consistent in patients with levels of LDL cholesterol above and below the median level and included favorable effects on mortality.

DOSAGE

Hypercholesterolemia and mixed dyslipidemia: The recommended initial dose is 10 or 20 mg once daily. Patients who require a large reduction in LDL cholesterol (>45%) may be initiated at 40 mg once daily. The dosage range is 10–80 mg administered as a single dose once daily, at any time of the day, with or without food. Dosage may be adjusted at intervals of 2–4 wk.

Heterozygous familial hypercholesterolemia in pediatric patients (10–17 years of age): The recommended initial dose is 10 mg/d; maximum recommended dose is 20 mg/d. Dosage may be adjusted at intervals of 4 wk or more.

Homozygous familial hypercholesterolemia: The recommended dosage is 10–80 mg/d. Use atorvastatin as an adjunct to other lipid-lowering treatments (*eg*, LDL apheresis) in these patients or if such treatments are unavailable.

Concomitant lipid-lowering therapy: Atorvastatin may be used in combination with a bile acid–binding resin for additive effect. Generally, avoid the combination of HMG-CoA reductase inhibitors and fibrates.

PHARMACOKINETICS AND PHARMACODYNAMICS

Duration of action:	4–6 wk after discontinuation
Onset of action:	within 2 wk
Peak effect:	within 4 wk
Bioavailability:	14%; systemic availability of HMG-CoA reductase inhibition: 30%
Effect of food:	food decreases rate and extent of absorption but does not impair efficacy
Protein binding:	≥98%
Metabolism:	extensive hepatic metabolism (most likely by CYP3A4) to active metabolites, which account for 70% of the clinical effect
Elimination:	primarily in bile
Elimination half-life:	14 h; 20–30 h half-life for HMG-CoA reductase inhibition

MONITORING

Plasma lipid profile, serum transaminases, signs and symptoms of muscle pain, tenderness, or weakness.

OVERDOSE

Treatment should be symptomatic and supportive. Atorvastatin is not removed by hemodialysis.

PATIENT INFORMATION

If you miss a dose, take it as soon as you remember. If it is about time for the next dose, take that dose only. Do not take two doses at once. If muscle pain, tenderness, or weakness occurs, notify your clinician. Follow your prescribed diet. This medication should not be taken during pregnancy because of possible harm to the fetus. Notify your clinician as soon as possible if you become pregnant or intend to become pregnant while taking this medication.

AVAILABILITY

Tablets, film coated—10 mg, 20 mg, 40 mg, 80 mg
Combination formulations:
Caduet—amlodipine/atorvastatin combination tablets
    5 mg/10 mg
    5 mg/20 mg
    5 mg/40 mg
    5 mg/80 mg
    10 mg/10 mg
    10 mg/20 mg
    10 mg/40 mg
    10 mg/80 mg

FLUVASTATIN (Lescol®, Lescol® XL)

In 1993, fluvastatin became the first entirely synthetic HMG-CoA reductase inhibitor approved for use in the United States. At initial dosages, fluvastatin is generally believed to produce the most modest reduction in cholesterol concentrations compared with other available HMG-CoA reductase inhibitors. However, one study showed the maximum dosage of 80 mg/d to decrease LDL cholesterol concentrations more than the maximum dosage of pravastatin (40 mg/d) in patients with type II hyperlipidemia. The least expensive HMG-CoA reductase inhibitor, fluvastatin may be the most cost-effective drug in this class for lowering cholesterol in patients with mild-to-moderate hypercholesterolemia. Because maximum dosages of fluvastatin would be expected to yield a 30%–35% reduction in LDL cholesterol, patients requiring greater LDL cholesterol lowering are likely to receive greater benefits from other HMG-CoA reductase inhibitors.

Fluvastatin has also been shown to slow the progression of CAD and may also promote atherosclerotic plaque regression. The Lipoprotein and Coronary Atherosclerosis Study showed a non–statistically significant reduction in clinical events (cardiac morbidity or any fatal event) and need for revascularization in hypercholesterolemic patients receiving fluvastatin compared with placebo. The Lescol in Severe Atherosclerosis Study demonstrated a 71% reduction in cardiac events (death from cardiovascular causes, MI, occurrence of unstable angina or coronary artery bypass surgery) with fluvastatin compared with placebo in 365 patients with elevated cholesterol and CAD.

Fluvastatin also appears to have unique antifungal activity (mechanism unknown), which may be clinically beneficial when combined with azole antifungal drugs.

SPECIAL GROUPS

Race: not evaluated
Children: safety and efficacy not established
Elderly: no dosage adjustment is required
Renal impairment: no dosage adjustment is required; use cautiously with severe renal impairment
Hepatic impairment: use cautiously because liver disease may increase plasma concentrations of fluvastatin; contraindicated in patients with active liver disease or unexplained persistent transaminase elevation
Pregnancy: category X; if the woman becomes pregnant while on fluvastatin, the drug should be discontinued
Breast-feeding: contraindicated

IN BRIEF

INDICATIONS
As adjunctive therapy to diet to reduce elevated total and LDL cholesterol concentrations, apo B, and triglyceride concentrations and to increase HDL cholesterol concentrations in patients with primary hypercholesterolemia and mixed dyslipidemia (types IIa and IIb hyperlipidemia)

To reduce the risk of undergoing coronary revascularization procedures in patients with CHD

To slow the progression of coronary atherosclerosis in patients with CHD as part of a treatment strategy to lower total and LDL cholesterol to target concentrations

CONTRAINDICATIONS
Active liver disease or persistent elevations of serum transaminases
Pregnancy
Breast-feeding
Hypersensitivity to product components

DRUG INTERACTIONS
Cyclosporine[4]
Fenofibrate[4]
Gemfibrozil[4]
Cholestyramine (when fluvastatin is given within 4 h after cholestyramine)[2]
Niacin[4]
Ritonavir[1]
Erythromycin[4]
Cimetidine[1]
Ranitidine[1]
Omeprazole[1]
Rifampin[2]
Digoxin[3,5]
Warfarin[3,5]

1 Effect/toxicity of fluvastatin may increase.
2 Effect of fluvastatin may decrease.
3 Fluvastatin may increase the effect/toxicity of this drug.
4 Concurrent use may increase the risk of myopathy and rhabdomyolysis.
5 The clinical significance of this interaction is unclear.

ADVERSE EFFECTS
CNS: dizziness (2%), insomnia (3%)
Respiratory: upper respiratory infections (16%) sinusitis (3%), rhinitis (5%)
GI: diarrhea (5%), nausea (3%), constipation (3%), dyspepsia (8%), flatulence (3%)
Skin: rash (2%)
Hepatic: serum transaminases >3 times upper limit of normal (0.2%–2.7%)
Musculoskeletal: myalgia (5%), arthritis (2%), myopathy, rhabdomyolysis (<1%)
Other: flulike symptoms (5%), abdominal pain (5%), headache (9%), fatigue (3%)

PHARMACOKINETICS AND PHARMACODYNAMICS
Duration of action: 4–6 wk after discontinuation
Onset of action: within 2 wk
Peak effect: 4 wk
Bioavailability: 24%
Effect of food: food decreases rate but not extent of absorption
Protein binding: 98%
Metabolism: extensive hepatic metabolism, primarily via CYP2C9; no active metabolites are present systemically
Elimination: about 90% eliminated in the feces as metabolites, <2% as unchanged drug
Elimination half-life: 2–3 h

FLUVASTATIN *(continued)*

DOSAGE

Patients requiring LDL cholesterol reduction to a goal of ≥25%: The recommended initial dose is 40 mg as 1 capsule, 80 mg as 1 tablet administered as a single dose in the evening, or 80 mg in divided doses of the 40 mg capsule given twice daily.

Patients requiring LDL cholesterol reduction to a goal of <25%: An initial dose of 20 mg may be used. The recommended dosing range is 20–80 mg/day. Dosage adjustments may be made at intervals of ≥4 wk.

Concomitant lipid-lowering therapy: Lipid-lowering effects on total cholesterol and LDL cholesterol are additive when IR fluvastatin is combined with a bile acid–binding resin or niacin. When administering a bile acid resin (*eg*, cholestyramine) and fluvastatin, administer fluvastatin at bedtime, at least 2 h following the resin to avoid a significant interaction because of drug binding to resin.

MONITORING

Plasma lipid profile, serum transaminases, signs and symptoms of muscle pain, tenderness, or weakness.

OVERDOSE

Treatment should be symptomatic and supportive.

PATIENT INFORMATION

Avoid prolonged exposure to the sun and other ultraviolet light. If the ER tablet is prescribed, swallow tablet whole with plenty of water (do not chew or crush). If you miss a dose, take it as soon as you remember. If it is about time for the next dose, take that dose only. Do not take two doses at once. If muscle pain, tenderness, or weakness occurs, notify your clinician. Follow your prescribed diet. This medication should not be taken during pregnancy because of possible harm to the fetus. Notify your clinician as soon as possible if you become pregnant or intend to become pregnant while taking this medication.

AVAILABILITY

Capsules (Lescol)—20 and 40 mg
Tablets, ER (Lescol XL)— 80 mg

LOVASTATIN
(Lovastatin, Altocor™, Mevacor®)

Lovastatin is an HMG-CoA reductase inhibitor derived from a strain of the fungus *Aspergillus terreus*. In 1987, lovastatin became the first HMG-CoA reductase inhibitor approved for use in the United States. Lovastatin itself is inactive but is hydrolyzed in vivo to the active beta-hydroxyacid metabolite. Starting dosages of 20 mg/d have been shown to decrease total cholesterol by a mean of 17%, decrease LDL by 24%, and increase HDL by 7%. Maximum dosages of 80 mg/d decrease total cholesterol by a mean of 29%, decrease LDL by 40%, and increase HDL by 10%. Triglycerides are decreased by a median of 10% and 19% at daily doses of 20 and 80 mg, respectively. Lovastatin has been shown to slow the progression of atherosclerosis in several trials as well as promote the regression of atherosclerotic plaques. Combining lovastatin with cholestyramine or ezetimibe results in additive cholesterol-lowering effects.

The Air Force/Texas Coronary Atherosclerosis Prevention Study (AFCAPS/TexCAPS) demonstrated the benefit of lovastatin in preventing coronary events in men and women with no prior history of atherosclerotic cardiovascular disease and a mean total cholesterol concentration of 221 mg/dL, LDL concentration of 150 mg/dL, and HDL concentration of 36 mg/dL for men and 40 mg/dL for women. After a mean follow-up of 5.2 years, the risk of MI, unstable angina, or sudden cardiac death was reduced by 37% with lovastatin treatment compared with placebo.

SPECIAL GROUPS

Race: not evaluated
Children: safety and efficacy not established in children <10 years of age
Elderly: no dosage adjustment is required
Renal impairment: dosages above 20 mg/d should be used cautiously in patients with CrCl <30 mL/min
Hepatic impairment: use cautiously in patients who consume substantial quantities of alcohol or have a past history of liver disease; contraindicated in patients with active liver disease or unexplained persistent transaminase elevation
Pregnancy: category X; if the woman becomes pregnant while on lovastatin, the drug should be discontinued
Breast-feeding: contraindicated

IN BRIEF

INDICATIONS
As adjunctive therapy to diet for reducing elevated total and LDL cholesterol concentrations in patients with primary hypercholesterolemia (types IIa and IIb hyperlipidemia)—IR only

To slow the progression of coronary atherosclerosis in patients with CHD as part of a treatment strategy to lower total and LDL cholesterol to target levels

Primary prevention of CHD in individuals without symptomatic cardiovascular disease who have average to moderately elevated total cholesterol and LDL cholesterol, and below-average HDL cholesterol

As adjunctive therapy to diet to reduce total and LDL cholesterol and apo B concentrations in adolescent boys and girls who are at least 1 y post menarche, 10–17 years of age, with heterozygous familial hypercholesterolemia if after an adequate trial of diet therapy, LDL cholesterol remains >189 mg/dL or if LDL cholesterol remains >160 mg/dL and there is a positive family history of premature cardiovascular disease or two or more other cardiovascular disease risk factors are present in the adolescent patient—IR only

As adjunctive therapy to diet for the reduction of elevated total and LDL cholesterol, apo B, and triglycerides and to increase HDL cholesterol in patients with primary hypercholesterolemia (heterozygous familial and nonfamilial) and mixed dyslipidemia (types IIa and IIb hyperlipidemia)—ER only

CONTRAINDICATIONS
Active liver disease or persistent elevations of serum transaminases
Pregnancy
Breast-feeding
Hypersensitivity to product components

DRUG INTERACTIONS
Cyclosporine[1,4]
FADs[4]
Niacin[4]
Macrolide antibiotics[1,4]
Nefazodone[1,4]
Azole antifungals[1,4]
Warfarin[3,5]
CYP3A4 inhibitors (eg, amiodarone, amprenavir, diltiazem)[1]
Verapamil[1]
Cholestyramine[2]
Levothyroxine[3]
Digoxin[3]
Norethindrone[3]
Ethinyl estradiol[3]

1 Effect/toxicity of lovastatin may increase.
2 Cholestyramine taken with lovastatin reduces lovastatin absorption and effect.
3 Lovastatin may increase the effect/toxicity of this drug.
4 Concurrent use may increase the risk of myopathy and rhabdomyolysis.
5 The clinical significance of this interaction is unclear.

ADVERSE EFFECTS
CNS: dizziness (1%–2%), headache (2%–10%)
GI: dyspepsia (1%–4%), diarrhea (2%–6%), nausea (2%–5%), constipation (2%–5%), flatulence (3%–6%), abdominal pain (2%–6%)
Skin: rash (1%–5%)
Hepatic: serum transaminases >3 times upper limit of normal (1.9%)
Musculoskeletal: myalgia (1%–3%), muscle cramps (1%), rhabdomyolysis (<1%)
Special senses: blurred vision (1%)
Other: asthenia (1%–2%)

LOVASTATIN (continued)

DOSAGE

IR: Usual initial dosage is 20 mg once daily for patients requiring ≥20% reductions in LDL cholesterol and 10 mg once daily for patients requiring LDL cholesterol reductions of <20%, administered with the evening meal. Dosage may be titrated every 4 wk or more up to 80 mg once daily or in 2 divided doses.

ER: Usual recommended initial dose is 20, 40, or 60 mg once daily given in the evening at bedtime. The recommended dosing range is 10–60 mg/d in single doses. An initial dose of 10 mg/d may be considered for patients requiring smaller reductions of LDL cholesterol. Adjust dosage at intervals of ≥4 wk.

Adolescents 10–17 years of age with heterozygous familial hypercholesterolemia (IR only): Usual initial dosage is 20 mg once daily for patients requiring ≥20% reductions in LDL cholesterol and 10 mg once daily for patients requiring LDL cholesterol reductions of <20%. The recommended dosing range is 10–40 mg/day. Adjust dosage at intervals of ≥4 wk.

Concomitant lipid-lowering therapy: If used in combination with fibrates or niacin, the dose of lovastatin should not exceed 20 mg/d.

Concomitant cyclosporine: Initiate lovastatin at 10 mg/d. Maximum dose is 20 mg/d as the risk of myopathy increases at higher doses.

Concomitant amiodarone or verapamil (IR only): In patients taking amiodarone or verapamil concurrently with lovastatin, the dose of lovastatin should not exceed 40 mg/d.

Renal function impairment: In patients with severe renal impairment (CrCl <30 mL/min), carefully consider dosage increases above 20 mg/d and, if deemed necessary; implement cautiously.

PHARMACOKINETICS AND PHARMACODYNAMICS

Duration of action: 4–6 wk after discontinuation
Onset of action: within 2 wk
Peak effect: 4–6 wk
Bioavailability: <5% because of extensive hepatic extraction
Effect of food: food increases bioavailability by 50%
Protein binding: >95%
Metabolism: extensive hepatic metabolism predominantly by CYP3A4 to active metabolites, most notably the beta-hydroxyacid metabolite
Elimination: 10% of a dose is excreted in the urine; 83% in the feces (biliary excretion and unabsorbed drug)
Elimination half-life: 1.1–1.7 h

MONITORING

Plasma lipid profile, serum transaminases, signs and symptoms of muscle pain, tenderness, or weakness.

OVERDOSE

Treatment should be symptomatic and supportive.

PATIENT INFORMATION

Take with food, preferably in the evening. If the ER tablet is prescribed, swallow tablet whole with plenty of water (do not chew or crush). If you miss a dose, take it as soon as you remember. If it is about time for the next dose, take that dose only. Do not take two doses at once. If blurred vision or muscle pain, tenderness, or weakness occurs, notify your clinician. Follow your prescribed diet. This medication should not be taken during pregnancy because of possible harm to the fetus. Notify your clinician as soon as possible if you become pregnant or intend to become pregnant while taking this medication.

AVAILABILITY

Tablets (Lovastatin, Mevacor)—10 mg, 20 mg, 40 mg
Tablets, ER (Altocor)—10 mg, 20 mg, 40 mg, 60 mg
Combination formulations:
 Advicor—niacin ER/lovastatin combination tablets
  500 mg/20 mg
  1000 mg/20 mg

PRAVASTATIN (Pravachol®)

Approved in 1991, pravastatin was the second HMG-CoA reductase inhibitor available for use in the United States. Unlike lovastatin and simvastatin, pravastatin is administered in the active form. Average reductions in LDL of 34% may be seen with pravastatin 40 mg once daily, and reductions of 50% or more may be achieved by combining pravastatin with cholestyramine. Pravastatin has been shown to slow the progression of atherosclerosis in several trials as well as reduce the risk of MI and death.

Pravastatin, in a dosage of 40 mg once daily, has been shown to decrease mortality in placebo-controlled studies in patients with a wide range of plasma cholesterol concentrations. The West of Scotland Coronary Prevention Study (WOSCOPS) demonstrated pravastatin to reduce the rate of MI or death by 31% in men with no prior history of MI and a mean total cholesterol concentration of 272 mg/dL. In patients with a history of MI and a mean total cholesterol concentration of 209 mg/dL, pravastatin yielded a 24% risk reduction for the same end point in the Cholesterol and Recurrent Events (CARE) trial. The Long-Term Intervention with Pravastatin in Ischaemic Disease (LIPID) study showed pravastatin to reduce the risk of death from CAD by 24% in patients with a history of MI or unstable angina and a total cholesterol concentration ranging between 155 and 271 mg/dL.

The Pravastatin in Elderly Individuals at Risk of Vascular Disease (PROSPER) study was a randomized, double-blind, placebo-controlled trial of 40 mg of pravastatin in elderly men and women (70 to 82 years of age) with a history of, or at risk for, vascular disease. Pravastatin given for 3 years reduced the risk of major adverse cardiovascular events by 15% ($P = 0.014$) in this population. The recent ALLHAT study showed no benefit of pravastatin on cardiovascular outcomes in hypertensive patients older than 55 years when compared with physician-guided therapy. However, the lack of benefit may be related to the 8% difference in LDL cholesterol lowering between the pravastatin and control groups.

SPECIAL GROUPS

Race: not evaluated

Children: safety and efficacy not established in children <8 years of age

Elderly: no dosage adjustment is required

Renal impairment: initiate with lower dose in patients with severe renal impairment; patients with renal impairment should be closely monitored

Hepatic impairment: use cautiously in patients who consume substantial quantities of alcohol or have a past history of liver disease; contraindicated in patients with active liver disease or unexplained persistent transaminase elevation

Pregnancy: category X; if the woman becomes pregnant while on pravastatin, the drug should be discontinued

Breast-feeding: contraindicated

IN BRIEF

INDICATIONS
Primary prevention of coronary events: In hypercholesterolemic patients without clinically evident CHD, to reduce the risk of MI; to reduce the risk of undergoing myocardial revascularization procedures; to reduce the risk of cardiovascular mortality with no increase in death from noncardiovascular causes.

Secondary prevention of cardiovascular events: In patients with clinically evident CHD, to reduce the risk of total mortality by reducing coronary death, MI, undergoing myocardial revascularization procedures, stroke, and stroke/transient ischemic attack, and to slow the progression of coronary atherosclerosis

As adjunctive therapy to diet for the reduction of elevated total and LDL cholesterol, apo B, and triglyceride concentrations and to increase HDL cholesterol in patients with primary hypercholesterolemia and mixed dyslipidemia (types IIa and IIb hyperlipidemia)

As adjunctive therapy to diet for the treatment of patients with elevated serum triglyceride concentrations (type IV hyperlipidemia)

For the treatment of patients with primary dysbetalipoproteinemia (type III hyperlipidemia) who do not respond adequately to diet

As adjunctive therapy to diet and lifestyle modification for treatment of heterozygous familial hypercholesterolemia in children and adolescents ≥8 years of age if after an adequate trial of diet, the following findings are present: 1) LDL cholesterol remains ≥190 mg/dL or 2) LDL cholesterol remains ≥160 mg/dL *and* a) there is a positive family history of premature cardiovascular disease or b) two or more other cardiovascular disease risk factors are present in the patient

CONTRAINDICATIONS
Active liver disease or persistent elevations of serum transaminases
Pregnancy
Breast-feeding
Hypersensitivity to product components

DRUG INTERACTIONS
Immunosuppressive drugs[3]
Gemfibrozil[3]
Niacin[3]
Cholestyramine[2]
Colestipol[2]
Erythromycin[3]
Itraconazole[1]
Ketoconazole[1]

1 Effect/toxicity of pravastatin may increase.

2 Concurrent administration may decrease pravastatin absorption; give pravastatin either ≥1 h before or ≥4 h following the resin.

3 Concurrent use may increase the risk of myopathy and rhabdomyolysis.

ADVERSE EFFECTS
Cardiac: cardiac chest pain (4%)
CNS: dizziness (3.3%), headache (6.2%)
GI: heartburn (2.9%), diarrhea (6.2%), nausea/vomiting (7.3%), constipation (4%), flatulence (3.3%), abdominal pain (5.4%)
Skin: rash (4%)
Hepatic: serum transaminases >3 times upper limit of normal (1.3%)
Musculoskeletal: myalgia (2.7%), localized pain (10%)
Respiratory: cough (2.6%), common cold (7%), rhinitis (4%)
Other: influenza (2.4%), chest pain (3.7%), fatigue (3.8%), lens opacity (<1%)

The information here is provided as guidance only. Prescribers should always consult the manufacturer's current prescribing information.

303

PRAVASTATIN (continued)

DOSAGE

Adults: The recommended initial dose is 40 mg once daily. If a daily dose of 40 mg does not achieve desired cholesterol concentrations, 80 mg once daily may be given. Dosage should be titrated based on response at 4-wk intervals. A lower initial dose of 10 mg is recommended for patients with significant renal or hepatic impairment. If used in combination with cyclosporine, therapy should begin with 10 mg pravastatin once daily at bedtime and generally should not exceed 20 mg/d. Dosage must be titrated with caution.

Children 8–13 years of age: The recommended dose is 20 mg once daily. Doses >20 mg have not been studied in this patient population.

Adolescents 14–18 years of age: The recommended initial dose is 40 mg once daily. Doses >40 mg have not been studied in this patient population.

PHARMACOKINETICS AND PHARMACODYNAMICS

Duration of action: 4–6 wk after discontinuation
Onset of action: within 2 wk
Peak effect: 4–6 wk
Bioavailability: 17% because of extensive hepatic extraction
Effect of food: food may decrease bioavailability somewhat, but does not diminish clinical efficacy
Protein binding: 50%
Metabolism: hepatic metabolism to inactive or weakly active metabolites. Pravastatin is not metabolized to a clinically significant extent by CYP3A4
Elimination: 20% of a dose is excreted in the urine; 70% in the feces (biliary excretion and unabsorbed drug)
Elimination half-life: 1.8 h

MONITORING

Plasma lipid profile, serum transaminases, signs and symptoms of muscle pain, tenderness, or weakness.

OVERDOSE

Treatment should be symptomatic and supportive.

PATIENT INFORMATION

Take at least 1 h before or 4 h after cholestyramine or colestipol. Take at bedtime for maximum effect. If you miss a dose, take it as soon as you remember. If it is about time for the next dose, take that dose only. Do not take two doses at once. If blurred vision or muscle pain, tenderness, or weakness occurs, notify your clinician. Follow your prescribed diet. This medication should not be taken during pregnancy because of possible harm to the fetus. Notify your clinician as soon as possible if you become pregnant or intend to become pregnant while taking this medication.

AVAILABILITY

Tablets—10 mg, 20 mg, 40 mg, 80 mg
Combination formulations:
Pravigard PAC—buffered aspirin/pravastatin combination tablets
    81 mg/20 mg
    81 mg/40 mg
    81 mg/80 mg
    325 mg/20 mg
    325 mg/40 mg
    325 mg/80 mg

ROSUVASTATIN (Crestor®)

Rosuvastatin is a new HMG-CoA reductase inhibitor with a number of favorable characteristics, including low lipophilicity, high hepatocyte selectivity, minimal metabolism, and a low propensity for cytochrome P450 drug interactions. Rosuvastatin has been studied at doses ranging from 1 to 80 mg. In comparative clinical trials, rosuvastatin given at 5 to 10 mg/d reduced LDL cholesterol to a significantly greater extent than atorvastatin 10 mg/d, pravastatin 20 mg/d, and simvastatin 20 mg/d. In addition, rosuvastatin exhibited beneficial effects on other lipid parameters, such as HDL cholesterol and triglycerides. In the United States, rosuvastatin is approved in daily dosages up to 40 mg; higher dosages may increase the risk of adverse effects (*eg*, myopathy, proteinuria, and hematuria). Further studies and clinical experience are needed to establish the long-term safety and efficacy of this drug.

SPECIAL GROUPS

Race: pharmacokinetic studies show an approximate twofold elevation in median exposure (area under the curve [AUC]) in Japanese subjects residing in Japan and in Chinese subjects residing in Singapore when compared with whites residing in North America and Europe. No studies directly examining Asian ethnic populations residing in the United States are available, so the contributions of environmental and genetic factors to the observed increases in rosuvastatin drug levels have not been determined.

Children: safety and efficacy have not been established

Elderly: no initial dosage adjustment is needed

Renal impairment: initiate with lower dose for patients with severe renal impairment; dosage should not exceed 10 mg once daily

Hepatic impairment: contraindicated in patients with active liver disease or unexplained persistent transaminase elevation

Pregnancy: category X; rosuvastatin is contraindicated in women who are or may become pregnant

Breast-feeding: rosuvastatin is contraindicated in nursing mothers

IN BRIEF

INDICATIONS
As adjunctive therapy to diet to reduce elevated total cholesterol, LDL cholesterol, apo B, non-HDL cholesterol, and triglyceride levels and to increase HDL cholesterol in patients with primary hypercholesterolemia (heterozygous familial and nonfamilial) and mixed dyslipidemia (Fredrickson types IIa and IIb)

As adjunctive therapy to diet for the treatment of patients with elevated serum triglyceride levels (Fredrickson type IV)

To reduce LDL cholesterol, total cholesterol, and apo B in patients with homozygous familial hypercholesterolemia as an adjunct to other lipid-lowering treatments (eg, LDL apheresis) or if such treatments are unavailable

CONTRAINDICATIONS
Hypersensitivity
Active liver disease or unexplained persistent elevations of serum transaminases
Pregnancy
Nursing mothers

DRUG INTERACTIONS
Antacids[2]
Cyclosporine[1]
Gemfibrozil[1]
Niacin[1]
Oral contraceptives[3]
Warfarin[3]

1 Effect/toxicity of rosuvastatin may increase.
2 Effect of rosuvastatin may decrease.
3 Rosuvastatin may increase the effect/toxicity of this drug.

ADVERSE EFFECTS
Cardiovascular: chest pain, hypertension, peripheral edema
CNS: headache (6%), depression, dizziness, insomnia
Dermatologic: rash
GI: pharyngitis (9%), abdominal pain, constipation, gastroenteritis
Neuromuscular and skeletal: myalgia (3%), arthritis, arthralgia, hypertonia, paresthesia, myositis (<1%), myopathy (<1%), rhabdomyolysis (<1%)
Respiratory: bronchitis, cough
Other: anemia, pain, proteinuria, hematuria, kidney failure (<1%)

PHARMACOKINETICS AND PHARMACODYNAMICS
Time to maximum therapeutic effect: ≈ 4 wk
Time to peak plasma concentration: 3–5 h
Bioavailability: 20% (high first-pass extraction by liver)
Effect of food: administration of rosuvastatin with food decreased the rate of drug absorption by 20% as assessed by maximum drug concentration (C_{max}). However, there was no effect on the extent of absorption as assessed by AUC.
Protein binding: 88%
Volume of distribution: 134 L
Metabolism: hepatic (10%), via CYP2C9 (1 active metabolite identified)
Elimination: feces (90%), primarily as unchanged drug
Half-life: 19 h

MONITORING
Total, LDL, and HDL cholesterol; liver function test should be determined at baseline and at 12 wk following both the initiation of therapy and any elevation of dose, and periodically thereafter; baseline creatinine phosphokinase (creatinine phosphokinase should be rechecked in patients with symptoms suggestive of myopathy).

ROSUVASTATIN (continued)

DOSAGE

Hypercholesterolemia and mixed dyslipidemia: The usual initial dose is 10 mg once daily. Initiation of therapy with 5 mg once daily may be considered for patients requiring less aggressive LDL cholesterol reductions or who have predisposing factors for myopathy. For patients with marked hypercholesterolemia (LDL cholesterol >190 mg/dL) and aggressive lipid targets, a 20 mg starting dose may be considered. The 40 mg dose should be reserved for patients who have not achieved goal LDL cholesterol at 20 mg. The dose range for rosuvastatin is 5 to 40 mg once daily.

Homozygous familial hypercholesterolemia: The recommended initial dose is 20 mg once daily in patients with homozygous familial hypercholesterolemia. The maximum daily dose is 40 mg. Rosuvastatin should be used in these patients as an adjunct to other lipid-lowering treatments (eg, LDL apheresis) or if such treatments are unavailable.

Concurrent use with cyclosporine: In patients taking cyclosporine, dose of rosuvastatin should be limited to 5 mg once daily.

Concomitant lipid-lowering therapy: If rosuvastatin is used in combination with gemfibrozil, the dose of rosuvastatin should be limited to 10 mg once daily.

Dosage in patients with renal insufficiency: No modification of dosage is needed for patients with mild to moderate renal impairment. For patients with severe renal impairment (CrCL <30 mL/min/1.73 m^2) not on hemodialysis, rosuvastatin should be initiated at 5 mg once daily and not exceed 10 mg once daily.

Note: The manufacturer recommends that rosuvastatin therapy be temporarily withheld in any patient with an acute, serious condition suggestive of myopathy or predisposing to the development of renal failure secondary to rhabdomyolysis (eg, sepsis; hypotension; major surgery; trauma; severe metabolic, endocrine, or electrolyte disorder; or uncontrolled seizures).

OVERDOSE

Treatment is supportive. Rosuvastatin is not removed by hemodialysis.

PATIENT INFORMATION

Rosuvastatin may be taken with or without food. If an antacid containing aluminum or magnesium hydroxide is used concurrently, the antacid should be taken at least 2 h after rosuvastatin. Report promptly unexplained muscle pain, tenderness, or weakness, particularly if accompanied by malaise or fever.

AVAILABILITY

Tablets—5 mg, 10 mg, 20 mg, 40 mg

SIMVASTATIN (Zocor®)

Simvastatin was the third HMG-CoA reductase inhibitor available for use in the United States, receiving approval from the FDA in 1991 immediately after pravastatin. Simvastatin, like lovastatin, is derived from the fungus *Aspergillus terreus* and is itself inactive, requiring in vivo hydrolysis to the active beta-hydroxyacid form for clinical effect. Lovastatin and simvastatin differ chemically by only a single methyl group.

Simvastatin has shown efficacy at reducing LDL cholesterol concentrations in patients with homozygous familial hypercholesterolemia, in which LDL receptor activity is absent or severely diminished. The Multicenter Anti-Atheroma Study showed simvastatin 20 mg daily to slow the progression of atherosclerosis, reduce the proportion of patients with new atherosclerotic lesions, and promote the regression of atherosclerotic plaques in hypercholesterolemic patients with CHD. Simvastatin is effective in reducing total and LDL cholesterol as monotherapy and in combination with other lipid-lowering agents, such as niacin or ezetimibe. A combination product containing simvastatin and ezetimibe (Vytorin™) has recently been approved for marketing in the United States.

Data supporting the use of simvastatin for the treatment of patients with CHD originated from the Scandinavian Simvastatin Survival Study (4S). This trial utilized 20 to 40 mg daily of simvastatin to reduce the risk of mortality by 30%, hospital-verified nonfatal MI by 37%, and myocardial revascularization by 37% compared with placebo in patients with a mean baseline total cholesterol concentration of 261 mg/dL, a mean LDL concentration of 188 mg/dL, and a history of angina or acute MI. Simvastatin also reduced the risk of fatal plus nonfatal cerebrovascular events (strokes and transient ischemic attacks [TIAs]) by 28%.

The HDL-Atherosclerosis Treatment Study (HATS) demonstrated simvastatin plus niacin to cause regression of atherosclerotic arterial plaques in patients with CAD, low HDL, and normal LDL cholesterol concentrations.

The Heart Protection Study (HPS) demonstrated that 40 mg daily of simvastatin significantly ($P = 0.0003$) reduced the primary end point of overall mortality by 13% compared with placebo in 20,536 patients with coronary disease, other occlusive arterial disease, or diabetes. Fatal or nonfatal vascular events were also significantly reduced with simvastatin treatment. The benefits of simvastatin were present in various patient subgroups, including those without diagnosed coronary disease who had cerebrovascular disease, peripheral arterial disease, or diabetes, and those who presented with low LDL cholesterol concentrations (<116 mg/dL).

The ongoing Study of Heart and Renal Protection (SHARP) is comparing simvastatin (20 mg daily) + ezetimibe (10 mg daily) with placebo in about 9000 patients with chronic kidney disease (dialysis or predialysis) without a history of MI or coronary revascularization. The study will have a follow-up period of at least 4 years with the primary endpoint being time to a first major vascular event.

IN BRIEF

INDICATIONS

Reductions in risk of CHD mortality and cardiovascular events: In patients at high risk of coronary events, to reduce the risk of total mortality by reducing CHD deaths; to reduce the risk of nonfatal MI and stroke; to reduce the need for coronary and noncoronary revascularization procedures

To reduce elevated total cholesterol, LDL cholesterol, apo B, and triglycerides, and to increase HDL cholesterol in patients with primary hypercholesterolemia (heterozygous familial and nonfamilial) and mixed dyslipidemia (types IIa and IIb)

Treatment of hypertriglyceridemia (type IV hyperlipidemia)

Treatment of primary dysbetalipoproteinemia (type III hyperlipidemia)

To reduce total cholesterol and LDL cholesterol in patients with homozygous familial hypercholesterolemia as an adjunct to other lipid-lowering treatments (eg, LDL apheresis) or if such treatments are unavailable

As adjunctive therapy to diet for reduction of elevated total cholesterol, LDL cholesterol, and apo B levels in adolescent boys and girls who are at least 1 year post menarche, 10–17 years of age, with heterozygous familial hypercholesterolemia if, after an adequate trial of diet therapy, the following findings are present: 1) LDL cholesterol remains ≥190 mg/dL or 2) LDL cholesterol remains ≥160 mg/dL *and* a) there is a positive family history of premature cardiovascular disease or b) two or more other cardiovascular disease risk factors are present in the adolescent patient

CONTRAINDICATIONS

Acute liver disease or persistent elevations of serum transaminases
Pregnancy
Breast-feeding
Hypersensitivity to product components

DRUG INTERACTIONS

Cyclosporine[1,4]
FADs[4]
Niacin[4]
Macrolide antibiotics[1,4]
Nefazodone[1,4]
Azole antifungals[1,4]
Warfarin[3,5]
Digoxin[3,5]
CYP3A4 inhibitors (eg, amiodarone, amprenavir, diltiazem)[1]
Grapefruit juice (large quantities; ie, >1 qt/d)[1]
Verapamil[1]
Cholestyramine[2]

1 Effect/toxicity of simvastatin may increase.
2 A decrease in absorption of simvastatin may occur when it is taken within 1 h before or up to 2 h after cholestyramine.
3 Simvastatin may increase the effect/toxicity of this drug.
4 Concurrent use may increase the risk of myopathy and rhabdomyolysis.
5 The clinical significance of this interaction is unclear.

ADVERSE EFFECTS

CNS: headache (3.5%)
GI: dyspepsia (1%), diarrhea (0.5%–2%), nausea (1%), constipation (2.3%), flatulence (1%–2%), abdominal pain (3.2%)
Skin: rash (0.6%), eczema (0.8%), pruritus (0.5%)
Hepatic: serum transaminases >3 times upper limit of normal (≈1%)
Musculoskeletal: myalgia, muscle cramps, rhabdomyolysis (<1%)
Respiratory: upper respiratory infection (2.1%)
Special senses: cataract (0.5%)
Other: asthenia (1.6%)

SPECIAL GROUPS

Race: not evaluated

Children: safety and efficacy not established in children <10 years of age

Elderly: dosages ≤20 mg daily are usually sufficient for maximum LDL reduction

Renal impairment: no dosage adjustment is required for patients with mild to moderate renal insufficiency. Patients with severe renal insufficiency should be started at 5 mg daily and closely monitored

Hepatic impairment: use cautiously in patients who consume substantial quantities of alcohol and/or have a past history of liver disease; contraindicated in patients with active liver disease or unexplained persistent transaminase elevation

Pregnancy: category X; if the woman becomes pregnant while on simvastatin, the drug should be discontinued

Breast-feeding: contraindicated

DOSAGE

Adults: The usual initial dose is 20–40 mg once daily in the evening. For patients at high risk for a CHD event due to existing CHD, diabetes, peripheral vessel disease, or history of stroke or other cerebrovascular disease, the recommended initial dose is 40 mg/d. Dosage adjustments may be made at intervals of ≥4 wk. The dosage range is 5–80 mg/d.

Patients with homozygous familial hypercholesterolemia: The recommended dosage is 40 mg/d in the evening or 80 mg/d in 3 divided doses of 20 mg, 20 mg, and an evening dose of 40 mg. Simvastatin may be used as an adjunct to other lipid-lowering treatments (eg, LDL apheresis) in these patients or if such treatments are unavailable.

Adolescents (10–17 years of age) with heterozygous familial hypercholesterolemia: The recommended initial dose is 10 mg once daily in the evening. The recommended dosing range is 10–40 mg/d. Dosage adjustments may be made at intervals of ≥4 wk.

Concomitant lipid-lowering therapy: If simvastatin is used in combination with gemfibrozil, the dose of simvastatin should not exceed 10 mg/d.

Concomitant cyclosporine: In patients taking cyclosporine concomitantly with simvastatin, therapy should begin with 5 mg/d and should not exceed 10 mg/d.

Concomitant amiodarone or verapamil: In patients taking amiodarone or verapamil concomitantly with simvastatin, the dose should not exceed 20 mg/d.

Renal function impairment: Exercise caution when simvastatin is administered to patients with severe renal insufficiency. Initiate therapy in such patients with 5 mg/d and monitor closely.

PHARMACOKINETICS AND PHARMACODYNAMICS

Duration of action: 4–6 wk after discontinuation

Onset of action: within 2 wk

Peak effect: 4–6 wk

Bioavailability: <5% because of extensive hepatic extraction

Effect of food: none

Protein binding: ≈95%

Metabolism: extensive hepatic metabolism, in part by CYP3A4, to active metabolites, most notably the beta-hydroxyacid metabolite

Elimination: 13% of a dose is excreted in the urine; 60% in the feces (biliary excretion and unabsorbed drug)

Elimination half-life: 1.9 h

MONITORING

Plasma lipid profile, serum transaminases, signs and symptoms of muscle pain, tenderness, or weakness.

OVERDOSE

Treatment should be symptomatic and supportive.

PATIENT INFORMATION

Take in the evening for maximum benefit. If you miss a dose, take it as soon as you remember. If it is about time for the next dose, take that dose only. Do not take two doses at once. If blurred vision or muscle pain, tenderness, or weakness occurs, notify your clinician. Follow your prescribed diet. This medication should not be taken during pregnancy because of possible harm to the fetus. Notify your clinician as soon as possible if you become pregnant or intend to become pregnant while taking this medication.

AVAILABILITY

Tablets, film coated—5 mg, 10 mg, 20 mg, 40 mg, 80 mg
Combination formulations:
Vytorin—ezetimibe/simvastatin combination tablets
    10 mg/10 mg
    10 mg/20 mg
    10 mg/40 mg
    10 mg/80 mg

Adkins JC, Faulds D: Micronised fenofibrate. A review of its pharmacodynamic properties and clinical efficacy in the management of dyslipidaemia. *Drugs* 1997, 54:615–633.

Albert MA, Danielson E, Rifai N, *et al.*: Effect of statin therapy on C-reactive protein levels. The Pravastatin Inflammation/CRP Evaluation (PRINCE): a randomised trial and cohort study. *JAMA* 2001, 286:64–70.

ALLHAT Officers and Coordinators: Major outcomes in moderately hypercholesterolemic patients randomized to pravastatin versus usual care. *JAMA* 2002, 288:2998–3007.

Anonymous: Choice of lipid-lowering drugs. *Med Lett Drugs Ther* 1998, 40:117–122.

Anonymous: Fenofibrate for hypertriglyceridemia. *Med Lett Drugs Ther* 1998, 40:68–69.

Ascah KJ, Rock GA, Wells PS: Interaction between fenofibrate and warfarin. *Ann Pharmacother* 1998, 32:765–768.

Austin MA, Hokanson JE, Edwards KL: Hypertriglyceridemia as a cardiovascular risk factor. *Am J Cardiol* 1998, 81(Suppl.):7B–12B.

Aviram M, Hussein O, Rosenblat M, *et al.*: Interactions of platelets, macrophages, and lipoproteins in hypercholesterolemia: antiatherogenic effects of HMG-CoA reductase inhibitor therapy. *J Cardiovasc Pharmacol* 1998, 31:39–45.

Ballantyne CM, Blazing MA, King TR, *et al.*: Efficacy and safety of ezetimibe co-administered with simvastatin compared with atorvastatin in adults with hypercholesterolemia. *Am J Cardiol* 2004, 93:1487–1494.

Bays HE, Dujovne CA, McGovern ME, *et al.*: Comparison of once-daily niacin extended-release/lovastatin with standard doses of atorvastatin and simvastatin (The Advicor versus Other Cholesterol-Modulating Agents Trial Evaluation (ADVOCATE). *Am J Cardiol* 2003, 91:667–672.

Bellosta S, Paoletti R, Corsini A: Safety of statins. Focus on clinical pharmacokinetics and drug interactions. *Circulation* 2004, 109(Suppl III):III50–III57.

Betteridge DJ, Bhatnager D, Bing RF, *et al.*: Treatment of familial hypercholesterolaemia. United Kingdom lipid clinics study of pravastatin and cholestyramine. *Br Med J* 1992, 304:1335–1338.

Blankenhorn DH, Azen SP, Dramsch DM, *et al.*: Coronary angiographic changes with lovastatin therapy. The Monitored Atherosclerosis Regression Study (MARS). *Ann Intern Med* 1993, 119:969–976.

Blankenhorn DH, Nessim SA, Johnson RL, *et al.*: Beneficial effects of combined colestipol-niacin therapy on coronary atherosclerosis and coronary venous bypass grafts. *JAMA* 1987, 257:3233–3240.

Bradford RH, Shear CL, Chremos AN, *et al.*: Expanded Clinical Evaluation of Lovastatin (EXCEL) study results. I. Efficacy in modifying plasma lipoproteins and adverse event profile in 8245 patients with moderate hypercholesterolemia. *Arch Intern Med* 1991, 151:43–49.

Brensike JF, Levy RI, Kelsey SF, *et al.*: Effects of therapy with cholestyramine on progression of coronary arteriosclerosis: results of the NHLBI Type II Coronary Intervention Study. *Circulation* 1984, 69:313–324.

Brown AS, Bakker-Arkema RG, Yellen L, *et al.*: Treating patients with documented atherosclerosis to National Cholesterol Education Program–recommended low-density-lipoprotein cholesterol goals with atorvastatin, fluvastatin, lovastatin, and simvastatin. *J Am Coll Cardiol* 1998, 32:665–673.

Brown BG, Zhao X-Q, Chait A, *et al.*: Simvastatin and niacin, antioxidant vitamins, or the combination for the prevention of coronary disease. *N Engl J Med* 2001, 345:1583–1592.

Brown G, Albers JJ, Fisher LD, *et al.*: Regression of coronary artery disease as a result of intensive lipid-lowering therapy in men with high levels of apolipoprotein B. *N Engl J Med* 1990, 323:1289–1298.

Brown WV: Niacin for lipid disorders. Indications, effectiveness, and safety. *Postgrad Med* 1995, 98:185–193.

Bucher HC, Griffith LE, Guyatt GH: Effect of HMG-CoA reductase inhibitors on stroke. A meta-analysis of randomized, controlled trials. *Arch Intern Med* 1998, 128:89–95.

Byington RP, Furberg CD, Crouse JR III, *et al.*: Pravastatin, Lipids, and Atherosclerosis in the Carotid Arteries (PLAC-II). *Am J Cardiol* 1995, 76(Suppl C):54C–59C.

Canner PI, Berge KG, Wenger NK, *et al.*: Fifteen year mortality in Coronary Drug Project patients: long-term benefit with niacin. *J Am Coll Cardiol* 1986, 8:1245–1255.

Cannon CP, Braunwald E, McCabe CH, *et al.*: Comparison of intensive and moderate lipid lowering with statins following acute coronary syndrome. *N Engl J Med* 2004, 350:1495–1504.

Carlson LA, Hamsten A, Asplund A: Pronounced lowering of serum levels of lipoprotein Lp(a) in hyperlipidaemic subjects treated with nicotinic acid. *J Intern Med* 1989, 226:271–276.

Carlson LA, Rosenhamer G: Reduction of mortality in the Stockholm Ischaemic Heart Disease Secondary Prevention Study by combined treatment with clofibrate and nicotinic acid. *Acta Med Scand* 1988, 223:405–418.

Cashin-Hemphill L, Mack WJ, Pogoda JM, *et al.*: Beneficial effects of colestipol-niacin on coronary atherosclerosis: a 4-year follow-up. *JAMA* 1990, 264:3013–3017.

Castelli WP, Garrison RJ, Wilson PWF, *et al.*: Incidence of coronary heart disease and lipoprotein cholesterol levels. *JAMA* 1986, 256:2835–2838.

Cheng-Lai A: Rosuvastatin: a new HMG-CoA reductase inhibitor for the treatment of hypercholesterolemia. *Heart Dis* 2003, 5:72–78.

Chien PC, Frishman WH: Lipid disorders. In *Current Diagnosis and Treatment in Cardiology* edn 2. Edited by Crawford MH. New York: McGraw Hill; 2002:15–30.

Chin NX, Weitzman I, Della-Latta P: In vitro activity of flu-vastatin, a cholesterol-lowering agent, and synergy with fluconazole and itraconazole against *Candida* species and *Cryptococcus neoformans*. *Antimicrob Agents Chemother* 1997, 41:850–852.

Collaborative Atorvastatin Diabetes Study (CARDS) Executive Committee. Presented at the 64th Scientific Sessions of the American Diabetes Association. Orlando, FL. June 6, 2004.

Committee of Principal Investigators: A co-operative trial in the primary prevention of ischaemic heart disease using clofibrate. *Br Heart J* 1978, 40:1069–1118.

Committee of Principal Investigators: WHO cooperative trial on primary prevention of ischaemic heart disease with clofibrate to lower serum cholesterol: final mortality fol-low-up. *Lancet* 1984, 2:600–604.

Consensus Development Conference: Treatment of hyper-triglyceridemia. *JAMA* 1984, 251:1196–1200.

Coronary Drug Project Research Group: Clofibrate and niacin in coronary heart disease. *JAMA* 1975, 231:360–381.

Corvol JC, Bouzamondo A, Sirol M, *et al.*: Differential effects of lipid-lowering therapies on stroke prevention. A meta-analysis of randomized trials. *Arch Intern Med* 2003, 163:669–676.

Crouse JR III, Lukacsko P, Niecestro R, and the Lovastatin Extended-Release Study Group: Dose response, safety and efficacy of an extended-release formulation of lovastatin in adults with hyper-cholesterolemia. *Am J Cardiol* 2002, 89:226–229.

Curran MP, Goa KL: Lovastatin extended release; a review of its use in the management of hyper-cholesterolemia. *Drugs* 2003, 63:685–699.

Dart A, Jerums G, Nicholson G, *et al.*: A multicenter, double-blind, one-year study comparing safety and efficacy of atorvastatin versus simvastatin in patients with hypercho-lesterolemia. *Am J Cardiol* 1997, 80:39–44.

Davignon J: Beneficial cardiovascular pleiotropic effects of statins. *Circulation* 2004, 109(Suppl III):III39–III43.

Diabetes Atherosclerosis Intervention Study (DAIS) Investigators: Effect of fenofibrate on progression of coro-nary artery disease in type 2 diabetes. *Lancet* 2001, 357:905–910.

Downs JR, Clearfield M, Weis S, *et al.*: Primary prevention of acute coronary events with lovastatin in men and women with average cholesterol levels. Results of AFCAPS/TexCAPS. *JAMA* 1998, 279:1615–1622.

Ellen RLB, McPherson R: Long-term efficacy and safety of fenofibrate and a statin in the treatment of combined hyperlipidemia. *Am J Cardiol* 1998, 81(Suppl 4A):60B–65B.

Ellis JJ, Erickson SR, Stevenson JG, *et al.*: Suboptimal statin adherence and discontinuation in primary and secondary prevention populations. *J Gen Intern Med* 2004, 19:638–645.

Ezetimibe/simvastatin combination reduces LDL cholesterol. *Formulary* 2004, 39:199–200.

Farmer JA: Economic implications of lipid-lowering trials: current considerations in selecting a statin. *Am J Cardiol* 1998, 82(Suppl):26M–31M.

Feldman T, Koren M, Insull W Jr., *et al.*: Treatment of high-risk patients with ezetimibe plus simvastatin co-adminis-tration versus simvastatin alone to attain National Cholesterol Education Program Adult Treatment Panel III low-density lipoprotein cholesterol goals. *Am J Cardiol* 2004; 93:1481–1486.

Figge HL, Figge J, Sonney PF, *et al.*: Nicotinic acid: a review of its clinical use in the treatment of lipid disor-ders. *Pharmacotherapy* 1988, 8:287–294.

Fonarow GC, Watson KE: High-density lipoprotein choles-terol as a therapeutic target to reduce cardiovascular events (editorial). *Am Heart J* 2004, 147:939–941.

Frick MH, Elo O, Haapa K, *et al.*: Helsinki Heart Study: pri-mary prevention trial with gemfibrozil in middle-aged men with dyslipidemia. *N Engl J Med* 1987, 317:1237–1245.

Frick MH, Heinonen OP, Huttunen JK, *et al.*: Efficacy of gemfibrozil in dyslipidaemic subjects with suspected heart disease. An ancillary study in the Helsinki Heart Study frame population. *Ann Med* 1993, 25:41–45.

Frick MH, Syvänne M, Nieminen MS, *et al.*: Prevention of the angiographic progression of coronary and vein-graft atherosclerosis by gemfibrozil after coronary bypass sur-gery in men with low levels of HDL cholesterol. *Circulation* 1997, 96:2137–2143.

Frishman WH, ed: *Medical Management of Lipid Disorders*. New York: Futura Publishing Co.; 1992.

Frishman WH, Choi AY, Guh A: Innovative medical approaches for the treatment of hyperlipidemia. In *Cardiovascular Pharmacotherapeutics*, edn 2. Edited by Frishman WH, Sonnenblick EH, Sica DA. New York: McGraw Hill; 2003:841–853.

Frishman WH, Rapier RC: Lovastatin: an HMG-CoA reduc-tase inhibitor for lowering cholesterol. *Med Clinics N Amer* 1989, 73:437–448.

Frishman WH, Sinatra ST, Kruger N: Nutriceuticals and cardiovascular disease. In *Complementary and Integrative Therapies for Cardiovascular Disease.* Edited by Frishman WH, Weintraub MI, Micozzi M. St. Louis: Elsevier; 2004, in press.

Frishman WH, Zuckerman AL: An amlodipine-atorvastatin combination: the first cross-risk factor polypill for the prevention and treatment of cardiovascular disease. *Exp Rev Cardiovasc Ther* 2004, in press.

Furberg CD, Pitt B, Byington RP, *et al.*: Reduction in coronary events during treatment with pravastatin. *Am J Cardiol* 1995, 76(Suppl C):60C–63C.

Gagne C, Bays HE, Weiss SR, *et al.*: Efficacy and safety of ezetimibe added to ongoing statin therapy for treatment of patients with primary hypercholesterolemia. *Am J Cardiol* 2002, 90:1084–1091.

Goldberg AC, Sapre A, Capece R, *et al.*: Efficacy and safety of ezetimibe coadministered with simvastatin in patients with primary hypercholesterolemia: a randomized, double-blind, placebo-controlled trial. *Mayo Clin Proc* 2004, 79:620–629.

Gotto AM, Farmer JA: Dyslipoproteinemias/atherosclerosis: pharmacologic therapy. In *Cardiovascular Therapeutics. A Companion to Braunwald's Heart Disease*, edn 2. Edited by Antman EM. Philadelphia: WB Saunders; 2001:567–588.

Gould AL, Rossouw JE, Santanello NC, *et al.*: Cholesterol reduction yields clinical benefit: impact of statin trials. *Circulation* 1998, 97:946–952.

Grundy SM, Cleeman JI, Bairey Merz CN, *et al.*: Implication of recent clinical trials for the National Cholesterol Education Program Adult Treatment Panel III guidelines. *Circulation* 2004, 110:227–239.

Grundy SM, Vega GL: Fibric acids: effects on lipids and lipoprotein metabolism. *Am J Med* 1987, 83(Suppl 5B):9–20.

Grundy SM, Vega GL, McGovern ME, *et al.*: Efficacy, safety and tolerability of once-daily niacin for the treatment of dyslipidemias associated with type 2 diabetes. Results of the Assessment of Diabetes Control and Evaluation of the Efficacy of Niaspan Trial. *Arch Intern Med* 2002, 162:1568–1576.

Gupta EK, Ito MK: Ezetimibe: the first in a novel class of selective cholesterol-absorption inhibitors. *Heart Dis* 2002, 4:399–409.

Gupta EK, Ito MK: Lovastatin and extended-release niacin combination product. The first drug combination for the treatment of hyperlipidemia. *Heart Dis* 2002, 4:124–137.

Guyton JR, Goldberg AC, Kreisberg RA, *et al.*: Effectiveness of once-nightly dosing of extended-release niacin alone and in combination for hypercholesterolemia. *Am J Cardiol* 1998, 82:737–743.

Halcox JPJ, Deanfield JE: Beyond the laboratory. Clinical implications for statin pleiotropy. *Circulation* 2004, 109(Suppl II):II42–II48.

Heart Protection Study Collaboration Group. MRC/BHF Heart Protection Study of cholesterol lowering with simvastatin in 20,536 high-risk individuals: a randomised placebo-controlled trial. *Lancet* 2002, 360:7–22.

Henderson RP, Solomon CP: Use of cholestyramine in the treatment of digoxin intoxication. *Arch Intern Med* 1988, 148:745–746.

Herd JA, Ballantyne CM, Farmer JA: Effects of fluvastatin on coronary atherosclerosis in patients with mild to moderate cholesterol elevations (Lipoprotein and Coronary Atherosclerosis Study [LCAS]). *Am J Cardiol* 1997, 80:278–286.

Hjermann I, Holme I, Velve Byre K, Leren P: Effect of diet and smoking intervention on the incidence of coronary heart disease. Report from the Oslo Study Group of a randomised trial in healthy men. *Lancet* 1981, ii:1303–1310.

Holme I: An analysis of randomized trials evaluating the effects of cholesterol reduction on total mortality and CHD incidence. *Circulation* 1990, 82:1916–1924.

Hunninghake D, Bakker-Arkema RG, Wigand JP, *et al.*: Treating to meet NCEP-recommended LDL cholesterol concentrations with atorvastatin, fluvastatin, lovastatin, or simvastatin in patients with risk factors for coronary heart disease. *J Fam Pract* 1998, 47:349–356.

Hunninghake DB, Peters JB: Effect of fibric acid derivatives on blood lipid and lipoprotein levels. *Am J Med* 1987, 83(Suppl 5B):44–49.

Illingworth DR, Rapp JH, Phillipson BE, Connor WE: Colestipol plus nicotinic acid in treatment of heterozygous familial hypercholesterolemia. *Lancet* 1981, 1:296–298.

Jacotot B, Benghozi R, Pfister P, Holmes D: Comparison of fluvastatin versus pravastatin treatment of primary hypercholesterolemia. *Am J Cardiol* 1995, 76(Suppl):54A–56A.

Jamal SM, Eisenberg MJ, Christopoulos S: Rhabdomyolysis associated with hydroxymethylglutaryl coenzyme A reductase inhibitors. *Am Heart J* 2004, 147:956–965.

Jen SL, Chen JW, Lee WL, Wang SP: Efficacy and safety of fenofibrate or gemfibrozil on serum lipid profiles in Chinese patients with type IIb hyperlipidemia: a single-blind, randomized, and cross-over study. *Chin Med J* 1997, 59:217–224.

Jeppesen J, Hein HO, Suadicani P, Gyntelberg F: Triglyceride concentration and ischemic heart disease. An eight-year follow-up in the Copenhagen Male Study. *Circulation* 1998, 97:1029–1036.

Jones PH, Davidson MH, Stein EA, *et al.*, for the STELLAR Study Group: Comparison of the efficacy and safety of rosuvastatin versus atorvastatin, simvastatin and pravastatin across doses trial. *Am J Cardiol* 2003, 93:152–160.

The information here is provided as guidance only. Prescribers should always consult the manufacturer's current prescribing information.

311

Jukema JW, Bruschke AVG, van Boven AJ, *et al.*: Effects of lipid lowering by pravastatin on progression and regression of coronary artery disease in symptomatic men with normal to moderately elevated serum cholesterol levels. The Regression Growth Evaluation Statin Study (REGRESS). *Circulation* 1995, 91:2528–2540.

Kane JP, Malloy MJ, Ports TA, Phillips NR, *et al.*: Regression of coronary atherosclerosis during treatment of familial hypercholesterolemia with combined drug regimens. *JAMA* 1990, 264:3007–3012.

Kane JP, Malloy MJ, Tun P, *et al.*: Normalization of low-density-lipoprotein levels in heterozygous familial hypercholesterolemia with a combined drug regimen. *N Engl J Med* 1981, 304:251–258.

Kidney Disease Outcomes Quality Initiative Clinical Practice Guidelines for Managing Dyslpidemias in Chronic Kidney Disease: II, Assessment of dyslipidemia. *Am J Kidney Dis* 2003, 41(Suppl 3):S22.

Knopp RH, Alagona P, Davidson M, *et al.*: Equivalent efficacy of a time-release form of niacin (Niaspan) given once-a-night versus plain niacin in the management of hyperlipidemia. *Metabolism* 1998, 47:1097–1104.

Kong SX, Crawford SY, Gandhi SK, *et al.*: Efficacy of 3-hydroxy-3-methylglutaryl coenzyme A reductase inhibitors in the treatment of patients with hypercholesterolemia: a meta-analysis of clinical trials. *Clin Ther* 1997, 19:778–797.

Kuo PT, Kostis JB, Moreyra AE, Hayes JA: Familial type II hyperlipoproteinemia with coronary heart disease. Effect of diet-colestipol-nicotinic acid treatment. *Chest* 1981, 79:286–291.

LaRosa J: Review of clinical studies of bile acid sequestrants for lowering plasma lipid levels. *Cardiology* 1989, 76(Suppl 1):55–64.

Lea AP, McTavish D: Atorvastatin. A review of its pharmacology and therapeutic potential in the management of hyperlipidaemias. *Drugs* 1997, 53:828–847.

Libby P, Aikawa M: Mechanisms of plaque stabilization with statins. *Am J Cardiol* 2003, 91(4A):4B.

Lipid Research Clinics Program: The Lipid Research Clinics Coronary Primary Prevention Trial results. I. Reduction in incidence of coronary heart disease. *JAMA* 1984, 251:351–364.

Lipid Research Clinics Program: The Lipid Research Clinics Coronary Primary Prevention Trial results. II. The relationship of reduction in incidence of coronary heart disease to cholesterol lowering. *JAMA* 1984, 251:365–374.

Lipid Research Clinics Investigators: The Lipid Research Clinics Coronary Primary Prevention Trial. Results of 6 years of post-trial follow-up. *Arch Intern Med* 1992, 152:1399–1410.

Long-Term Intervention with Pravastatin in Ischaemic Disease (LIPID) Study Group: Prevention of cardiovascular events and death with pravastatin in patients with coronary heart disease and a broad range of initial cholesterol levels. *N Engl J Med* 1998, 339:1349–1357.

MAAS Investigators: Effect of simvastatin on coronary atheroma: the Multicentre Anti-Atheroma Study (MAAS). *Lancet* 1994, 334:633–638.

Mach F: Statins as immunomodulatory agents. *Circulation* 2004, 109(Suppl II):II15–II17.

Malloy MJ, Kane JP, Kunitake ST, *et al.*: Complementarity of colestipol, niacin, and lovastatin in treatment of severe familial hypercholesterolemia. *Ann Intern Med* 1987, 107:616–623.

Mason RP, Walter MF, Jacob RF: Effects of HMG-CoA reductase inhibitors on endothelial function. Role of microdomains and oxidative stress. *Circulation* 2004, 109(Suppl II):II34–II41.

McFarlane SI, Muniyappa R, Francisco R, Sowers JR. Pleiotropic effects of statins: lipid reduction and beyond. *J Clin Endocrinol Metab* 2002, 87:1451–1458.

McKenney J: New perspectives on the use of niacin in the treatment of lipid disorders. *Arch Intern Med* 2004, 164:697–705.

National Cholesterol Education Program (NCEP) Expert Panel on Detection, Evaluation, and Treatment of High Blood Cholesterol in Adults (Adult Treatment Panel III): Third report of the National Cholesterol Education Program (NCEP) Expert Panel on Detection, Evaluation, and Treatment of High Blood Cholesterol in Adults (Adult Treatment Panel III): final report. *Circulation* 2002, 106:3143–3421.

Nissen SE, Tuzcu EM, Schoenhagen P, *et al.*: Effect of intensive compared with moderate lipid-lowering therapy on progression of coronary atherosclerosis: a randomized controlled trial. *JAMA* 2004, 291:1071–1080.

Otto CM: Aortic stenosis and hyperlipidemia: establishing a cause-effect relationship [editorial]. *Am Heart J* 2004, 147:761–763.

Payne VW, Secter RA, Noback RK: Use of colestipol in a patient with digoxin intoxication. *Drug Intell Clin Pharm* 1981, 15:902–903.

Pearson TA: EASE (Ezetimibe add-on-to-statin for effectiveness trial. Presented at the 53rd Annual Scientific Sessions of the American College of Cardiology. New Orleans, LA; 2004.

Pitt B, Mancini GBJ, Ellis SG, *et al.*: Pravastatin limitation of atherosclerosis in the coronary arteries (PLAC I): reduction in atherosclerosis progression and clinical events. *J Am Coll Cardiol* 1995, 26:1133–1139.

Pitt B, Waters D, Brown WV, *et al.*: Aggressive lipid-lowering therapy compared with angioplasty in stable coronary artery disease. *N Engl J Med* 1999, 341:70–76.

PPP Project Investigators: Design, rationale, and baseline characteristics of the Prospective Pravastatin Pooling (PPP) Project: a combined analysis of three large-scale randomized trials: Long-term Intervention with Pravastatin in Ischemic Disease (LIPID), Cholesterol and Recurrent Events (CARE), and West of Scotland Coronary Prevention Study (WOSCOPS). *Am J Cardiol* 1995, 76:899–905.

Prevention of cardiovascular events and death with pravastatin in patients with coronary heart disease and a broad range of initial cholesterol levels: the Long-term Intervention with Pravastatin in Ischaemic Disease (LIPID) Study Group. *N Engl J Med* 1998, 339:1349–1357.

Probstfield JL, Margitic SE, Byington RP, *et al.*: Results of the primary outcome measure and clinical events from the asymptomatic carotid artery progression study. *Am J Cardiol* 1995, 76(Suppl.):47C–53C.

Report from the Committee of Principal Investigators: A cooperative trial in the primary prevention of ischaemic heart disease using clofibrate. *Br Heart J* 1978, 40:1069–1118.

Rubins HB, Robins SJ, Collins D, *et al.*: Gemfibrozil for the secondary prevention of coronary heart disease in men with low levels of high-density lipoprotein cholesterol. *N Engl J Med* 1999, 341:410–418.

Sacks FM, Pfeffer MA, Moye LA, *et al.*: The effect of pravastatin on coronary events after myocardial infarction in patients with average cholesterol levels. *N Engl J Med* 1996, 335:1001–1009.

Salonen R, Nyyssönen K, Porkkala E, *et al.*: Kuopio Atherosclerosis Prevention Study (KAPS). *Circulation* 1995, 92:1758–1764.

Scandinavian Simvastatin Survival Study Group: Randomised trial of cholesterol lowering in 4444 patients with coronary heart disease: the Scandinavian Simvastatin Survival Study (4S). *Lancet* 1994, 344:1383–1389.

Schneck DW, Birmingham BK, Zalikowski JA, *et al.*: The effect of gemfibrozil on the pharmacokinetics of rosuvastatin. *Clin Pharmacol Ther* 2004, 75:455–463.

Schönbeck U, Libby P: Inflammation, immunity, and HMG-CoA reductase inhibitors. Statins as anti-inflammatory agents? *Circulation* 2004, 109(Suppl II):II18–II26.

Schwartz GG, Oliver MF, Ezekowitz MD, *et al.*: Rationale and design of the myocardial ischemia reduction with aggressive cholesterol lowering (MIRACL) study that evaluates atorvastatin in unstable angina pectoris and in non–Q-wave acute myocardial infarction. *Am J Cardiol* 1998, 81:578–581.

Serruys PWJC, deFeyter P, Macaya C, *et al.*, for the Lescol Intervention Prevention Study (LIPS) Investigators: Fluvastatin for prevention of cardiac events following successful first percutaneous coronary intervention. A randomized controlled trial. *JAMA* 2002, 287:3215–3222.

Sever PS, Dahlof B, Poulter NR, *et al.*: Prevention of coronary and stroke events with atorvastatin in hypertensive patients who have average or lower than average cholesterol concentrations, in the Anglo-Scandinavian Cardiac Outcomes Trial-Lipid Lowering Arm (ASCOT-LLA): a multicentre randomised controlled trial. *Lancet* 2003, 361:1149–1158.

Shachter NS, Frishman WH: Lipid-lowering drugs. In *Cardiovascular Pharmacotherapeutics Manual,* edn 2. Edited by Frishman WH, Sonnenblick EH, Sica DA. New York: McGraw Hill; 2004:328–376.

Shachter NS, Zimetbaum P, Frishman WH: Lipid-lowering drugs. In *Cardiovascular Pharmacotherapeutics*, edn 2. Edited by Frishman WH, Sonnenblick EH, Sica DA. New York: McGraw Hill; 2003:317–353.

Shepherd J, Blauw GJ, Murphy MB, *et al.*: Pravastatin in elderly individuals at risk for vascular disease (PROSPER): a randomised controlled trial. PROspective Study of Pravastatin in the Elderly at Risk. *Lancet* 2002, 360:1623–1630.

Shepherd J, Cobbe SM, Ford I, *et al.*: Prevention of coronary heart disease with pravastatin in men with hypercholesterolemia. *N Engl J Med* 1995, 333:1301–1307.

Simon A, Drewe E, van der Meer JWM, *et al.*: Simvastatin treatment for inflammatory attacks of the hyper-immunoglobulinemia D and periodic fever syndrome. *Clin Pharmacol Ther* 2004, 75:476–483.

Slater EE, MacDonald JS: Mechanism of action and biological profile of HMG-CoA reductase inhibitors. A new therapeutic alternative. *Drugs* 1988, 36:72–82.

Stein EA, Lane M, Laskarzewski P: Comparison of statins in hypertriglyceridemia. *Am J Cardiol* 1998, 81(Suppl 4A):66B–69B.

The Long-Term Intervention with Pravastatin in Ischaemic Disease (LIPID) Study Group: Prevention of cardiovascular events and death with pravastatin in patients with coronary heart disease and a broad range of initial cholesterol levels. *N Engl J Med* 1998, 339:1349–1357.

Todd PA, Ward A: Gemfibrozil: a review of its pharmacodynamic and pharmacokinetic properties and therapeutic use in dyslipidaemia. *Drugs* 1988, 36:314–339.

Vega GL, Grundy SM: Mechanisms of primary hypercholesterolemia in humans. *Am Heart J* 1987, 112:493–502.

Wadham C, Albanese N, Roberts J, *et al.*: High-density lipoproteins neutralize C-reactive protein proinflammatory activity. *Circulation* 2004, 109:2116–2122.

Waehre T, Yndestad A, Smith C, *et al.*: Increased expression of interleukin-1 in coronary artery disease with downregulatory effects of HMG-CoA reductase inhibitors. *Circulation* 2004, 109:1966–1972.

Walker JF: HMG-CoA reductase inhibitors: current clinical experience. *Drugs* 1988, 36(Suppl 3):83–86.

Warshafsky S, Packard D, Marks SJ, *et al.*: Efficacy of the HMG-CoA reductase inhibitors for prevention of fatal and nonfatal stroke: a meta-analysis. *J Gen Intern Med* 1999, 14:763–774.

Waters D, Higginson L, Gladstone P, *et al.*: Effects of monotherapy with an HMG-CoA reductase inhibitor on the progression of coronary atherosclerosis as assessed by serial quantitative arteriography. The Canadian Coronary Atherosclerosis Intervention Trial. *Circulation* 1994, 89:959–968.

Watts GF, Lewis B, Brunt JNH, *et al.*: Effects on coronary artery disease of lipid-lowering diet, or diet plus cholestyramine, in the St Thomas' Atherosclerosis Regression Study (STARS). *Lancet* 1992, 339:563–569.

Wiegman A, Hutten BA, de Groot E, *et al.*: Efficacy and saftey of statin therapy in children with familial hypercholesterolemia. A randomized controlled trial. *JAMA* 2004, 292:331–337.

Wild SH, Fortmann SP, Marcovina SM: A prospective case-control study of lipoprotein (a) levels and Apo (a) size and risk of coronary heart disease in Stanford Five-city Project participants. *Arterioscler Thromb Vasc Biol* 1997, 17:239–245.

Willerson JT, Ridker PM: Inflammation as a cardiovascular risk factor. *Circulation* 2004, 109(Suppl II):II2–I10.

Wilt TJ, Bloomfield HE, MacDonald R, *et al.*: Effectiveness of statin therapy in adults with coronary heart disease. *Arch Intern Med* 2004, 164:1427–1436.

Wolfe SM: Dangers of rosuvastatin identified before and after FDA approval [correspondence]. *Lancet* 2004, 363:2189–2190.

Wong NN: Colesevelam: a new bile acid sequestrant. *Heart Dis* 2001, 3:63–70.

XIII International Symposium on Drugs Affecting Lipid Metabolism, Florence, Italy, June 2, 1998.

Zimetbaum P, Frishman WH, Ooi WL, *et al.*: Plasma lipids and lipoproteins and the incidence of cardiovascular disease in the old: The Bronx Longitudinal Aging Study. *Arteriol Thromb* 1992, 12:416–423.

12

NEURONAL AND GANGLIONIC BLOCKERS

Some of the earliest antihypertensive treatments involved the use of neuronal and ganglionic blockers, but they proved to have numerous unpleasant side effects. As a result, these blockers are now used as third- or fourth-line agents in the management of severe hypertension when the combination of better-tolerated agents has failed to achieve adequate blood pressure (BP) control. **Trimethaphan** has been used for the reduction of BP during surgery and the treatment of hypertensive emergencies. However, this drug was discontinued by the manufacturer in the United States.

EFFICACY AND USE

Guanethidine is an adrenergic neural blocking drug that is effective for the treatment of high BP, but it is rarely used today. Because of its ability to reduce BP by decreasing the degree of vasoconstriction that accompanies increased sympathetic activity on moving to an upright posture, it tends to cause orthostatic hypotension. Because prolonged standing, excessive heat, alcohol, or exercise may increase the risk for orthostatic hypotension, its use is now restricted. **Guanadrel**, structurally and pharmacologically similar to **guanethidine**, inhibits sympathetic vasoconstriction by inhibiting norepinephrine release from neuronal storage sites in response to nerve stimulation. Depletion of norepinephrine causes a relaxation of vascular smooth muscle, which decreases total peripheral resistance and venous return. Thus, **guanadrel** is effective in reducing BP, and it is indicated for the treatment of hypertension in patients not responding adequately to a thiazide-type diuretic.

Mecamylamine is a potent oral ganglionic blocker. Although its antihypertensive effect is predominantly orthostatic, supine blood pressure is also significantly reduced. **Mecamylamine** is indicated for the management of moderately severe to severe essential hypertension as well as uncomplicated malignant hypertension. **Reserpine**, a rau-wolfia alkaloid, is one of the oldest drugs used to treat hypertension, and has been available for almost 50 years. Recently, it was shown to be effective in relatively low dosages as an adjunct therapy in older patients with isolated systolic hypertension. It is commonly used as a second- or third-line agent to treat refractory mild-to-moderate hypertension. It is fairly well tolerated, especially when used in low doses and concomitantly with a diuretic agent. Its use is limited primarily by its side effect profile; depression and other central nervous system (CNS) effects in particular may be a significant problem.

Although systemic vascular resistance is depressed in patients undergoing treatment with ganglionic blockers, the response of individual organ beds is variable. Splanchnic and cerebral blood flow may be reduced slightly, whereas the blood flow in skin may increase. Attempting to exploit these differential effects, **reserpine** has been used with mixed success in the treatment of Raynaud's phenomenon and migraine headaches. The renal effects of ganglionic blockade are of particular importance because of the association of severe hypertension with renal disease. In normotensive and some hypertensive subjects, ganglionic blockade may lead to a fall in glomerular filtration rate (GFR) and renal blood flow (RBF) and an increase in renal vascular resistance (RVR). These effects occur acutely but may also persist. In some hypertensive patients, RBF is unchanged or may increase, whereas RVR is reduced. Apart from the peripheral effects of ganglionic blockers (Table 12.1), those that penetrate the CNS may produce prominent unwanted effects, such as mental confusion.

MODE OF ACTION

Guanethidine and **guanadrel** interfere with the release of norepinephrine from postganglionic adrenergic nerve endings. They are taken up and stored in the neuron via the

Site	Predominant tone	Effect of ganglionic blockade
Arterioles	Sympathetic (adrenergic)	Vasodilation; increased peripheral blood flow; hypotension
Veins	Sympathetic (adrenergic)	Dilation: peripheral pooling of blood; decreased venous return; decreased cardiac output
Heart	Parasympathetic (cholinergic)	Tachycardia
Iris	Parasympathetic (cholinergic)	Mydriasis
Ciliary muscle	Parasympathetic (cholinergic)	Cycloplegia
Gastrointestinal tract	Parasympathetic (cholinergic)	Reduced tone and motility; constipation; decreased gastric and pancreatic secretions
Urinary bladder	Parasympathetic (cholinergic)	Urinary retention
Salivary glands	Parasympathetic (cholinergic)	Xerostomia
Sweat glands	Sympathetic (cholinergic)	Anhidrosis
Genital tract	Sympathetic and parasympathetic	Decreased stimulation

TABLE 12.1 SITE OF ACTION AND PREDOMINANT NEURAL TONE WITH CONSEQUENT EFFECTS OF AUTONOMIC GANGLIONIC BLOCKADE

Adapted from Taylor P: Agents acting on the neuromuscular junction and autonomic ganglia. In *Goodman & Gilman's The Pharmacological Basis of Therapeutics*, edn 10. Edited by Hardman JG, Limbird LE. New York: McGraw Hill; 2001:211.

same mechanisms by which norepinephrine is handled. Reduced catecholamine release results in reduced arteriolar vasoconstriction and reduction in the reflex increase in sympathetic activity that accompanies a change in position. **Guanethidine** also causes depletion of norepinephrine from nerve endings and structural changes that are slow to reverse. **Guanethidine** has a long duration of action; its effects are observable for 1 to 3 weeks after discontinuation of treatment. Peak effect occurs within 8 hours after a single oral dose. However, full therapeutic effects are not observed until 1 to 3 weeks after initiation of therapy. By contrast, guanadrel has a rapid onset of action, reaching its peak effect in 4 to 6 hours.

Reserpine acts by depleting catecholamines and serotonin in the brain and in many other organs. It exerts its antihypertensive effect by reducing sympathetic peripheral vasoconstriction and by reducing cardiac output with chronic administration. Depletion of biogenic amines may be inhibited by the action of monoamine oxidase inhibitor

(MAOI) agents, which in turn would limit the effectiveness of **reserpine** to reduce BP. **Reserpine** has a long duration of action, and when taken chronically, exerts additive effects through progressive catecholamine depletion. This depletion has been implicated in the unwanted occurrence of mental depression and the deregulation of pituitary hormone synthesis and secretion, yielding increased serum prolactin levels. **Mecamylamine** is a very potent oral ganglionic blocker, its effect being predominantly orthostatic.

The ganglionic blockers produce widespread effects in the body (Table 12.1). Changes in cardiac rate following ganglionic blockade depend primarily on the concurrent vagal tone: mild tachycardia usually accompanies the fall in BP. In patients with normal cardiac function, ganglionic blockers often reduce cardiac output because venous dilatation diminishes venous return. In patients with congestive heart failure (CHF), ganglionic blockers frequently increase cardiac output because peripheral resistance is reduced, thus decreasing afterload.

INDICATIONS

	Guanadrel	Guanethidine	Mecamylamine	Reserpine
Unresponsive moderate to severe hypertension	+	+	+	+
Malignant hypertension			+	
Renal hypertension		+		
Psychosis				+

+ — FDA-approved indication.

GUANADREL (Hylorel®)

Guanadrel sulfate blocks the efferent peripheral sympathetic pathways selectively. It suppresses sympathetic vasoconstriction by inhibiting norepinephrine release from neuronal storage sites in response to stimulation of the nerve. Guanadrel also causes depletion of norepinephrine from the nerve ending, resulting in relaxation of vascular smooth muscle. This in turn decreases total peripheral vascular resistance and decreases venous return, both of which decrease the ability to maintain BP in the upright position.

Guanadrel reduces systolic BP more than diastolic BP. Because this agent can reduce or eliminate cardiovascular reflexes, greater reductions of BP are observed when patients are upright than when they are supine. Renal blood flow and glomerular filtration usually are unchanged when patients are in the supine position, but may be reduced by 30% to 40% when they are in the upright position.

Given the equal antihypertensive effectiveness of guanethidine and guanadrel, guanadrel's shorter duration of action may make it preferable to limit the duration of possible unwanted side effects. Postural and postexercise hypotension is common in patients receiving this drug. Heat-induced vasodilation may also increase the hypotensive effect of guanadrel. However, tolerance to the hypotensive effect of guanadrel may also result during prolonged therapy because of sodium and water retention induced by this agent. For this reason, the concurrent use of a diuretic with this agent is recommended.

SPECIAL GROUPS

Race: no differences in response
Children: not recommended; safety and effectiveness have not been established
Elderly: lower dosages are recommended; elderly are more susceptible to hypotensive effects of the drug
Renal impairment: may increase plasma half-life and diminish clearance; recommend dose reduction or use prolonged dosing intervals, especially with a creatinine clearance of <60 mL/min
Hepatic impairment: not known
Pregnancy: category B; no adequate and well-controlled studies in pregnant women have been performed
Breast-feeding: not recommended; may be excreted in breast milk

DOSAGE

Initially, give 5 mg twice daily. Adjust dosage weekly or monthly until BP is controlled.
Maintenance dose is usually 20–75 mg/d in two to four divided doses. For patients with creatinine clearance of 30–60 mL/min, initiate therapy with 5 mg every 24 h. For patients with creatinine clearance of <30 mL/min, increase dosage interval to 48 h. Dosage increments should be made cautiously at intervals ≥7 d for patients with moderate renal insufficiency and ≥14 d for patients with severe renal insufficiency.

NEURONAL AND GANGLIONIC BLOCKERS

IN BRIEF

INDICATIONS
Hypertension

CONTRAINDICATIONS
Hypersensitivity
Pheochromocytoma
Concurrent treatment or within 1 week of treatment with MAOIs
Frank CHF

DRUG INTERACTIONS
Beta-blockers[1]
Hypotension-producing medications[1]
MAOIs[2]
Phenothiazines[2]
Sympathomimetic agents[2,3]
Tricyclic antidepressants[2]
Vasodilators[1]

1 Effect/toxicity of guanadrel may increase.
2 Effect of guanadrel may decrease.
3 Guanadrel may increase the effect/toxicity of this drug.

ADVERSE EFFECTS
Cardiovascular: chest pain; orthostatic hypotension; peripheral edema
CNS: fatigue; headache; drowsiness
GI/GU: increased bowel movements; dry mouth; dry throat; nocturia; ejaculation disturbances
Respiratory: shortness of breath
Others: excessive weight gain/loss

PHARMACOKINETICS AND PHARMACODYNAMICS
Duration of action: 9 h (range, 4–14 h) after single dose
Onset of action: 2 h
Peak effect: 4–6 h
Bioavailability: rapidly and almost completely absorbed from the gastrointestinal tract
Effect of food: not known
Protein binding: ≈20%
Metabolism: hepatic
Elimination: 85% renal (≈40% as unchanged drug)
Plasma half-life: 10 h; increased in renal impairment

MONITORING
Because guanadrel may cause orthostatic hypotension, monitor both supine and standing pressures, especially during dosage adjustments. In addition to the contraindications listed above, use with extreme caution in patients with diabetes mellitus, regional vascular disease, asthma, recent myocardial infarction (MI), angina pectoris, history of peptic ulcer, sinus bradycardia, cerebrovascular insufficiency, diarrhea, fever, salt depletion, anemia, or Addison's disease.

OVERDOSE
Usually produces dizziness and blurred vision; patient should lie down until symptoms subside. Treatment should be supportive. Persistent, excessive hypotension may require intensive therapy to support vital functions. Vasoconstrictors will counteract guanadrel's effects; use with caution.

PATIENT INFORMATION
Postural hypotension is greatest in the morning and on standing up. Avoid getting up suddenly from a lying or sitting position. Hypotension may be heightened by fever, heat, exercise, prolonged standing, and alcohol use. Sit or lie down at the first sign of dizziness. Notify physician if persistent side effects occur. Consult physician before taking nonprescription remedies for colds, allergies, or asthma. Take medication as prescribed; do not discontinue therapy without physician's advice.

AVAILABILITY
Tablets—10 mg, 25 mg

GUANETHIDINE (Ismelin®)

Guanethidine is a postganglionic adrenergic-blocking agent that is structurally and pharmacologically related to guanadrel. Guanethidine acts by displacing norepinephrine from terminal vesicle storage sites and by inhibiting norepinephrine release and reuptake. Consequently, guanethidine exerts its antihypertensive effects by reducing peripheral sympathetic vasoconstriction. Although rarely used, it is indicated for the treatment of moderate to severe hypertension in addition to other, better-tolerated drugs when those, in combination, have failed to achieve adequate BP control. Absorption of guanethidine varies considerably among patients, necessitating individualization of dosage.

Because of its long duration of action, guanethidine may be taken on a once-daily regimen, which may be considered an advantage over guanadrel if patient compliance is a significant concern. Similar to guanadrel, guanethidine decreases systolic BP more than diastolic BP. Because guanethidine reduces or eliminates cardiovascular reflexes, further lowering of BP is observed when patients are upright than when they are supine.

Postural and postexercise hypotension is common in patients receiving guanethidine. Guanethidine is most effective in treating hypertension when used in conjunction with a diuretic to avoid tolerance from salt and fluid retention.

Other uses of guanethidine include effective treatment of refractory variant angina that has failed to be controlled by nitrates and calcium channel blockers. Guanethidine has also been used successfully to control hyperreflexic bladders in spinal cord trauma patients.

SPECIAL GROUPS

Race: no differences in response
Children: use with caution; safety and effectiveness have not been established
Elderly: may be more sensitive to hypotensive effect
Renal impairment: because decreased BP may further compromise renal function, use with extreme caution in hypertensive patients with renal dysfunction
Hepatic impairment: reduced metabolism and excessive accumulation of guanethidine may occur; lower doses or increased dosage interval may be required
Pregnancy: category C; safety for use during pregnancy has not been established
Breast-feeding: not recommended; guanethidine is excreted in breast milk

DOSAGE

Adult: Initially, give 10 or 12.5 mg/d orally; increase gradually according to response (10–12.5 mg increments at weekly intervals). Usual maintenance dose is 25–50 mg/d. Dosage may be increased more rapidly and with larger dosage increments under careful hospital supervision.
Elderly: Use lower dose.
Children: Initially, give 0.2 mg/kg body weight orally once a day. Daily dose may be increased by 0.2 mg/kg body weight at 7–10 d intervals, up to five to eight times the initial daily dose.

IN BRIEF

INDICATIONS
Moderate to severe hypertension
Renal hypertension

CONTRAINDICATIONS
Hypersensitivity
Pheochromocytoma
Concurrent or recent treatment with MAOIs
Frank CHF

DRUG INTERACTIONS
Anorexiants[2]
Haloperidol[2]
MAOIs[2]
Methylphenidate[2]
Minoxidil[1]
Phenothiazines[2]
Sympathomimetics[2,3]
Thioxanthenes[2]
Tricyclic antidepressants[2]

1 Effect/toxicity of guanethidine may increase.
2 Effect of guanethidine may decrease.
3 Guanethidine may increase the effect/toxicity of this drug.

ADVERSE EFFECTS
Cardiovascular: bradycardia; orthostatic hypotension; peripheral edema; angina
CNS: fatigue; weakness; syncope; headache; mental depression; blurred vision
GI/GU: nausea; vomiting; dry mouth; diarrhea; increase in bowel movements; inhibition of ejaculation
Respiratory: dyspnea; nasal congestion
Others: myalgia; weight gain; dermatitis; alopecia

PHARMACOKINETICS AND PHARMACODYNAMICS
Duration of action: 24–48 h (BP returns gradually to pretreatment levels within 1–3 wk after discontinuing therapy)
Onset of action: 0.5–2 h
Peak effect: within 8 h after single dose. The full effect may not be noticed until 1–3 wk after initiation of therapy.
Bioavailability: 3%–30% (varies tenfold)
Effect of food: not known
Protein binding: not known
Metabolism: partially metabolized by the liver to three metabolites that are less active than the parent drug
Elimination: 25%–60% of a dose excreted in urine as unchanged drug
Plasma half-life: 1.5 d (alpha), 4–8 d (beta)

MONITORING
Monitor BP and other vital signs. In addition to the contraindications listed above, use guanethidine with extreme caution in patients with cerebrovascular insufficiency, cardiac ischemia, and peptic ulcers.

OVERDOSE
Gastric lavage may be useful for very recent ingestion. Treatment should be symptomatic and supportive.

PATIENT INFORMATION
This medication may cause gastrointestinal side effects (particularly diarrhea), headache, blurred vision, fatigue, and dizziness. If severe, do not drive or operate machinery. Notify physician if persistent side effects occur. Consult physician before taking nonprescription remedies for colds, allergies, or asthma. Avoid alcohol use. Take medication as prescribed; do not discontinue therapy without physician's advice.

AVAILABILITY
Tablets—10 mg, 25 mg

MECAMYLAMINE

(Inversine®)

Mecamylamine is a very potent oral ganglionic blocker used in the treatment of moderately severe or severe hypertension and uncomplicated malignant hypertension. It is rarely used now except as additional therapy when better-tolerated agents have failed to achieve the desired level of BP control. Other uses for mecamylamine include the treatment of hyperreflexia in patients with spinal cord injuries and the promotion of smoking cessation. The latter effect occurs by mecamylamine inhibiting central nicotinic cholinergic receptors. Despite an initial increase in the number of cigarettes smoked, continued use of this medication may lead to conditioning that suppresses the nicotine craving. Adequate studies to exclude the contribution of a placebo effect must be performed to clarify this issue.

SPECIAL GROUPS

Race: no differences in response
Children: not recommended; safety and effectiveness have not been established
Elderly: may be more sensitive to hypotensive effect
Renal impairment: excretion may be reduced; reduce dose
Hepatic impairment: little, if any, impact on elimination; dose reduction unnecessary
Pregnancy: category C; not recommended; may decrease intestinal motility in fetus, resulting in meconium or paralytic ileus
Breast-feeding: not recommended; may be excreted in breast milk

DOSAGE

Initially, give 2.5 mg twice daily; increase in increments of 2.5 mg at intervals of at least every 2 d according to response. Smallest dose should be taken in the mornings to limit the orthostatic adverse effects of the drug. Maintenance dose is usually 25 mg/d in three divided doses.

Note: It is recommended that mecamylamine be administered at consistent times in relation to meals because hypotension may occur after a meal. Mecamylamine ingestion with meals may slow the drug's absorption and thereby produce desired gradual correction of severe hypertension. Discontinuation of mecamylamine in an abrupt manner may result in severe rebound hypertension, especially in patients being treated for malignant hypertension. Gradual withdrawal is recommended when mecamylamine therapy is discontinued, and the substitution of another antihypertensive therapy may be necessary.

IN BRIEF

INDICATIONS
Essential hypertension, moderately severe
Essential hypertension, severe
Malignant hypertension, uncomplicated

CONTRAINDICATIONS
Hypersensitivity
Recent MI
Recent cardiac ischemia
Recent cerebrovascular accident
Glaucoma
Organic pyloric stenosis
Uremia
Concurrent use of sulfonamides or antibiotics that cause neuromuscular blockade
Uncooperative patients

DRUG INTERACTIONS
Alcohol[1]
Anesthetic agents[1]
Antibiotics that cause neuromuscular blockade[1]
Bethanechol[1]
Drugs that increase urinary pH (eg, sodium bicarbonate, acetazolamide)[1]
Hypotensive agents[1]
Sulfonamides[1]

[1] Effect/toxicity of mecamylamine may increase.

ADVERSE EFFECTS
Cardiovascular: orthostatic hypotension; syncope
CNS: fatigue; weakness; blurred vision; paresthesia; tremor; choreiform movements; mental changes (confusion, excitement, depression); convulsions
GI/GU: anorexia; dry mouth; nausea; vomiting; constipation; ileus; impotence; urinary retention
Respiratory: nasal congestion; interstitial pulmonary edema; fibrosis

PHARMACOKINETICS AND PHARMACODYNAMICS
Duration of action: 6–12 h
Onset of action: 0.5–2 h
Peak effect: 3–5 h
Bioavailability: not known
Effect of food: administration of mecamylamine after meals may provide more gradual control of BP than that produced when the drug is given on an empty stomach
Protein binding: not known
Metabolism: little hepatic metabolism
Elimination: renal, largely unchanged (clearance is decreased in alkaline urine and is increased in acidic urine)
Plasma half-life: not known

MONITORING
Monitor BP and observe for tolerance. Additional diuretic treatment may be required. In addition to the contraindications listed above, use mecamylamine with caution in patients with prostatic hypertrophy, bladder neck obstruction, and urethral stricture because urinary retention may occur.

OVERDOSE
Treatment should be symptomatic and supportive. Pressor agents may be required, but sensitivity to their effects may be exaggerated.

PATIENT INFORMATION
Take mecamylamine after meals. This medication may cause gastrointestinal side effects, urinary retention, CNS effects, weakness, vision problems, drowsiness, and dizziness. If affected, do not drive or operate machinery. You may experience dizziness when getting up from a sitting or lying position; do this slowly. Do not take antacids, especially those containing sodium bicarbonate. Do not take other medications without consulting your physician. If any unusual effects appear, consult your physician immediately. Avoid alcohol use. Take medication as prescribed; do not discontinue therapy without physician's advice.

AVAILABILITY
Tablets—2.5 mg

RESERPINE (Reserpine, Serpalan®)

Reserpine, a rauwolfia alkaloid, is one of the earliest drugs that was used effectively for the treatment of systemic hypertension. It acts at postganglionic sympathetic nerve endings and causes a depletion of CNS stores of catecholamines and serotonin. With repeated administration, depletion of catecholamine stores happens slowly, causing a gradual decrease in peripheral vascular resistance and BP, which is usually associated with bradycardia. With prolonged therapy, venous dilation decreases venous return to the heart and causes a reduction of cardiac output. Reserpine is the least expensive nondiuretic, antihypertensive agent available and is fairly well tolerated when used in low doses (0.1 to 0.2 mg daily) in combination with a diuretic agent. Depression and other CNS effects were very common when high doses of reserpine were used. The drug is found in many combination products, which include diuretics and hydralazine. Reserpine was one of the drugs used in the National Institutes of Health–sponsored Systolic Hypertension in the Elderly program to treat isolated systolic hypertension.

By depleting catecholamine stores in sympathetic nerve terminals, reserpine diminishes adrenergic vasoconstriction in cutaneous blood vessels. Consequently, reserpine may be useful in Raynaud's syndrome by reducing both the severity and frequency of vasospastic episodes. A placebo effect may account for the limited success noted in using reserpine for this indication. Similarly, reserpine has been used with variable success in the treatment of migraine headaches by reducing cerebral vasoconstriction. Reserpine may also be used as a second-line agent to control the cardiovascular and neurologic symptoms associated with hyperthyroidism in patients who are resistant to propranolol or in whom beta-blockade is contraindicated.

SPECIAL GROUPS

Race:	no differences in response
Children:	safety and effectiveness have not been established; however, there is experience with the use of reserpine in children
Elderly:	more sensitive to the hypotensive and CNS effects
Renal impairment:	no dosage adjustment is necessary; avoid use with severe impairment
Hepatic impairment:	reduce dose in severe impairment
Pregnancy:	category C; not recommended. Reserpine crosses the placental barrier. Increased respiratory tract secretions, nasal congestion, cyanosis, and anorexia may occur in neonates of reserpine-treated mothers.
Breast-feeding:	not recommended; possible adverse reactions in infants from reserpine in breast milk

IN BRIEF

INDICATIONS
Hypertension
Psychotic disorders

CONTRAINDICATIONS/WARNINGS
Hypersensitivity
Active peptic ulcer disease
Ulcerative colitis
Gallstones
Electroconvulsive therapy
Mental depression

DRUG INTERACTIONS
Digitalis glycosides[3]
Hypotension-producing agents[1]
MAOIs[5]
Quinidine[3]
Sympathomimetics, direct-acting (eg, epinephrine, isoproterenol, phenylephrine)[3]
Sympathomimetics, indirect-acting (eg, ephedrine, amphetamines)[4]
Tricyclic antidepressants[2]

[1] Effect/toxicity of reserpine may increase.
[2] Effect of reserpine may decrease.
[3] Reserpine may increase the effect/toxicity of this drug.
[4] Reserpine may decrease the effect of this drug.
[5] Avoid concurrent use of reserpine with MAOIs.

ADVERSE EFFECTS
Cardiovascular: bradycardia; arrhythmias; hypotension; syncope; edema
CNS: drowsiness; fatigue; lethargy; mental depression; headache; dizziness; nervousness; anxiety; nightmares; Parkinsonian syndrome and other extrapyramidal tract symptoms (rare)
GI/GU: abdominal cramps; diarrhea; nausea; vomiting; anorexia; dryness of mouth; hypersecretion; pseudolactation; impotence; dysuria
Respiratory: dyspnea; epistaxis; nasal congestion
Others: purpura; rash; pruritus; weight gain; muscular aches; deafness (rare); optic atrophy (rare); glaucoma (rare)

PHARMACOKINETICS AND PHARMACODYNAMICS
Duration of action:	1–6 wk
Onset of action:	several days to 3 wk
Peak effect:	3–6 wk
Bioavailability:	≈50%
Effect of food:	not known
Protein binding:	96%
Metabolism:	hepatic; inactive metabolites
Elimination:	renal; fecal, 60% unchanged
Plasma half-life:	4.5 h, initial; 45–168 h, terminal

MONITORING
Monitor BP. In addition to the contraindications listed above, reserpine should be used with extreme caution in patients with cardiac arrhythmias, epilepsy, CHF, Parkinson's disease, or pheochromocytoma.

OVERDOSE
Treat with immediate evacuation of stomach and installation of an activated charcoal slurry. Use vasopressors if necessary to support BP (norepinephrine, phenylephrine). Observe for at least 72 h.

PATIENT INFORMATION
Take reserpine with food or milk. This medication may cause gastrointestinal side effects (dry mouth, stomach pains), mental depression, drowsiness, or dizziness. If severe, do not drive or operate machinery. Avoid alcohol use. Take medication as prescribed; do not discontinue therapy without physician's advice.

RESERPINE (continued)

DOSAGE

Adults: For hypertension, the usual initial dosage is 0.5 mg daily for 1 or 2 weeks in patients not receiving other antihypertensive therapy. The usual maintenance dose is 0.1–0.25 mg/d, taken with meals to avoid gastric irritation.

AVAILABILITY

Tablets—0.1 mg, 0.25 mg
Combination formulations:
Diupres—Reserpine/chlorothiazide combination tablets
  0.125 mg/250 mg
  0.125 mg/500 mg
Regroton—Reserpine/chlorthalidone combination tablets
  0.25 mg/50 mg
Demi-Regroton—Reserpine/chlorthalidone combination tablets
  0.125 mg/25 mg
Hydropres—Reserpine/hydrochlorothiazide combination tablets
  0.125 mg/25 mg
  0.125 mg/50 mg
Salutensin—Reserpine/hydroflumethiazide combination tablets
  0.125 mg/50 mg
Diutensen-R—Reserpine/methyclothiazide combination tablets
  0.1 mg/2.5 mg
Metatensin—Reserpine/trichlormethiazide combination tablets
  0.1 mg/2 mg
  0.1 mg/4 mg
Renese-R—Reserpine/trichlormethiazide combination tablets
  0.25 mg/2 mg
Hydrap-ES
Marpres
Ser-Ap-Es
Tri-Hydroserpine
Unipres—Reserpine/hydrochlorothiazide/hydralazine HCl
  combination tablets
  0.1 mg/15 mg/25 mg

SELECTED BIBLIOGRAPHY

Bonelli S, Conoscente F, Movilia PG, *et al.*: Regional intravenous guanethidine versus stellate ganglion blocker in reflex sympathetic dystrophies. A randomized trial. *Pain* 1983, 16:297–307.

Braddom RL, Johnson EW: Mecamylamine in control of hyperreflexia. *Arch Phys Med Rehab* 1969, 50:448–456.

Cheah JS: A double blind trial of reserpine in small doses as an adjunct in the treatment of hyperthyroidism. *Med J Aus* 1972, 1:322.

Driessen JJ, van der Werken C, Nicolai JPA, *et al.*: Clinical effects of regional intravenous guanethidine (Ismelin) in reflex sympathetic dystrophy. *Acta Anaesthesiol Scand* 1983, 27:505–509.

Eriksen S: Duration of sympathetic blockade: stellate ganglion versus intravenous regional guanethidine block. *Anaesthesia* 1981, 36:768–771.

Frenneaux M, Kaski JC, Brown M, *et al.*: Refractory variant angina relieved by guanethidine and clonidine. *Am J Cardiol* 1988, 62:832–833.

Frolich ED: Other adrenergic inhibitors and the direct-acting smooth muscle vasodilators. In *Hypertension. A Companion to Brenner & Rector's The Kidney*. Edited by Oparil S, Weber MA. Philadelphia: WB Saunders Co.; 2000:637–643.

Glynn CJ, Basedow RW, Walsh JA: Pain relief following post-ganglionic sympathetic blockade with IV guanethidine. *Br J Anaesth* 1981, 53:1297–1302.

Halstenson CE, Opsahl JA, Abraham PA, *et al.*: Disposition of guanadrel in subjects with normal and impaired renal function. *J Clin Pharmacol* 1989, 29:128–132.

Kaplan NM: Treatment of hypertension: drug therapy. In *Kaplan's Clinical Hypertension*, edn 8. Philadelphia: Lippincott Williams & Wilkins; 2002:237–338.

Keller S, Frishman WH, Epstein J: Neuropsychiatric manifestations of cardiovascular drug therapy. *Heart Dis* 1999, 1:241–254.

Krakoff LR: Antiadrenergic drugs with central action, ganglionic blockers and neuron depletors. In *Cardiovascular Pharmacotherapeutics*, edn 2. Edited by Frishman WH, Sonnenblick EH, Sica DA. New York: McGraw Hill; 2003:215–219.

Krakoff LR, Frishman WH: Antiadrenergic drugs with central action and neuron depletors. In *Cardiovascular Pharmacotherapeutics Manual*. Edited by Frishman WH, Sonnenblick EH, Sica DA. New York: McGraw Hill 2004:201–208.

Martin BR, Onaivi ES, Martin TJ: What is the nature of mecamylamine's antagonism of the central effects of nicotine? *Biochem Pharmacol* 1989, 38:3391–3397.

Materson BJ: Central and peripheral sympatholytics. In *Hypertension Primer*, edn 3. Edited by Izzo JL Jr, Black HR. Dallas: American Heart Association; 2003:423–425.

Miller R, Toth C, Silva DA, *et al.*: Nitroprusside versus a nitroprusside-trimethaphan mixture: a comparison of dosage requirements and hemodynamic effects during induced hypotension for neurosurgery. *Mt. Sinai J Med* 1987, 54:308–312.

Nattero G, Lisino F, Brandi G, *et al.*: Reserpine for migraine prophylaxis. *Headache* 1976, 15:279–281.

Nunn-Thompson CL, Simon PA: Pharmacotherapy for smoking cessation. *Clin Pharm* 1989, 8:710–720.

Phillips WA, Hensinger RN: Control of blood loss during scoliosis surgery. *Clin Orthop* 1988, 229:88–93.

Pomerleau CS, Pomerleau OF, Majchrzak MJ: Mecamylamine pretreatment increases subsequent nicotine self-administration as indicated by changes in plasma nicotine level. *Psychopharmacology* 1987, 91:391–393.

Rose JE, Sampson A, Levin ED, *et al.*: Mecamylamine increases nicotine preference and attenuates nicotine discrimination. *Pharmacol Biochem Behav* 1989, 32:933–938.

Samuels AH, Taylor AJ: Reserpine withdrawal psychosis. *Aust NZ J Psych* 1989, 23:129–130.

SHEP Cooperative Research Group: Prevention of stroke by antihypertensive drug treatment in older persons with isolated systolic hypertension: Final results of the Systolic Hypertension in the Elderly Program (SHEP). *JAMA* 1991, 265:3255–3264.

Siegel RC, Fried JF: Intraaterially administered reserpine and saline in scleroderma. *Arch Intern Med* 1974, 134:515–518.

Stolerman IP. Could nicotine antagonists be used in smoking cessation? *Br J Addict* 1986, 81:47–53.

Stumph JL: Drug therapy of hypertensive crises. *Clin Pharmacol* 1988, 7:582–591.

Taylor P: Agents acting on the neuromuscular junction and autonomic ganglia. In *Goodman & Gilman's The Pharmacological Basis of Therapeutics*, edn 10. Edited by Hardman JG, Limbird LE. New York: McGraw Hill; 2001:193–213.

Tindall JP, Whalen RE, Burton EE Jr: Medical uses of intraarterial injections of reserpine. Treatment of Raynaud's syndrome and of some vascular insufficiencies of the lower extremities. *Arch Dermatol* 1974, 110:233–237.

13

VASODILATORS (OTHER AGENTS AND DRUG CLASSES)

In addition to the angiotensin II receptor blockers, the angiotensin-converting enzyme (ACE) inhibitors, and the calcium channel blockers, which are discussed in other chapters, there are other peripheral vasodilators that include a wide variety of compounds with different mechanisms of action. These drugs also differ enormously in their effects on small and large arteries and in their differential vasodilatory actions on arterial and venous vessels. Several drugs have poorly defined pharmacologic profiles, and many nonspecific agents have little clinical usefulness despite having been available for many years, but some drugs in this broad group have a valuable place in cardiovascular therapy.

EFFICACY AND USE

Hydralazine and **minoxidil** are two potent and effective arterial vasodilators. Because of their unfavorable side effect profiles (possible drug-induced lupus with **hydralazine** and possible pericardial effusion with **minoxidil**), they are used as second-, third-, and fourth-line drugs in complicated or resistant hypertension. **Minoxidil** is reserved for the management of severe hypertension that is symptomatic or associated with target organ damage. **Hydralazine** and **minoxidil** have been shown to be ineffective in reversing left ventricular hypertrophy, possibly because of volume overload and the stimulation of growth factors such as angiotensin II and catecholamines.

Nitrates have, for many years, been the mainstay of treatment of angina, as well as other cardiovascular problems. They are useful in the acute reduction of blood pressure (BP) and for the relief of heart failure. Combination vasodilator therapy is particularly valuable. A useful combination is that of **hydralazine** and **isosorbide dinitrate**, as used in the Veterans Administration Heart Failure Trial (VHeFT-I). This demonstrated a decrease in mortality in patients with New York Heart Association (NYHA) class II–III congestive heart failure (CHF) receiving **isosorbide-hydralazine** compared with those given **prazosin**. Mortality reduction, however, was lower in patients on the combination than in patients on **enalapril**. **Diazoxide** is a powerful and fast-acting vasodilator that, like **nitroprusside**, is used for situations in which rapid reduction in BP is desired. **Nitroprusside** is also useful when swift unloading of the heart is required, as in acute heart failure.

Fenoldopam is a selective dopamine$_1$ agonist that is available in intravenous (IV) form and approved for the short-term management of severe hypertension and for patients with malignant hypertension having end-organ dysfunction. The drug has hemodynamic effects similar to **nitroprusside**, but unlike **nitroprusside**, it may also induce both a diuresis and natriuresis and does not cause cyanide toxicity. **Epoprostenol** is a naturally occurring prostaglandin approved for IV use in patients having advanced primary pulmonary hypertension. The drug may be used long term as a continuous chronic infusion therapy.

Pentoxifylline and **cilostazol** are both approved for use in patients with intermittent claudication. **Papaverine** is a vasodilator approved for relief of cerebral and peripheral ischemia associated with arterial spasm and myocardial ischemia complicated by arrhythmias. **Isoxsuprine**, an oral vasodilator that now has limited use, is indicated for relieving symptoms associated with cerebral vascular insufficiency and peripheral vascular disease. **Alprostadil** (prostaglandin E$_1$) produces vasodilation, inhibits platelet aggregation, and stimulates intestinal and uterine smooth muscle. This agent is indicated for palliative therapy to temporarily maintain the patency of the ductus arteriosus until corrective or palliative surgery can be performed in neonates who have congenital heart defects. **Alprostadil** has also been used for the treatment of erectile dysfunction of vasculogenic, psychogenic, or neurogenic etiology. **Nesiritide** mimics the actions of endogenous B-type natriuretic peptide. Clinical studies using the IV infusion of **nesiritide** in patients with acute decompensated heart failure have demonstrated that it exerts dose-related vasodilation that is rapid in onset and sustained for the duration of infusion. **Nesiritide** was shown to reduce pulmonary capillary wedge pressure and improve dyspnea in patients with acutely decompensated CHF. **Bosentan** is the first endothelin (ET) receptor antagonist approved by the Food and Drug Administration (FDA) for the management of pulmonary arterial hypertension. **Treprostinil** is a direct dilator of both pulmonary and systemic arterial vascular beds. Similar to **bosentan**, **treprostinil** is indicated for the treatment of pulmonary arterial hypertension.

MODE OF ACTION

Hydralazine exerts a peripheral vasodilating effect through a direct relaxant action on arterial smooth muscle. Its main activity appears to be via interference with the cellular calcium movements responsible for initiating or maintaining a contractile state. **Minoxidil** also produces vasodilation by direct relaxation of arteriolar smooth muscle. In contrast to **hydralazine** and **minoxidil**, relaxation of vascular smooth muscle (via stimulation of intracellular cyclic guanosine monophosphate [cGMP] production) is the principal pharmacologic action of nitrates. **Diazoxide**, a nondiuretic antihypertensive agent, is structurally related to the thiazides. It reduces BP rapidly by relaxing smooth muscle in the peripheral arterioles. **Nitroprusside** is a potent IV antihypertensive agent. The principal action of **nitroprusside** is relaxation of vascular smooth muscle and consequent dilation of peripheral arteries and veins. **Nitroprusside** is more active on veins than on arteries. However, this selectivity is much less discernible than that of **nitroglycerin**. **Fenoldopam** is a selective postsynaptic dopamine agonist (D$_1$-receptors) that exerts hypotensive effects by decreasing peripheral vasculature resistance with increased renal blood flow, diuresis, and natriuresis. This agent is about six times as potent as **dopamine** in producing renal vasodilatation and has minimal adrenergic effects. **Epoprostenol** and **treprostinil** are direct dilators of both pulmonary and systemic arterial vascular beds. These agents also inhibit platelet aggregation.

Pentoxifylline and **cilostazol** are both indicated for the management of intermittent claudication. **Pentoxifylline** appears to reduce blood viscosity and improve blood flow by altering the rheology of red blood cells. **Cilostazol** is a selective phosphodiesterase III inhibitor that suppresses cyclic adenosine monophosphate (cAMP) degradation, with a resultant elevation of cAMP in blood platelets and blood vessels, thus leading to an inhibition of platelet aggregation and vasodilation. **Papaverine** directly relaxes the tonus of various smooth muscles, especially when it has been spasmodically contracted. Vasodilation may be related to its ability to inhibit cyclic nucleotide phosphodiesterase, thus increasing levels of intracellular cAMP. **Isoxsuprine** is a vasodilator that acts primarily on blood vessels within skeletal muscle. In healthy subjects, resting blood flow in skeletal muscle is increased whereas cutaneous blood flow is usually not affected. At high doses, this agent lowers blood viscosity and inhibits platelet aggregation. **Alprostadil** causes vasodilation by means of direct effect on vascular and ductus arteriosus smooth muscle. **Alprostadil** also relaxes trabecular smooth muscle by dilation of cavernosal arteries when this drug is injected along the penile shaft, allowing blood flow to and entrapment in the lacunar spaces of the penis.

The pharmacologic effects of **nesiritide** are mediated via the same receptor that mediates the effects of atrial natriuretic peptide, guanylyl cyclase A (GC-A). It binds to the GC-A receptors on the cell surface of vascular smooth muscle and endothelial cells. This receptor binding triggers intracellular activation of the secondary messenger cGMP, and this causes relaxation of vascular smooth muscle and vasodilation. Some vasodilating effects of **nesiritide** may also derive from the peptide's ability to inhibit the production of vasoconstrictive peptide, ET-1, secreted by endothelial cells. **Bosentan** is a specific and competitive antagonist of ET-1 receptors (ET_A and ET_B). ET_A receptors are present on smooth muscle cells and are responsible for the contractile response to ET-1. ET_B receptors were first described on endothelial cells, and their stimulation may lead to transient vasodilation. However, ET_B receptors are also present on vascular smooth muscle cells, where their activation produces vasoconstriction. The affinity of **bosentan** for the ET_A receptor is about 100 times greater than for the ET_B receptor in cultured cells. Therefore, administration of **bosentan** causes vascular smooth muscle relaxation and vasodilation.

INDICATIONS*

	Alpros	Bos	Cilos	Diaz	Epo	Fenold	Hydral	Minox	Nesir	Nitrates	Nitrop	Pentox	Trep
Angina pectoris (prevention and/or treatment)										+			
Cerebrovascular insufficiency												(+)	
Congestive heart failure							(+)‡		+¶	(+)‡	+**		
Controlled hypotension during surgery										+§	+		
Ductus arteriosus	+†												
Erectile dysfunction	+												
Essential hypertension							+‡						
Severe hypertension/hypertensive crises				+		+	+§	+‡		(+)§	+		
Peripheral vascular disease			+									+	
Pulmonary hypertension		+			+								+

*Refer to individual drug monographs for more detailed information.

†Alprostadil is indicated for palliative, not definitive, therapy to temporarily maintain the patency of the ductus arteriosus until corrective or palliative surgery can be performed in neonates who have congenital heart defects and who depend on the patent ductus for survival.

‡Oral formulation.

§Parenteral formulation.

¶Nesiritide is indicated for the management of acutely decompensated congestive heart failure.

**Nitroprusside is indicated for use in acute congestive heart failure.

+—FDA approved; (+)—clinical use, not FDA approved; Alpros—alprostadil; Bos—bosentan; Cilos—cilostazol; Diaz—diazoxide; Epo—epoprostenol; Fenold—fenoldopam; Hydral—hydralazine; Minox—minoxidil; Nesir—nesiritide; Nitrop—nitroprusside; Pentox—pentoxifylline; Trep—treprostinil.

The information here is provided as guidance only. Prescribers should always consult the manufacturer's current prescribing information.

ALPROSTADIL
(Alprostadil, Caverject® Injection, Edex® Injection, Muse® Pellet, Prostin VR Pediatric® Injection)

Alprostadil is a naturally occurring prostaglandin E_1. It is a vasodilator and a platelet-aggregation inhibitor. Alprostadil has been used for the treatment of erectile dysfunction in adult males and for temporary maintenance of patency of the ductus arteriosus in neonates. Alprostadil causes erection by relaxing trabecular smooth muscle and dilating cavernosal arteries. This leads to a process referred to as the corporeal veno-occlusive mechanism, in which lacunar spaces expand and blood becomes entrapped as a result of compression of venules against the tunica albuginea. When alprostadil is given by intracavernosal injection, there is no significant rise in levels of prostaglandin E_1 in the systemic circulation. Alprostadil is metabolized by the lungs with a short half-life of 30 seconds to 10 minutes, which may explain the low rate of priapism associated with intracavernosal injection with this agent.

In neonates with a closing ductus arteriosus, alprostadil relaxes and therefore may reopen the ductus. By maintaining ductal patency, alprostadil may improve blood flow and oxygenation in neonates with congenital heart defects who depend on the patent ductus for survival until corrective or palliative surgery can be performed.

SPECIAL GROUPS
Race: no differences in response
Children: has been used as palliative therapy to temporarily maintain the patency of the ductus arteriosus until corrective or palliative surgery can be performed in neonates who have congenital heart defects
Elderly: initiate with low dose; individualize dose according to response
Renal impairment: initiate with low dose; individualize dose according to response
Hepatic impairment: initiate with low dose; individualize dose according to response
Pregnancy: category X; not indicated for use in women

IN BRIEF

INDICATIONS
Erectile dysfunction (Caverject Injection, Edex Injection, Muse Pellet)
Temporary maintenance of the patency of the ductus arteriosus until corrective or palliative surgery can be performed in neonates who have congenital heart defects and who depend on the patent ductus for survival (alprostadil, Prostin VR Pediatric Injection)

CONTRAINDICATIONS/PRECAUTIONS
Hypersensitivity
Respiratory distress syndrome (hyaline membrane disease)
Conditions that might predispose patients to priapism (in adult males)
Patients with anatomic deformation of the penis (in adult males)
Patients with penile implants (in adult males)
Use in women
For sexual intercourse with a pregnant woman unless the couple uses a condom barrier
Use in men for whom sexual activity is inadvisable

DRUG INTERACTIONS
Anticoagulants[1]
Antihypertensives[1]
Ethanol[2]
1 Alprostadil may increase the effect/toxicity of this drug.
2 Avoid concurrent use because of alcohol's vasodilating effect.

ADVERSE EFFECTS
Cardiovascular: flushing (10%, more common after intra-arterial dosing), bradycardia, hypotension, tachycardia, cardiac arrest, edema
CNS: fever, headache, dizziness, seizures
GI: diarrhea
Respiratory: apnea (12%), upper respiratory infection, flu syndrome, sinusitis, bronchial wheezing, nasal congestion, respiratory depression, cough
GU (intracavernosal injection): penile pain, prolonged erection, penile fibrosis, injection site hematoma, penile disorder

PHARMACOKINETICS AND PHARMACODYNAMICS
Onset of action: rapid
Duration of action: the dose of alprostadil that is selected for self-injection treatment should provide patient with an erection that is sufficient for sexual intercourse and that is maintained for no longer than 1 h (adults). Closure of the ductus arteriosus usually begins within 1–2 h after the discontinuation of infusion (neonates)
Protein binding: ≈80% to albumin
Metabolism: pulmonary. In patients with normal respiratory function, up to 80% of a dose may be metabolized in one pass through the lungs
Elimination: metabolites excreted in urine (90% within 24 h)
Elimination half-life: 30 sec to 10 min

MONITORING
For adults: degree of penile pain, length of erection, signs of infection.
For neonates: arterial blood gases, arterial blood pH, blood pressure, heart rate, respiratory rate, temperature, respiratory status, renal output.

ALPROSTADIL *(continued)*

DOSAGE

Adults: For erectile dysfunction, initiate with low dose and individualize dose by careful titration. Refer to manufacturer's package insert for details on dosage and administration.

Neonates: The preferred administration route is continuous IV infusion into a large vein. Alternatively, alprostadil may be given through an umbilical artery catheter placed at the ductal opening. Alprostadil must be diluted in the appropriate amount of sodium chloride injection or dextrose injection prior to infusion. Initiate infusion with 0.05–0.1 µg/kg/min. After a therapeutic response is achieved (increased pO_2 in infants with restricted pulmonary blood flow or increased systemic blood pressure and blood pH in infants with restricted systemic blood flow), reduce the infusion rate to the lowest dosage that maintains the response. This may be achieved by lowering the dosage from 0.1 to 0.05 to 0.025 to 0.01 µg/kg/min. If response to 0.05 µg/kg/min is inadequate, dosage may be increased gradually up to 0.4 µg/kg/min. However, infusion rates higher than 0.1 µg/kg/min generally do not produce greater response.

OVERDOSE

If intracavernous overdose occurs, monitor patient until any systemic effects have resolved or until penile detumescence has occurred. Symptomatic treatment of any systemic symptoms would be appropriate. Symptoms of overdose when treating patent ductus arteriosus include apnea, bradycardia, pyrexia, hypotension and flushing. If apnea or bradycardia occurs, discontinue alprostadil infusion and provide appropriate medical therapy. Use caution in restarting the infusion. If pyrexia or hypotension occurs, decrease the infusion rate until symptoms subside. Flushing is usually a result of incorrect intra-arterial catheter placement; repositioning the catheter may help.

PATIENT INFORMATION

For adult patients using alprostadil for erectile dysfunction, refer to manufacturer's patient package literature for proper administration and storage of alprostadil. Do not change the dose of alprostadil established in the physician's office without consulting the physician. Erection may be expected within 5 to 20 minutes after administration of medication. Do not use alprostadil if the female partner is pregnant, unless a condom barrier is used. Inform physician as soon as possible if any new penile pain, nodules, hard tissue, or signs of infection develop. The risk of transmission of blood-borne disease is increased with the use of alprostadil injections because a small amount of bleeding at the injection site is possible. Do not share this medication or needles/syringes. Do not drive or operate heavy machinery within 1 hour of administration.

AVAILABILITY

Caverject Injection (injection, powder for reconstitution)—
10 µg, 20 µg, 40 µg
Edex Injection—10 µg, 20 µg, 40 µg
Muse (pellet)—125 µg, 250 µg, 500 µg, 1000 µg
Alprostadil, Prostin VR Pediatric (injection)—500 µg/mL
(1 mL ampule)

BOSENTAN (Tracleer®)

Bosentan is the first ET receptor antagonist approved by the FDA for the management of pulmonary arterial hypertension (PAH) in patients with World Health Organization class III or IV symptoms. In these patients, bosentan has been demonstrated to improve dyspnea and exercise tolerance. ET also plays an important role in the pathophysiology of different vascular diseases. Therefore, bosentan may have the potential to alter the outcome of many other diseases, such as heart failure, hypertension, ischemic heart disease, renal disease, and cerebrovascular disorders. Because of the rarity and the poor prognosis of patients with PAH, as well as the potential for bosentan to cause liver dysfunction and teratogenic effects, close monitoring is required for patients who receive this medication. Bosentan is currently available only through a special access program and is distributed by selected pharmacies. Patients who are receiving bosentan should be taught to recognize early signs and symptoms of liver dysfunction and possible pregnancy. In addition, bosentan is a substrate as well as an inducer of cytochrome P-450 (CYP)3A4 and CYP2C9. Therefore, a number of drug interactions may occur with bosentan. Patients should be advised to consult with their physicians or pharmacists when new prescription or nonprescription medications are needed.

SPECIAL GROUPS

Race: no information

Children: safety and effectiveness have not been established

Elderly: use usual dose with caution

Renal impairment: use usual dose

Hepatic impairment: caution should be exercised during the use of bosentan in patients with mildly impaired liver function; bosentan generally should be avoided in patients with moderate or severe hepatic impairment

Pregnancy: category X; bosentan is expected to cause fetal harm if administered to pregnant women

Breast-feeding: not recommended; may be excreted in breast milk

DOSAGE

Initiate at 62.5 mg twice daily for 4 wk and then increase to the maintenance dose of 125 mg twice daily. Doses >125 mg twice daily do not appear to confer additional benefit sufficient to offset the increased risk of liver injury. In patients weighing <40 kg but older than 12 years, the recommended initial and maintenance dose is 62.5 mg twice daily. Refer to Tracleer package insert for recommendations on dosage adjustment and monitoring in patients developing aminotransferase abnormalities during therapy.

Note: Because of potential liver injury and in an effort to make the chance of fetal exposure to bosentan as small as possible, bosentan may be prescribed only through the Tracleer Access Program.

IN BRIEF

INDICATIONS
Treatment of PAH in patients with World Health Organization class III or IV symptoms to improve exercise ability and decrease the rate of clinical worsening

CONTRAINDICATIONS/WARNINGS
Hypersensitivity
Pregnancy
Coadministration with cyclosporine or glyburide
Moderate or severe hepatic impairment

DRUG INTERACTIONS
Cyclosporine[1,3,4]
Glyburide[2,3,4]
Hormonal contraceptives[4]
Hydroxy-methylglutaryl coenzyme A reductase inhibitors[4]
Ketoconazole[1]
Warfarin[4,5]

1 Effect/toxicity of bosentan may increase.
2 Effect of bosentan may decrease.
3 Coadministration of this agent with bosentan is contraindicated.
4 Bosentan may decrease the effect of this drug.
5 The clinical significance of this interaction is unclear.

ADVERSE EFFECTS
Cardiovascular: flushing (7%–9%), edema (lower limb, 8%; generalized, 4%), hypotension (7%), palpitations (5%)
CNS: headache (16%–22%), fatigue (4%)
Dermatologic: pruritus (4%)
GI: dyspepsia (4%)
Hematologic: decreased hemoglobin (≥1 g/dL in up to 57%, usually during first 6 wk of therapy), anemia (3%)
Hepatic: increased serum transaminases (>3 times upper limit of normal; up to 11%), abnormal hepatic function (6%–8%)
Respiratory: nasopharyngitis (11%)

PHARMACOKINETICS AND PHARMACODYNAMICS
Time to peak plasma concentration: 3–5 h
Bioavailability: ≈50%
Protein binding: >98%
Volume of distribution: ≈18 L
Metabolism: hepatic via CYP2C9 and 3A4 to three primary metabolites (one having pharmacologic activity)
Elimination: feces (as metabolites); urine (<3% as unchanged drug)
Elimination half-life: 5 h, prolonged with heart failure and possibly in PAH

MONITORING
Serum transaminase (aspartate aminotransferase and alanine aminotransferase) should be obtained prior to initiation of therapy and at monthly intervals thereafter. If elevated liver function tests are observed, changes in monitoring and treatment must be initiated. Monitor for clinical signs and symptoms of liver injury. Pregnancy test for a woman of childbearing potential must be negative prior to the initiation of therapy and monthly thereafter. Hemoglobin and hematocrit should be measured at baseline, at 1 mo, and 3 mo of treatment, and every 3 mo thereafter.

OVERDOSE
Massive overdosage may result in pronounced hypotension requiring active cardiovascular support.

PATIENT INFORMATION
This medication may be taken with or without food. Report unusual fatigue, nausea, vomiting, abdominal pain, and/or yellowing of the skin/eyes to physician immediately. Do not get pregnant while taking this medication. A woman of childbearing potential must use an effective nonhormonal method of contraception during treatment with this medication.

AVAILABILITY
Tablets—62.5 mg, 125 mg

The information here is provided as guidance only. Prescribers should always consult the manufacturer's current prescribing information.

327

CILOSTAZOL (Pletal®)

Cilostazol is a phosphodiesterase III inhibitor demonstrated to be effective for the management of intermittent claudication. It suppresses cAMP degradation, with a resultant elevation of cAMP in blood platelets and blood vessels, thus leading to vasodilation and an inhibition of platelet aggregation.

For additional information on cilostazol, please refer to the chapter on antithrombotic therapy.

DIAZOXIDE
(Diazoxide, Hyperstat® I.V., Proglycem®)

Diazoxide is structurally related to the thiazides. It is used orally for the treatment of intractable hypoglycemia and intravenously for the acute management of hypertensive crisis. In contrast to the thiazide diuretics, diazoxide causes sodium and water retention. This may result in expansion of plasma and extracellular fluid volume, edema, and CHF, especially during prolonged therapy. The sodium- and water-retaining effects may be prevented by concurrent administration of diazoxide with a diuretic. The hyperglycemic effect is primarily a result of the inhibition of insulin release from the pancreas, as well as an extrapancreatic (catecholamine-induced) effect.

Diazoxide is an extremely useful drug for the emergency management of high BP, as in patients with hypertensive encephalopathy. It offers the advantage of rapidly and consistently lowering the arterial pressure toward normal values, but rarely achieves values below normal. In comparison with nitroprusside, diazoxide has the advantage that constant patient monitoring is not necessary, but it lacks nitroprusside's advantage of immediate dose adjustability. Its diabetogenic effect limits its usefulness, and enthusiasm for its use has declined because of occasional episodes of profound BP reduction.

SPECIAL GROUPS

Race: no differences in response

Children: diazoxide-induced edema occurs most frequently in infants given the oral form; may lead to CHF; no problems seen with parenteral diazoxide in children

Elderly: may require reduction in dose or lengthening of dosage interval

Renal impairment: reduced dose may be necessary, especially with repeated administration

Hepatic impairment: administer with caution; lower doses may be needed

Pregnancy: category C; to be used only when condition may put the mother's life at risk; crosses placenta; may cause harm to fetus; safety is not established

Breast-feeding: not recommended; diazoxide may be excreted in breast milk

IN BRIEF

INDICATIONS
Hypertensive emergencies (IV)

Hypoglycemia related to islet cell adenoma, carcinoma, hyperplasia, adenomatosis, nesidioblastosis, leucine sensitivity, or extrapancreatic malignancy (oral)

CONTRAINDICATIONS/WARNINGS
Hypersensitivity to diazoxide, other thiazides, or other sulfonamide-derived drugs

Compensatory hypertension, such as that associated with aortic coarctation or arteriovenous shunt

Hypertension caused by pheochromocytoma

Dissecting aortic aneurysm

Coronary or cerebral insufficiency

Diabetes mellitus

Inadequate cardiac reserve (*ie*, uncompensated CHF)

DRUG INTERACTIONS
Hydantoins[3]

Hypotension-producing medications[1]

Sulfonylureas[3]

Thiazide diuretics[1]

Warfarin[2]

1 Effect/toxicity of diazoxide may increase.
2 Diazoxide may increase the effect/toxicity of this drug.
3 Diazoxide may decrease the effect of this drug.

ADVERSE EFFECTS
Cardiovascular: hypotension (7%), sodium and water retention, myocardial ischemia, atrial and ventricular arrhythmias, ECG changes
CNS: dizziness/weakness (2%), cerebral ischemia, convulsions, confusion, headache
GI: nausea, vomiting (4%), abdominal discomfort, anorexia, alterations in taste, dry mouth, constipation, diarrhea
Others: hyperglycemia, dyspnea, cough, choking sensation, hirsutism, tinnitus, neutropenia, leukopenia, thrombocytopenia, hyperuricemia, decreased libido

PHARMACOKINETICS AND PHARMACODYNAMICS
Duration of action: 2–12 h (IV)
Onset of action: 1 min (IV)
Time to peak effect: 2–5 min (after IV push)
Bioavailability: oral formulation is readily absorbed
Effect of food: not known
Protein binding: >90%
Metabolism: hepatic
Elimination: approximately 50% excreted unchanged in the urine
Elimination half-life: 9–24 h (children), 20–36 h (adults), >30 h (end-stage renal disease)

MONITORING
BP, blood glucose, serum uric acid. Cardiac and BP monitoring are required for IV administration.

OVERDOSE
May result in hyperglycemia (which responds to insulin); monitor patient for up to 7 d while blood sugar concentration stabilizes. Severe hypotension responds to vasopressor treatment.

DIAZOXIDE (continued)

DOSAGE

Hypertension: Adults—IV, give 1–3 mg/kg body weight or up to 150 mg every 5–15 min if necessary to obtain desired response. Further doses may be administered every 4–24 h as needed to maintain desired BP until oral antihypertensive medication is effective, usually within 4–5 d. Do not use for more than 10 d.

Note: IV injection should be administered only into a peripheral vein. Because the alkalinity of the solution is irritating to tissue, avoid extravascular injection or leakage. Treatment is most effective if IV administration is completed within 10–30 sec. Patient should remain recumbent during and for 15–30 min after administration.

Children—IV 1–3 mg/kg body weight or 30–90 mg/m² body surface area (maximum dose for a single injection is 150 mg), every 5–15 min as necessary to obtain desired response. Further doses may be given every 4–24 h as needed to maintain desired BP until oral antihypertensive medication is effective. Injection should be rapid and not exceed 30 sec.

Elderly—may require reduction in dose or lengthening of dosage interval.

Hypoglycemia: Adults and children—oral, initially 1 mg/kg of body weight every 8 h, adjusted according to clinical response. For maintenance, 3–8 mg/kg of body weight a day, divided into 2 or 3 equal doses every 12 or 8 h, respectively.

Neonates and infants—oral, 3.3 mg/kg body weight every 8 h, adjusted according to clinical response. For maintenance, 8–15 mg/kg of body weight a day divided into 2 or 3 equal doses every 12 or 8 h, respectively.

Elderly—more likely to have age-related renal function impairment, which may require a reduction in dosage and/or longer dosing interval.

PATIENT INFORMATION

If the suspension has been prescribed, shake well before using. Check blood glucose carefully. This medication may cause dizziness, headache, edema, weakness, nausea, and vomiting. Notify physician if persistent side effects occur. Do not discontinue therapy without your physician's advice.

AVAILABILITY

Injection (Hyperstat I.V.)—15 mg/mL (20 mL)
Suspension, oral (Proglycem)—50 mg/mL (30 mL)

EPOPROSTENOL (Flolan®)

Epoprostenol, a metabolite of arachidonic acid, is a naturally occurring prostaglandin. It causes direct vasodilation of pulmonary and systemic arterial vascular beds, inhibits platelet aggregation, and has antiproliferative effects. Epoprostenol is rapidly hydrolyzed in the blood, with a half-life of approximately 6 minutes. A 12-week controlled trial in 81 patients with severe primary pulmonary hypertension showed that the addition of epoprostenol to conventional treatment was associated with better exercise capacity, fewer symptoms, and no deaths among 40 patients, compared with eight deaths among 41 patients treated with conventional therapy alone. In a study involving 27 patients with advanced primary pulmonary hypertension, McLaughlin et al., found that long-term (>1 year) therapy with epoprostenol lowered pulmonary vascular resistance beyond the level achieved in the short term with IV adenosine.

The use of epoprostenol in patients with CHF, however, has not been very successful, as demonstrated by the FIRST trial, in which the combination of epoprostenol infusion and standard therapy was compared with standard therapy alone in 471 patients with class IIIB/IV CHF and decreased left ventricular ejection fraction. Although epoprostenol infusion was associated with a significant increase in cardiac index, a decrease in pulmonary capillary wedge pressure, and a decrease in systemic vascular resistance, this trial was terminated early because of a strong trend toward decreased survival in the patients treated with epoprostenol. Hence, the manufacturer of epoprostenol states that this medication should not be used on a chronic basis in patients with CHF due to severe left ventricular systolic dysfunction.

SPECIAL GROUPS

Race: not studied
Children: safety and effectiveness have not been established
Elderly: use with caution; reduced doses may be needed
Renal impairment: use with caution; the metabolites of epoprostenol are excreted in the urine
Hepatic impairment: use with caution
Pregnancy: category B; this drug should be used during pregnancy only if clearly indicated
Breast-feeding: not recommended; epoprostenol may be excreted in breast milk

IN BRIEF

INDICATIONS
Primary pulmonary hypertension (epoprostenol is indicated for the long-term IV treatment of primary pulmonary hypertension in NYHA class III and IV patients).

CONTRAINDICATIONS
Hypersensitivity
Chronic use in patients with CHF due to severe left ventricular systolic dysfunction

DRUG INTERACTIONS
Antiplatelet agents[1,2]
Anticoagulants[1,2]
Diuretics[1]
Other vasodilators[1]
1 Epoprostenol may increase the effect/toxicity of this drug.
2 The clinical significance of this interaction is unclear.

ADVERSE EFFECTS
Cardiovascular: tachycardia, hypotension, chest pain, bradycardia
CNS: dizziness, headache, anxiety, nervousness, hyperesthesia, paresthesia
GI: nausea, vomiting, diarrhea, abdominal pain
Musculoskeletal: jaw pain, myalgia, nonspecific musculoskeletal pain
Others: flushing, chills, fever, catheter-associated sepsis, flulike symptoms, hemorrhage, dyspnea

PHARMACOKINETICS AND PHARMACODYNAMICS
Duration of action: 5 min (cardiovascular effects), 2 h (platelet aggregation inhibition)
Time to steady-state concentration: 15 min (continuous infusion)
Metabolism: rapidly hydrolyzed at neutral pH in blood and is also subjected to enzymatic degradation. Epoprostenol is metabolized to two primary metabolites, both of which have pharmacologic activity orders of magnitude less than the parent drug in animal test systems.
Elimination: metabolites of epoprostenol are found mainly in the urine
Half-life: ≤6 min

MONITORING
Monitor for improvements in pulmonary function and dose-related adverse effects. Adjust infusion rate accordingly. Pump device and catheters should be checked frequently to avoid system-related failure.

OVERDOSE
Signs and symptoms of excessive doses of epoprostenol during clinical trials are the expected dose-limiting pharmacologic effects of epoprostenol, including flushing, headache, hypotension, tachycardia, nausea, vomiting, and diarrhea. Treatment will ordinarily require dose reduction of epoprostenol. One patient with secondary pulmonary hypertension accidentally received 50 mL of an unknown concentration of epoprostenol. The patient vomited and became unconscious with an initially unrecordable BP. Epoprostenol was discontinued, and the patient regained consciousness within seconds.

EPOPROSTENOL (continued)

DOSAGE

Acute dose-ranging: The infusion rate is initiated at 2 ng/kg/min and increased in increments of 2 ng/kg/min every 15 min or longer until dose-limiting pharmacologic effects occur. The most common dose-limiting pharmacologic effects are nausea, vomiting, headache, hypotension, and flushing. During acute dose-ranging in clinical trials, the mean maximum dose that did not result in dose-limiting pharmacologic effects was 8.6 ± 0.3 ng/kg/min.

Note: Epoprostenol must be reconstituted only with sterile diluent for epoprostenol. Reconstituted solutions of epoprostenol must not be diluted or administered with other parenteral solutions or medications.

Continuous chronic infusion: Chronic infusions of epoprostenol should be initiated at 4 ng/kg/min less than the maximum-tolerated infusion rate determined during acute dose-ranging. If the maximum-tolerated infusion rate is <5 ng/kg/min, the chronic infusion should be started at one-half the maximum-tolerated infusion rate. During clinical trials, the mean initial chronic infusion rate was 5 ng/kg/min.

Note: Chronic continuous infusion of epoprostenol should be administered through a central venous catheter. Temporary peripheral IV infusions may be used until central access is established.

Dosage adjustments: Alterations in the chronic infusion rate should be based on persistence, recurrence, or worsening of the patient's symptoms of primary pulmonary hypertension and the occurrence of adverse events due to excessive doses of epoprostenol. In general, increases in dose from the initial chronic dose should be expected. Increments in dose should be considered if symptoms of primary pulmonary hypertension persist or recur after improving. The infusion should be increased by 1–2 ng/kg/min increments at intervals sufficient to allow assessment of clinical response; these intervals should be at least 15 min. In contrast, decreased dosage of epoprostenol should be considered when dose-related pharmacologic events occur. Dosage decreases should be made gradually in 2 ng/kg/min decrements every 15 min or longer until the dose-limiting adverse effects resolve.

Note: Abrupt withdrawal of epoprostenol or sudden large reductions in infusion rates should be avoided except in life-threatening situations, such as unconsciousness or collapse. Consult manufacturer's package insert for detailed information on administration and reconstitution of epoprostenol.

PATIENT INFORMATION

Epoprostenol must be reconstituted only with sterile diluent for epoprostenol. Epoprostenol is infused continuously through a permanent indwelling central venous catheter via a small, portable infusion pump. Therefore, therapy with epoprostenol requires commitment by the patient to drug reconstitution, drug administration, and care of the permanent central venous catheter. Sterile technique must be followed in preparing the drug and in the care of the catheter. Even brief interruptions in the delivery of epoprostenol may result in rapid symptomatic deterioration. Base the decision to receive epoprostenol for primary pulmonary hypertension on the understanding that there is a high likelihood that therapy with this medication will be needed for prolonged periods, possibly years. Infusion rates of epoprostenol should be adjusted only under the direction of a physician.

AVAILABILITY

Powder for reconstitution—0.5 mg, 1.5 mg (mannitol, NaCl; in 17 mL flint glass vials)

FENOLDOPAM (Corlopam® I.V.)

Fenoldopam mesylate is a dopamine agonist that induces peripheral vasodilation through stimulation of dopamine$_1$ receptors. Fenoldopam also causes renal vasculature vasodilation, which leads to an increase in renal blood flow. Fenoldopam has been compared with sodium nitroprusside in the management of patients with hypertensive urgencies and emergencies.

Treatment with fenoldopam was demonstrated to be as effective as treatment with sodium nitroprusside in a randomized, open-label, multicenter trial involving 153 severely hypertensive patients with diastolic BP of 120 mm Hg or higher. A dose-dependent reduction in arterial pressure for up to 24 hours without evidence of tolerance, rebound on withdrawal, or significant changes in heart rate was observed with IV infusion of fenoldopam.

Fenoldopam has also been shown to be an appropriate alternative to sodium nitroprusside for patients who develop hypertension after coronary artery bypass graft surgery. Additional evidence has demonstrated fenoldopam to be effective in treating hypertension after noncardiac surgery. The adverse event profiles of fenoldopam and sodium nitroprusside were generally comparable in comparative trials. In contrast to sodium nitroprusside, fenoldopam produces a dose-related modest increase in intraocular pressure and may be associated with a lower incidence of hypotension. In addition, IV fenoldopam may offer advantages over sodium nitroprusside because it can induce both a diuresis and natriuresis, is not light sensitive, and is not associated with cyanide toxicity.

SPECIAL GROUPS

Race: no differences in response
Children: safety and effectiveness have not been established
Elderly: dosage adjustments are generally not necessary
Renal impairment: dosage adjustments are generally not necessary
Hepatic impairment: dosage adjustments are generally not necessary; use with caution in patients with cirrhosis
Pregnancy: category B; fenoldopam should be used in pregnancy only if clearly indicated
Breast-feeding: not recommended; fenoldopam may be excreted in breast milk

IN BRIEF

INDICATIONS
Short-term management of severe hypertension
Malignant hypertension associated with deteriorating end-organ function

CONTRAINDICATIONS/PRECAUTIONS
Hypersensitivity to fenoldopam and sodium metabisulfite
Use with caution in patients with glaucoma or intraocular hypertension

DRUG INTERACTIONS
Formal drug–drug interaction studies using IV fenoldopam have not been performed.
Acetaminophen[1]
Beta-blockers[1,2]

1 Effect/toxicity of fenoldopam may increase.
2 Concurrent use of fenoldopam with a beta-blocker should be avoided; beta-blockers may increase the risk of hypotension.

ADVERSE EFFECTS
Cardiovascular: hypotension (>5%), palpitations, tachycardia, bradycardia, edema, heart failure, ischemic heart disease, myocardial infarction (MI), angina pectoris
CNS: headache (>5%), dizziness
GI: nausea (>5%), vomiting, diarrhea
Others: flushing (>5%), hypokalemia, increased intraocular pressure, dyspnea, elevated blood urea nitrogen (BUN), elevated serum glucose, elevated transaminase, leukocytosis, bleeding, limb cramp, oliguria, pyrexia

PHARMACOKINETICS AND PHARMACODYNAMICS
Duration of action: ≈1 h (IV)
Onset of action: ≈5 min (IV)
Time to steady-state plasma concentration: ≈20 min
Metabolism: hepatic to inactive metabolites
Elimination: renal (90%), fecal (10%); only 4% of a dose is eliminated as unchanged drug
Half-life: ≈5 min

MONITORING
Monitor BP and heart rate at frequent intervals (ie, every 15 min) to avoid hypotension and rapid reductions of BP. Electrolytes should also be monitored frequently (electrolytes were monitored at intervals of 6 h during clinical trials).
Fenoldopam may increase intraocular pressure; administer with caution in patients with glaucoma or intraocular hypertension.

OVERDOSE
Intentional fenoldopam overdosage has not been reported. The most likely reaction would be excessive hypotension, which should be managed with drug discontinuation and appropriate supportive measures.

FENOLDOPAM (continued)

DOSAGE

The initial dose of fenoldopam is chosen according to the desired magnitude and rate of BP reduction in a given clinical situation. In general, there is a greater and more rapid BP reduction as the initial dose is increased. Lower initial doses (0.03–0.1 µg/kg/min) titrated slowly have been associated with less reflex tachycardia than have higher initial doses (≥0.3 µg/kg/min). The recommended increments for titration are 0.05–0.1 µg/kg/min at intervals of ≥15 min. Doses below 0.1 µg/kg/min have very modest effects and appear to be only marginally useful in patients with severe hypertension. Fenoldopam infusion can be abruptly discontinued or gradually tapered prior to discontinuation. Oral antihypertensive agents can be added during fenoldopam infusion (after BP is stable) or following its discontinuation. Patients in clinical trials have received IV fenoldopam for a maximum of 48 h.

Note: Fenoldopam should be administered by continuous IV infusion only. A bolus dose should not be used. The fenoldopam injection ampule concentrate must be diluted with the appropriate amount of 0.9% sodium chloride or 5% dextrose before infusion. See fenoldopam package insert for details on proper dilution.

PATIENT INFORMATION

This drug is used for short-term management of severe hypertension. Adverse effects such as headache, flushing, nausea, and dizziness may occur.

AVAILABILITY

Injection, concentrate—10 mg/mL (5 mL ampules)

HYDRALAZINE
(Hydralazine, Apresoline®)

The predominant effect of hydralazine is direct vasodilatation of arterioles, with only slight effect on veins. Hydralazine reduces peripheral vascular resistance, an action probably important in its antihypertensive effect. The increase in cardiac output, decrease in systemic resistance, and reduction in afterload may explain its efficacy in treating CHF, where, in combination with nitrates, it has been shown to reduce mortality more than prazosin. This combination, however, has since been shown to be less effective in reducing mortality than an ACE inhibitor.

Apparent tolerance to the antihypertensive effects of hydralazine may develop with chronic administration. Concurrent diuretic therapy may decrease this tendency and enhance the antihypertensive effects. Hydralazine does not appear to reverse left ventricular hypertrophy. Lupus erythematosus is a recognized adverse effect that is apparently more frequent in those who are slow to form acetyl derivatives. Despite this effect, the drug is well tolerated when used as a third drug after the concomitant use of a diuretic agent and a beta-blocker.

SPECIAL GROUPS

Race: no differences in response

Children: safety and efficacy have not been established; however, there is experience with the use of hydralazine in children

Elderly: may require reduction in dose or lengthening of dosage interval

Renal impairment: in severe renal impairment, interval between doses should be prolonged to avoid accumulation

Hepatic impairment: may require reduction in dose or lengthening of dosage interval

Pregnancy: category C; use only when potential benefits outweigh potential hazards to the fetus. However, IV hydralazine has been used effectively and generally is considered the parenteral hypotensive agent of choice for the management of hypertensive emergencies associated with pregnancy (*eg*, pre-eclampsia, eclampsia).

Breast-feeding: not recommended; hydralazine is excreted in breast milk

IN BRIEF

INDICATIONS
Essential hypertension (oral formulation)

Severe essential hypertension when the drug cannot be given orally or when the need to lower BP is urgent (parenteral formulation)

CONTRAINDICATIONS/PRECAUTIONS
Hypersensitivity to hydralazine or any of its components, such as tartrazine and sulfites

Mitral valve rheumatic heart disease

Coronary artery disease (use with caution; hydralazine has been implicated in the production of MI)

DRUG INTERACTIONS
Beta-blockers (metoprolol, propranolol)[1,3]

Indomethacin[2]

Monoamine oxidase (MAO) inhibitors[4]

1 Effect/toxicity of hydralazine may increase.
2 Effect of hydralazine may decrease.
3 Hydralazine may increase the effect/toxicity of this drug.
4 Concurrent use may cause a significant decrease in BP.

ADVERSE EFFECTS
Cardiovascular: palpitations, tachycardia, hypotension, angina pectoris

CNS: headache, peripheral neuritis, numbness and tingling, dizziness, tremors, depression, anxiety

GI: nausea, vomiting, anorexia, diarrhea, constipation, paralytic ileus

Hematologic: blood dyscrasias, leukopenia, agranulocytosis and purpura, lymphadenopathy, splenomegaly

Others: nasal congestion, flushing, edema, muscle cramps, dyspnea, urination difficulty, lupuslike syndrome, rash, urticaria, fever, arthralgia, eosinophilia, hepatitis (rare)

PHARMACOKINETICS AND PHARMACODYNAMICS
Duration of action: 6–12 h (oral), 2–4 h (IV)
Onset of action: 45 min (oral), 10–20 min (IV)
Time to peak effect: 1 h (oral), 15–30 min (IV)
Bioavailability: 30%–50%
Effect of food: administration with food results in higher plasma hydralazine concentrations
Protein binding: 87%
Metabolism: hepatic, extensive
Elimination: in urine as active drug (12%–14%) and metabolites
Half-life: 3–7 h

MONITORING
BP, heart rate, antinuclear antibody (ANA) titer determinations, CBC. In addition to the contraindications/precautions listed above, hydralazine should be used with extreme caution in patients with cerebrovascular accidents, pulmonary hypertension, or severe renal damage.

OVERDOSE
Symptoms of overdose include hypotension, tachycardia, headache, and generalized skin flushing. Complications can include myocardial ischemia and subsequent MI, cardiac arrhythmias, and shock. Treatment is primarily supportive and symptomatic. In acute overdose, perform gastric lavage as soon as possible. Supportive measures include the administration of IV fluids. In hypotension, raise pressure without increasing or aggravating tachycardia. Avoid adrenaline use. Tachycardia responds to beta-blockers. Digitalization may be necessary.

HYDRALAZINE (continued)

DOSAGE

Oral: Adults—for hypertension, give 40 mg/d for the first 2–4 d, 100 mg/d for the balance of week 1, and 200 mg/d for week 2 and subsequent weeks in 4 divided daily doses. Maintain dose at lowest effective level. Maximum dose is 300 mg/d. Higher doses have been used in the treatment of CHF.

Children—for hypertension, give 750 µg (0.75 mg)/kg body weight per day divided into 4 doses; increase gradually over 3–4 wk as needed. Maximum dose is 7.5 mg/kg of body weight or 200 mg/d.

Parenteral: Adults—for hypertension, give 10–40 mg IV or intramuscularly (IM); repeat as needed.

Note: Hydralazine injection should be used immediately after the vial is opened. Hydralazine injection should not be added to infusion solutions. Hydralazine injection may discolor upon contact with metal; discolored solutions should be discarded.

Children—for hypertension, give 0.1–0.2 mg/kg/dose IV or IM every 4–6 h as needed.

PATIENT INFORMATION

Take hydralazine with meals. Because this medication may cause dizziness, use caution when driving or performing other activities that require alertness. Notify physician if side effects such as tiredness, fever, muscle or joint aches, or chest pain occur. Do not discontinue therapy without your physician's advice.

AVAILABILITY

Tablets—10 mg, 25 mg, 50 mg, 100 mg
Injection—20 mg/mL (1 mL)
Combination formulations:
Apresazide—hydralazine HCl/hydrochlorothiazide (HCTZ)
  combination capsules
     25 mg/25 mg
     50 mg/50 mg
     100 mg/50 mg
Hydra-Zide—hydralazine HCl/HCTZ combination capsules
  25 mg/25 mg
  50 mg/50 mg
  100 mg/50 mg
Hydrap-ES
Marpres
Ser-Ap-Es
Tri-Hydroserpine
Unipres—reserpine/HCTZ/hydralazine HCl combination tablets
  0.1 mg/15 mg/25 mg

ISOSORBIDE DINITRATE
(Isosorbide dinitrate, Isordil®, Sorbitrate®, Dilatrate®-SR)

Isosorbide dinitrate is an important member of the organic nitrate ester family. Although the exact mechanism of action of the nitrates is not fully known, the principal pharmacologic action of these agents is relaxation of vascular smooth muscle, resulting in generalized vasodilation. Nitrates are well established in the treatment of various cardiovascular disorders, most notably angina pectoris. Attenuation of hemodynamic effects may occur with all long-acting nitrates. Continuous administration tends to promote this tolerance, whereas intermittent administration appears to maintain efficacy.

Isosorbide dinitrate reduces left ventricular preload and afterload because of venous (predominantly) and arterial dilatation, with a more efficient redistribution of blood flow within the myocardium. Because of its venodilatory action, it has been advantageously combined with hydralazine, an arterial vasodilator, to produce a balanced effect leading to a greater reduction in mortality in heart failure than has been seen with prazosin but less of an effect than that seen with ACE inhibitors. Isosorbide dinitrate is available in various formulations. Slow-release formulations are available for prophylaxis, and chewable forms are available to provide rapid absorption and relief of symptoms. Isosorbide dinitrate is indicated for the prophylaxis and treatment of angina. Low-dose nitrate treatment has been regarded as well tolerated in the treatment of acute MI. It improves left ventricular performance, possibly limiting infarct size and reducing complications. However, nitrates should be used under close clinical observation and with hemodynamic monitoring in acute MI. A short-acting form should be used in this setting because its effects can be terminated rapidly should excessive hypotension or tachycardia develop.

SPECIAL GROUPS

Race: no differences in response
Children: safety and effectiveness have not been established
Elderly: lower doses may be required
Renal impairment: dosage adjustment is usually not necessary. Use with caution in severe renal impairment.
Hepatic impairment: lower doses may be advisable; avoid use in severe hepatic impairment
Pregnancy: category C; use only when clearly needed and when potential benefits outweigh potential hazards to the fetus
Breast-feeding: not recommended; nitrates may be excreted in breast milk

IN BRIEF

INDICATIONS
Angina pectoris (treatment and prevention of angina pectoris)

CONTRAINDICATIONS
Hypersensitivity or idiosyncrasy to nitrates
Severe anemia
Closed-angle glaucoma (intraocular pressure may be increased)
Postural hypotension
Head trauma or cerebral hemorrhage (nitrates may increase intracranial pressure)
Concurrent use with phosphodiesterase-5 inhibitors (eg, sildenafil, tadalafil, vardenafil)

DRUG INTERACTIONS
Alcohol[3]
Aspirin[1]
Calcium channel blockers[3]
Dihydroergotamine[2]
Sildenafil[4]
Tadalafil[4]
Vardenafil[4]

1 Effect/toxicity of isosorbide dinitrate may increase.
2 Effect of isosorbide dinitrate may decrease.
3 Concurrent use may increase the risk of hypotension.
4 Concurrent use with nitrates is contraindicated; significant reduction of BP may occur.

ADVERSE EFFECTS
Cardiovascular: hypotension, tachycardia, retrosternal discomfort, palpitations, syncope, arrhythmias, edema
CNS: headache, lightheadedness, dizziness, weakness, anxiety, confusion, insomnia
GI: nausea, vomiting, diarrhea, dyspepsia, dry mouth
Dermatologic: drug rash, pruritus, exfoliative dermatitis, cutaneous vasodilation with flushing
Others: flushing, arthralgia, dysuria, impotence, urinary frequency, hemolytic anemia, asthenia, blurred vision, methemoglobinemia (rare, usually with overdose)

PHARMACOKINETICS AND PHARMACODYNAMICS
Duration of action: oral, 4–6 h; sublingual, 1–2 h; chewable, 0.5–2 h; sustained release, 6–8 h
Onset of action: oral, 20–40 min; sublingual, 2–5 min; chewable, 2–5 min; sustained release, 30 min–4 h
Bioavailability: sublingual, 59%; oral, 22%
Effect of food: for faster absorption, administer oral nitrates on an empty stomach with a glass of water
Protein binding: minimal
Metabolism: hepatic (very rapid and nearly complete) and in blood (enzymatically). Two active metabolites are isosorbide-5-mononitrate and isosorbide-2-mononitrate
Elimination: renal, as metabolites
Half-life: oral, 4 h; sublingual, 1 h

MONITORING
BP, heart rate.

OVERDOSE
Gastric lavage may be useful if the medication has only recently been swallowed. If excessive hypotension occurs, elevate legs to aid venous return. Administer oxygen and artificial ventilation if needed. Monitor methemoglobin concentrations as indicated.

The information here is provided as guidance only. Prescribers should always consult the manufacturer's current prescribing information.

337

ISOSORBIDE DINITRATE *(continued)*

DOSAGE

Oral tablets, short acting (isosorbide dinitrate, Isordil Titradose, Sorbitrate): As an antianginal agent, give 5–20 mg in tablet form 3 times daily; adjust as needed and tolerated. Usual dosage range is 10–40 mg 3 times daily. Elderly may be more sensitive to hypotensive effect. Use with caution in those with impaired hepatic and renal functions; a reduction in dosage may be required.

Note: A daily nitrate-free interval of at least 14 h is advisable to minimize tolerance. The optimal interval will vary with the individual patient, dose, and regimen.

Oral tablets and capsules, sustained-release (isosorbide dinitrate, Dilatrate-SR, Isordil Tembids): Administer sustained-release preparations once daily or twice daily in doses given 6 h apart (*ie*, 8 am and 2 pm). Do not exceed 160 mg/d.

Sublingual and chewable tablets (isosorbide dinitrate, Isordil, Sorbitrate): For angina pectoris, the usual starting dose is 2.5–5 mg for sublingual tablets and 5 mg for chewable tablets. Titrate upward until angina is relieved or when dose-related adverse effects occur. For acute prophylaxis, administer 5–10 mg sublingual or chewable tablets every 2–3 h or 15 minutes before expected activity.

Note: Limit use of sublingual or chewable isosorbide dinitrate for terminating an acute anginal attack in patients intolerant of or unresponsive to sublingual nitroglycerin.

AVAILABILITY

Oral tablets, short acting (isosorbide dinitrate)—5 mg, 10 mg, 20 mg, 30 mg

Oral tablets, short acting (Isordil Titradose, Sorbitrate)—5 mg, 10 mg, 20 mg, 30 mg, 40 mg

Tablets, sublingual (isosorbide dinitrate, Isordil)—2.5 mg, 5 mg, 10 mg

Tablets, sublingual (Sorbitrate)—2.5 mg, 5 mg

Tablets, chewable (Sorbitrate)—5 mg, 10 mg

Tablets, sustained release (isosorbide dinitrate, Isordil Tembids)—40 mg

Capsules, sustained release (Dilatrate-SR, Isordil Tembids)—40 mg

ISOSORBIDE MONONITRATE
(Isosorbide mononitrate, Ismo®, Monoket®, Imdur®)

The active metabolite of isosorbide dinitrate, isosorbide-5-mononitrate, is available for the prophylaxis of angina pectoris. Because it is not subjected to first-pass metabolism in the liver, its bioavailability is almost complete. With an eccentric dosing regimen, the tolerance problem with nitrates may be less prominent, and rebound (early-morning worsening of angina) is less of a problem. Regular formulations for twice-daily dosing and a once-daily extended-release formulation are available. In a placebo-controlled outcomes study, ISIS-4, there was no demonstrable effect of mononitrates on survival in patients with acute MI. The effects of isosorbide mononitrate are difficult to terminate rapidly. Therefore, the use of these agents should be avoided in patients with acute MI or CHF.

SPECIAL GROUPS

Race: no differences in response

Children: safety and effectiveness have not been established

Elderly: lower doses are not usually required. However, older patients may be more susceptible to risks for hypotension.

Renal impairment: dosage adjustment is usually not necessary; use with caution in severe renal impairment

Hepatic impairment: dosage adjustment is usually not necessary; use with caution in severe hepatic impairment

Pregnancy: category C; use only when clearly needed and when potential benefits outweigh potential hazards to the fetus

Breast-feeding: not recommended; nitrates may be excreted in breast milk

DOSAGE

For angina prophylaxis, tablets should be swallowed whole. Administer 20 mg (isosorbide mononitrate tablet, Ismo, Monoket) twice daily with doses given 7 h apart. An initial dose of 5 mg twice daily may be appropriate for persons of small stature. Imdur or isosorbide mononitrate extended-release tablets may be initiated at 30 or 60 mg once daily. Dosage of Imdur or isosorbide mononitrate extended-release tablet may be increased to 120 mg once daily after several days if necessary.

IN BRIEF

INDICATIONS
Angina pectoris (prevention of angina pectoris)

CONTRAINDICATIONS
Hypersensitivity or idiosyncrasy to nitrates

Acute MI with low filling pressures

Severe anemia

Closed-angle glaucoma (intraocular pressure may be increased)

Postural hypotension

Head trauma or cerebral hemorrhage (nitrates may increase intracranial pressure)

Concurrent use with phosphodiesterase-5 inhibitors (eg, sildenafil, tadalafil, vardenafil)

DRUG INTERACTIONS

Alcohol[3]	Sildenafil[4]
Aspirin[1]	Tadalafil[4]
Calcium channel blockers[3]	Vardenafil[4]
Dihydroergotamine[2]	

1 Effect/toxicity of isosorbide mononitrate may increase.

2 Effect of isosorbide mononitrate may decrease.

3 Concurrent use may increase the risk of hypotension.

4 Concurrent use with nitrates is contraindicated; significant reduction of BP may occur.

ADVERSE EFFECTS
Cardiovascular: hypotension, tachycardia, retrosternal discomfort, palpitations, syncope, arrhythmias, edema

CNS: headache, lightheadedness, dizziness, weakness, anxiety, confusion, insomnia

GI: nausea, vomiting, diarrhea, dyspepsia

Dermatologic: drug rash, pruritus, exfoliative dermatitis, cutaneous vasodilation with flushing

Others: flushing, arthralgia, dysuria, impotence, urinary frequency, hemolytic anemia, asthenia, blurred vision, methemoglobinemia (rare, usually with overdose)

PHARMACOKINETICS AND PHARMACODYNAMICS

Duration of action: 1–10 h (Ismo, Monoket); ≈12 h (Imdur). Duration of action may vary because of development of tolerance.

Onset of action: 30–60 min

Time to peak plasma concentration: 30–60 min (Ismo, Monoket); 3–4 h (Imdur)

Bioavailability: ≈100%

Effect of food: concomitant food intake may decrease the rate but not the extent of absorption of isosorbide mononitrate

Protein binding: minimal, <5%

Metabolism: hepatic

Elimination: renal, mainly as inactive metabolites.

Elimination half-life: ≈5 h (Ismo, Monoket); ≈6 h (Imdur)

MONITORING
BP, heart rate.

OVERDOSE
Gastric lavage may be useful if the medication has only recently been swallowed. If excessive hypotension occurs, elevate legs to aid venous return. Administer oxygen and artificial ventilation if needed. Monitor methemoglobin concentrations as indicated.

PATIENT INFORMATION
Extended-release tablets should not be chewed or crushed and should be swallowed together with a half-glassful of fluid. Avoid alcohol. This medication may cause headache, dizziness, flushing, blurred vision, or dry mouth. Notify physician if persistent side effects occur. Do not discontinue therapy without your physician's advice.

AVAILABILITY
Tablets (isosorbide mononitrate, Ismo)—20 mg

Tablets (Monoket)—10 mg, 20 mg

Extended-release tablets (isosorbide mononitrate)—60 mg

Extended-release tablets (Imdur)—30 mg, 60 mg, 120 mg

The information here is provided as guidance only. Prescribers should always consult the manufacturer's current prescribing information.

339

ISOXSUPRINE
(Isoxsuprine, Vasodilan®, Voxsuprine®)

Isoxsuprine is a vasorelaxant that stimulates beta-receptors in the vascular wall. Isoxsuprine produces peripheral vasodilatation through a direct effect on vascular smooth muscle, primarily within skeletal muscle, with a smaller effect on cutaneous blood flow. This drug also causes cardiac stimulation (increased contractility, heart rate, and cardiac output) and uterine relaxation. At high doses, it lowers blood viscosity and inhibits platelet aggregation. Isoxsuprine has been recommended for the treatment of cerebrovascular insufficiency or peripheral vascular disease, but data supporting these claims are very weak. Isoxsuprine has also been used in the management of dysmenorrhea, threatened abortion, and premature labor. However, the efficacy of this agent in the treatment of these conditions has not been established.

SPECIAL GROUPS

Race: no differences in response
Children: safety and efficacy have not been established
Elderly: risk for hypotension may be increased with isoxsuprine; initiate with lower doses
Renal impairment: lower doses may be needed
Hepatic impairment: lower doses may be needed
Pregnancy: category C; use only if the potential benefit justifies the potential risk to the fetus
Breast-feeding: not recommended; isoxsuprine may be excreted in breast milk.

DOSAGE

The usual adult dose is 10–20 mg 3–4 times daily.
Medication may be given with meals to reduce gastrointestinal irritation.

IN BRIEF

INDICATIONS
Relief of symptoms associated with cerebral vascular insufficiency (possibly effective)
Peripheral vascular disease (possibly effective)

CONTRAINDICATIONS
Hypersensitivity
Immediately postpartum; in the presence of arterial bleeding

DRUG INTERACTIONS
Hypotensive agents[1]
1 Concurrent use may increase the risk of hypotension.

ADVERSE EFFECTS
Cardiovascular: hypotension, tachycardia, chest pain
CNS: dizziness, weakness
GI: nausea, vomiting, abdominal distress
Others: rash

PHARMACOKINETICS AND PHARMACODYNAMICS
Time to peak
plasma concentration: within 1 h
Bioavailability: ≈100%
Effect of food: not known
Protein binding: not known
Metabolism: partially conjugated in the liver
Elimination: primarily in urine
Half-life: 1.25 h

MONITORING
BP, heart rate.

OVERDOSE
Symptoms of overdose include hypotension, flushing, and vasodilation. Treat with intravenous fluids. Alpha-adrenergic pressors may be required.

PATIENT INFORMATION
This medication may cause dizziness, use caution when driving or performing other activities that require alertness. Notify physician if persistent side effects occur.

AVAILABILITY
Tablets—10 mg, 20 mg

MINOXIDIL (Minoxidil, Loniten®, Rogaine®)

Minoxidil is a direct-acting peripheral vasodilator. Although minoxidil is indicated for the treatment of hypertension, it has serious side effects and is, therefore, not considered a primary agent in treating essential hypertension. It is recommended for use only in patients with symptomatic or organ-damaging hypertension not responsive to other treatment. Its exact mechanism of action is unknown, but some of its action may be the result of the opening of potassium channels in smooth muscle cells. Its predominant effect is direct vasodilatation of arterioles, with marginal effects on veins. Minoxidil reduces peripheral resistance and causes a reflex increase in heart rate and cardiac output. It should not be used as the sole agent to initiate therapy. Rather, it should be given in conjunction with both a diuretic, to control salt and water retention, and a beta-blocker, to control reflex tachycardia.

SPECIAL GROUPS

Race:	no differences in response
Children:	safety and efficacy have not been established; however, there is experience with the use of minoxidil in children
Elderly:	may be more sensitive to hypotensive effects; lower doses may be required
Renal impairment:	lower doses may be required
Hepatic impairment:	dosage adjustment is usually not necessary
Pregnancy:	category C; use only when clearly needed and when potential benefits outweigh potential hazards to the fetus
Breast-feeding:	not recommended; minoxidil is excreted in breast milk

DOSAGE

Oral: Adults and children 12 years of age or older—usual initial dose is 5 mg/d as a single dose; may be increased by 10 mg every 3 d (seldom necessary to exceed 50 mg/d). Usual maintenance dose is 10–40 mg/day in 1–2 divided doses. Maximum dose is 100 mg/d.

Children—for children under 12 y, the usual initial dose is 0.1–0.2 mg/kg once daily; maximum initial dose is 5 mg/d. Increase gradually every 3 d as needed and tolerated. Usual maintenance dose is 0.25–1 mg/kg/d in 1–2 divided doses. Maximum dose is 50 mg/d.

Topical: Apply 1 mL to affected areas of the scalp twice daily (morning and night). Wash hands after applying.

IN BRIEF

INDICATIONS
Severe hypertension (oral formulation)
Resistant or refractory hypertension (oral formulation)
Male-pattern baldness of the vertex of the scalp (topical formulations)

CONTRAINDICATIONS
Hypersensitivity
Pheochromocytoma
Acute MI
Dissecting aortic aneurysm

DRUG INTERACTIONS
Guanethidine[1]
Other hypotensive agents[2]

1 Concurrent use may result in profound orthostatic hypotension.
2 Concurrent use may cause additive hypotensive effect.

ADVERSE EFFECTS
Cardiovascular: ECG changes, tachycardia, CHF, hypotension, edema, pericardial effusion and tamponade (<1%)
CNS: headache, fatigue
GI: nausea, vomiting
Hematologic: transient hematocrit and hemoglobin decrease, thrombocytopenia (<1%), leukopenia (rare)
Others: rash, breast tenderness, hypertrichosis, fluid and electrolyte imbalance

PHARMACOKINETICS AND PHARMACODYNAMICS
Duration of action:	up to 100 h (oral)
Onset of action:	30 min (oral)
Time to peak effect:	within 2–8 h (oral)
Bioavailability:	90% (oral); 1%–4% (topical)
Effect of food:	not known
Protein binding:	not significant
Metabolism:	hepatic, 90%; predominantly by conjugation with glucuronic acid; metabolites exert much less pharmacologic effect than the parent drug (oral)
Elimination:	primarily in the urine (12% as unchanged drug)
Elimination half-life:	4.2 h

MONITORING
BP, heart rate, CBC, electrolytes, body weight.

OVERDOSE
If marked hypotension occurs, give normal saline intravenously.
Avoid epinephrine and norepinephrine because of their stimulant effects on the heart.
Use vasopressors such as phenylephrine, vasopressin, and dopamine only if a vital organ is underperfused.

PATIENT INFORMATION
If the topical formulation of this product is prescribed, apply to affected areas of the scalp twice daily. Wash hands after applying. Hair growth usually takes 4 mo. The oral formulation of this medication may cause dizziness, use caution when performing tasks that require alertness. Get up slowly from a sitting or lying position. Notify physician if persistent side effects occur (ie, increased heart rate; rapid weight gain; unusual swelling of extremities, face, or abdomen; breathing difficulty, especially when lying down; chest pain). Do not discontinue therapy without your physician's advice.

AVAILABILITY
Tablets—2.5 mg, 10 mg
Topical solution—2% (60 mL), 5% (60 mL)

The information here is provided as guidance only. Prescribers should always consult the manufacturer's current prescribing information.

341

NESIRITIDE (Natrecor®)

Nesiritide is a recombinant form of human brain natriuretic peptide (BNP) that is structurally and biochemically identical to endogenously produced BNP. The pharmacodynamic effects of nesiritide mimic the biologic effects of BNP. Clinical studies on patients who had acute decompensated heart failure demonstrated rapid-onset dose-related vasodilatory effects. In the Vasodilation in the Management of Acute Congestive Heart Failure (VMAC) study, nesiritide was shown to decrease pulmonary capillary wedge pressure to a greater extent compared with nitroglycerin and placebo in hospitalized patients with acutely decompensated CHF. Although nesiritide led to improvement in dyspnea compared with placebo at 3 hours post initiation of study treatments, there was no significant difference in dyspnea or global clinical status with nesiritide compared with nitroglycerin.

Nesiritide decreases preload and afterload and suppresses the renin-angiotensin-aldosterone axis and the release of norepinephrine. In addition, nesiritide promotes diuresis and has no proarrhythmic effects. Nesiritide appears to be a valuable therapeutic option in the treatment of patients hospitalized for decompensated heart failure. Further studies are needed to evaluate nesiritide's effects on long-term morbidity and mortality as well as any potential pharmacoeconomic benefits in heart failure management.

SPECIAL GROUPS

Race: clearance is not influenced significantly by race/ethnicity
Children: safety and effectiveness have not been established
Elderly: no dosage adjustment is required
Renal impairment: no dosage adjustment is required
Hepatic impairment: cirrhotic patients with ascites and avid sodium retention were shown to have blunted natriuretic response to low-dose BNP
Pregnancy: category C; use only if potential benefit justifies potential risk to the fetus
Breast-feeding: not recommended; may be excreted in breast milk

DOSAGE

The recommended dose of nesiritide is an IV bolus of 2 µg/kg followed by a continuous infusion of 0.01 µg/kg/min. Nesiritide should not be initiated at a dose that is above the recommended dose. The dose-limiting side effect is hypotension. BP should be monitored closely during administration. If hypotension occurs during the administration of nesiritide, the dose should be reduced or discontinued and other measures to support BP should be started (IV fluids, changes in body position). In the VMAC trial, when symptomatic hypotension occurred, nesiritide was discontinued and subsequently could be restarted at a dose that was reduced by 30% (with no bolus administration) once the patient was stabilized.

In the VMAC trial, there was limited experience with increasing the dose of nesiritide above the recommended dose. In those patients, the infusion dose of nesiritide was increased by 0.005 µg/kg/min (preceded by a bolus of 1 µg/kg), no more frequently than every 3 h up to a maximum dose of 0.03 µg/kg/min.

IN BRIEF

INDICATIONS
Treatment of patients with acutely decompensated CHF who have dyspnea at rest or with minimal activity.

CONTRAINDICATIONS/WARNINGS
Hypersensitivity
Cardiogenic shock
Systolic BP <90 mm Hg
Low cardiac filling pressures

DRUG INTERACTION
ACE inhibitors[1]

1 Concomitant therapy may cause an increase in symptomatic hypotension.

ADVERSE EFFECTS
Cardiovascular: hypotension (11%), ventricular tachycardia (3%), ventricular extrasystoles (3%), angina pectoris (2%), bradycardia (1%), tachycardia, atrial fibrillation, atrioventricular (AV) node conduction abnormalities
CNS: headache (8%), dizziness (3%), insomnia (2%), anxiety (3%)
GI: nausea (4%), abdominal pain, vomiting
Respiratory: cough (increased), hemoptysis, apnea
Dermatologic: pruritus, rash
Neuromuscular and skeletal: back pain (4%), leg cramps
Renal: increased serum creatinine

PHARMACOKINETICS AND PHARMACODYNAMICS
Duration of action: 0.5–2 h (hemodynamic improvement)
Onset of action: 15–30 min (hemodynamic improvement)
Volume of distribution: 0.19 L/kg (at steady state)
Elimination: Human BNP is cleared from the circulation via 1) binding to cell surface clearance receptors with subsequent cellular internalization and lysosomal proteolysis; 2) proteolytic cleavage of the peptide by endopeptidases, such as neutral endopeptidase; 3) renal filtration.
Elimination half-life: 18 min (terminal elimination half-life)

MONITORING
BP, hemodynamic responses (pulmonary capillary wedge pressure, right atrial pressure, cardiac index)

OVERDOSE
The expected reaction would be excessive hypotension, which should be treated with drug discontinuation or reduction and appropriate measures.

PATIENT INFORMATION
This medication is administered intravenously. The patient will be closely monitored during and following infusion, and told to remain in bed until advised otherwise. Immediately report headache, dizziness, chest pain, palpitations, and/or other side effects if they occur.

AVAILABILITY
Sterile lyophilized powder—1.5 mg single-use vials

NITROGLYCERIN

(Nitroglycerin, Tridil®, Nitro-Bid®, Nitrostat®, Nitrolingual®, Nitrong®, Minitran®, Nitro-Dur®, Nitro-Time®)

Nitroglycerin has been the mainstay in the acute management of angina pectoris for many years. It reduces left ventricular preload and afterload because of venous (predominantly) and arterial dilatation, with a beneficial redistribution of blood flow within the myocardium. It may be successfully combined with other vasodilators and is available as parenteral, capsule, tablet, topical, sublingual, aerosol, ointment, and transdermal formulations. As with all other nitrate formulations, nitroglycerin is associated with pharmacologic tolerance and with continued use, must be administered intermittently. Low-dose treatment with IV nitroglycerin has been regarded as safe and effective for use after MI. Its use results in reduced infarct size and improved left ventricular performance.

SPECIAL GROUPS

Race: no differences in response
Children: safety and effectiveness have not been established
Elderly: lower doses may be required
Renal impairment: dosage adjustment is usually not necessary; use with caution in severe renal impairment
Hepatic impairment: lower doses may be advisable; avoid use in severe hepatic impairment
Pregnancy: category C; use only when clearly needed and when potential benefits outweigh potential hazards to the fetus
Breast-feeding: not recommended; nitrates may be excreted in breast milk

DOSAGE

Sublingual tablets (Nitrostat): Dissolve one tablet under the tongue or in the buccal pouch (between cheek and gum) at first sign of an acute anginal attack. Repeat approximately every 5 min until relief is obtained. No more than 3 tablets should be taken in 15 min. If pain persists, notify physician or get to emergency room immediately. Sublingual tablets also may be used prophylactically 5–10 min prior to activities that might trigger an acute attack.

Note: Although the traditional recommendation is for patients to take 1 nitroglycerin dose sublingually, 5 minutes apart, for up to 3 doses before calling for emergency evaluation, this recommendation has been modified to encourage earlier contacting of emergency medical services (EMS) by patients with symptoms suggestive of ST-elevation myocardial infarction. According to the American College of Cardiology/American Heart Association guidelines for the management of patients with ST-elevation myocardial infarction (published in 2004), healthcare providers should instruct patients for whom nitroglycerin has been prescribed previously to take ONE nitroglycerin dose sublingually in response to chest discomfort/pain. If chest discomfort/pain is unimproved or worsening 5 minutes after 1 sublingual nitroglycerin dose has been taken, it is recommended that the patient or family member/friend call 9-1-1 immediately to access EMS.

IN BRIEF

INDICATIONS
Prevention of angina pectoris (oral sustained-release tablets and capsules, transdermal system)
Prevention and treatment of angina pectoris (sublingual tablets, translingual spray, topical ointment)
Control of BP in perioperative hypertension (IV)
CHF associated with acute MI (IV)
Angina pectoris unresponsive to recommended doses of organic nitrates or beta-blockers (IV)
Controlled hypotension during surgical procedures (IV)

CONTRAINDICATIONS
Hypersensitivity or idiosyncrasy to nitrates
Severe anemia
Closed-angle glaucoma (intraocular pressure may be increased)
Postural hypotension
Head trauma or cerebral hemorrhage (nitrates may increase intracranial pressure)
Increased intracranial pressure
Concurrent use with phosphodiesterase-5 inhibitors (eg, sildenafil, tadalafil, vardenafil)
Hypotension or uncorrected hypovolemia (IV)
Cerebral ischemia (IV)
Constrictive pericarditis (IV)
Pericardial tamponade (IV)

DRUG INTERACTIONS
Alcohol[3]
Aspirin[1]
Calcium channel blockers[3]
Dihydroergotamine[2]
Heparin[5]
Sildenafil[4]
Tadalafil[4]
Vardenafil[4]

1 Effect/toxicity of nitroglycerin may increase.
2 Effect of nitroglycerin may decrease.
3 Concurrent use may increase the risk of hypotension.
4 Concurrent use with nitrates is contraindicated; significant reduction of BP may occur.
5 The effect of heparin may decrease.

ADVERSE EFFECTS
Cardiovascular: hypotension, tachycardia, retrosternal discomfort, palpitations, syncope, arrhythmias, edema
CNS: headache, lightheadedness, dizziness, weakness, anxiety, confusion, insomnia
GI: nausea, vomiting, diarrhea, dyspepsia
Dermatologic: drug rash, pruritus, exfoliative dermatitis, contact dermatitis (transdermal systems), cutaneous vasodilation with flushing
Others: flushing, arthralgia, dysuria, impotence, urinary frequency, hemolytic anemia, asthenia, blurred vision, methemoglobinemia (rare, usually with overdose)

The information here is provided as guidance only. Prescribers should always consult the manufacturer's current prescribing information.

343

NITROGLYCERIN (continued)

DOSAGE (continued)

Translingual spray (Nitrolingual): At the onset of an attack, spray 1–2 metered doses into mouth under the tongue. No more than 3 metered doses should be administered within 15 min. If chest pain continues, seek immediate medical attention. Translingual spray also may be used prophylactically 5–10 min before engaging in activities that might trigger an acute attack. Do not inhale spray. Please also see **Note** under sublingual tablets.

Sustained-release capsules (nitroglycerin, Nitro-Time): Initiate with 2.5 mg 3 times daily. Titrate upward to an effective dose or until dose-related adverse effects occur.

Note: Tolerance may develop when nitroglycerin is administered without a nitrate-free interval. Consider administering on a reduced schedule (once or twice daily).

Sustained-release tablets (Nitrong): Initiate with 2.6 mg 3 times daily. Titrate upward to an effective dose or until dose-related adverse effects occur.

Note: Tolerance may develop when nitroglycerin is administered without a nitrate-free interval. Consider administering on a reduced schedule (once or twice daily).

Topical ointment (nitroglycerin, Nitro-Bid): Initiate at 7.5 mg (one-half in) every 8 h, increasing by one-half inch per application every 6 h to a maximum of 75 mg (5 in) per application every 4 h.

Note: Any regimen of nitroglycerin ointment administration should include a daily nitrate-free interval of about 10–12 h to avoid tolerance. To apply the ointment using the dose-measuring paper applicator, place the applicator on a flat surface, printed side down. Squeeze the necessary amount of ointment from the tube onto the applicator, place the applicator (ointment side down) on the desired area of skin (usually on nonhairy skin of chest or back), and tape the applicator into place. Do not rub in.

Transdermal systems (nitroglycerin transdermal, Minitran, Nitro-Dur): Initiate with a 0.1 or 0.2 mg/h patch. Apply patch for 12–14 h; remove for 10–12 h before applying a new patch. Patch should be applied to clean, dry, hairless skin of chest, inner upper arm, or shoulder. Avoid placing below knee or elbow. Vary site of placement to decrease skin irritation. Apply a new patch if the first patch loosens or falls off.

IV (nitroglycerin I.V., Tridil I.V., Nitro-Bid I.V., nitroglycerin in 5% dextrose): Initiate IV infusion at 5 μg/min; increase by increments of 5 μg/min at 3–5 min intervals until desired effect is obtained or to 20 μg/min. Dosage may be increased beyond 20 μg/min by 10 μg/min increments at 3–5 min intervals, then by 20 μg/min increments until desired effect is reached. Reduce dosage increments and frequency of dosage increments as partial effect is noted. There is no fixed optimum dose. Continuously monitor physiologic parameters such as BP and heart rate and other measurements, such as pulmonary capillary wedge pressure, to achieve accurate dose. Maintain adequate blood and coronary perfusion pressures.

Note: IV infusion is not direct, but must be given through a special nonpolyvinylchloride (non-PVC) IV infusion set or infusion pump. Refer to manufacturer's package insert for instructions on dilution and administration of IV nitroglycerin. Do not administer with other medications.

PHARMACOKINETICS AND PHARMACODYNAMICS

Dosage form	Onset of action	Duration
Sublingual tablet	1–3 min	30–60 min
Translingual spray	2 min	30–60 min
Sustained release	20–45 min	3–8 h
Topical ointment	15–60 min	2–12 h
Transdermal system	30–60 min	8–24 h
IV	Immediate	3–5 min

Note: The duration of action of nitroglycerin may vary because of development of tolerance.

Bioavailability: variable
Effect of food: not known
Protein binding: 60%
Metabolism: hepatic (very rapid and nearly complete) and in blood (enzymatically). Oral dosage forms undergo extensive first-pass metabolism
Elimination: renal, as metabolites
Elimination half-life: 1–4 min

MONITORING
BP, heart rate.

OVERDOSE
Gastric lavage may be useful if the medication has only recently been swallowed. Treat severe hypotension and reflex tachycardia by elevating the legs and administering IV fluids. The rapid metabolism of nitroglycerin usually makes additional measures unnecessary. However, if additional correction of severe hypotension is needed, administration of an IV alpha-adrenergic agonist such as methoxamine or phenylephrine may be considered. Epinephrine should be avoided because it aggravates the shocklike reaction. Methemoglobin concentrations in blood should be monitored and methemoglobinemia treated with high-flow oxygen and IV methylene blue.

PATIENT INFORMATION
Do not chew or crush sustained-release dosage form.
Do not swallow or chew sublingual form. To avoid falling, use sublingual tablets or translingual spray only when sitting or lying down. Keep tablets and capsules in original container; keep tightly closed. Do not change from one brand of this drug to another without consulting your physician or pharmacist. Avoid alcohol. This medication may cause headache, dizziness, flushing, blurred vision, or dry mouth. Notify physician if persistent side effects occur. Do not discontinue therapy without your physician's advice.
(In addition, please look under the dosage section for administration instructions for various nitroglycerin dosage forms.)

AVAILABILITY
Sublingual tablets (Nitrostat)—0.15 mg, 0.3 mg, 0.4 mg, 0.6 mg
Translingual spray (Nitrolingual)—0.4 mg per metered dose
Capsules, sustained release (nitroglycerin, Nitro-Time)—2.5 mg, 6.5 mg, 9 mg
Tablets, sustained release (Nitrong)—2.6 mg, 6.5 mg, 9 mg
Topical ointment (nitroglycerin, Nitro-Bid)—2% in a lanolin petrolatum base
Transdermal systems (nitroglycerin)—0.2 mg/h, 0.4 mg/h, 0.6 mg/h
Transdermal system (Nitro-Dur)—0.3 mg/h
Transdermal systems (Minitran, Nitro-Dur)—0.1 mg/h, 0.2 mg/h, 0.4 mg/h, 0.6 mg/h
Transdermal systems (Nitro-Dur)—0.8 mg/h
IV (nitroglycerin I.V., Nitro-Bid I.V., Tridil I.V.)—5 mg/mL (1, 5, and 10 mL vials)
IV (Tridil I.V.)—0.5 mg/mL, 10 mL ampules
IV (nitroglycerin in 5% dextrose)—25 mg in 250 mL, 50 mg in 250 and 500 mL, 100 mg in 250 mL, 200 mg in 500 mL)

SODIUM NITROPRUSSIDE
(Sodium nitroprusside, Nitropress®)

Nitroprusside is a potent and rapidly acting vasodilator. It is effective only when given intravenously and is used for the acute management of hypertensive crises, heart failure, or during surgery when elective hypotension is desirable. It acts on both peripheral arterial and venous vessels. Its effects are dose related and depend on the preexisting hemodynamic state of the patient. In hypertensive and normotensive patients, a slight increase in heart rate is observed with a slight reduction in cardiac output. In those with heart failure, substantial improvements in left ventricular performance are seen, together with a slight reduction in heart rate and a reduction in arrhythmias.

Because nitroprusside is metabolized rapidly to cyanogen (cyanide radical) and then to thiocyanate in the liver, care must be taken to ensure that the dosage rate does not exceed the capacity of the body to remove the cyanide radical; if this happens, toxicity manifest as coma, dilated pupils, pink coloration of the skin, and weak vital signs may result. For this reason, thiocyanate concentrations should be monitored periodically in patients with renal insufficiency and in those receiving prolonged infusion of sodium nitroprusside (>48–72 h).

SPECIAL GROUPS

Race: no differences in response

Children: appropriate studies have not been performed; however, pediatric-specific problems that would limit the usefulness of this agent in children are not expected

Elderly: may be more sensitive to hypotensive effects; age-related renal impairment is also more likely to exist; use with caution

Renal impairment: dosage may have to be reduced because excretion of thiocyanate is reduced; use with caution

Hepatic impairment: dosage may have to be reduced because hepatic enzymes are involved in the metabolism of cyanide; use with caution

Pregnancy: category C; administer to a pregnant woman only if clearly needed; use only when potential benefits outweigh potential hazards to the fetus

Breast-feeding: not recommended; nitroprusside and its metabolites may be excreted in breast milk

IN BRIEF

INDICATIONS
Hypertensive crises
Controlled hypotension during surgery to reduce bleeding into the surgical field
Acute CHF

CONTRAINDICATIONS/PRECAUTIONS
Hypersensitivity
To produce hypotension during surgery in patients with known inadequate cerebral circulation or in moribund patients coming to emergency surgery
Increased intracranial pressure (use with extreme caution)
Treatment of compensatory hypertension (arteriovenous shunting, coarctation of the aorta)
Congenital (Leber's) optic atrophy
Tobacco amblyopia
Acute CHF associated with reduced peripheral vascular resistance, such as high-output heart failure that may be seen in endotoxic sepsis

DRUG INTERACTIONS
Hypotension-producing medications[1]
[1] Concurrent use may increase the risk of hypotension.

ADVERSE EFFECTS
Cardiovascular: hypotension, palpitations, substernal distress, ECG changes, bradycardia, tachycardia
CNS: disorientation, headache, dizziness, restlessness
GI: nausea, vomiting, abdominal pain
Hematologic: decreased platelet aggregation, methemoglobinemia
Others: flushing, diaphoresis, irritation at the infusion site, hypothyroidism, increased intracranial pressure, tinnitus, muscle twitching, thiocyanate toxicity

PHARMACOKINETICS AND PHARMACODYNAMICS
Duration of action: 1–10 min after infusion is stopped
Onset of action: almost immediate
Time to peak effect: almost immediate
Protein binding: not known
Metabolism: nitroprusside is metabolized by an enzyme present in red blood cells to cyanide ions with subsequent metabolism in the liver and the kidney, by the enzyme rhodanase, to thiocyanate
Elimination: thiocyanate is eliminated renally
Elimination half-life: parent drug: 3–4 min
thiocyanate: 3–4 d with normal renal function; half-life increases as renal function decreases

MONITORING
BP, heart rate, ECG, acid–base status, serum thiocyanate concentrations (during prolonged infusion or in patients with renal impairment), serum cyanide concentrations (in patients with decreased hepatic function), methemoglobin concentrations.

OVERDOSE
Signs of excessive hypotension usually disappear if infusion rate is slowed or temporarily discontinued.
If signs and symptoms of thiocyanate toxicity occur, discontinue drug therapy.
Treat massive overdose and signs and symptoms of cyanide toxicity immediately. Serum cyanide concentrations may be reduced by IV infusions of sodium nitrate and sodium thiosulfate.

SODIUM NITROPRUSSIDE *(continued)*

AVAILABILITY
Injection, solution—25 mg/mL (2 mL)

DOSAGE

Adults: The usual initial dose is 0.3 µg/kg/min (range, 0.1–0.5 µg/kg/min) IV infusion; may be adjusted slowly in increments of 0.5 µg/kg/min according to response. Usual dose is 3 µg/kg/min. The maximum recommended infusion rate is 10 µg/kg/min. Infusion at the maximum dose rate (10 µg/kg/min) should never last for more than 10 min. To keep the steady-state thiocyanate concentration below 1 mmol/L, the rate of a prolonged infusion should not exceed 3 µg/kg/min (1 µg/kg/min in anuric patients). When >500 µg/kg of nitroprusside is administered faster than 2 µg/kg/min, cyanide is generated faster than the unaided patient can eliminate it.

Note: After reconstitution with appropriate diluent, sodium nitroprusside injection is not suitable for direct injection. The reconstituted solution must be further diluted in the appropriate amount of sterile 5% dextrose injection before infusion. Protect the diluted solution from light by promptly wrapping the medication container with the supplied opaque sleeve, aluminum foil, or other opaque material. Sodium nitroprusside should not be infused through an ordinary IV apparatus, regulated only by gravity and mechanical clamps. Only an infusion pump, preferably a volumetric pump, should be used. Refer to manufacturer's package insert for complete prescribing information.

PAPAVERINE (Papaverine, Para-Time SR®)

Papaverine hydrochloride is a benzylisoquinoline alkaloid. It may be prepared synthetically or derived from opium. In contrast to morphine, the principal opium alkaloid, papaverine usually does not lead to tolerance or addiction. Papaverine has little effect on the central nervous system, although large doses may cause sedation and sleepiness in some patients. The major therapeutic action of papaverine is its spasmolytic effect on smooth muscles, which is most pronounced on blood vessels including the coronary, cerebral, pulmonary, and peripheral arteries. By depressing cardiac conduction, prolonging the refractory period, and depressing the excitability of the myocardium, papaverine induces relaxation of the cardiac muscle. Papaverine also relaxes smooth muscles of the bronchi, gastrointestinal tract, ureters, and biliary system. At present, the oral formulation of papaverine is indicated for the relief of cerebral and peripheral ischemia associated with arterial spasm and myocardial ischemia complicated by arrhythmias.

SPECIAL GROUPS

Race: no differences in response
Children: safety and efficacy have not been established
Elderly: lower doses may be required
Renal impairment: lower doses may be required
Hepatic impairment: lower doses may be required
Pregnancy: category C; use only when clearly needed and when the potential benefits outweigh the potential harm to the fetus
Breast-feeding: not recommended; papaverine may be excreted in breast milk

DOSAGE

Oral, sustained release: 150 mg every 12 h; 150 mg every 8 h or 300 mg every 12 h may be given in difficult cases
Note: It is uncertain if effective plasma concentrations are maintained for 12 h with sustained-release preparations. In the past, the FDA has recommended that papaverine products be withdrawn from the market.

IN BRIEF

INDICATIONS
Oral formulations: Relief of peripheral and cerebral ischemia associated with arterial spasm and myocardial ischemia complicated by arrhythmias

CONTRAINDICATIONS
Hypersensitivity to papaverine or its components
Complete AV heart block

DRUG INTERACTIONS
Levodopa[1]

1 Effect of levodopa may decrease.

ADVERSE EFFECTS
Cardiovascular: tachycardia, arrhythmia, mild hypertension
CNS: vertigo, drowsiness, sedation, headache
GI: nausea, abdominal discomfort, anorexia, constipation, diarrhea
Others: flushing, sweating, skin rash, malaise, hepatic hypersensitivity, chronic hepatitis

PHARMACOKINETICS AND PHARMACODYNAMICS
Duration of action: up to 12 h (sustained release)
Onset of action: rapid
Time to peak plasma concentration: 1–2 h
Bioavailability: 30%–54%
Effect of food: not known
Protein binding: 90%
Metabolism: hepatic
Elimination: papaverine is excreted in the urine primarily as inactive metabolites
Elimination half-life: estimates of papaverine's biologic half-life vary widely; however, reasonably constant plasma concentrations can be maintained after 4 d with regular administration at 6 h intervals

MONITORING
BP, heart rate, ECG, liver function test. Use with caution in patients with glaucoma.

OVERDOSE
In case of papaverine overdose, the patient's airway should be protected and ventilation and perfusion supported. Carefully monitor vital signs, blood gases, and blood chemistry values. If seizures occur, they may be managed with diazepam, phenytoin, or phenobarbital. Administration of IV fluids and/or a vasopressor and elevation of the patient's legs may be used to treat hypotension. Calcium gluconate may be useful for the treatment of papaverine-induced adverse cardiac effects. Plasma calcium concentrations and ECG should be monitored. It is not known if papaverine is removed by hemodialysis.

PATIENT INFORMATION
The sustained-release capsules must be swallowed whole, without crushing, dividing, or chewing. This medication may cause dizziness, drowsiness, nausea, flushing, and headache. Use caution when driving or performing other tasks that require alertness. Avoid alcohol intake. Notify physician if persistent side effects occur.

AVAILABILITY
Capsules, sustained release—150 mg

PENTOXIFYLLINE
(Pentoxifylline, Pentoxil®, Trental®)

Pentoxifylline is thought to decrease blood viscosity and improve erythrocyte flexibility, microcirculatory flow, and tissue oxygen concentrations. Improvement in erythrocyte flexibility appears to be caused by inhibition of phosphodiesterase and a resultant increase in cAMP in red blood cells. Reduction in blood viscosity may be the result of decreased plasma fibrinogen concentrations and inhibition of red blood cells and platelet aggregation. Pentoxifylline has modest efficacy in improving treadmill exercise performance in patients with intermittent claudication. Before the approval of cilostazol, this agent was the only approved claudication drug in the United States.

SPECIAL GROUPS
Race: no differences in response
Children: safety and efficacy have not been established
Elderly: use usual dose with caution; dose reduction may be necessary
Renal impairment: lower doses may be required
Hepatic impairment: dosage adjustment is usually not necessary
Pregnancy: category C; use only when clearly needed and when potential benefits outweigh potential hazards to the fetus
Breast-feeding: not recommended; pentoxifylline and its metabolites are excreted in breast milk

DOSAGE
Usual initial dose is 400 mg 3 times daily with meals, reduced to 400 mg twice daily if gastrointestinal or central nervous system side effects occur. Although therapeutic effects may be observed within 2–4 wk, continue treatment for ≥8 wk.

IN BRIEF

INDICATIONS
Intermittent claudication

CONTRAINDICATIONS
Hypersensitivity, intolerance to pentoxifylline or methylxanthines (eg, caffeine, theophylline)
Recent cerebral and/or retinal hemorrhage

DRUG INTERACTIONS
Antihypertensive agents[2]
Cimetidine[1]
Theophylline[2]
Warfarin[2]

1 Effect/toxicity of pentoxifylline may increase.
2 Pentoxifylline may increase the effect/toxicity of this drug.

ADVERSE EFFECTS
Cardiovascular: angina/chest pain, edema, hypotension, arrhythmia (rare)
CNS: dizziness, headache, seizures (<1%)
GI: dyspepsia, nausea, vomiting

PHARMACOKINETICS AND PHARMACODYNAMICS
Duration of action: not known
Onset of action: multiple doses, 2–4 wk
Bioavailability: 20%
Effect of food: food intake delays absorption, but does not affect total absorption
Protein binding: bound to erythrocyte membrane, 45%
Metabolism: liver, extensive; erythrocytes, minor
Elimination: primarily in urine
Elimination half-life: 24–48 min, parent drug; 60–96 min, metabolites

MONITORING
BP, heart rate, maximal walking distance.

OVERDOSE
Symptoms of overdose include hypotension, flushing, seizures, somnolence, loss of consciousness, agitation, bradycardia, and AV block. Treatment is supportive and symptomatic.

PATIENT INFORMATION
Take this medication with food or meals. If gastrointestinal or central nervous system side effects (ie, dizziness, headache, indigestion, nausea, and vomiting) continue, contact physician. Although improvement may be experienced in 2–4 wk, continue treatment for at least 8 wk. Do not discontinue therapy without your physician's advice.

AVAILABILITY
Tablets, controlled release (Trental)—400 mg
Tablets, extended release (pentoxifylline, Pentoxil)—400 mg

TREPROSTINIL (Remodulin™)

Treprostinil is a direct dilator of both pulmonary and systemic arterial vascular beds; it also inhibits platelet aggregation. This agent has recently been approved for the treatment of pulmonary arterial hypertension (PAH). Treprostinil is a tricyclic benzidine analog of epoprostenol. This alteration in chemical structure resulted in an increase in half-life, the ability for subcutaneous delivery, and stability at room temperature. Pooled results from two 12-week clinical trials involving 469 patients with PAH showed that patients who received treprostinil had a lesser reduction in exercise performance and greater improvement in hemodynamic parameters compared with patients who received placebo. The most common adverse events, experienced by 80% to 90% of patients receiving treprostinil in clinical trials, consisted of infusion site pain, infusion site reactions, and bleeding or bruising at the site of the reaction. No significant drug interactions have been observed with treprostinil. However, the effects of agents that may reduce BP or the effects of anticoagulants may be potentiated by treprostinil.

SPECIAL GROUPS

Race: no data
Children: safety and efficacy have not been established
Elderly: use usual dose with caution
Renal impairment: use usual dose with caution. No specific dosage adjustment is recommended.
Hepatic impairment: initiate therapy with lower dose in patients with mild or moderate hepatic insufficiency. Treprostinil has not been studied in patients with severe hepatic insufficiency.
Pregnancy: category B; use during pregnancy only if clearly needed
Breast-feeding: not recommended; may be excreted in breast milk

DOSAGE

Treprostinil is administered by continuous subcutaneous infusion. The infusion rate is initiated at 1.25 ng/kg/min. If this initial dose is not tolerated, the infusion rate should be reduced to 0.625 ng/kg/min. Increase the infusion rate in increments of no more than 1.25 ng/kg/min/wk for the first 4 wk and then no more than 2.5 ng/kg/min/wk for the remaining duration of infusion, based on clinical response. There is little experience with doses >40 ng/kg/min. Avoid abrupt withdrawal or sudden large reductions in dosage of treprostinil, as they may result in worsening of PAH symptoms. In patients with mild or moderate hepatic impairment, decrease the initial dose to 0.625 ng/kg/min ideal body weight and increase cautiously. This drug has not been studied in patients with severe hepatic insufficiency.

IN BRIEF

INDICATIONS
As a continuous subcutaneous infusion for the treatment of PAH in patients with NYHA class II–IV symptoms to diminish symptoms associated with exercise.

CONTRAINDICATIONS/WARNINGS
Hypersensitivity, use caution in patients with renal or hepatic impairment

DRUG INTERACTIONS
Anticoagulants[1]
Antihypertensive agents[2]
Diuretics[2]
Vasodilators[2]

1 Treprostinil may increase the effect/toxicity of this drug.
2 May increase the risk of hypotension.

ADVERSE EFFECTS
Cardiovascular: vasodilation (11%), edema (9%), hypotension (4%)
CNS: headache (27%), dizziness (9%)
Dermatologic: rash (14%), pruritus (8%)
GI: diarrhea (25%), nausea (22%)
Local: infusion site pain (85%), infusion site reaction (83%)
Others: jaw pain (13%)

PHARMACOKINETICS AND PHARMACODYNAMICS
Absorption: subcutaneous: relatively rapid and complete
Bioavailability: ≈100%
Protein binding: 91%
Volume of distribution: 14 L/70 kg ideal body weight
Metabolism: hepatic (enzymes unknown); forms metabolites
Elimination: urine (4% as unchanged drug; 64% as metabolites); feces (13%)
Elimination half-life: 2–4 h

MONITORING
Dyspnea, fatigue, and activity tolerance.
Note: Treprostinil is a potent pulmonary and systemic vasodilator. Initiation of treprostinil must be performed in a setting with adequate personnel and equipment for physiologic monitoring and emergency care.

OVERDOSE
Signs and symptoms of overdose with treprostinil during clinical trials are extensions of its dose-limiting pharmacologic effects and include flushing, headache, hypotension, nausea, vomiting, and diarrhea. Most events were self-limiting and resolved with reduction or withholding of treprostinil.

PATIENT INFORMATION
Treprostinil is infused continuously through a subcutaneous catheter, via an infusion pump. Treprostinil therapy will be needed for prolonged periods, possibly years. Carefully consider the patient's ability to accept, place, and care for a subcutaneous catheter and to use an infusion pump.

AVAILABILITY
Injection—1 mg/mL, 20 mL; 2.5 mg/mL, 20 mL; 5 mg/mL, 20 mL; 10 mg/mL, 20 mL

Abrams J, Frishman WH, Bates SM, *et al.*: Pharmacologic options for treatment of ischemic disease. In *Cardiovascular Therapeutics*, edn 2. Edited by Antman EM. Philadelphia: WB Saunders Co.; 2002:97–153.

Antman EM, Anbe DT, Armstrong PW, *et al.*: ACC/AHA guidelines for the management of patients with ST-elevation myocardial infarction: executive summary: a report of the American College of Cardiology/American Heart Association task force on practice guidelines (Committee to revise the 1999 guidelines on the management of patients with acute myocardial infarction). *J Am Coll Cardiol* 2004, 44:671–719.

Badesch DB, Abman SH, Ahearn GS, *et al.*: Medical therapy for pulmonary arterial hypertension. ACCP evidence-based clinical practice guidelines. *Chest* 2004, 126:35s–62s.

Barst RJ, Rubin LJ, Long WA, *et al.*: A comparison of continuous intravenous epoprostenol (prostacyclin) with conventional therapy for primary pulmonary hypertension. The Primary Pulmonary Hypertension Study Group. *N Engl J Med* 1996, 334:296–302.

Brogden RN, Markham A: Fenoldopam: a review of its pharmacodynamic and pharmacokinetic properties and intravenous clinical potential in the management of hypertensive urgencies and emergencies. *Drugs* 1997, 54:634–650.

Califf RM, Adams KF, McKenna WJ, *et al.*: A randomized controlled trial of epoprostenol therapy for severe congestive heart failure: The Flolan International Randomized Survival Trial (FIRST). *Am Heart J* 1997, 134:44–54.

Campese VM: Minoxidil: a review of its pharmacological properties and therapeutic use. *Drugs* 1981, 22:237–278.

Cheng JWM: The use of cilostazol for the management of intermittent claudication. *Heart Dis* 1999, 1:182–186.

Cheng JWM. Nesiritide: review of clinical pharmacology and role in heart failure management. *Heart Dis* 2002, 4:199–203.

Cheng JWM. Bosentan. *Heart Dis* 2003, 5:161–169.

Colucci WS, Elkayam U, Horton DP, *et al.*: Intravenous nesiritide, a natriuretic peptide, in the treatment of decompensated congestive heart failure. Nesiritide Study Group. *N Engl J Med* 2000, 343:246–253.

Cohn JN, Archibald DG, Ziesche S, *et al.*: Effect of vasodilator therapy on mortality in chronic congestive heart failure. Results of a Veterans Administration Cooperative Study. *N Engl J Med* 1986, 314:1547–1552.

Cohn JN, Johnson G, Ziesche S, *et al.*: A comparison of enalapril with hydralazine-isosorbide dinitrate in the treatment of chronic congestive heart failure. *N Engl J Med* 1991, 325:303–310.

Dawson DL, Cutler BS, Meissner MH, Strandness DE: Cilostazol has beneficial effects in treatment of intermittent claudication: results from a multicenter, randomized, prospective, double-blind trial. *Circulation* 1998, 98:678–686.

deLemos JA, McGuire DK, Drazner MH: B-type natriuretic peptide in cardiovascular disease. *Lancet* 2003, 362:316–322.

Eberhardt RT, Coffman JD: Drug treatment of peripheral vascular disease. In *Cardiovascular Pharmacotherapeutics*, edn 2. Edited by Frishman WH, Sonnenblick EH, Sica DA. New York: McGraw Hill; 2003:919–934.

Frishman WH: Tolerance, rebound and time-zero effect of nitrate therapy. *Am J Cardiol* 1992, 70(Suppl 17): 43G–48G.

Frishman WH, Azizad M, Agarwal Y, Kang DW: Use of prostacyclin and its analogues in the treatment of pulmonary hypertension and other cardiovascular diseases. In *Cardiovascular Pharmacotherapeutics*, edn 2. Edited by Frishman WH, Sonnenblick EH, Sica DA. New York: McGraw Hill; 2003:429–442.

Frishman WH, Azizad M, Agarwal Y, Kang DW: Prostacyclin and its analogues. In *Cardiovascular Pharmacotherapeutics Manual*, edn 2. Edited by Frishman WH, Sonnenblick EH, Sica DA. New York: McGraw Hill; 2004:403–411.

Frishman WH, Cheng JWM: Endothelin inhibitors: bosentan. In *Cardiovascular Pharmacotherapeutics Manual*, edn 2. New York: McGraw Hill; 2004:421–432.

Frishman WH; Hotchkiss H: Selective and nonselective dopamine receptor agonist. In *Cardiovascular Pharmacotherapeutics Manual*, edn 2. Edited by Frishman WH, Sonnenblick EH, Sica DA. New York: McGraw Hill; 2004:396–402.

Frishman WH, Hotchkiss J: Selective and non-selective dopamine receptor agonists. In *Cardiovascular Pharmacotherapeutics*, edn 2. Edited by Frishman WH, Sonnenblick EH, Sica DA. New York: McGraw Hill; 2003:443–449.

Frishman WH, Sica DA, Cheng JWM: Natriuretic peptides: neseritide. In *Cardiovascular Pharmacotherapeutics Manual*, edn 2. Edited by Frishman WH, Sonnenblick EH, Sica DA. New York: McGraw Hill; 2004:412–420.

Frohlich ED: Other adrenergic inhibitors and the direct-acting smooth muscle vasodilators. In *Hypertension: A Companion to Brenner & Rector's The Kidney*. Philadelphia: WB Saunders Co.; 2000:637–643.

Kaplan NM: *Kaplan's Clinical Hypertension*, edn 8. Philadelphia: Lippincott Williams & Wilkins; 2002.

Keating GM, Goa KL: Nesiritide: a review of its use in acute decompensated heart failure. *Drugs* 2003, 63:47–70.

Khot UN, Novaro GM, Popvic ZB, *et al.*: Nitroprusside in critically ill patients with left ventricular dysfunction and aortic stenosis. *N Engl J Med* 2003, 348:1756–1763.

Koch Weser J: Diazoxide. *N Engl J Med* 1976, 294:1271–1274.

LeJemtel TH, Sonnenblick EH, Frishman WH: Diagnosis and management of heart failure. In *Hurst's The Heart*, edn 11. Edited by Fuster V, Alexander RW, O'Rourke RA. New York: McGraw Hill; 2004:723–762.

Levin E: Endothelins. *N Engl J Med* 1995, 333:356–363.

Mansoor GA, Frishman WH: Comprehensive management of hypertensive emergencies and urgencies. *Heart Dis* 2002, 4:358–371.

McLaughlin VV, Genthner DE, Panella MM, Rich S: Reduction in pulmonary vascular resistance with long-term epoprostenol (prostacyclin) therapy in primary pulmonary hypertension. *N Engl J Med* 1998, 338:273–277.

Money SR, Herd JA, Isaacsohn JL, *et al.*: Effect of cilostazol on walking distances in patients with intermittent claudication caused by peripheral vascular disease. *J Vasc Surg* 1998, 27:267–274.

Murphy MB, Murray C, Shorten GD: Fenoldopam: a selective peripheral dopamine receptor agonist. *N Engl J Med* 2001, 345:1548–1557.

Parker JD, Gori G: Tolerance to the organic nitrates: new ideas, new mechanisms, continued mystery. *Circulation* 2001, 104:2263–2265.

Pass SE, Dusing ML: Current and emerging therapy for primary pulmonary hypertension. *Ann Pharmacother* 2002, 36:1414–1423.

Phillips BB, Gandhi AJ: Epoprostenol in the treatment of congestive heart failure. *Am J Health Sys Pharm* 1997, 54:2613–2615.

Post JB, Frishman WH: Fenoldopam: a new dopamine agonist for the treatment of hypertensive urgencies and emergencies. *J Clin Pharmacol* 1998, 38:2–13.

Prakash A, Markham A: Long-acting isosorbide mononitrate. *Drugs* 1999, 57:93–99.

Ram CVS, Fenves A: Direct vasodilators. In *Hypertension Primer*, edn 3. Edited by Izzo JL Jr, Black HR. Dallas: American Heart Assn; 2003:437–439.

Rubin LJ, Badesch DB, Barst RJ, *et al.*: Bosentan therapy for pulmonary arterial hypertension. *N Engl J Med* 2002, 346:896–903.

Thadani U: Nitrate tolerance, rebound, and their clinical relevance in stable angina pectoris, unstable angina, and heart failure. *Cardiovasc Drugs Ther* 1997, 10:735–742.

The VAMC Investigators. Intravenous nesiritide vs nitroglycerin for treatment of decompensated congestive heart failure: a randomized controlled trial. *JAMA* 2002, 287:1531–1540.

Vidt DG: Treatment of hypertensive emergencies and urgencies. In *Hypertension Primer*, edn 3. Edited by Izzo JL Jr, Black HR. Dallas: American Heart Assn; 2003:452–455.

Zineh I, Schofield RS, Johnson JA: The evolving role of nesiritide in advanced or decompensated heart failure. *Pharmacotherapy* 2003, 23:1266–1280.

The information here is provided as guidance only. Prescribers should always consult the manufacturer's current prescribing information.

351

APPENDIX I. GUIDE TO CARDIOVASCULAR DRUGS USED IN PREGNANCY AND IN NURSING

Drugs	Pregnancy	Lactation	Pregnancy category*
α-Adrenergic antagonists			
Doxazosin	Weigh benefits vs risk	Breastfeeding not recommended; excretion in milk unknown	C
Phenoxybenzamine	Weigh benefits vs risk	Breastfeeding not recommended; excretion in milk unknown	C
Phentolamine	Weigh benefits vs risk	Breastfeeding not recommended; excretion in milk unknown	C
Prazosin	Weigh benefits vs risk	Breastfeed with caution; drug excreted in breast milk	C
Terazosin	Weigh benefits vs risk	Breastfeeding not recommended; excretion in milk unknown	C
α₂-Adrenergic agonists			
Clonidine	Weigh benefits vs risk	Breastfeeding not recommended; drug excreted in breast milk	C
Guanabenz	Weigh benefits vs risk	Breastfeeding not recommended; excretion in milk unknown	C
Guanfacine	Use only if clearly indicated	Breastfeeding not recommended; excretion in milk unknown	B
Methyldopa	Weigh benefits vs risk	Breastfeed with caution; drug excreted in breast milk	B (PO), C (IV)
Angiotensin converting enzyme inhibitors			
Benazepril	Use of ACE inhibitors during the second and third trimesters of pregnancy has been associated with fetal and neonatal injury, including hypotension, neonatal skull hypoplasia, anuria, reversible or irreversible renal failure, and death	Breastfeeding not recommended; excretion in milk unknown	C (first trimester) D (second, third trimesters)
Captopril		Breastfeeding not recommended; drug excreted in breast milk	
Enalapril		Breastfeeding not recommended; drug excreted in breast milk	
Fosinopril		Breastfeeding not recommended; drug excreted in breast milk	
Lisinopril		Breastfeeding not recommended; excretion in milk unknown	
Moexipril		Breastfeeding not recommended; excretion in milk unknown	
Perindopril		Breastfeeding not recommended; excretion in milk unknown	
Quinapril		Breastfeeding not recommended; drug excreted in breast milk	
Ramipril		Breastfeeding not recommended; excretion in milk unknown	
Trandolapril		Breastfeeding not recommended; excretion in milk unknown	
Angiotensin II receptor blockers			
Candesartan	Use of medications that act directly on the renin angiotensin system during the second and third trimesters of pregnancy has been associated with fetal and neonatal injury, including hypotension, neonatal skull hypoplasia, anuria, reversible or irreversible renal failure, and death	Breastfeeding not recommended; excretion in milk unknown	C (first trimester) D (second, third trimesters)
Eprosartan		Breastfeeding not recommended; excretion in milk unknown	
Irbesartan		Breastfeeding not recommended; excretion in milk unknown	
Losartan		Breastfeeding not recommended; excretion in milk unknown	
Olmesartan		Breastfeeding not recommended; excretion in milk unknown	
Telmisartan		Breastfeeding not recommended; excretion in milk unknown	
Valsartan		Breastfeeding not recommended; excretion in milk unknown	
Antiarrhythmic agents			
Class IA			
Disopyramide	Weigh benefits vs risk	Breastfeeding not recommended; drug excreted in breast milk	C
Procainamide	Weigh benefits vs risk	Breastfeeding not recommended; drug excreted in breast milk	C
Quinidine	Weigh benefits vs risk	Breastfeeding not recommended; drug excreted in breast milk	C
Class IB			
Lidocaine	Use only if clearly indicated	Breastfeed with caution; drug excreted in breast milk	B
Mexiletine	Weigh benefits vs risk	Breastfeeding not recommended; drug excreted in breast milk	C
Tocainide	Weigh benefits vs risk	Breastfeeding not recommended; drug excreted in breast milk	C
Class IC			
Flecainide	Weigh benefits vs risk	Breastfeeding not recommended; drug excreted in breast milk	C

The information here is provided as guidance only. Prescribers should always consult the manufacturer's current prescribing information.

Drugs	Pregnancy	Lactation	Pregnancy category*
Class IC (continued)			
Moricizine	Use only if clearly indicated	Breastfeeding not recommended; drug excreted in breast milk	B
Propafenone	Weigh benefits vs risk	Breastfeeding not recommended; excretion in milk unknown	C
Class II (β blockers)			
Acebutolol	Use only if clearly indicated	Breastfeeding not recommended; drug excreted in breast milk	B
Atenolol	Not recommended	Breastfeeding not recommended; drug excreted in breast milk	D
Betaxolol	Weigh benefits vs risk	Breastfeeding not recommended; drug excreted in breast milk	C
Bisoprolol	Weigh benefits vs risk	Breastfeeding not recommended; excretion in milk unknown	C
Carteolol	Weigh benefits vs risk	Breastfeeding not recommended; excretion in milk unknown	C
Carvedilol	Weigh benefits vs risk	Breastfeeding not recommended; excretion in milk unknown	C
Esmolol	Weigh benefits vs risk	Breastfeeding not recommended; excretion in milk unknown	C
Labetalol	Weigh benefits vs risk	Breastfeed with caution; drug excreted in breast milk	C
Metoprolol	Weigh benefits vs risk	Breastfeeding not recommended; drug excreted in breast milk	C
Nadolol	Weigh benefits vs risk	Breastfeeding not recommended; drug excreted in breast milk	C
Penbutolol	Weigh benefits vs risk	Breastfeeding not recommended; excretion in milk unknown	C
Pindolol	Use only if clearly indicated	Breastfeeding not recommended; drug excreted in breast milk	B
Propranolol	Weigh benefits vs risk	Breastfeed with caution; drug excreted in breast milk	C
Timolol	Weigh benefits vs risk	Breastfeeding not recommended; drug excreted in breast milk	C
Class III			
Amiodarone	Not recommended	Breastfeeding not recommended; drug excreted in breast milk	D
Bretylium	Weigh benefits vs risk	Breastfeeding not recommended; excretion in milk unknown	C
Dofetilide	Weigh benefits vs risk	Breastfeeding not recommended; excretion in milk unknown	C
Ibutilide	Weigh benefits vs risk	Breastfeeding not recommended; excretion in milk unknown	C
Sotalol	Use only if clearly indicated	Breastfeeding not recommended; drug excreted in breast milk	B
Class IV (calcium antagonists)†			
Amlodipine	Weigh benefits vs risk	Breastfeeding not recommended; excretion in milk unknown	C
Bepridil	Weigh benefits vs risk	Breastfeeding not recommended; drug excreted in breast milk	C
Diltiazem	Weigh benefits vs risk	Breastfeeding not recommended; drug excreted in breast milk	C
Felodipine	Weigh benefits vs risk	Breastfeeding not recommended; excretion in milk unknown	C
Isradipine	Weigh benefits vs risk	Breastfeeding not recommended; excretion in milk unknown	C
Nicardipine	Weigh benefits vs risk	Breastfeeding not recommended; excretion in milk unknown	C
Nifedipine	Weigh benefits vs risk	Breastfeeding not recommended; drug excreted in breast milk	C
Nimodipine	Weigh benefits vs risk	Breastfeeding not recommended; excretion in milk unknown	C
Nisoldipine	Weigh benefits vs risk	Breastfeeding not recommended; excretion in milk unknown	C
Verapamil	Weigh benefits vs risk	Breastfeeding not recommended; drug excreted in breast milk	C
Antithrombotic agents			
Anticoagulants			
Argatroban	Use only if clearly indicated	Breastfeeding not recommended; excretion in milk unknown	B
Bivalirudin	Use only if clearly indicated	Breastfeeding not recommended; excretion in milk unknown	B
Dalteparin	Use only if clearly indicated	Breastfeeding not recommended; excretion in milk unknown	B
Desirudin	Weigh benefits vs risk	Breastfeeding not recommended; excretion in milk unknown	C
Enoxaparin	Use only if clearly indicated	Breastfeeding not recommended; excretion in milk unknown	B
Fondaparinux	Use only if clearly indicated	Breastfeeding not recommended; excretion in milk unknown	B
Heparin	Weigh benefits vs risk	Not excreted in breast milk	C

The information here is provided as guidance only. Prescribers should always consult the manufacturer's current prescribing information.

353

Drugs	Pregnancy	Lactation	Pregnancy category*
Lepirudin	Use only if clearly indicated	Breastfeeding not recommended; excretion in milk unknown	B
Tinzaparin	Use only if clearly indicated	Breastfeeding not recommended; excretion in milk unknown	B
Warfarin	Contraindicated	Breastfeeding not recommended; drug excreted in breast milk	X
Antiplatelets			
Abciximab	Weigh benefits vs risk	Breastfeeding not recommended; excretion in milk unknown	C
Aspirin	Avoid in third trimester	Breastfeed with caution; drug excreted in breast milk	D
Cilostazol	Weigh benefits vs risk	Breastfeeding not recommended; excretion in milk unknown	C
Clopidogrel	Use only if clearly indicated	Breastfeeding not recommended; excretion in milk unknown	B
Dipyridamole	Use only if clearly indicated	Breastfeed with caution; drug excreted in breast milk	B
Eptifibatide	Use only if clearly indicated	Breastfeeding not recommended; excretion in milk unknown	B
Ticlopidine	Use only if clearly indicated	Breastfeeding not recommended; excretion in milk unknown	B
Tirofiban	Use only if clearly indicated	Breastfeeding not recommended; excretion in milk unknown	B
Thrombolytics			
Alteplase (tPA)	Weigh benefits vs risk	Breastfeeding not recommended; excretion in milk unknown	C
Reteplase	Weigh benefits vs risk	Breastfeeding not recommended; excretion in milk unknown	C
Streptokinase	Weigh benefits vs risk	Breastfeeding not recommended; excretion in milk unknown	C
Tenecteplase	Weigh benefits vs risk	Breastfeeding not recommended; excretion in milk unknown	C
Urokinase	Use only if clearly indicated	Breastfeeding not recommended; excretion in milk unknown	B
Diuretics			
Loop			
Bumetanide	Weigh benefits vs risk	Breastfeeding not recommended; excretion in milk unknown	C
Ethacrynic acid	Use only if clearly indicated	Breastfeeding not recommended; excretion in milk unknown	B
Furosemide	Weigh benefits vs risk	Breastfeeding not recommended; drug excreted in breast milk	C
Torsemide	Use only if clearly indicated	Breastfeeding not recommended; excretion in milk unknown	B
Thiazides			
Bendroflumethiazide	Weigh benefits vs risk	Breastfeed with caution; drug excreted in breast milk	C
Benzthiazide	Weigh benefits vs risk	Breastfeed with caution; drug excreted in breast milk	C
Chlorothiazide	Use only if clearly indicated	Breastfeed with caution; drug excreted in breast milk	B
Chlorthalidone	Use only if clearly indicated	Breastfeeding not recommended; drug excreted in breast milk	B
Hydrochlorothiazide	Use only if clearly indicated	Breastfeeding not recommended; drug excreted in breast milk	B
Hydroflumethiazide	Weigh benefits vs risk	Breastfeeding not recommended; drug excreted in breast milk	C
Indapamide	Use only if clearly indicated	Breastfeeding not recommended; excretion in milk unknown	B
Methyclothiazide‡	Use only if clearly indicated	Breastfeeding not recommended; drug excreted in breast milk	B
Metolazone	Use only if clearly indicated	Breastfeeding not recommended; drug excreted in breast milk	B/D
Polythiazide	Not recommended	Breastfeed with caution; drug excreted in breast milk	D
Quinethazone	Not recommended	Breastfeed with caution; drug excreted in breast milk	D
Trichlormethiazide	Weigh benefits vs risk	Breastfeed with caution; drug excreted in breast milk	C
Potassium sparing			
Amiloride	Use only if clearly indicated	Breastfeeding not recommended; excretion in milk unknown	B
Eplerenone	Use only if clearly indicated	Breastfeeding not recommended; excretion in milk unknown	B
Spironolactone	Weigh benefits vs risk	Breastfeeding not recommended; drug excreted in breast milk	C/D
Triamterene	Use only if clearly indicated	Breastfeeding not recommended; excretion in milk unknown	B/D

The information here is provided as guidance only. Prescribers should always consult the manufacturer's current prescribing information.

Drugs	Pregnancy	Lactation	Pregnancy category*
Inotropic and vasopressor agents			
Digoxin	Weigh benefits vs risk	Breastfeed with caution; drug excreted in breast milk	C
Dobutamine	Use only if clearly indicated	Breastfeeding not recommended; excretion in milk unknown	B
Dopamine	Weigh benefits vs risk	Breastfeeding not recommended; excretion in milk unknown	C
Epinephrine	Weigh benefits vs risk	Breastfeed with caution; excretion in milk unknown	C
Inamrinone	Weigh benefits vs risk	Breastfeeding not recommended; excretion in milk unknown	C
Isoproterenol	Weigh benefits vs risk	Breastfeeding not recommended; excretion in milk unknown	C
Metaraminol	Weigh benefits vs risk	Breastfeeding not recommended; excretion in milk unknown	C
Methoxamine	Weigh benefits vs risk	Breastfeeding not recommended; excretion in milk unknown	C
Midodrine	Weigh benefits vs risk	Breastfeeding not recommended; excretion in milk unknown	C
Milrinone	Weigh benefits vs risk	Breastfeeding not recommended; excretion in milk unknown	C
Norepinephrine	Weigh benefits vs risk	Breastfeeding not recommended; excretion in milk unknown	C
Phenylephrine	Weigh benefits vs risk	Limited absorption in gastrointestinal tract; excretion in milk unknown	C
Vasopressin	Weigh benefits vs risk	Breastfeed with caution; drug excreted in breast milk	C
Lipid-lowering agents			
Bile acid sequestrants			
Cholestyramine	Weigh benefits vs risk	Breastfeed with caution; excretion in breast milk unknown	C
Colesevelam	Use only if clearly indicated	Breastfeed with caution; excretion in breast milk unknown	B
Colestipol	Weigh benefits vs risk	Breastfeed with caution; excretion in breast milk unknown	Not evaluated
Cholesterol absorption inhibitor			
Ezetimibe	Weigh benefits vs risk	Breastfeeding not recommended; excretion in milk unknown	C
Fibric acid derivatives			
Fenofibrate	Weigh benefits vs risk	Breastfeeding not recommended; excretion in milk unknown	C
Gemfibrozil	Weigh benefits vs risk	Breastfeeding not recommended; excretion in milk unknown	C
Nicotinic acid	Weigh benefits vs risk	Breastfeed with caution; excretion in breast milk unknown	C
HMG-CoA reductase inhibitors			
Atorvastatin	Contraindicated	Contraindicated	X
Fluvastatin	Contraindicated	Contraindicated	X
Lovastatin	Contraindicated	Contraindicated	X
Pravastatin	Contraindicated	Contraindicated	X
Rosuvastatin	Contraindicated	Contraindicated	X
Simvastatin	Contraindicated	Contraindicated	X
Neuronal and ganglionic blockers			
Guanadrel	Use only if clearly indicated	Breastfeeding not recommended; excretion in milk unknown	B
Guanethidine	Weigh benefits vs risk	Breastfeeding not recommended; drug excreted in breast milk	C
Mecamylamine	Weigh benefits vs risk	Breastfeeding not recommended; excretion in milk unknown	C
Reserpine	Weigh benefits vs risk	Breastfeeding not recommended; drug excreted in breast milk	C
Vasodilators			
Alprostadil	Contraindicated	Not indicated for use in women	X
Bosentan	Contraindicated	Breastfeeding not recommended; excretion in milk unknown	X
Diazoxide	Weigh benefits vs risk	Breastfeeding not recommended; excretion in milk unknown	C
Epoprostenol	Use only if clearly indicated	Breastfeeding not recommended; excretion in milk unknown	B
Fenoldopam	Use only if clearly indicated	Breastfeeding not recommended; excretion in milk unknown	B
Hydralazine	Weigh benefits vs risk	Breastfeeding not recommended; drug excreted in breast milk	C

Drugs	Pregnancy	Lactation	Pregnancy category*
Isosorbide dinitrate	Weigh benefits vs risk	Breastfeeding not recommended; excretion in milk unknown	C
Isosorbide mononitrate	Weigh benefits vs risk	Breastfeeding not recommended; excretion in milk unknown	C
Isoxsuprine	Weigh benefits vs risk	Breastfeeding not recommended; excretion in milk unknown	C
Minoxidil	Weigh benefits vs risk	Breastfeeding not recommended; drug excreted in breast milk	C
Nesiritide	Weigh benefits vs risk	Breastfeeding not recommended; excretion in milk unknown	C
Nitroglycerin	Weigh benefits vs risk	Breastfeeding not recommended; excretion in milk unknown	C
Nitroprusside	Weigh benefits vs risk	Breastfeeding not recommended; excretion in milk unknown	C
Papaverine	Weigh benefits vs risk	Breastfeeding not recommended; excretion in milk unknown	C
Pentoxifylline	Weigh benefits vs risk	Breastfeeding not recommended; drug excreted in breast milk	C
Treprostinil	Use only if clearly indicated	Breastfeeding not recommended; excretion in milk unknown	B

*Pregnancy categories/US Food and Drug Administration Pregnancy Risk Classification:

B: Either animal-reproduction studies have not demonstrated a fetal risk but there are no controlled studies in pregnant women, or animal-reproduction studies have shown an adverse effect (other than a decrease in fertility) that was not confirmed in controlled studies in women in the first trimester and there is no evidence of a risk in later trimesters.

C: Either animal studies have revealed adverse effects (teratogenic or embryocidal) but there are no confirmatory studies in women, or studies in both animals and women are not available. Because of the potential risk to the fetus, drugs should be given only if justified by potentially greater benefits.

D: Evidence of human fetal risk is available. Despite the risk, benefits from use in pregnant women may be justifiable in select circumstances (eg, if the drug is needed in a life-threatening situation and no other safer, more acceptable drugs are effective). An appropriate warning statement will appear on the labeling.

X: Studies in animals or human beings have demonstrated fetal abnormalities or there is evidence of fetal risk based on human experience, or both, and the risk of the use of the drug in pregnant women clearly outweighs any possible benefit. The drug is contraindicated in women who are or may become pregnant.

†Only diltiazem and verapamil are indicated for arrhythmias.

‡The pregnancy category of methyclothiazide has ranged from B to D.

ACE—angiotensin converting enzyme; HMG-CoA—hydroxymethylglutaryl coenzyme A; IV—intravenous; PO—by mouth.

Adapted from Cheng-Lai A, Frishman WH, Spiegel A, Charney P: Appendix 3: Guide to Cardiovascular drugs used in pregnancy and with nursing. In Cardiovascular Pharmacotherapeutics, edn 2. Edited by Frishman WH, Sonnenblick EH, Sica DA. New York: McGraw Hill; 2003:1015–1019.

APPENDIX II. DOSING RECOMMENDATIONS OF CARDIOVASCULAR DRUGS IN PATIENTS WITH HEPATIC DISEASE AND/OR CONGESTIVE HEART FAILURE

Drug	Cirrhosis	Congestive heart failure
α-Adrenergic antagonists		
Doxazosin	Initiate with lower dose	Usual dose with frequent monitoring
Phenoxybenzamine	Usual dose with frequent monitoring	Usual dose with frequent monitoring
Phentolamine	Usual dose with frequent monitoring	Usual dose with frequent monitoring
Prazosin	Initiate with lower dose	Usual dose with frequent monitoring
Terazosin	Initiate with lower dose	Usual dose with frequent monitoring
α₂-Adrenergic agonists		
Clonidine	Usual dose with frequent monitoring	Usual dose with frequent monitoring
Guanabenz	Initiate with lower dose	Usual dose with frequent monitoring
Guanfacine	Initiate with lower dose	Usual dose with frequent monitoring
Methyldopa	Initiate with lower dose	Usual dose with frequent monitoring
Angiotensin converting enzyme inhibitors		
Benazepril	Usual dose with frequent monitoring	Usual dose with frequent monitoring
Captopril	Usual dose with frequent monitoring	Usual dose with frequent monitoring
Enalapril	Usual dose with frequent monitoring	Usual dose with frequent monitoring
Fosinopril	Usual dose with frequent monitoring	Usual dose with frequent monitoring
Lisinopril	Usual dose with frequent monitoring	Usual dose with frequent monitoring
Moexipril	Dose reduction may be necessary	Usual dose with frequent monitoring
Perindopril	Usual dose with frequent monitoring	Usual dose with frequent monitoring
Quinapril	Usual dose with frequent monitoring	Usual dose with frequent monitoring
Ramipril	Usual dose with frequent monitoring	Usual dose with frequent monitoring
Trandolapril	Initiate with lower dose	Usual dose with frequent monitoring
Angiotensin II receptor antagonists		
Candesartan	Usual dose with frequent monitoring	Usual dose with frequent monitoring
Eprosartan	Usual dose with frequent monitoring	Usual dose with frequent monitoring
Irbesartan	Usual dose with frequent monitoring	Usual dose with frequent monitoring
Losartan	Initiate with lower dose	Usual dose with frequent monitoring
Olmesartan	Usual dose with frequent monitoring	Usual dose with frequent monitoring
Telmisartan	Dose reduction may be necessary; consider alternative treatment	Dose reduction may be necessary
Valsartan	Usual dose with frequent monitoring	Usual dose with frequent monitoring
Antiarrhythmics		
Adenosine	Usual dose with frequent monitoring	Usual dose with frequent monitoring
Amiodarone	Usual dose with frequent monitoring	Usual dose with frequent monitoring
Atropine	Usual dose with frequent monitoring	Usual dose with frequent monitoring
Bretylium	Usual dose with frequent monitoring	Usual dose with frequent monitoring
Disopyramide	Initiate with lower dose	Dose reduction may be necessary
Dofetilide	Usual dose with frequent monitoring	Usual dose with frequent monitoring
Flecainide	Use lower dose or alternative treatment	Use with caution, dose reduction may be necessary
Ibutilide	Usual dose with frequent monitoring	Usual dose with frequent monitoring
Lidocaine	Initiate with lower dose	Initiate with lower dose
Mexiletine	Initiate with lower dose	Initiate with lower dose
Moricizine	Use lower dose or alternative treatment	Dose reduction may be necessary

Drug	Cirrhosis	Congestive heart failure
Procainamide	Dose reduction is necessary	Use with caution, dose reduction may be necessary
Propafenone	Initiate with lower dose	Contraindicated in uncontrolled CHF
Quinidine	Reduce maintenance dose and monitor serum concentration*	May precipitate or exacerbate CHF
Sotalol	Usual dose with frequent monitoring	Contraindicated in uncontrolled CHF
Tocainide	Initiate with lower dose; limit dose to 1200 mg/d	Use with caution, dose reduction may be necessary
Antithrombotic agents		
Anticoagulants		
Argatroban	Initiate with lower dose	Usual dose with frequent monitoring
Bivalirudin	Usual dose with frequent monitoring	Usual dose with frequent monitoring
Dalteparin	Usual dose with frequent monitoring	Usual dose with frequent monitoring
Desirudin	Usual dose with frequent monitoring	Usual dose with frequent monitoring
Enoxaparin	Usual dose with frequent monitoring	Usual dose with frequent monitoring
Fondaparinux	Usual dose with frequent monitoring	Usual dose with frequent monitoring
Heparin	Dose reduction may be necessary; titrate dose based on coagulation test result	Usual dose with frequent monitoring
Lepirudin	Usual dose with frequent monitoring	Usual dose with frequent monitoring
Tinzaparin	Usual dose with frequent monitoring	Usual dose with frequent monitoring
Warfarin	Initiate at lower dose	Dose reduction may be necessary
Antiplatelets		
Abciximab	Usual dose with frequent monitoring	Usual dose with frequent monitoring
Aspirin	Usual dose with frequent monitoring	Usual dose with frequent monitoring
Cilostazol	Usual dose with frequent monitoring	Contraindicated
Clopidogrel	Usual dose with frequent monitoring	Usual dose with frequent monitoring
Dipyridamole	Reduce dose with biliary obstruction	Usual dose with frequent monitoring
Eptifibatide	Usual dose with frequent monitoring	Usual dose with frequent monitoring
Ticlopidine	Contraindicated in severe liver dysfunction	Usual dose with frequent monitoring
Tirofiban	Usual dose with frequent monitoring	Usual dose with frequent monitoring
Thrombolytics		
Alteplase	Usual dose with frequent monitoring	Usual dose with frequent monitoring
Streptokinase	Usual dose with frequent monitoring	Usual dose with frequent monitoring
Urokinase	Dose reduction may be necessary	Usual dose with frequent monitoring
Reteplase	Usual dose with frequent monitoring	Usual dose with frequent monitoring
Tenecteplase	Use usual dose with caution; risk of bleeding may increase	Usual dose with frequent monitoring
β-Adrenergic blockers		
Nonselective		
Nadolol	Usual dose with frequent monitoring	Usual dose with frequent monitoring[†]
Propranolol	Initiate with lower dose	Usual dose with frequent monitoring[†]
Timolol	Initiate with lower dose	Usual dose with frequent monitoring[†]
β_1-Selective		
Atenolol	Usual dose with frequent monitoring	Usual dose with frequent monitoring[†]
Betaxolol	Usual dose with frequent monitoring	Usual dose with frequent monitoring[†]
Bisoprolol	Initiate with lower dose	Usual dose with frequent monitoring[†]
Esmolol	Usual dose with frequent monitoring	Usual dose with frequent monitoring[†]
Metoprolol	Dose reduction may be necessary	Usual dose with frequent monitoring[†]

Drug	Cirrhosis	Congestive heart failure
With ISA: nonselective		
Carteolol	Usual dose with frequent monitoring	Usual dose with frequent monitoring[†]
Penbutolol	Dose reduction may be necessary	Usual dose with frequent monitoring[†]
Pindolol	Dose reduction may be necessary	Usual dose with frequent monitoring[†]
With ISA: β_1-selective		
Acebutolol	Usual dose with frequent monitoring	Usual dose with frequent monitoring[†]
Dual acting		
Carvedilol	Initiate with lower dose; contraindicated in patients with active liver disease	Initiate at lower dose; contraindicated in severely decompensated CHF
Labetalol	Dose reduction may be necessary	Contraindicated in patients with overt heart failure
Calcium channel blockers		
Amlodipine	Initiate with lower dose	Usual dose with frequent monitoring
Bepridil	Dose reduction may be necessary	Contraindicated in uncompensated cardiac insufficiency
Diltiazem	Dose reduction may be necessary	Usual dose with frequent monitoring
Felodipine	Dose reduction may be necessary	Usual dose with frequent monitoring
Isradipine	Dose reduction may be necessary	Usual dose with frequent monitoring
Nicardipine	Initiate with lower dose	Usual dose with frequent monitoring
Nifedipine	Dose reduction may be necessary	Usual dose with frequent monitoring
Nimodipine	Initiate with lower dose	Usual dose with frequent monitoring
Nisoldipine	Initiate with lower dose	Usual dose with frequent monitoring
Verapamil	Initiate with lower dose	Contraindicated in patients with severe left ventricular dysfunction and in patients with severe CHF (unless secondary to a supraventricular tachycardia amenable to verapamil therapy)
Diuretics		
Loop		
Bumetanide	Dose reduction is probably not necessary; titrate dosage based on clinical response	Usual dose with frequent monitoring
Ethacrynic Acid		
Furosemide		
Torsemide		
Thiazide		
Bendroflumethiazide	Dosage adjustment is probably not required in hepatic impairment; titrate dosage based on clinical response	Usual dose with frequent monitoring
Benzthiazide		
Chlorthalidone		
Chlorothiazide		
Hydrochlorothiazide		
Hydroflumethiazide		
Methyclothiazide		
Metolazone		
Polythiazide		
Quinethazone		
Trichlormethiazide		
Indapamide	Dose reduction may be necessary	Usual dose with frequent monitoring

The information here is provided as guidance only. Prescribers should always consult the manufacturer's current prescribing information.

359

Drug	Cirrhosis	Congestive heart failure
K+-sparing		
Amiloride	Usual dose with frequent monitoring	Usual dose with frequent monitoring
Eplerenone	Usual dose with frequent monitoring	Usual dose with frequent monitoring
Spironolactone	Usual dose with frequent monitoring	Usual dose with frequent monitoring
Triamterene	Initiate with lower dose; contraindicated in severe liver disease	Usual dose with frequent monitoring
Inotropic and vasopressor agents		
Digoxin	Usual dose with frequent monitoring	Usual dose with frequent monitoring
Dobutamine	Usual dose with frequent monitoring	Usual dose with frequent monitoring
Dopamine	Usual dose with frequent monitoring	Usual dose with frequent monitoring; initiate dopamine at lower dose in patients with chronic heart failure
Epinephrine	Usual dose with frequent monitoring	Usual dose with frequent monitoring
Inamrinone	Dose reduction may be necessary	Usual dose with frequent monitoring
Isoproterenol	Usual dose with frequent monitoring	Usual dose with frequent monitoring
Metaraminol	Usual dose with frequent monitoring	Usual dose with frequent monitoring
Methoxamine	Usual dose with frequent monitoring	Usual dose with frequent monitoring
Midodrine	Usual dose with frequent monitoring	Usual dose with frequent monitoring
Milrinone	Usual dose with frequent monitoring	Usual dose with frequent monitoring
Norepinephrine	Usual dose with frequent monitoring	Usual dose with frequent monitoring
Phenylephrine	Usual dose with frequent monitoring	Usual dose with frequent monitoring
Vasopressin	Lower doses may be sufficient	Usual dose with frequent monitoring
Lipid lowering agents		
Bile acid sequestrants		
Cholestyramine	Contraindicated in total biliary obstruction	Usual dose with frequent monitoring
Colesevelam	Ineffective in total biliary obstruction	Usual dose with frequent monitoring
Colestipol	Ineffective in total biliary obstruction	Usual dose with frequent monitoring
Cholesterol absorption inhibitors		
Ezetimibe	Not recommended in patients with moderate or severe hepatic impairment	Usual dose with frequent monitoring
Fibric acid derivatives		
Fenofibrate	Contraindicated in clinically significant hepatic dysfunction including primary biliary cirrhosis and patients with unexplained persistent transaminase elevation	Unknown
Gemfibrozil	Contraindicated in clinically significant hepatic dysfunction including primary biliary cirrhosis	Unknown
HMG-CoA reductase inhibitors		
Atorvastatin, Fluvastatin, Lovastatin, Pravastatin, Rosuvastatin, Simvastatin	Start at lowest dose and titrate cautiously; contraindicated in patients with active liver disease or unexplained persistent transaminase elevation	Usual dose with frequent monitoring
Nicotinic acid	Use with caution; contraindicated in patients with active liver disease or unexplained persistent transaminase elevation	Usual dose with frequent monitoring
Neuronal and ganglionic blockers		
Guanadrel	Usual dose with frequent monitoring	Contraindicated in frank CHF
Guanethidine	Dose reduction may be necessary	Contraindicated in frank CHF

Drug	Cirrhosis	Congestive heart failure
Mecamylamine	Usual dose with frequent monitoring	Usual dose with frequent monitoring
Reserpine	Dose reduction may be necessary	Usual dose with frequent monitoring
Vasodilators		
Alprostadil	Usual dose with frequent monitoring	Usual dose with frequent monitoring
Bosentan	Caution should be exercised during the use of bosentan in patients with mildly impaired liver function; bosentan generally should be avoided in patients with moderate or severe hepatic impairment	Usual dose with frequent monitoring
Diazoxide	Dose reduction may be necessary	Contraindicated in uncompensated CHF
Epoprostenol	Usual dose with frequent monitoring	Chronic use in patients with CHF due to severe left ventricular systolic dysfunction is contraindicated
Fenoldopam	Usual dose with frequent monitoring	Usual dose with frequent monitoring
Hydralazine	Dose reduction may be necessary	Higher doses have been used
Isosorbide dinitrate	Use lower dose; avoid in severe hepatic impairment	Used in combination with hydralazine
Isosorbide mononitrate	Caution in severe hepatic impairment	Avoid in acute CHF
Isoxsuprine	Dose reduction may be necessary	Usual dose with frequent monitoring
Minoxidil	Usual dose with frequent monitoring	Usual dose with frequent monitoring
Nesiritide	Cirrhotic patients with ascites and avid sodium retention were shown to have blunted natriuretic response to low-dose brain natriuretic peptide	Usual dose with frequent monitoring
Nitroglycerin	Dose reduction may be necessary; avoid in severe hepatic impairment	Usual dose with frequent monitoring
Sodium Nitroprusside	Initiate with lower dose	Usual dose with frequent monitoring; contraindicated in CHF associated with reduced peripheral vascular resistance
Papaverine	Dose reduction may be necessary	Usual dose with frequent monitoring
Pentoxifylline	Usual dose with frequent monitoring	Unknown
Treprostinil	Reduce initial dose in patients with mild-moderate hepatic impairment; use of treprostinil has not been studied in patients with severe hepatic impairment	Usual dose with frequent monitoring

*Due to an increased volume of distribution, a larger loading dose of quinidine may be indicated.

†Contraindicated with overt/severe CHF.

CHF—congestive heart failure; HMG-CoA—hydroxymethylglutaryl coenzyme A; ISA—intrinsic sympathomimetic activity.

Adapted from Cheng-Lai A, Frishman WH, Spiegel A, Charney P: Appendix 4: dosing recommendations of cardiovascular drugs in patients with hepatic disease and/or congestive heart failure. In Cardiovascular Pharmacotherapeutics, edn 2. Edited by Frishman WH, Sonnenblick EH, Sica DA. New York: McGraw Hill, 2003:1021–1024.

The information here is provided as guidance only. Prescribers should always consult the manufacturer's current prescribing information.

361

APPENDIX III. DOSE ADJUSTMENT IN PATIENTS WITH RENAL INSUFFICIENCY			
Drug	**Creatinine clearance 30 to 60 mL/min**	**Creatinine clearance less than 30 mL/min**	**Dialyzability (hemodialysis)**
α-Adrenergic antagonists			
Doxazosin	Use usual dose	Use usual dose	No
Phenoxybenzamine	Use usual dose	Use usual dose	No
Phentolamine	Use usual dose	Use usual dose	No
Prazosin	Use usual dose	Start with low dose and titrate based on response	No
Terazosin	Use usual dose	Use usual dose	No
α₂-Adrenergic agonists			
Clonidine	Use usual dose	Start with low dose and titrate based on response	No
Guanabenz	Use usual dose	Use usual dose with caution	Unknown
Guanfacine	Use usual dose	Start with low dose and titrate based on response	No
Methyldopa	Use usual dose	Start with low dose and titrate based on response	Yes
Angiotensin converting enzyme inhibitors			
Benazepril	Use usual dose	Start with low dose and titrate based on response	No†
Captopril	Start with low dose and titrate based on response	Start with low dose and titrate based on response	Yes
Enalapril	Use usual dose	Start with low dose and titrate based on response	Yes
Fosinopril	Use usual dose	Start with low dose and titrate based on response	No
Lisinopril	Use usual dose	Start with low dose and titrate based on response	Yes
Moexipril	For patients with CrCl of 40 mL/min or less, start with low dose and titrate based on response	Start with low dose and titrate based on response	Unknown
Perindopril	Start with low dose and titrate based on response	The use of this drug is not recommended because of significant perindoprilat accumulation	Yes
Quinapril	Start with low dose and titrate based on response	Start with low dose and titrate based on response	No
Ramipril	For patients with CrCl less than 40 mL/min, start with low dose and titrate based on response	Start with low dose and titrate based on response. Up to a max of 5 mg/d	Unknown
Trandolapril	Use usual dose	Start with low dose and titrate based on response	Yes (trandolaprilat)
Angiotensin II receptor blockers			
Candesartan	Use usual dose	Use usual initial dose with caution	No
Eprosartan	Use usual dose	Use usual initial dose	No
Irbesartan	Use usual dose	Use usual initial dose	No
Losartan	Use usual dose	Use usual initial dose	No
Olmesartan	Use usual dose	Use usual initial dose	Unknown
Telmisartan	Use usual dose	Use usual initial dose	No

Drug	Creatinine clearance 30 to 60 mL/min	Creatinine clearance less than 30 mL/min	Dialyzability (hemodialysis)
Valsartan	Use usual dose	Use usual dose with caution	No
Antiarrhythmic agents			
Adenosine	Use usual dose	Use usual dose	No
Atropine	Use usual dose with caution	Use usual dose with caution	No
Class IA			
Disopyramide	Decrease loading dose by 25% to 50%	Decrease loading dose by 50% to 75%	No[†]
	Decrease maintenance dose by 25% or give 100 mg (nonsustained release) every 6 to 8 h	Decrease maintenance dose by 50% to 75% or give 100 mg (nonsustained release) every 12 to 24 h	
Procainamide	Increase dosing interval to every 4 to 6 h (immediate-release oral formulation)	Increase dosing interval to every 8 to 24 h (immediate-release oral formulation)	Yes (Give maintenance dose after dialysis or supplement with 250 mg post hemodialysis)
Quinidine	Use usual dose	Use usual dose with caution: decrease maintenance dose by 25% if CrCl <10 mL/min	Yes (Give maintenance dose after dialysis or supplement with 200 mg post hemodialysis)
Class IB			
Lidocaine	Use usual dose	Use usual dose with caution	No
Mexiletine	Use usual dose	Use usual dose with caution	No
Tocainide	Use usual dose	Decrease dose by 25% to 50% or increase dosing interval to every 24 h	Yes (Give maintenance dose after dialysis or supplement with 25% of maintenance dose post hemodialysis)
Class IC			
Flecainide	Use usual dose	Initiate with 100 mg every 24 h or 50 mg every 12 h; titrate based on response	No
Moricizine	Use usual dose	Start with low dose and titrate based on response	No
Propafenone	Use usual dose	Use usual dose with caution	No
Class II (β-adrenergic antagonists)			
Acebutolol	Decrease dose by 50% when CrCl is <50 mL/min	Decrease dose by 75% when CrCl is <25 mL/min	Yes (acebutolol and diacetolol)
Atenolol	Use a maximum dose of 50 mg/d in patients with CrCl of 15–35 mL/min	Use lower dose	Yes
Betaxolol	Use usual dose with caution	Initiate with lower dose	No
Bisoprolol	Use usual dose with caution	Start with low dose and titrate based on response	No
Carteolol	Increase dosing interval to every 48 h	Increase dosing interval to every 48 to 72 h	No
Carvedilol	Use usual dose with caution	Start with low dose and titrate based on response	No
Esmolol	Use usual dose	Use usual dose	No
Labetalol	Use usual dose	Increase dosing interval	No
Metoprolol	Use usual dose	Use usual dose	No
Nadolol	Use usual dose with caution	Increase dosing interval based on CrCl	Yes
Penbutolol	Use usual dose	Use usual dose	No

The information here is provided as guidance only. Prescribers should always consult the manufacturer's current prescribing information.

363

Drug	Creatinine clearance 30 to 60 mL/min	Creatinine clearance less than 30 mL/min	Dialyzability (hemodialysis)
Pindolol	Use usual dose	Use usual dose with caution	No
Propranolol	Use usual dose	Use usual dose with caution	No
Timolol	Use usual dose	Use usual dose with caution	No
Class III			
Amiodarone	Use usual dose	Use usual dose	No
Bretylium	Decrease 50%	Decrease 50% to 75%	No
Dofetilide	Start with lower dose	Start with lower dose; dofetilide is contraindicated in patients with CrCl of <20 mL/min	Unknown
Ibutilide	Use usual dose	Use usual dose with caution	Unknown (probably no)
Sotalol	Increase dosing interval to every 24 h; Betapace AF is contraindicated in patients with CrCl <40 mL/min	Increase dosing interval to every 36 to 48 h; individualize dosage for patients with ventricular arrhythmias and CrCl below 10 mL/min; use of Betapace AF is contraindicated	Yes (Give maintenance dose after dialysis or supplement with 80 mg post hemodialysis)
Class IV (calcium antagonists*)			
Amlodipine	Use usual dose	Use usual dose with caution	No
Bepridil	Use usual dose	Use usual dose with caution	No
Diltiazem	Use usual dose	Use usual dose with caution	No
Felodipine	Use usual dose	Use usual dose	No
Isradipine	Use usual dose	Use usual dose with caution	No
Nicardipine	Use usual dose	Use usual dose; titrate dose carefully	No
Nifedipine	Use usual dose	Use usual dose	No
Nimodipine	Use usual dose	Use usual dose	No
Nisoldipine	Use usual dose	Use usual dose	No
Verapamil	Use usual dose	Use usual dose with caution	No
Antithrombotic agents			
Antiplatelets			
Abciximab	Use usual dose	Use usual dose with caution	No
Aspirin	Use usual dose	Use usual dose with caution	Yes
Cilostazol	Use usual dose	Use usual dose with caution; patients on hemodialysis have not been studied	No
Clopidogrel	Use usual dose	Use usual dose	No
Dipyridamole	Use usual dose	Use usual dose	No
Eptifibatide	Use lower dose if SCr is above 2 mg/dL or CrCl <50 mL/min	Use lower dose if SCr is above 2 mg/dL or CrCl <50 mL/min	Yes
Ticlopidine	Use usual dose	Use with caution; dose reduction may be required	No
Tirofiban	Use usual dose with caution	Decrease dose by 50%	Yes
Anticoagulants			
Argatroban	Use usual dose	Use usual dose	Unknown
Bivalirudin	Reduce infusion dose by ≈20%	Reduce infusion dose by 60%–90%	Yes (≈25% removed)
Dalteparin	Use usual dose	Use usual dose with caution; specific recommendations on dosage adjustment are not available	No

Drug	Creatinine clearance 30 to 60 mL/min	Creatinine clearance less than 30 mL/min	Dialyzability (hemodialysis)
Desirudin	Use lower dose	Use lower dose	Probable
Enoxaparin	Use usual dose	Use lower dose	No
Fondaparinux	Use usual dose with caution	Contraindicated	Yes
Heparin	Use usual dose	Use usual dose with caution	No
Lepirudin	Bolus dose: 0.2 mg/kg; initial infusion rate: 30% to 50% of usual dose	Bolus dose: 0.2 mg/kg; initial infusion rate: 15% of usual dose; avoid use if SCr is above 6 mg/dL or CrCl <15 mL/min	Yes
Tinzaparin	Use usual dose	Use usual dose with caution; specific recommendations on dosage adjustments are not available	No
Warfarin	Use usual dose	Use usual dose with caution	No

Thrombolytics

Alteplase	Use usual dose with caution	Use usual dose with caution	No
Reteplase	Use usual dose with caution	Use usual dose with caution	No
Streptokinase	Use usual dose with caution	Use usual dose with caution	No
Tenecteplase	Use usual dose with caution	Use usual dose with caution	No
Urokinase	Use usual dose with caution	Use usual dose with caution	No

Diuretics (contraindicated in anuric patients)

Loop

Bumetanide	Use usual dose	Use usual dose with caution	No
Ethacrynic acid	Use usual dose	Use usual dose with caution	No
Furosemide	Use usual dose	Use usual dose with caution	No
Torsemide	Use usual dose	Use usual dose with caution	No

Thiazide

Chlorthalidone	Use usual dose with caution	Ineffective	No
Hydrochlorothiazide and similar agents	Use usual dose with caution	Ineffective	No
Indapamide	Use usual dose with caution	Ineffective if CrCl below 15 mL/min	No
Metolazone	Use usual dose with caution	Use usual dose with caution	No

Potassium-sparing

Amiloride	Lower dose may be necessary; do not use with BUN >30 mg/dL or SCr >1.5 mg/dL	Do not use with BUN >30 mg/dL or SCr >1.5 mg/dL	Unknown
Eplerenone	Contraindicated for treatment of hypertension in patients with CrCl <50 mL/min	Contraindicated in patients with CrCl ≤30 mL/min	No
Spironolactone	Lower dose may be necessary	Contraindicated	No
Triamterene	Use usual dose with caution; contraindicated with progressive kidney disease	Contraindicated	Unknown

The information here is provided as guidance only. Prescribers should always consult the manufacturer's current prescribing information.

365

Drug	Creatinine clearance 30 to 60 mL/min	Creatinine clearance less than 30 mL/min	Dialyzability (hemodialysis)
Inotropic and vasopressor agents			
Digoxin	Use usual dose and titrate based on response	Start with low dose, many patients only need a dose every 48 to 72 h (if loading dose is indicated, decrease 25%)	No
Dobutamine	Use usual dose and titrate based on response	Use usual dose and titrate based on response	Unknown
Dopamine	Use usual dose and titrate based on response	Use usual dose and titrate based on response	No
Epinephrine	Use usual dose with caution	Use usual dose with caution	Unknown
Inamrinone	Start with low dose and titrate based on response	Start with low dose and titrate based on response	No
Isoproterenol	Use usual dose with caution	Use usual dose with caution	Unknown
Metaraminol	Start with low dose and titrate to response	Start with low dose and titrate to response	Unknown
Methoxamine	Use usual dose with caution	Use usual dose with caution	Unknown
Midodrine	Start with low dose and titrate based on response	Start with low dose and titrate based on response	Yes (midodrine and desglymidodrine)
Milrinone	Reduce initial infusion rate based on CrCl; start with low dose and titrate based on response	Reduce initial infusion rate based on CrCl; start with low dose and titrate based on response	Unknown
Norepinephrine	Use usual dose with caution	Use usual dose with caution	Yes
Phenylephrine	Use usual dose with caution	Use usual dose with caution	Unknown
Vasopressin	Use usual dose	Use usual dose with caution	Unknown
Lipid-lowering agents			
Bile acid sequestrants			
Cholestyramine	Possibility of hyperchloremic acidosis is increased in patients with renal insufficiency; use usual dose with caution	Possibility of hyperchloremic acidosis is increased in patients with renal insufficiency; use usual dose with caution	
Colesevelam			
Colestipol			
Cholesterol absorption inhibitor			
Ezetimibe	Use usual dose	Use usual dose	Unknown (probably no)
Fibric acid derivatives			
Fenofibrate	Start with low dose and titrate based on response	Start with low dose and titrate based on response	No
Gemfibrozil	Use usual dose with caution	Use usual dose with caution	No
HMG-CoA reductase inhibitors			
Atorvastatin	Use usual dose	Use usual dose	No
Fluvastatin	Use usual dose	Use usual dose with caution	No
Lovastatin	Use usual dose	Use usual dose with caution	No
Pravastatin	Use usual dose	Start with lower dosage; titrate based on response	No
Rosuvastatin	Use usual dose	Start with low dose (5 mg once daily) and titrate; not to exceed 10 mg once daily	No
Simvastatin	Use usual dose	Start with low dose and titrate based on response	No

Drug	Creatinine clearance 30 to 60 mL/min	Creatinine clearance less than 30 mL/min	Dialyzability (hemodialysis)
Nicotinic acid	Start with low dose and titrate based on response; use with caution	Start with low dose and titrate based on response; use with caution	Unknown
Neuronal and ganglionic blockers			
Guanadrel	Increase dosing interval to every 24 h; dosage increments should be made cautiously at intervals of 7 or more days	Increase dosing interval to every 48 h; dosage increments should be made cautiously at intervals of 14 days or more	Unknown (probably no)
Guanethidine	Start with low dose and titrate based on response	Start with low dose and titrate based on response; use with caution	Unknown
Mecamylamine	Start with low dose and titrate based on response	Start with low dose and titrate based on response; use with caution, if at all	Unknown
Reserpine	Use usual dose	Use usual dose with caution; avoid use if CrCl is below 10 mL/min	No
Vasodilators			
Alprostadil	Individualize dose	Individualize dose	Unknown
Bosentan	Use usual dose	Use usual dose	Unknown (probably no)
Diazoxide	Start with low dose and titrate based on response	Start with low dose and titrate based on response; use with caution	No
Epoprostenol	Individualize dose	Individualize dose	Unknown
Fenoldopam	Individualize dose	Individualize dose	Unknown
Hydralazine	Increase dosing interval to every 6 to 8 h	Increase dosing interval to every 8 to 24 h	No
Isosorbide dinitrate	Use usual dose	Start with low dose and titrate based on response; use with caution	Unknown
Isosorbide mononitrate	Use usual dose	Use usual dose with caution	No
Isoxsuprine	Start with low dose and titrate based on response	Start with low dose and titrate based on response; use with caution	Unknown
Minoxidil	Use usual dose	Start with low dose and titrate based on response	No
Nesiritide	Use usual dose	Use usual dose with caution	Unknown (probably no)
Nitroglycerin	Use usual dose	Use usual dose with caution	No
Nitroprusside	Start with low dose and titrate based on response; use with caution	Start with low dose and titrate based on response; use with caution	Yes (thiocyanate)
Papaverine	Use usual dose	Lower doses may be required	Unknown
Pentoxifylline	Lower doses may be required	Lower doses may be required; use with caution	Unknown
Treprostinil	Use with caution; no studies have been performed in patients with renal insufficiency	Use with caution; no studies have been performed in patients with renal insufficiency	Unknown

* *Only diltiazem and verapamil are indicated for arrhythmias.*

†*Hemodialysis does not remove appreciable amounts of this drug. However, dialysis may be considered in overdosed patients with severe renal impairment.*

CrCl—creatinine clearance; HMG-CoA—hydroxymethylglutaryl coenzyme A; SCr—serum creatinine.

The information here is provided as guidance only. Prescribers should always consult the manufacturer's current prescribing information.

367

APPENDIX IV. PHARMACOKINETIC CHANGES, ROUTE(S) OF ELIMINATION, AND DOSAGE ADJUSTMENT OF CARDIOVASCULAR DRUGS IN THE ELDERLY

Drug	Half-life	Volume of distribution	Clearance	Primary route(s) of elimination	Dosage adjustment
α-Adrenergic antagonists					
Doxazosin	Increase	Increase	Increase*	Hepatic	Initiate at lowest dose; titrate to response
Phenoxybenzamine	—	—	—	Hepatic	Initiate at lowest dose; titrate to response
Phentolamine	—	—	—	Hepatic/renal	No initial dose adjustment is needed
Prazosin	Increase	—	—	Hepatic	Initiate at lowest dose; titrate to response
Terazosin	Increase	—	—	Hepatic	Initiate at lowest dose; titrate to response
α₂-Adrenergic agonists					
Clonidine	—	—	—	Hepatic/renal	Initiate at lowest dose; titrate to response
Guanabenz	—	—	—	Hepatic	Initiate at lowest dose; titrate to response
Guanfacine	Increase	—	Decrease	Hepatic/renal	Initiate at lowest dose; titrate to response
Methyldopa	—	—	—	Hepatic	Initiate at lowest dose; titrate to response
Angiotensin converting enzyme inhibitors					
Benazepril	Increase	—	Decrease	Renal	No initial dosage adjustment is needed
Captopril	NS	—	Decrease	Renal	Initiate at lowest dose; titrate to response
Enalapril	—	—	—	Renal	Initiate at lowest dose; titrate to response
Fosinopril	—	—	—	Hepatic/renal	No initial dosage adjustment is needed
Lisinopril	Increase	NS	Decrease	Renal	Initiate at lowest dose; titrate to response
Moexipril	—	—	—	Hepatic/renal	Initiate at lowest dose; titrate to response
Perindopril	—	—	Decrease	Renal	Initiate at lowest dose; titrate to response
Quinapril	—	—	—	Renal	Initiate at lowest dose; titrate to response
Ramipril	—	—	—	Renal	Initiate at lowest dose; titrate to response
Trandolapril	—	—	—	Hepatic/renal	Initiate at lowest dose; titrate to response
Angiotensin II receptor blockers					
Candesartan	—	—	—	Hepatic/renal	No initial dosage adjustment is needed
Eprosartan	—	—	—	Hepatic/biliary/renal	No initial dosage adjustment is needed
Irbesartan	NS	—	—	Hepatic	No initial dosage adjustment is needed
Losartan	—	—	—	Hepatic	No initial dosage adjustment is needed
Olmesartan	—	—	—	Renal/biliary	No initial dosage adjustment is needed
Telmisartan	—	—	—	Hepatic/biliary	No initial dosage adjustment is needed
Valsartan	Increase	—	—	Hepatic	No initial dosage adjustment is needed
Antiarrhythmic agents					
Class I					
Disopyramide	Increase	—	Decrease	Renal	Initiate at lowest dose; titrate to response
Flecainide	Increase	Increase	Decrease	Hepatic/renal	Initiate at lowest dose; titrate to response
Lidocaine	Increase	Increase	NS	Hepatic	Initiate at lowest dose; titrate to response
Mexiletine	—	—	—	Hepatic	No dosage adjustment is needed
Moricizine	—	—	—	Hepatic	No dosage adjustment is needed
Procainamide	—	—	Decrease	Renal	Initiate at lowest dose; titrate to response
Propafenone	—	—	—	Hepatic	No dosage adjustment is needed
Quinidine	Increase	NS	Decrease	Hepatic	Initiate at lowest dose; titrate to response
Tocainide	Increase	—	Decrease	Hepatic/renal	No dosage adjustment is needed

Drug	Half-life	Volume of distribution	Clearance	Primary route(s) of elimination	Dosage adjustment
Class II (*see* β blockers)					
Class III					
Amiodarone	—	—	—	Hepatic/biliary	No dosage adjustment needed
Bretylium	—	—	—	Renal	Initiate at lowest dose; titrate to response
Dofetilide	—	—	—	Renal	Adjust dose based on renal function
Ibutilide	—	—	—	Hepatic	No adjustment needed
Sotalol	—	—	—	Renal	Adjust dose based on renal function
Class IV (*see* calcium channel blockers)					
Other antiarrhythmics					
Adenosine	—	—	—	Erythrocytes/vascular endothelial cells	No adjustment needed
Atropine	—	—	—	Hepatic/renal	Use usual dose with caution
Antithrombotic agents					
Anticoagulants					
Argatroban	—	—	—	Hepatic/biliary	Use usual dose with caution
Bivalirudin	—	—	—	Renal/proteolytic cleavage	Adjust dose based on renal function
Dalteparin	—	—	—	Renal	Use usual dose with caution
Desirudin	—	—	—	Renal	Adjust dose based on renal function
Enoxaparin	—	—	—	Renal	Adjust dose based on renal function
Fondaparinux	Increase	—	Decrease	Renal	Use usual dose with caution
Heparin	—	—	—	Hepatic/reticuloendothelial system	Use usual dose with caution
Lepirudin	Increase	—	Decrease	Renal	Adjust dose based on renal function
Tinzaparin	—	—	—	Renal	Use usual dose with caution
Warfarin	NS	NS	NS	Hepatic	Initiate at lowest dose; titrate to response
Antiplatelets					
Abciximab	—	—	—	Unknown	Use usual dose with caution
Aspirin	—	—	Decrease	Hepatic/renal	Use usual dose with caution
Cilostazol	—	—	—	Hepatic	No adjustment necessary
Clopidogrel	NS	—	—	Hepatic	Use usual dose with caution
Dipyridamole	—	—	—	Hepatic/biliary	Use usual dose with caution
Eptifibatide	—	—	—	Renal/plasma	Use usual dose with caution
Ticlopidine	—	—	Decrease	Hepatic	Use usual dose with caution
Tirofiban	Increase	—	Decrease	Renal	Use usual dose with caution
Thrombolytics					
Alteplase	—	—	—	Hepatic	Use usual dose with caution
Reteplase	—	—	—	Hepatic	Use usual dose with caution
Streptokinase	—	—	—	Circulating antibodies/reticuloendothelial system	Use usual dose with caution
Tenecteplase	—	—	—	Hepatic	Use usual dose with caution
Urokinase	—	—	—	Hepatic	Use usual dose with caution
β-Adrenergic blockers					
Nonselective without ISA					
Nadolol	NS	—	—	Renal	Initiate at lowest dose; titrate to response

The information here is provided as guidance only. Prescribers should always consult the manufacturer's current prescribing information.

369

Drug	Half-life	Volume of distribution	Clearance	Primary route(s) of elimination	Dosage adjustment
Propranolol	Increase	NS	Decrease	Hepatic	Initiate at lowest dose; titrate to response
Timolol	—	—	—	Hepatic	Initiate at lowest dose; titrate to response
β₁-Selective without ISA					
Atenolol	Increase	NS	Decrease	Renal	Initiate at lowest dose; titrate to response
Betaxolol	—	—	—	Hepatic	Initiate at lowest dose; titrate to response
Bisoprolol	—	—	—	Hepatic/renal	Initiate at lowest dose; titrate to response
Esmolol	—	—	—	Erythrocytes	Use usual dose with caution
Metoprolol	NS	NS	NS	Hepatic	Initiate at lowest dose; titrate to response
β₁-Selective with ISA					
Acebutolol	Increase	Decrease	—	Hepatic/biliary	Initiate at lowest dose; titrate to response
Nonselective with ISA					
Carteolol	—	—	—	Renal	Initiate at lowest dose; titrate to response
Penbutolol	—	—	—	Hepatic	Initiate at lowest dose; titrate to response
Pindolol	—	—	—	Hepatic/renal	Initiate at lowest dose; titrate to response
Dual acting					
Carvedilol	—	—	—	Hepatic/biliary	Initiate at lowest dose; titrate to response
Labetalol	—	—	NS	Hepatic	Initiate at lowest dose; titrate to response
Calcium channel blockers					
Amlodipine	Increase	—	Decrease	Hepatic	Initiate at lowest dose; titrate to response
Bepridil	—	—	—	Hepatic	Use usual dose with caution
Diltiazem	Increase	NS	Decrease	Hepatic	Initiate at lowest dose; titrate to response
Felodipine	—	NS	Decrease	Hepatic	Initiate at lowest dose; titrate to response
Isradipine	—	—	—	Hepatic	Initiate at lowest dose; titrate to response
Nicardipine	NS	—	—	Hepatic	No initial dosage adjustment is needed
Nifedipine	Increase	NS	Decrease	Hepatic	Initiate at lowest dose; titrate to response
Nimodipine	—	—	—	Hepatic	Use usual dose with caution
Nisoldipine	—	—	—	Hepatic	Initiate at lowest dose; titrate to response
Verapamil	Increase	NS	Decrease	Hepatic	Initiate at lowest dose; titrate to response
Diuretics					
Loop					
Bumetanide	—	NS	—	Renal/hepatic	No initial dosage adjustment is needed
Ethacrynic Acid	—	—	—	Hepatic	No initial dosage adjustment is needed
Furosemide	Increase	NS	Decrease	Renal	No initial dosage adjustment is needed
Torsemide	—	—	—	Hepatic	No initial dosage adjustment is needed
Thiazides					
Bendroflumethiazide	—	—	—	Renal	No initial dosage adjustment is needed
Benzthiazide	—	—	—	Unknown	No initial dosage adjustment is needed
Chlorothiazide	—	—	—	Renal	No initial dosage adjustment is needed
Chlorthalidone	—	—	—	Renal	No initial dosage adjustment is needed
Hydrochlorothiazide	—	—	Decrease	Renal	No initial dosage adjustment is needed
Hydroflumethiazide	—	—	—	Unknown	No initial dosage adjustment is needed
Indapamide	—	—	—	Hepatic	No initial dosage adjustment is needed

Drug	Half-life	Volume of distribution	Clearance	Primary route(s) of elimination	Dosage adjustment
Methyclothiazide	—	—	—	Renal	No initial dosage adjustment is needed
Metolazone	—	—	—	Renal	No initial dosage adjustment is needed
Polythiazide	—	—	—	Unknown	No initial dosage adjustment is needed
Quinethazone	—	—	—	Unknown	No initial dosage adjustment is needed
Trichlormethiazide	—	—	—	Unknown	No initial dosage adjustment is needed
Potassium sparing					
Amiloride	—	—	Decrease	Renal	No initial dosage adjustment is needed
Eplerenone	—	—	—	Hepatic	No initial dosage adjustment is needed
Spironolactone	—	—	—	Hepatic/biliary/renal	No initial dosage adjustment is needed
Triamterene	Increase	—	—	Hepatic/renal	Initiate at lowest dose; titrate to response
Inotropic and vasopressor agents					
Inamrinone	—	—	—	Hepatic/renal	Initiate at lowest dose; titrate to response
Digoxin	Increase	Decrease	Decrease	Renal	Initiate at lowest dose; titrate to response
Dobutamine	—	—	—	Hepatic/tissue	Initiate at lowest dose; titrate to response
Dopamine	—	—	—	Renal/hepatic/plasma	Initiate at lowest dose; titrate to response
Epinephrine	—	—	—	Sympathetic nerve endings/hepatic	Initiate at lowest dose; titrate to response
Isoproterenol	—	—	—	Renal	Initiate at lowest dose; titrate to response
Metaraminol	—	—	—	Hepatic/biliary/renal	Initiate at lowest dose; titrate to response
Methoxamine	—	—	—	Unknown	Initiate at lowest dose; titrate to response
Midodrine	—	—	—	Tissue/hepatic/renal	No initial dosage adjustment is needed
Milrinone	—	—	—	Renal	Adjust based on renal function
Norepinephrine	—	—	—	Sympathetic nerve endings/hepatic	Initiate at lowest dose; titrate to response
Phenylephrine	—	—	—	Hepatic/intestinal	Initiate at lowest dose; titrate to response
Vasopressin	—	—	—	Hepatic	Adjust based on hepatic function and response
Lipid-lowering agents					
Bile acid sequestrants					
Cholestyramine	—	—	—	Not absorbed from GI tract	No adjustment needed
Colesevelam	—	—	—	Not absorbed from GI tract	No adjustment needed
Colestipol	—	—	—	Not absorbed from GI tract	No adjustment needed
Cholesterol absorption inhibitor					
Ezetimibe	—	—	—	Small intestine/hepatic/biliary	No adjustment needed
Fibric acid derivatives					
Fenofibrate	—	—	—	Renal	Initiate at lowest dose; titrate to response
Gemfibrozil	—	—	—	Hepatic/renal	No adjustment necessary
Nicotinic acid	—	—	—	Hepatic/renal	No initial dosage adjustment is needed
HMG-CoA reductase inhibitors					
Atorvastatin	Increase	—	—	Hepatic/biliary	No initial dosage adjustment is needed
Fluvastatin	—	—	—	Hepatic	No initial dosage adjustment is needed
Lovastatin	—	—	—	Hepatic/fecal	No initial dosage adjustment is needed
Pravastatin	—	—	—	Hepatic	No initial dosage adjustment is needed
Rosuvastatin	—	—	—	Hepatic/fecal	No initial dosage adjustment is needed
Simvastatin	—	—	—	Hepatic/fecal	Initiate at lowest dose; titrate to response

The information here is provided as guidance only. Prescribers should always consult the manufacturer's current prescribing information.

371

Drug	Half-life	Volume of distribution	Clearance	Primary route(s) of elimination	Dosage adjustment
Neuronal and ganglionic blockers					
Guanadrel	—	—	—	Hepatic/renal	Initiate at lowest dose; titrate to response
Guanethidine	—	—	—	Hepatic/renal	Initiate at lowest dose; titrate to response
Mecamylamine	—	—	—	Renal	Initiate at lowest dose; titrate to response
Reserpine	—	—	—	Hepatic/fecal	Initiate at lowest dose; titrate to response
Vasodilators					
Alprostadil	—	—	—	Pulmonary/renal	Initiate at lowest dose; titrate to response
Bosentan	—	—	—	Hepatic/biliary	Use usual dose with caution
Diazoxide	—	—	—	Hepatic/renal	Initiate at lowest dose; titrate to response
Epoprostenol	—	—	—	Hepatic/renal	Initiate at usual dose with caution
Fenoldopam	—	—	—	Hepatic	No adjustment necessary
Hydralazine	—	—	—	Hepatic	Initiate at lowest dose; titrate to response
Isosorbide dinitrate	—	—	—	Hepatic	Initiate at lowest dose; titrate to response
Isosorbide mononitrate	NS	—	NS	Hepatic	No adjustment necessary
Isoxsuprine	—	—	—	Renal	Initiate at lowest dose; titrate to response
Minoxidil	—	—	—	Hepatic	Initiate at lowest dose; titrate to response
Nesiritide	—	—	—	Cellular internalization and lysosomal proteolysis/ proteolytic cleavage/renal filtration	Use usual dose with caution
Nitroglycerin	—	—	—	Hepatic	Initiate at lowest dose; titrate to response
Nitroprusside	—	—	—	Hepatic/renal/erythrocytes	Use usual dose with caution
Papaverine	—	—	—	Hepatic	Initiate at lowest dose; titrate to response
Pentoxifylline	—	—	Decrease	Hepatic/renal	Use usual dose with caution; dose reduction may be necessary
Treprostinil	—	—	—	Hepatic/renal	Use usual dose with caution; dose reduction may be necessary

*Increase in clearance is small compared to increase in volume of distribution.

GI—gastrointestinal; ISA—intrinsic sympathomimetic activity; NS—no significant change; — —no information or not relevant; HMG-CoA—hydroxymethylglutaryl coenzyme A.

Adapted from Cheng-Lai A, Frishman WH, Spiegel A, Charney P: Appendix 7: Pharmacokinetic changes, route of elimination, and dosage adjustment of selected cardiovascular drugs in the elderly. In Cardiovascular Pharmacotherapeutics, edn 2. Edited by Frishman WH, Sonnenblick EH, Sica DA. New York: McGraw Hill; 2003: 1033–1036.

The information here is provided as guidance only. Prescribers should always consult the manufacturer's current prescribing information.

373

Congestive heart failure, *continued*
  digitalis, 272
  digoxin, 272–274
  diuretics, 214, 216, 226, 244. *See also* specific drugs
  dobutamine, 257, 259
  dopamine, 257, 260
  enalapril, 20, 25
  eplerenone, 244, 246–247
  ethacrynic acid, 216, 219–220
  fosinopril, 20
  furosemide, 216, 221–222
  hydralazine, 3, 20, 324, 335–336
  inamrinone, 254–255
  isoproterenol, 257
  isosorbide dinitrate, 3, 20, 323–324
  lisinopril, 34–35
  milrinone, 254, 256
  nesiritide, 323–324, 342
  nitroglycerin, 343–344
  prazosin, 3, 6
  quinapril, 20, 40
  ramipril, 20, 42
  sodium nitroprusside, 324, 345–346
  spironolactone, 248–249
  torsemide, 216, 223
  triamterene, 250
Coronary angioplasty
  argatroban, 101
  bivalirudin, 105
  heparin, 99, 101
Coronary artery disease
  aspirin, 120–121
  colestipol, 292
  fluvastatin, 299–300
  lovastatin, 292, 301–302
  nicotinic acid, 292–294
  perindopril, 22
  pravastatin, 303–304
  simvastatin, 292, 307–308
Coronary revascularization
  fluvastatin, 299–300
Coronary stent placement
  clopidogrel, 126–127
  ticlopidine, 128–129

D

Death
  risk of cardiovascular
    ramipril, 22, 25, 42–43
Deep venous thrombosis
  prophylaxis of
    dalteparin, 99, 106–107
    desirudin, 108
  treatment of
    enoxaparin, 99, 109–110
    streptokinase, 142
    tinzaparin, 99
Dermal necrosis

phentolamine, 9
Diabetes insipidus
  vasopressin, 270–271
Diabetic nephropathy
  captopril, 22, 25, 28–29
  irbesartan, 48–50, 54
  losartan, 48, 50, 55–56
  valsartan, 48
Dialysis
  heparin, 102
Disseminated intravascular coagulation
  heparin, 101–103
Ductus arteriosus patency
  alprostadil, 323–324, 325–326
Dysbetalipoproteinemia
  atorvastatin, 297–298
  pravastatin, 303–304
  simvastatin, 307–308
Dyslipidemia
  mixed. *See* Mixed dyslipidemia

E

Edema
  amiloride, 244–245
  bendroflumethiazide, 226–228
  benzthiazide, 226, 229
  bumetanide, 216–218
  chlorothiazide, 226, 230–231
  chlorthalidone, 226, 232–233
  diuretics, 214, 216, 226, 244. *See also* specific drugs
  ethacrynic acid, 216, 219–220
  furosemide, 216, 221–222
  hydrochlorothiazide, 226, 234–235
  hydroflumethiazide, 226, 236
  indapamide, 226, 237
  methylclothiazide, 226, 238
  metolazone, 226, 239
  polythiazide, 226, 240–241
  quinethazone, 226, 242
  spironolactone, 244, 248–249
  torsemide, 216, 223
  triamterene, 244, 250
  trichlormethiazide, 226, 243
Erectile dysfunction
  alprostadil, 323–324, 325–326
Esophageal varices
  vasopressin, 270–271
Essential hypertension. *See* Hypertension
Essential tremor
  propranolol, 156, 158–159
Extracorporeal circulation
  heparin, 101–102

F

Fallot's tetralogy
  propranolol, 155
Familial hypercholesterolemia

ezetimibe, 287
lovastatin, 301–302
pravastatin, 303–304
rosuvastatin, 305–306
simvastatin, 307–308
Familial sitosterolemia
  ezetimibe, 287

H

Heart block
  epinephrine, 262
  isoproterenol, 261
Heart disease
  coronary. *See* Coronary artery disease
Heart failure. *See also* Congestive heart failure
  captopril, 25, 28–29
  enalapril, 25, 30–31
  fosinopril, 25, 32–33
  indapamide, 226, 237
  lisinopril, 25, 34–35
  metoprolol, 164, 170–171
  quinapril, 25, 40–41
  ramipril, 22, 25, 42–43
  trandolapril, 25, 44–45
  valsartan, 50, 59–60
Heart surgery
  heparin, 99, 101–103
Hemodialysis
  aspirin, 120
Hemodynamic imbalance
  dopamine, 260
Hemorrhage
  hypotension in
    metaraminol, 264
  subarachnoid
    nimodipine, 190, 205–206
Heparin-induced thrombocytopenia
  argatroban, 99, 101, 104
  lepirudin, 99, 101, 112
Hepatic cirrhosis
  ethacrynic acid, 219–220
  furosemide, 221
  spironolactone, 248
  torsemide, 223
  triamterene, 250
Hip replacement surgery
  thromboembolic prophylaxis in
    dalteparin, 106–107
    desirudin, 108
    enoxaparin, 109–110
    fondaparinux, 111
Hyperaldosteronism
  spironolactone, 244, 248–249
  triamterene, 244, 250
Hypercholesterolemia. *See also* Hyperlipoproteinemia
  atorvastatin, 297–298
  colesevelam, 285

INDEX TO PROPRIETARY NAMES

tirofiban hydrochloride, 118, 134–135
Antithrombotic therapy, 98–146. *See also* specific drugs
    anticoagulants, 99–116
    antiplatelet agents, 117–135
    fibrinolytic agents, 136–146
    hemostasis and, 98
    overview of, 98
Argatroban, 99–101, 104
Aspirin, 117–122
Atenolol, 152, 154, 163–166
Atropine, 91, 93

B

Benazepril, 25–27
Bendroflumethiazide, 226–228
Benzthiazide, 226, 229
Bepridil, 187, 189–190, 193–194
Beta-adrenergic blockers, 152–183
    beta$_1$-selective without ISA
        atenolol, 163–166
        betaxolol, 164, 167
        bisoprolol, 164, 168
        efficacy and use of, 163–164
        esmolol, 80, 164, 169
        indications for, 164
        metoprolol succinate, 164, 170–171
        metoprolol tartrate, 164, 170–171
        mode of action of, 164
    classification of, 154
    in congestive heart failure, 179
    dual-acting
        carvedilol, 179–181
        efficacy and use of, 179
        indications for, 179
        labetalol, 179, 182–183
        mode of action of, 179
    hemodynamic effects of, 154
    with ISA
        acebutolol, 173–174
        carteolol, 173, 175
        efficacy and use of, 172–173
        indications for, 173
        mode of action of, 173
        penbutolol, 173, 176
        pindolol, 172–173, 177–178
    mode of action of, 152, 154
    nonselective without ISA
        efficacy and use of, 155
        indications for, 156
        mode of action of, 155–156
        nadolol, 154–157
        propranolol, 80, 152, 154–156, 158–159
        sotalol, 81–82, 89, 154–156, 160
        timolol, 154–156, 161–162
    overview of, 152
    receptor type and, 153
    in supraventricular tachycardia, 79–80

Betaxolol, 164, 167
Bile acid sequestrants, 281–288
    cholestyramine, 281–284
    colesevelam, 281–282, 285
    colestipol, 281–282, 286, 292
    efficacy and use of, 281–282
    ezetimibe, 281–282, 287–288
    indications for, 282
    mode of action of, 282
    overview of, 281
    in type II hyperlipoproteinemia, 281
Bisoprolol, 164, 168
Bivalirudin, 99–101, 105
Bosentan, 323–324, 327
Breast-feeding
    ACE inhibitors and, 26, 28, 30, 32, 34, 36, 38, 40, 42, 44
    alpha$_2$-adrenergic agonists and, 13, 15–17
    alpha-adrenergic blockers and, 5–9
    angiotensin II receptor blockers and, 52–54, 56–58, 60
    antiarrhythmics and, 66–68, 70, 72, 74, 76, 78, 84–86, 88–89, 92, 93, 273
    anticoagulants and, 102, 104–106, 108–109, 111–113, 115
    antiplatelet agents and, 121, 123, 125–126, 128, 131–132, 135
    beta-blockers and, 157–158, 161, 165, 168–170, 174–177, 180, 182
    calcium antagonists and, 191, 193, 195, 197, 199, 201, 204–205, 207, 210
    diuretics and, 217, 220–221, 223, 227, 229–230, 232, 234, 236–240, 242–243, 245–246
    fibrinolytic agents and, 139–140, 142, 144, 146
    inotropic and vassopressors and, 25–256, 259–262, 264–268, 271–273
    lipid-lowering drugs and, 283, 285–287, 290–291, 293, 297, 299, 301, 303, 305, 308
    neuronal and ganglionic blockers and, 317–320
    vasodilators and, 325, 327–329, 331, 333, 335, 337, 339–343, 345, 347–349
Bretylium tosylate, 81–82, 85
Bumetanide, 216–218

C

Calcium antagonists, 187–211
    amlodipine, 187–192
    bepridil, 187, 189–190, 193–194
    diltiazem, 80, 90, 187, 189–190, 195–196
    efficacy and use of, 187–189

felodipine, 187, 190, 197–198
    hemodynamic effects of, 189
    indications for, 190
    isradipine, 187, 190, 199–200
    mode of action of, 188–189
    nicardipine, 187, 190, 201–202
    nifedipine, 155, 163, 187, 189–190, 203–204
    nimodipine, 187, 190, 205–206
    nisoldipine, 187, 190, 207–208
    overview of, 187
    in supraventricular tachycardia, 80
    verapamil, 80, 90, 187–190, 209–211
Candesartan cilexetil, 50–52
Captopril, 20, 22–23, 25, 28–29
Cardiac glycosides, 80, 90–91, 272–275
    digoxin immune Fab dosing guidelines, 275
    efficacy and use of, 272
    indications for, 272
    mode of action of, 272
Carteolol, 154–155, 173, 175
Children
    ACE inhibitors in, 26, 28, 30, 32, 34, 36, 38, 40, 42, 44
    alpha$_2$-adrenergic agonists in, 13, 15–17
    alpha-adrenergic blockers in, 5–9
    angiotensin II receptor blockers in, 52–54, 56–58, 60
    antiarrhythmics in, 66–68, 70, 72, 74, 76, 78, 84–86, 88–89, 92, 93, 273
    anticoagulants in, 102, 104–106, 108–109, 111–113, 115
    antiplatelet agents in, 121, 123, 125–126, 128, 131–132, 135
    beta-blockers in, 157–158, 161, 165, 168–170, 174–177, 180, 182
    calcium antagonists and, 191, 193, 195, 197, 199, 201, 204–205, 207, 210
    diuretics in, 217, 220–221, 223, 227, 229–230, 232, 234, 236–240, 242–243, 245–246, 248
    fibrinolytic agents in, 139–140, 142, 144, 146
    inotropic and vassopressors in, 25–256, 259–262, 264–268, 271–273
    lipid-lowering drugs in, 283, 285–287, 290–291, 293, 297, 299, 301, 303, 305, 308
    neuronal and ganglionic blockers in, 317–320
    vasodilators in, 325, 327–329, 331, 333, 335, 337, 339–343, 345, 347–349
Chlorothiazide, 226, 230–231
Chlorthalidone, 224–226, 232–233
Cholesterol absorption inhibitors, 281–288. *See also* Bile acid sequestrants

The information here is provided as guidance only. Prescribers should always consult the manufacturer's current prescribing information.

381